THE LOST ONES

"... these people are not sick.
They have lost their way."
Pai Cambini

THE
LOST ONES

SOCIAL FORCES
AND MENTAL ILLNESS
IN RIO DE JANEIRO

EUGENE B. BRODY

With the Collaboration of

José Leme Lopes

Jurema Alcides Cunha

Manoel Wilson Penna

Roberto Alexandre Correa

Jayme Bisker

Maria Ampares de Dante

Lucia de Marques

INTERNATIONAL UNIVERSITIES PRESS, INC.

New York   New York

Library of Congress Cataloging in Publication Data
Brody, Eugene B
    The lost ones; social forces and mental illness
in Rio de Janeiro.

    Bibliography: p.
    1. Social psychiatry—Brazil—Rio de Janeiro.
I. Title.   [DNLM: 1. Mental disorders—Etiology.
2. Socioeconomic factors. [WM100 B864L 1973]
RC455.B76   362.2′0981′5   72-8794
ISBN 0-8236-3050-1

Manufactured in the United States of America

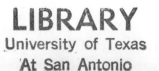

CONTENTS

PREFACE

THE IDEA for this book began in June of 1962 when I was invited to address the meeting of the Latin American Congress of Psychoanalysis in Rio de Janeiro. At that time I met Professor José Leme Lopes, Director of the Psychiatric Institute of the Federal University of Rio de Janeiro (formerly the University of Brazil) and visited the Institute. I also had the opportunity to become acquainted with the Brazilian National Mental Health System and to visit a number of mental hospitals in Rio de Janeiro and elsewhere in Brazil. Professor Jurema Alcides Cunha of Pôrto Alegre, one of the area's leading psychologists, was planning a visit to the United States as a traveling Fulbright scholar and spent several weeks at The Psychiatric Institute of the University of Maryland in 1963. This circumstance, along with other visits to Brazil, concomitant with attendance at the conference of the Pan American Association of Medical Schools in Valparaiso, Chile in 1962 and the WHO/PAHO mental health conference in Buenos Aires in 1963, made it possible to plan for a research project in the field of social psychiatry. Support was given by the Foundations Fund for Research in Psychiatry through two grants. One was made to Friends of Psychiatric Research, the administering agency for the Baltimore staff; the other to the Federal University of Rio de Janeiro for the support of the Rio de Janeiro staff.

On-site organization for data gathering began in Rio de Janeiro in April, 1964. Form construction and the training of interviewers recruited by Professor Leme Lopes, along with the gathering of preliminary data, later to be discarded, progressed at a slow pace. The beginning of the final data-gathering phase was not initiated until early 1965 and was completed in late 1966. Professor Cunha served as a consultant and planning advisor throughout; she also carried out psychological testing on many of the patients. We are grateful to the Secretary of Education of the state of Rio Grande do Sul for granting Professor Cunha time to participate in the project. Dr. Roberto Correa and Dr. Jayme Bisker conducted the patient interviewing. Miss Maria Ampares de Dante and Miss Lucia de Marques, social workers, interviewed the families. Dr. Manoel Wilson Penna of Belém and São Paulo, later on the staff of the University of Maryland, supervised the basic organization of data as it was mailed from Rio de Janeiro to Baltimore. During this period Professor Leme Lopes kept in regular touch with the staff while I made frequent visits to the hospitals where data gathering was in progress, observing interviews and collecting background material. I initiated the process of data analysis which continued in Baltimore during 1967.

In 1968 the Commonwealth Fund made it possible for me to return to Brazil during a sabbatical leave to complete the study of the context in which the patients lived, and to devote time after my return to the United States to completing the manuscript. I worked in Rio de Janeiro from the first of July to mid-September with the invaluable collaboration of Dr. Penna and the institutional support of an appointment as Visiting Professor of Psychiatry at the Federal University. This last was made possible by Professor Leme Lopes, who had been designated Dean of the Medical School.

Professor Leme Lopes deserves special mention for his generosity in providing the institutional base without which this work would have been impossible. His sympathetic interest in work for which his own demanding schedule did not allow intimate participation was reassuring and essential to progress. A special *homenagem* is due him for his broad vision and willingness to depart from traditional viewpoints in order to advance the health and education of his countrymen and his students.

We are indebted to four United States institutions. The Foundations Fund for Research in Psychiatry and the Commonwealth

Fund provided the necessary financial resources. Friends of Psychiatric Research, with their understanding administrative policies, facilitated continuation of work at long distance, often under adverse conditions. The University of Maryland deserves particular mention. Its generous leave policy permitted me the freedom to explore new areas of research and international collaboration. In this respect the forbearance and patience of my own faculty during my frequent absences from the country were equally essential and appreciated.

The members of the Brazilian research staff, each in his own way, have been far more than clinical technicians. Each was a friend, an unstinting source of information about the people and culture of his country, and a source of emotional and intellectual support. Finally, I owe a debt of gratitude to the patients, their families, the staffs of the hospitals to which they came for help, and to the innumerable unnamed individuals upon whom a visitor to a strange land must depend for many things he takes for granted at home. All displayed the warmth, the helpfulness, and the generosity which I have come to love and to regard as characteristically Brazilian.

E.B.B.

INTRODUCTION

THIS BOOK IS about people who have become psychiatric patients and how their thoughts, feelings, and actions have been influenced by sociocultural forces and contexts. It deals with three overlapping subject areas. The first area concerns symptomatic behavior: thinking, feeling, and acting sufficiently deviant from social norms to be defined as psychiatrically disturbed. What is the character of such behavior? What are the sociocultural factors which shape it? Which sociocultural factors diminish or increase the likelihood of its occurrence? How is it related to what is considered natural, proper, or desirable in the socioculture? The main focus is on the nature of a person's participation in an ongoing social process.

The second area concerns aspects of the socioculture which are encountered in behavioral settings throughout the world. These aspects include socioeconomic status, institutions of socialization and social control, and a range of demographic and related variables. They encompass sociocultural change, including development and modernization. From this second standpoint the individual's sick behavior may be viewed as indicative of the evolving state of the socioculture in which he lives. This is true as well for the process of labeling behavior as sick or deviant, for the transformation of freely moving individuals into patients, and for the availability of certain types of isolating or behavior-modifying mechanisms such as mental hospitals or clinics.

The third area concerns unique aspects of the behavioral setting. In a significant sense this is a study of present-day Brazil. It approaches the current Brazilian (and to some extent Latin

American) reality through its focus on sociocultural statuses, the mental health system, and psychiatric behavior. It assumes that a major path to understanding a nation lies in studying the individuals who live within its borders and who, in aggregate, constitute it as a social system. It further assumes, along with Freud, that the study of pathology is one of the best ways to learn about the normal; the disordered behavior of individuals throws the usually quiet and unnoticed aspects of the ordered into sharp relief. Similarly, an understanding of any society and its culture may be approached through a study of its mentally ill. Institutions for the mentally ill, and institutionalized ways of dealing with people so defined, are key aspects of any complex socioculture.

The frequency and form of palpably maladaptive behavior reflect in part the quality of a society's organization or disorganization. It mirrors its values and belief systems and its socially transmitted blueprint for living as Kluckhohn (1944) referred to culture. The same is true for the way in which unhappy or destructive people become labeled as sick. The socioculture molds the expected behavior patterns and sanctions which make up the sick role as well as the processes of transforming a defined sick person into a patient; these last bring him into a therapeutically oriented relationship with a societally designated helping individual or agency.

This book's view of Brazil is seen through the window of Rio de Janeiro, the former capital and still the cultural focus and *cidade maravillhosa* of Brazilians. It concerns the *cariocas* born or migrated into a city of contradictions, where the beauty of a lavish natural setting helps to hide the often staggering daily burdens of many of its residents, and the pride of a wealthy capital obscures the degree to which it has become a noncommunity. In this respect too, Rio's problems and those of the *cariocas* transcend national and cultural boundaries. In varying measures and qualities they may be recognized as similar to those of New York, Baltimore, Washington, or San Francisco. Baltimore and Washington, in particular, without the leavening impact of mountains or beaches, struggle under the weight of overwhelming migrant populations, mainly black, underemployed, and partly literate. In their humid sinks beaten down by sullen, subtropical summer heat, the tension has climbed to points of violent eruption not yet reached by Rio's swollen population. Here lies a historically interesting question. How long will the culturally reinforced passivity of these Brazilians, their physical fatigue, their exclusion from a social participation, and their outlets through religion, music, and the worship of natural beauty, continue to outweigh their gradually developing collective sense of self and outrage and keep them from the violence now described by their educated compatriots as so characteristically "North American?"

Rio de Janeiro is one of the great terminal points for the long migratory streams from vast areas of the nation's East and Northeast. While it is a metropolis with some of the most densely packed urban districts in the world, it contains rural pockets and small farms. The slums or *favelas* which house approximately one-quarter of its population retain more of the character of the country than the city; and the *favelados* who inhabit them do not yet constitute a true urban proletariat. Yet the city's factories are growing. Its people are evermore acutely aware of what they are missing and what they want. Education is penetrating the barrier of their illiteracy, if not through the written word then by way of the transistor radio. In short, the problems of the nation, and those of most of the world's urban peoples, may be seen in microcosm in Rio de Janeiro.

The present study combines aspects of social psychiatry and psychiatric sociology. Limiting itself to people already defined as patients, it cannot deal with the broad question of incidence, that is, the frequency with which certain types of behavior occur in the general population at large. The study of people admitted for the first time to mental hospitals does permit, however, the investigation of particular points. It allows the accumulation of data about why they were considered hospitalizable, how they arrived at the institutions, and what their families thought about it all. More importantly, it makes possible the study of relationships between behavior and psychiatric symptomatology on the one hand, and the presence of major social processes or tendencies on the other. The study of such relationships also makes it possible to draw inferences about the occurrence and etiology of deviant, disturbed, maladaptive, or subjectively uncomfortable ways of thinking, feeling, and acting.

Any study of psychiatric patients must pay attention to the devices used by a society to deal with its deviant or anxious members. Hospitals and clinics are part of the social control system. The frequency of hospitalization is positively influenced by the ready availability and public acceptance of conventional medical facilities. It is negatively affected by the availability and public acceptance of such naturally occurring sources of support as religious-healing sects. Social welfare agencies also play a role. They make it possible for many people with psychiatric problems to continue, however marginally, in the community but at the same time, as representatives of the Western health oriented segment of the community, social workers act as gate keepers for mental hospitals and other control agencies.

The most visible social forces in modern Brazil are those at work in all "developing" countries as well as in the less developed regions of technologically advanced nations such as the United States. But in Brazil the sheer size of the country and the vast numbers of individuals involved dramatize these forces as nowhere else in the Western Hemisphere. Migration involves the movement of millions from the rural interior to urban centers without the capacity to receive them. Illiteracy and partial literacy influence the perception and behavior of more than one-half the population past the age when reading skills could have been acquired. Despite Brazil's much vaunted "ethnic democracy" the confrontation between the races is latently present, ever closer to the surface, and color itself is a social force. This is a country in which rapid industrialization is creating a new labor force but in which the service occupations, a high proportion of agricultural workers, and the drive for independence as a small entrepreneur still characterize the occupational scene. Yet the increasing self-awareness of industrial operators as members of a collectivity is a new social force in Brazil. Inadequate housing is the rule rather than the exception, and this, along with the development in urban areas of large geographically bounded slums with subcultures of their own, constitutes a social phenomenon with as yet unrealized implications for individual behavior including those of a political nature. Age in a country characterized by high infant mortality and disease rates has a special significance. Brazil is a country of the young and a country in which ill health is a norm.

Sex or gender status also has special significance in an area in which women have been a minority group and are just now in the process of emancipation.

All these factors: age, sex, color, migration, education, literacy, occupation, housing, the *favelas,* and religion, as well as the nature of the city and its mental health facilities, constitute a matrix for individual behavior. Sometimes the subjectively reported or publicly observed behavior of the individual seems clearly a function of his place and role in this matrix. Often it is impossible to do more than describe the individual as he exists in his social context and assume a probable but so far unvalidated relationship between them. The development of articulating concepts between the individual and the social, the intrapsychic and interpersonal, remains a major and only partly solved preoccupation which will be discussed from varying standpoints in the chapters which follow.

CHAPTER 1

THE PATIENT PROCESSING SYSTEM—
MENTAL HEALTH SERVICES
IN RIO DE JANEIRO

BECOMING A PATIENT—ENTERING THE MENTAL HEALTH SYSTEM

THE PEOPLE whose behavior is described in the main section of this book are patients. At the time of the study they were in a systematic care-receiving relationship with a societally designated help-giving (labeling, sequestering, and behavior-modifying) agency, the psychiatric hospital. Almost all were accompanied to the hospital by family members. All these patients and their families, then, whose behavior was sampled by the project interviewers, were among Brazilians who turned to doctors and conventional medical facilities for help with upsetting personal experience or the deviant behavior of others. This implies they knew about such facilities and found them both physically and psychologically accessible. It suggests respect for what the facilities can offer, willingness (in some cases) to pay money for their assistance and to subject oneself to externally imposed restrictions, and a value system in which health and psychological well-being have sufficient priority to warrant the expenditure of effort. Further, these were patients who upon consultation were judged by the doctors to be sufficiently disturbed to warrant hospital admission. Relatively few are so judged. In the first half of 1968 for example, only 5.2 per cent of all patients seen in the psychiatric clinics of the INPS (social security system) and 29.1 per cent of those seen in the Pronto Socorro (first-aid station) were hospitalized. (Seventy-six per cent of the sample were hospitalized under INPS auspices.)

Conventional mental health services, however, entrap only a certain proportion of the casualties or adaptive fallout of any social system. Others may indefinitely avoid the net. Their social behavior does not reveal their inner turmoil; they live alone so that their problems do not make others anxious or create an intensifying spiral of mutually reinforced tension, or their families shelter them against the rest of the world. The extended family in Latin America may provide a refuge for considerable numbers of quietly psychotic persons, especially unmarried females whose economic contributions are not needed by the family. In the United States, Jaco's (1960) finding of the lowest psychosis rates for Spanish-American women in Texas may reflect the way in which prevalence figures are obscured by just this kind of family protection. In Baltimore's inner city, mental hospitalization for the poor black population was often delayed for prolonged periods because families regarded paranoid behavior as adaptive in a social context in which suspicious hostility against white power holders was a norm (Brody, Derbyshire, & Schleifer, 1967).

Some mentally-ill isolates undoubtedly die of intercurrent infection or disease developing on a substratum of chronic malnutrition before hospitalization becomes inevitable. In Brazil, the numbers of socially isolated floaters, especially in the *favelas,* sleeping on sidewalks in the central city or residing in the cheap rooming house districts, are uncounted. Similarly, the number of those excluded from their families and regarded by them as *pessoas mortes* (dead persons) who are part of the unstable migrant stream between country and city is unknown.

This study presents no data on the total numbers of persons with subjective states or overt behavior identical to those of patients who have been so labeled. It does, however, describe certain services and experiences which are alternatives to the official mental health system. These include psychological counseling centers in the public schools and the Federal Youth Guidance Service (in the chapters on education and literacy and age); medical and psychiatric services or their equivalents offered by Spiritist and cult centers (in the chapter on religion); and those for transients (in the chapter on migration) and beggars (in the chapter on occupation). No information is available on the degree to which medical and surgical services of general hospitals and clinics in Rio de Janeiro deal with essentially psychiatric problems. The influence of medicine in the culture is seen, though, in the prevalence of self-treatment; according to one saying, "Every Brazilian is his own doctor." The pharmacist is a traditional source of help in the urban centers, and in many interior communities he continues to fit glasses, give injections, dispense his own brand of counseling, and even on occasion pull teeth. This practice has been facilitated by the absence of prescription regulations for many drugs, although in recent years more effective regulation is being established. Still, an injection apparatus remains part of the ordinary home equipment for most urban families of middle-class and above.

Some light was thrown on self-medication practices by Iutaka's (1966) 1962 survey of 1,810 Botafogo dwellings (the only one of its kind so far). Of the 40 per cent of the inhabitants who declared they had been sick or suffered from some symptom in the month preceding the survey, 42 per cent and 44 per cent of the higher and middle class respectively (categories I-II and III-IV as defined in the chapter on occupation) obtained drugs and medicated themselves without a prescription, in preference to consulting a physician or clinic. The figure was only 28 per cent for the lowest class (categories V-VI). The difference between classes appeared due to upper-class persons' greater self-confidence, information, and influential relationship with pharmacists, as well as to their greater ability to pay. Only 14 per cent of the group did nothing at all about their complaints, suggesting a relatively high value placed on general health. It was not possible, however, to estimate the number of those without complaints who might have been suffering from disorders underlying such socially common and often, therefore, unlabeled states as chronic weakness, fatigue, cough, mild diarrhea, or underweight (all of which may be part of a depressive syndrome).

In general, identification as mentally ill and transformation into the role of patient appear less probable for persons with deviant behavior in areas where the basic problems of nutrition and infectious disease have not been solved than in the more developed regions. In these areas the relative absence of conventional medical-psychiatric facilities and the expectation that psychological changes may be the result of physical disease reduce the likelihood of their being labeled mentally ill.

Rio de Janeiro along with São Paulo has the highest concentration of conventional psychiatric services in Brazil. It may be assumed, therefore, that the likelihood is greater here than in most of the country of an emotionally disturbed or behaviorally deviant person becoming identified as a psychiatric case. This chapter describes the facilities in which such persons are segregated in Rio, the training of Brazilian psychiatrists, the labeling system which they use, and the nature of the labeled population as revealed by available statistics. In order to indicate the general health service context of which mental health facilities are a part, it also offers data on mental hospitals and general health throughout the nation.

GENERAL HEALTH AND HEALTH SERVICES IN BRAZIL

As in most unevenly developed countries, facilities and personnel are concentrated in the large urban centers and are among the "pull" factors drawing migrants to the cities. Since municipal services are unable to accommodate the influx, newcomers often suffer from the same lack of potable water supplies, sewage disposal, and medical care characterizing the rural areas from which they came. Lack of literacy and education in the lower-class urban as well as rural populations also contribute to a failure to use available hygienic and dietary measures. While they may value good health, their expectations of and demands upon the health system appear to be low.

Recent data on death rates and causes in various areas of Brazil are illustrative. Table 1* indicates the tremendous range in infant mortality rates among state capitals with the overwhelmingly highest rates in the Northeast. Similar although less marked differences are present for general death rates. It is only in the two metropolitan centers of Rio de Janeiro and São Paulo that some relative mastery and stability may have been attained. The expectation of illness or early death verbalized by many of the poorest patients in this study can be understood as a reflection of social reality as well as of intrapsychic difficulty. In 1968, the Brazilian Health Minister, commenting on the fatalistic attitude of the Northeastern poor toward infant mortality, told the story of an older boy forced by his mother to return a rubber pacifier to his infant brother. "All right," the boy declared, "but when baby brother dies the pacifier is for me." (de Onis, 1968). Campbell (1967), on the basis of 1964 data, pointed out that only 72 of every 100 *Nordestinos* could be expected to reach the age of 20. He noted the translation of parental frustration, pain, and insecurity into "an increased effort to beat the vicious circle by having more and more children . . . [leading to] a . . . gambler's mentality." An alternative to a gambler's mentality and the passive fatalism noted above is migration; the opportunity to rear a healthy family has been regarded as an important determinant of the vast migratory movements away from the Northeast. It was estimated in 1964 (Leiby) that a third of the pregnancies of mothers in the lowest socioeconomic group in Recife were artificially terminated under nonhygienic conditions with much ensuing infection so that they could "raise those [children] who already have been born (p. 1211)." Out-of-wedlock pregnancies accounted for a negligible number of these. The culture of this region also includes a historical preoccupation with the plight of the refugees from recurrent droughts and famines, the *retirantes* who sometimes walked hundreds of miles in search of relief. The gradual dehumanization and the ubiquitousness of death are reflected in Joao Cabral de Mello Netos' poem, *Pernambuco Cemeteries* (de Castro, 1966): "The dead, never one of them here / Come decked out in a coffin / They are not buried / But dumped into the ground." Again, this perception is reflected in the stereotype of the *Nordestino* as sad, passive, withdrawn, and vulnerable to promises of mystical help.

Some of the major causes of death throughout the nation are shown in Table 2. The prevalence of infections of all kinds is in striking contrast to that in the United States and Western Europe. In Recife, as recently as 1961 almost one-third of the deaths were considered attributable to readily preventable causes, and the greatest killer in the adult group was tuberculosis, the characteristic disease of the slums. Powerlessness in the face of illness continues as a salient feature of life. A survey of 5,538 persons in 16 communities of six Northeastern states showed a high prevalence of anemias, reflecting almost universal parasitic infestation,

---

*All tables will be found at the end of the book.

protein and vitamin deficiency, all of which produce feelings of depression, weakness, and fatigue (Leiby, 1964). Rates are lowest in Rio de Janeiro and São Paulo, although they are increased by patients with serious diseases of later life who come from other parts of the country for medical treatment. Chronically ill or impaired persons migrating into Rio de Janeiro, then, include many who are ready to make contact with medical facilities.

Within the city itself the 1962 survey (Iutaka, 1966) revealed expected social class-related differences in reported disease. While 12.6 per cent and 13.3 per cent of the higher and middle classes respectively reported two diseases, this was true for 25.4 per cent or approximately twice the proportion of the lower class. A similar though not so marked difference was found in reporting chronic disease. Of the nonmanual category, 28.8 per cent reported continuing or recurring illness with an acute exacerbation during the study period, in contrast to 36.7 per cent of the manual workers. Medical expenses surpassed or required major modifications in monthly expenditures for other causes in 46.6 per cent of the manual, as compared to 18.6 per cent of nonmanual, workers. The additional expense was dealt with by a reduction of the amount spent for food by 45.3 per cent of the manual, as compared with 9.7 per cent of the nonmanual, workers.

A comparative view of Brazil's health status by regions in relation to Mexico and the United States is given in Tables 1 and 3. It is clear that the highest infant and adult mortality rates are in regions with the lowest per capita income. Levels of illness and mortality are also reciprocally related to levels of health manpower. This is shown in Table 4, which demonstrates that almost 70 per cent of the nation's physicians are concentrated in the "golden triangle" of the Southeast which includes only 44 per cent of the population. More than half the East Zone physicians reside within the limits of Guanabara state itself. In 1965 this included 8,913 physicians or 236.5 per 100,000 inhabitants. The numbers of physicians are growing although not in proportion to population growth. There is great pressure to increase the number of medical schools, and by 1966 there were 40, 28 of which had been opened since 1950 and 12 since 1960. Twenty-eight of the 40 schools were associated with universities, of which 19 were under federal sponsorship. The average number of graduates per year as of 1969 was about 2,000. An informal estimate by the Health Ministry put the total number of graduate physicians at 40,000 in 1968; a ratio of one for every 2,140 inhabitants. While, as previously noted, the great majority are in urban centers, a number are available to man local public health service stations or *postos de saude*. Approximately 6500 doctors and 2000 nurses are employed in the public health services. The Ministry listed, however, 743 municipalities (equivalent to United States counties) totaling 18 million people with no local public health service at all. The situation is further complicated by the lack of technical and auxiliary personnel, ranging from X-ray assistants and laboratory technicians to social work assistants and practical nurses. In the United States these are in the ratio of 10 to 15 for each physician; the ratio in Brazil is only from two to five per physician (Pinho, 1968).

Approximately 60 per cent of all health facilities are administered by private organizations, including church groups. The oldest hospitals are the *santas casas* established by priests of the Catholic Church; they offer "free" beds to those who cannot afford to pay and private rooms for those who can. Like other hospitals, they may provide major teaching services for local medical schools. Free beds in other private hospitals are often operated under contract by one of the branches of the *Instituto Nacional de Previdencia Social* (National Social Welfare Institute), which operate on the basis of a social security arrangement. This system, described in more detail below, does not cover the large masses of those not regularly employed.

Of the remaining 40 per cent of health facilities, more than half are operated by state governments. All the hospitals under governmental and philanthropic auspices maintain outpatient departments or *ambulatórios*, and many of these have *Pronto Socorros*, or first aid or emergency rooms, as well. Approximately two-thirds of the total number of beds are considered free; the patient is not requested to pay, but in the general hospitals the proportion of free beds is somewhat less at 59 per cent.

Table 5 lists comparative bed and personnel statistics for hospitals in five areas, from the Northeast to the South. In Guanabara itself there are by latest official count (Anuário Estatística, 1967) 173 hospitals including 89 general hospitals. Five of these are

teaching hospitals associated with the medical schools. Of the
173, 67 are governmentally operated (one-half state, a fourth federal, and a fourth autonomous state-sponsored agencies), and 106
privately operated (approximately two-thirds profit-making and a
third nonprofit philanthropic). Most districts have their own government operated outpatient clinic or health post, sometimes but
not always associated with one of the hospitals. Several privately
operated Pronto Socorros are available with their own ambulances
for around-the-clock emergency care.

In summary, these data suggest several probable characteristics
of the lower-class population from which the psychiatric study-
sample is largely drawn. Approximately a third may be expected to have chronic or recurrent physical disease of sufficient
severity to be diagnosed, and this is most prevalent among the
poorest manual workers. Most, and especially the approximately
one-half who have migrated into Rio de Janeiro from rural areas,
have low expectations regarding health care and their own bodily
integrity and longevity; this is in spite of the evidence that they
place a high value on health and are willing to reduce food expenditures in order to obtain medical care. They have experienced relative powerlessness in the face of physical illness of a
potentially preventible nature (although those of higher socioeconomic status are more apt to have engaged in systematic
self-medication with the advice of a pharmacist). Their chronic
physical symptoms tend to be those, such as fatigue and weakness, characteristic of depressive syndromes. In these respects they
resemble a sample of United States blacks in urban ghettos and
Appalachian whites in rural areas, nearly two-thirds of whom
reported that "feeling sick" was their usual condition. Similarly,
two-thirds of these last were worried about getting money to pay
for a doctor or for medication (Harris, 1968).

PSYCHIATRIC SERVICES

The establishment and maintenance of standards, national
supervision of services, and overall program development has for
several years been in the hands of the National Service of Mental
Disease, a department of the Ministry of Health. Of the 172 psychiatric hospitals in the country, 119 are labeled "neuropsy-

chiatric" and 53 "mental disease." Within this last category are included the large public mental hospitals and colonies. Their distribution by state and territory is shown in Table 6. The large majority are in Minas Gerais, Guanabara, and São Paulo.

Table 7 lists psychiatric beds and psychiatric dispensaries per population unit according to region. The South has the highest density of beds per population; its lead over the East is attributable largely to the number of private hospitals.

Nine of the 58 public mental hospitals in the country are maintained by the federal government and located in Guanabara. The other 49, distributed among 20 states, are maintained by the state government. The profit-making private psychiatric hospitals also depend indirectly on governmental support, inasmuch as the major payments for patient care come through the Instituto Nacional da Previdencia Social.

THE PRODUCTION OF PSYCHIATRICALLY TRAINED PHYSICIANS— THE OFFICIAL HELPERS

Aside from lack of money, the major obstacle to the development and effectiveness of facilities is a shortage of trained personnel. The personnel problem is made particularly severe by the lack of paramedical workers such as specialized nurses, social workers, and others whose capacity to carry major responsibilities has markedly extended the effectiveness of the inadequate supply of physicians in the United States. Only two medical schools (the federal universities of Rio de Janeiro and São Paulo) administer their own psychiatric hospitals and clinics. The others utilize wards in public hospitals and occasionally in general hospitals associated with the school. Some have only dispensary facilities.

Medical education begins after 12 years of schooling (five primary, four secondary, and three of *colégio*, equivalent to the last three years of United States high school but more concentrated and specialized). This means the student starts his medical training at an age when many United States students are becoming college freshmen. Education in medicine occupies six years, the last of which is usually devoted to practical experience in the field the student expects to specialize in. In addition, students may work in hospitals in their spare time throughout the six years. In spite of the many opportunities for part-time hospital jobs the educational programs themselves tend to emphasize theoretical and academic issues with little laboratory or closely supervised clinical experience. This stems in part from the precarious economic infrastructure which demands that most professors devote a major portion of their time to private practice in order to support their families, and in part from the still important European tradition which stresses lectures and large classes with promotion dependent upon written examinations which may be repeated in another year once failed. As part of this tradition many senior professors are still reluctant to engage in any interchange of ideas with students, and their material is presented in a form which discourages questioning. Identification by the student with this authoritarian role-model might well be expected to increase his already considerable social distance from lower-class patients.

There are reasonably well-developed departments of psychiatry in a few of the 40 medical schools. These are mainly in Rio de Janeiro, São Paulo, Recife, Pôrto Alegre, and Ribeirão Preto; progress is being made in this direction in Salvador do Bahia, Belo Horizonte, and elsewhere. In some schools the departments are represented only by a part-time professor who gives an occasional lecture. The usual approach is classical-descriptive, with emphasis on fixed clinical syndromes. Teaching from the psychodynamic point of view or in relation to the contribution of the social and behavioral sciences is rare. The professors are lifetime occupants of their positions, *catedráticos,* and in most schools other faculty members regardless of age and experience still tend to be regarded as their assistants and are expected to follow their lead. The best known professors are often impressive scholars in the European literature of the field and may pride themselves, as well, on their encyclopedic knowledge of certain other fields, e.g., literature, as they bear on human behavior. Outpatient treatment is mainly dependent upon drugs; on the inpatient services drugs are supplemented with electroshock or insulin. Some efforts are being made in Ribeirão Preto in the State of São Paulo and in Brasilia to introduce public health, preventive, and ecological viewpoints into psychiatric teaching, but these are in early stages of development. Residency training as it is known in the United States does not exist although part-time programs of one or two years have been established in Rio de Janeiro and São Paulo, and beginnings in this direction have been made elsewhere.

A student who is interested in intensive individual psychotherapy has little choice but to become a candidate in a psychoanalytic institute. In Rio there are two such institutes, affiliated with the International Psychoanalytic Association, which follow a line intermediate between Freud and Melanie Klein. Their training is highly doctrinaire, involving a prolonged personal analysis, supervision, and seminars. Once finished, their graduates engage in a life of private practice confined to the affluent and educated classes, having much in common with their counterparts in the major cities of Europe or the United States. A third group, unaffiliated with the International Psychoanalytic Association, is the Institute of Psychological Medicine which follows the general point of view of the William Alanson White Institute in New York City. Its brand of psychoanalysis is less rigidly constrained and more akin to the intensive psychoanalytically oriented psychotherapy practiced widely in the United States. This pays considerable attention to current interpersonal factors as well as to unfolding the individual biography and is less concerned than classical Freudian analysis with reconstructing the important forgotten elements of childhood experience.

One or two centers show considerable interest in group psychotherapy, particularly in the use of "sensitivity groups" for training, but the interest is limited and has little impact on training or treatment in general. Similarly, though much is written and said about the use of "therapeutic communities," the term seems used mainly to refer to those conventional psychiatric units able to operate with better than average facilities and personnel. There are psychoanalytic institutes and societies in São Paulo and Pôrto Alegre as well as Rio de Janeiro. The one in Pôrto Alegre is unique in that one of its senior members was, until his death in early 1969, the *catedrático* of the Rio Grande do Sul medical school which in consequence offers more psychodynamically and psychotherapeutically oriented teaching than do most of the other universities.

Formal training in psychiatric social work is limited to the large urban centers and so few are trained in this field that they exert no real impact on mental health care over the country as a whole. Psychiatric nursing has not yet developed as an academic specialty. Clinical psychologists are hardly represented in the psychiatric services. There are many, however, who have or who are obtaining diplomas in this field. Ph.D. programs comparable to those in the United States are not yet available, and the training includes almost nothing of an experimental and research nature. It is often more oriented to psychotherapy of a relationship type with psychoanalytic flavoring, projective and intelligence testing, and educational and developmental psychology. In comparison with the United States a considerably larger proportion of psychologists are women associated with various school systems. As noted in the chapter on education and literacy, the major counseling services for young people in Rio de Janeiro, which are strongly influenced by psychoanalytic thinking, are operated by female psychologists.

PRIVATE PRACTICE

Informed estimates indicate that between 700 and 1,000 (perhaps 2.5%) of the nation's physicians confine their practices to psychiatry, usually with some neurology as well. Approximately a third of these are believed to have had some special training in the field, and no more than half of these latter have had some training or supervised experience in psychotherapy. These include the psychoanalysts as well as a small number of psychiatrists who have been trained abroad.

Many of the members of psychoanalytic societies, all of whom engage in private practice, are not physicians. Rather, in the tradition of pre-World-War-II United States (before organized psychoanalysis became dominated by medically trained psychiatrists), they are often creative workers in literature and the arts, social scientists, social workers, and psychologists.

Three styles of private practice prevail. By far the largest number of practitioners, probably 85 per cent or more, operate within the medical tradition, depending heavily upon the use of drugs or other organic methods and seeing considerable numbers of patients for brief visits. In their private *consultórios* as well as when making rounds on their hospitalized patients their manner is paternalistic and benevolent. Long consultations are occasionally required in order to resolve tangled situational problems. The doctor's manner and self-percept fit the patient's cultural stereotype of the educated professional man as a wise father upon whom one may be safely dependent and from whom one expects directives, advice, and pills rather than a collaborative interchange. Private patients are admitted to 23 hospitals in Guanabara. This may be because of behavior disturbing to the family, the doctor's feeling that a "rest" of some kind is needed, or for the administration of electroshock, insulin coma, prolonged sleep (with a mixture of barbiturates and tranquilizers), or other therapy requiring nursing care. The sections of these hospitals occupied mainly by non-INPS patients are clean and well kept. Since so many are in old buildings constructed in the colonial tradition they may have impressive chandeliers, fireplaces, and highly polished wooden floors. The physical surroundings and the nursing sisters who are often in charge of floors all contribute to an aura of respectful and trusting dependence upon the authoritative yet kind figure of the physician, who is linked with tradition, religion, material substance, and knowledge. All factors, including the doctor's own set, combine to reinforce an unquestioning acceptance of the physician's point of view.

The second style of private practice is psychoanalytic. Here too, in spite of a rather anxious public adherence to approved format by members of the two affiliates of the International Association, the private interaction appears to be less cool and impersonal than that maintained by "classical" analysts in the United States. The "analytic incognito" is not maintained with such rigor; patient and analyst, both creatures of the same culture, seem to relate with more overt expressiveness and more in terms of reality factors in their own lives than in the United States.

The third style of practice is more conventionally psychotherapeutic as it is known in the United States. The very few in this category tend to be the English-speaking psychiatrists, educated abroad, who are often the therapists for members of the local American and English colonies.

All three types of practitioners may occasionally utilize the services of clinical psychologists, especially for projective and intelligence testing. This is relatively rare, however, and depends mainly upon the existence of a personal contact. As indicated above, the psychologists in the city, mainly female, have been educated in the therapeutic-educational tradition, often with strong psychoanalytic overtones. They engage in private psychotherapy and are more apt to be viewed by the psychiatrists as competitors than as helpers. Similarly, the use of a privately practicing social worker is most uncommon.

Newspapers carry advertisements of physicians announcing themselves as specialists in "nervous diseases" as well as in the other fields. One clinic described itself as having a staff of both physicians and psychologists and offered "global treatment," using all modalities for every type of complaint. While advertising does not mean that the doctor in question is unethical or has a poor reputation, it may be noted that no doctor associated with academic or established private institutions engages in this practice.

THE INSTITUTO NACIONAL DA PREVIDENCIA SOCIAL*

This organization, the national health social security system, is the largest supporter and purveyor of psychiatric aid in Brazil aside from the system of public mental hospitals. It began in 1923, with a Legislative Act creating an Office of Retirement and Pensions to deal with benefits for railroad-company workers. At first there was one such organization for each individual company. Later separate Institutes were organized to deal with different occupations: workers in industry, banks, transportation, commerce, railroad and utilities combined, and government employees for a total of six private and governmental Institutes. In 1966 the whole system was organized into a single entity, called the National Institute of Social Welfare (Instituto Nacional da Previdencia Social—INPS). All employees, including those in management, professionals, and self-employed persons (with the exception of rural workers) are required by law to make contributions to the INPS and are thus eligible for its benefits. The contributions are a percentage of the monthly salary of each worker plus the same amount paid by the employer. The federal government is also expected to pay an amount equivalent to these con-

*The section on the INPS was written by Dr. Manoel Wilson Penna.

tributions. Benefits include pensions, sick leave payments, and medical care.

A National Health Plan was proposed as a substitute for the INPS in 1968. Its primary feature would be the assumption by private organizations of all health activities now being carried out by the federal government. Although the plan met opposition from many physicians and medical associations, a pilot project was established in the town of Friburgo. Which system will prevail in the future is uncertain.

This report deals primarily with the delivery of psychiatric care by the INPS in the State of Guanabara. Besides the author's own experience in the system, it is based on information from interviews with INPS physicians and psychiatrists. Drs. Luis Cerqueira and Isaac Charan provided valuable information.

Celso Barroso Leite and Luiz Paranhos Velloso (1963) state that in 1962 about 15 million people (over one-fifth of the Brazilian population), including workers and their families, were associated with the INPS. In the same year over a million and a half received some sort of benefit from the INPS. In 1969, including both workers and their dependents, at least 18 million were probably associated with the system. It should be emphasized, however, that though the Brazilian population is still predominantly rural the INPS is primarily an urban organization. In Guanabara, which is almost wholly urban, about 80 per cent of the population or between three and four million people are associated with INPS. This is approximately the proportion of patients in the present sample hospitalized under INPS auspices. Most of the others are not employed with sufficient regularity to have such coverage.

The INPS is probably the single most important source of medical care in Guanabara. It works through a network of outpatient clinics and a few hospitals of its own. It also has agreements with other hospitals to provide medical and surgical treatment. Its clinics, however, including the psychiatric, are overcrowded, and the bulk of medical care is of poor quality. Whenever possible, people look for help in other institutions where they feel they can be better served. A small fraction who can afford it go to private physicians despite their INPS coverage.

Reports on the chief complaints of patients who seek treatment in the general medical clinics are not adequate but physicians at the clinics state that many patients have psychophysiologic complaints related to emotional or situational problems. This corroborates a view of the outpatient clinics as important sources of support for the working population with social and emotional difficulties.

In Guanabara the INPS employs approximately 70 psychiatrists and maintains seven psychiatric outpatient clinics and one psychiatric first aid station or emergency facility, a *Pronto Socorro*. In theory, psychiatrists are hired to work six hours daily, but salaries are low and they actually work less than a half day, an average of two or three hours. Patients are hospitalized in private psychiatric hospitals, such as the *Casa Eiras,* which have a contract with the INPS. Admission is based on the judgment of the INPS' own psychiatrists at the time of outpatient or emergency evaluation. Once admitted, however, patients are treated by the private hospital's own staff.

In 1967, 137,493 patients were seen in the INPS Guanabara psychiatric outpatient clinics, a daily average of eight patients for each psychiatrist. A patient is seldom seen for more than 10 or 15 minutes, and disposition is most often the prescription of medication. This appears to fit the expectations of patients who are not accustomed to speaking at length about themselves to strangers and have great faith in the powers of medicine. On December 31, 1967 there were 3,735 patients from the INPS in psychiatric hospitals in the State of Guanabara, their average hospital stay was approximately 280 days. These high figures can be partly accounted for by the fact that insulin coma, electroshock, and psychotropic drugs are the mainstay of hospital treatment programs with little attention paid to social and psychological factors. They also reflect the lack of well-defined channels of communication between the hospital staff and the INPS psychiatrists.

Few data are available on the demographic and psychiatric characteristics of INPS patients. Charan, in a personal communication to the author, described patients attending one of the seven INPS psychiatric outpatient clinics from December 1 to 27, 1965. In his sample of 148, all factory workers or their families, 54 per cent were female and 46 per cent male, a reversal of the public inpatient facility sex ratio described below. Seventy per cent were white, 17 per cent black and 13 per cent brown, making a higher proportion of whites than in the public hospital. Their average age was 33–34 years. About half were married. Fifty-two per cent were either illiterate or had little education; 33 per cent had completed primary school. Most had migrated with two-thirds born outside the State of Guanabara. The largest single group, about 40 per cent of all the patients, presented a chief complaint of depressive symptoms often with hypochondriacal components. Twenty-nine per cent suffered from seizures associated with some emotional difficulty. Nineteen per cent complained of anxiety. Only eight per cent were classified as schizophrenic and four per cent as alcoholic. These last figures probably reflect the fact that INPS clinics deal with a regularly employed working population, one which has been reasonably well socialized and has considerable adaptive capacity.

Some of the most frequent difficulties met by the INPS in providing psychiatric care for its associates are as follows:

1. Administrators question the development of a mental health program when some primary needs such as employment, housing, education, and general health are still to be met. This is despite the finding that the number of people coming to the INPS psychiatric clinics and the level of absenteeism due to emotional difficulties are of themselves high enough to make the issue an important one. Health education is badly needed, and it is here that INPS could make an important contribution. The system, however, has allowed practically no opportunity for preventive work.

2. The low income of the great majority of the population is a serious problem. Even when the patient does not have to pay the physician he often cannot afford to buy the prescribed medication, so that treatment is delayed and jeopardized.

3. Psychiatric care provided by the INPS does not allow for continuity. Treatment alternatives are either outpatient visits (usually to have a drug prescribed) or hospitalization. Communication between the clinic and the hospital is minimal; sharing information and experience throughout the patient's treatment is rare.

4. The INPS psychiatrist uses traditional methods of psychiatric care to deal with large numbers of people; outpatient clinics are operated almost exclusively by psychiatrists who have but a

few minutes to obtain a history and make a disposition. This situation calls for a reevaluation of present methods, particularly as they relate to personnel and training. A new approach, perhaps making better use of social workers and trained mental health aides, must be designed. INPS has no training programs and the training of most psychiatrists working in the system does not give them the necessary sophistication to cope with the problems they encounter. It is of utmost importance, therefore, that it carry out a detailed investigation of its problems and attempt to organize its approaches in accordance with the findings.

Patients and doctors always belong to different social classes and have different subcultural backgrounds, an important variable of which the psychiatrist seldom appears aware. This makes communication between them troublesome and reduces the physician's therapeutic value, thus seeming to create the most common misunderstandings between doctors and patients at the INPS clinics.

Each month a percentage of the worker's salary is taken by the INPS. He often feels he deserves something for what he has been paying and may go to the INPS clinic for almost any reason, expecting some sort of benefit. The level and quality of the client's expectations will obviously be important determinants of the outcome of his encounter with the physician. Unfortunately, they are not often recognized and dealt with and thus have a negative effect on relationships with both the physician and the Institute. Similar factors have been noted in United States patients coming to Veteran's Administration psychiatric facilities (Brody & Fishman, 1960).

It is well known that INPS clinics are always crowded and that doctors do not spend enough time with their patients. Thus the patient approaches the consultation already feeling some resentment toward the Institute and the doctor. Furthermore, he displaces onto the latter his anger at having a fraction of his already small salary taken away from him to support his medical care.

The patients' attitudes toward illness and their interpretation of the disease process are important. Common among these is a feeling of "weakness" for which patients request calcium injections and vitamins, or a feeling that one is suffering "from his liver" associated with a request for liver extracts. Even though some of these symptoms are related to malnutrition, emotional difficulties play an important role in them. Patients' self-treatment also creates conflicts with the physician, aggravating an already tense relationship.

The families' attitudes toward illness and their views of how the patient should be treated create problems. Physicians and social workers frequently state that families abandon patients who are very troublesome, such as alcoholics, or very disorganized, such as psychotics. If the problem is a general one, it clearly makes treatment more difficult and creates an additional burden for an all too busy organization. This is an issue which deserves serious investigation.

The INPS observations suggest how few of the disturbed or unhappy population at large actually become mental hospital patients. Those complaining of weakness and associated symptoms are more apt to consult nonpsychiatric physicians on the basis of their self-diagnosis, though the symptoms may be part of a depressive or psychoneurotic syndrome. Those who do seek or are referred for psychiatric assistance at INPS centers (which provide the majority of referrals to the hospitals from which the present study population was drawn) have been well adapted to the point of finding and engaging in regular paid work for at least two years. Health care is universally regarded as a benefit of employment, and INPS membership for which the potential patient pays fosters an attitude of ambivalent dependence upon the doctors, reinforcing a cultural attitude of the lower classes toward the *patroes* or those in power. Many who are alcoholic, seriously disorganized, or whose reality testing is severely impaired are apt to be abandoned by their families and to become vagrants. The likelihood, therefore, of their becoming mental-hospital patients is much decreased. As noted later, some of these come eventually to migrant centers, *favela* rehabilitation centers, and particularly to the beggars' service. Those who end up in public psychiatric facilities are referred from these agencies or are brought directly to a Pronto Socorro.

CHARACTERISTICS OF PSYCHIATRIC PATIENTS IN GUANABARA

Thirty-four psychiatric hospitals, 11 public (all administered by the federal government) and 23 private, function in the state.

They include those which are part of the Centro Psiquiatrico
Pedro II in the district of Engenho de Dentro. The Pronto Socorro
for the North Zone of the city, which supplied most of the
non-INPS patients for the present study, is part of this center,
which also includes the Hospital Neuro-Psiquiatria Infantil
(occupied mainly by mentally defective, severely deteriorated psychotic, or brain-damaged children) and several other units. Also
among the public hospitals are the Colonia Juliano Moreira with
several thousand patients in essentially domiciliary care, located
in Jacarepagua; a hospital specializing in forensic and criminal
problems; the psychiatric units of the army, navy, and air force;
the Psychiatric Institute of the Federal University, which supplied
several cases described in the chapter on religion; and the Hospital Pinel. The emergency service of this last, in physical approximation with the medical school and used for its teaching, is described in greater detail below.

Among the private hospitals are the Casa de Saude Dr. Eiras,
and the Sanatorio Botafogo, both sources of patients for the present study. As indicated above, a large proportion of the patients
at the Casa Eiras, as it is commonly called, which supplied the
majority of the study cases, as well as most other private hospitals, are supported by INPS. A few, such as the Sanatorio Botafogo, place somewhat greater emphasis on the development of ac-
commodations and care for more affluent patients who prefer to
pay their own way. The Hospital Espirita Pedro de Alcantara,
described in the chapter on religion, is also listed among the private institutions. The private hospitals are all located within
heavily urbanized areas: four each are in Botafogo, Tijúca, Gavea, and Jacarepagua, two are in the Centro, and Rio Comprido,
Bomsucesso, and Meier each have one.

In 1966, the most recent year for which data are available,
there were 11,687 first admissions and 11,166 readmissions to the
Guanabara psychiatric hospitals, with a total hospital population
at year's end of 10,350. According to official reports, about half of
those discharged were regarded as improved, and a quarter each
as cured or unchanged. These statistics resemble those issued by
most conventional facilities in Western countries including the
United States. Table 8 shows considerable differences, however,
reflecting social class lines, between the populations of public and

private psychiatric hospitals. These are not so much due to a large number of affluent people who can afford private hospitalization as they are to INPS-financed care in private hospitals being available to most regularly employed persons in Guanabara. This means that the people most likely to become public hospital patients are those who have not been regularly employed for at least two years: recent migrants, the young, the least educated and adequate, and those with chronic or recurrent mental or emotional difficulties interfering with their ability to work. The differences between the public and private groups are, however, reduced to some degree by the inclusion in the former of the military hospitals and the university Psychiatric Institute. Additionally, there is some evidence that many patients in the Center Pedro II, especially those admitted through its associated Pronto Socorro, are covered by INPS but do not take advantage of it.

As shown in Table 8, the patients in private hospitals in comparison with those in public hospitals are more often white, older, admitted for the first time, and discharged as "cured." In both public and private institutions almost two-thirds are male. This may reflect a cultural tendency to maintain mentally ill women at home, the less intense economic demand upon them, and the fact that they are less inclined to violence when psychotic. Table 9 shows no difference in age distribution of first admissions according to color and sex.

Table 10 lists the official diagnostic classifications for all Guanabara mental hospitals. The private hospital population had twice the proportion of the public of exotoxic psychoses (mainly alcoholic, and almost entirely in men), neuroses, manic-depressive psychoses (predominantly melancholias), and psychoses with cerebral lesions (predominantly arteriosclerotic and senile). The public patient population included considerably higher proportions of schizophrenia and a somewhat higher proportion of epileptic-associated disturbances, situational (psychogenic) psychotic reactions, and psychopathic states of various types. The discrepancy in admission for alcoholic psychoses appears to reflect greater social tolerance for disturbance among the poor and unemployed, since there is no reason to suspect a higher incidence of alcoholism in the private population. The comments of many patients and relatives make it clear that for most of the manual workers and unemployed the behavioral disturbances associated with acute or chronic alcoholism are regarded as expected concomitants of heavy drinking rather than as illness requiring hospital care. The discrepancy in age-related psychoses probably reflects a greater concern for elderly relatives and ability to do something about it, as well as greater longevity in the more stable and economically secure groups. The comments of the poorest patients about senility symptoms indicate that these too are regarded as the inevitable concomitants of a certain stage in the life cycle rather than as symptoms of disease requiring hospitalization. In this respect the attitudes of these people at the periphery of the social power system resemble those of primitive tribesmen such as the Yoruba (Leighton, 1963).

In both the private and public populations approximately a third of those diagnosed as manic-depressive were male and two-thirds female. Marked differences were present, however, in the proportion of manic to melancholic states between the two groups. In the private group three times as many males and one-third again as many females were classified as melancholic in proportion to manic; in the public group, in contrast, the proportions were the same for males and twice as many females were classified as manic than melancholic. In other words, the more economically secure patients showed a relative predominance of depressive psychoses, most marked among the male, and the less secure, a predominance of manic psychoses, more marked among the female. In the presence of other data suggesting the ubiquitousness of depressive symptoms among the poor, these differences may reflect either the more serious evaluation of such symptoms when appearing among the well-to-do not suffering from gross socioeconomic stress, or the rapid development of depression to a psychotic level when it does finally appear in the more secure group. The relative prominence of manic psychoses among the most deprived suggests the operation of denial mechanisms, distractive activity, and the substitution of pleasanter fantasies for unsatisfying and powerless reality.

In the private group approximately 55 per cent of those diagnosed neurotic were female. Whether or not this reflects a labeling bias or a tendency for higher-class females to be admitted for less severely disturbed behavior than higher-class males or lower-class females is uncertain. Almost 40 per cent of these female neurotics in contrast to 17 per cent of the males fell into the hysterical-conversion category. In the other subgroupings males were predominant or proportionally equal to females.

The larger proportion of public than private male patients diagnosed as neurotic is due to a relatively higher incidence of anxious, neurasthenic, or mixed (i.e., "other") forms; the use of these subcategories, especially the last, suggests a relatively high prevalence of fluctuating symptoms of anxiety, depression, weakness, and fatigue which might under other circumstances have been diagnosed as "manic-depressive, melancholic." In other words, the label "neurotic" among male public hospital admissions appears to have masked a high prevalence of nonpsychotic or prepsychotic depressive states.

Table 11 presents diagnostic data from patients seen during 1967 in 19 outpatient clinics in Guanabara. This distribution, with the heaviest emphasis on neuroses, is not unexpected, although psychiatric complaints related to epilepsy are more prominent than in the developed countries. This last may be plausibly related to the higher frequency among the lower socioeconomic groups of sequelae of head injuries and infection as well as to the presence of conversion seizures labeled as "epilepsy" in the absence of adequate laboratory diagnostic facilities.

PRONTO SOCORRO PSIQUIATRICO PINEL—ZONA SUL

This is a unit of the National Service of Mental Disease and is the only Psychiatric First Aid Station in urban Guanabara besides that in the Engenho de Dentro. It is given special mention here as an example of what is considered best in present-day Brazilian public psychiatry. Its patients, coming from throughout the South Zone, offer another sample of the social and behavior characteristics of the Carioca who seeks psychiatric help for himself or, because of his disturbed acts, is sent by the authorities or brought by his family without his own decision.

The Pronto Socorro is located in a modern structure completed in late 1966 in connection with the old Federal Neurosyphilis Hospital, which was established in 1935. It is adjacent to the school of

medicine and has been in full operation since the beginning of
1967. The unit, its history, organization, and program have been
described in detail by Moraes (1967). Its administrators consider
it an example of a "modern psychiatric community." In addition
to the usual organic treatments, it is interested in providing some
forms of individual and group psychotherapy, especially in work
as therapy in the sense of re-education, and whatever methods of
resocialization may be developed.

The director estimated that as of July, 1968, approximately 25
patients were coming through the service daily. All were acutely
disturbed, and most were sent out on the same day, although
some remained for the 72-hour residence limit. Those who could
not be returned to the community were transferred to the wards
of the Pinel Hospital, the University Psychiatric Institute, the
Pedro II, or, if they were covered, to various INPS-supported
services. A number of alcoholics were sent home to return to the
day-treatment unit of the Pinel Hospital. The clients included a
few who could afford private care as well as some foreigners with
no other place to go. Nonetheless, the service was free to everyone, although explorations were in progress about the possibility
of tying it in to the INPS, with the aim of at least obtaining
payment for the so far undetermined but probably significant
segment of patients already having such coverage.

Patients are most often brought to the Pronto Socorro by family
members. Some come with the police who usually telephone first
to make arrangements, and others are sent by ambulance from
various INPS hospitals. Records are brief, occupying a four-by-six
card, part of which includes a photograph, fingerprint, and X-ray
and tuberculin report. A few sentences describe the patient's chief
complaint and physical status. This is partly because of the emphasis on rapid disposition and partly because of lack of personnel time. The unit functions under the immediate direction of a
single physician on call for 24 hours once weekly. With social
work and nursing assistants and the help of some medical students, he is responsible for record keeping and dispositional decisions.

The statistics for 1967, the first year of operation, indicate the
variety of people requiring emergency psychiatric assistance. During this period the patients included 1,192 women, 358 of whom

were readmitted on at least one occasion, and 1,569 men, 517 of whom were readmitted at least once. Table 12 indicates some demographic features by sex. By far the largest proportion are in the young adult range from ages 20 through 39. Whites, although constituting the majority of the sample, are somewhat under represented in terms of the general population. Similarly, fewer than would be expected for the Guanabara population have had no or only primary schooling (the proportion completing primary school being unspecified). It is likely that those about whom educational information was not available were unschooled. The proportion of married patients is less than half of what would be expected for this age group. Surveys in most Western countries indicate that relatively more male than female psychiatric patients are never married, and the Pinel data are similar. The difference is usually attributed to the greater demands upon the males for activity and the relatively greater opportunities for passive adaptation in a marital situation of a mentally ill or inadequate female. This difference in a gender role is probably more marked in Brazil than in the United States.

Table 13 indicates the patients' birthplaces. Approximately three-fourths originated elsewhere than Guanabara, and approximately a quarter of the total came from Minas Gerais or other eastern states. The Northeast, traditional source of migrants, contributed approximately the same number as surrounding Rio State. This may in part reflect the fact that the largest number of *Nordestinos* live in the North Zone and use the Pronto Socorro in Engenho de Dentro.

Occupational data on the females are unclear because fully 75 per cent are listed as *doméstica,* including both those who work as maids and those who confine themselves to their own homes. It also seems likely that patients whose occupations were unknown were lumped together in this group. The largest additional categories, including two per cent of the female population, are commercial employee, government clerk (*funcionário público*), seamstress, and student, with the next largest category of primary-school teacher accounting for one per cent of the group. The remaining 16 per cent are divided among a host of individual positions mainly at the technical or skilled manual level, although a number list themselves as servants, kitchen workers, or waitresses. Some of the other specific jobs listed are nurse, governess, masseuse, cashier, typist, telephone operator, manicurist, and dancer. One physician and one lawyer are included.

The occupational status of 20 per cent of the male patients is unknown; 17 per cent are listed as "without occupation," and four per cent are *biscateiros,* i.e., they depend upon odd jobs. The other major categories are commercial employees with five per cent of the patients, servant and *funcionário público* with four per cent each, and student with three per cent. Of the remaining 43 per cent, the majority are in the various building trades, factory, or mechanical shop work. From five to 15 individuals each are listed as office boy, truck driver's helper, butcher, cook, carpenter, typist, stevedore, cleaning man, waiter, auto guard, gardener, journalist, radio technician, telegraph operator, and doorman. Twenty-one are taxi drivers. The professional classes are represented by nine lawyers, an architect, and five physicians. These latter probably came from the nearby School of Medicine.

Diagnoses are listed in Table 14. The largest number are unclassified, evidently a reflection of the amorphous nature of the clinical pictures encountered as well as of the limited time available for study. The larger proportion of unclassified females is balanced by the larger proportion of males diagnosed as alcoholic psychotic reactions. The "exotoxic" psychoses constitute a large group, which, on the basis of qualifications added to the official diagnostic term and of personal experience, may include many chronically psychotic or severely neurotic people for whom a crisis resulting in hospital admission is precipitated by the use of drugs or alcohol.

Excessive drinking is generally regarded by professionals as widespread among the lower classes. Whether or not this purported incidence rather than social tolerance and selection methods or a bias in diagnosing is truly a central issue in the large number classified as alcoholic psychoses remains unclear. Data from the National Service for Mental Illnesses (Ribeiro, 1968) indicate a gradual increase in the proportion of total mental hospital admissions for alcoholism from 9.4 per cent in 1953 to 13.2 per cent in 1960 with a relative plateau since that time. On the average, 92 per cent of these were men and eight per cent women with little change from year to year. The only reported alcoholism-incidence survey in Brazil was carried out in Ribeirão Preto in São Paulo State in 1962 (Azoubel, 1967). Eighty-eight men and 115 women, almost the total population of one district, were interviewed. Approximately a third of the women and a fifth of the men claimed to be teetotalers. Seventy per cent said they drank to some degree. An analysis of this 70 per cent by degree of drinking activity revealed the following: moderate drinkers, 48 per cent of the men and 52 per cent of the women; excessive drinkers, 17 per cent of the men and 10 per cent of the women; pathological drinkers, 14 per cent of the men and one per cent of the women.

In summary, both public and private mental hospitals in Rio de Janeiro admit more male than female patients and include a proportional overrepresentation of never-married. The public hospitals are somewhat overrepresented with nonwhites and migrants. Fewer public hospital patients are diagnosed as alcoholic and more as schizophrenic, psychotic, and generally psychopathic (including seizure-related behavior). More exhibit manic psychotic behavior and nonpsychotic depressive states masked under a variety of neurotic labels. The largest proportion of more advantaged females with neurotic diagnoses were in the hysterical-conversion category. The hospitals attract a broad cross-section of the population and appear to be psychologically accessible as well as physically available to those in need.

HEALTH- AND MENTAL HEALTH-RELATED SERVICES OF SOCIAL AGENCIES

These constitute one series of alternatives to the mental hospitals, especially for those who are not regularly employed and are not labeled by themselves or relatives as mentally sick. Their value for individuals who are potential patients may be considered more supportive than curative. The major social welfare activities of the Guanabara Secretariat of Social Services are conducted through the Fundação Leao XIII. Established in 1947, it maintains social service centers and elementary schools in seven *favelas*. The schools provide regular primary instruction, while the centers offer personal counseling, vocational training of various types, help in community organization, and education in home economics and personal hygiene. They also provide limited medi-

cal and dental care including free prescriptions as well as sup-
plying legal aid. The center in the *favela* of Jacarezinho, described
in the chapter on housing is the largest of these. They are not oriented to mental illness as such, and informal inquiry suggests
that they are rarely instrumental in referring potential patients to
psychiatric facilities. Nonetheless, their support does make it possible for many inadequate or chronically disturbed persons to
function, however marginally, in the *favelas,* without having to be
extruded into a hospital.

By far the largest and most effective privately sponsored agency
in Rio de Janeiro is the Banco da Providencia which operates the
Emaus Community, described in the chapter on occupation. This
was organized by Dom Elder Camara when he was Archbishop of
Rio de Janeiro. The original community development teams he
founded came to be viewed as a social danger and were dissolved,
he then interested upper-class women, the wives of powerful businessmen, in a church-sponsored organization. This was acceptable
because it would operate in the familiar tradition if not in the
actual manner of religious charities. The Banco, functioning since
1960, is financed by private and business contributions and an
annual fair, which is one of the city's social as well as charitable
events.

Emaus was created to fill a social psychological need; in the
words of one of its directors, "to drain off disturbing marginal
people." These, often with a police record, came looking for help
to the Banco's other services at the rate of 50 to 60 a month.
They were described as frequently aggressive, some with knives on
their persons, mostly "alcoholic," and without families. It is still
not possible to handle them all. In 1967 Emaus had to refuse 600
applications because of lack of space. Discussions and written
reports regularly mention alcoholism as a problem among the
men, but the figures are vague. The latest report of the Banco da
Providencia (1968) stated that about a quarter of the alcoholic
men who come to Emaus are considered recovered and that the
outlook of an additional third is improved. Aside from this,
Emaus gives its goals and results in clear "mental health" terms
(optimal function, improved adaptation, and coping). By 1967 it
claimed to have achieved since its inception "a total of 766 men

completely re-educated, who have returned to society and are working normally" (p. 6).

The Banco is subdivided into four services and six *carteiras* (literally, desks) or sections. Emaus is one of the services. Another is concerned with the establishment and maintenance of Centros da Providencia. Four centers presently exist in slum areas of Catumbí, Engenho Novo, Campo Grande, and Copacabana. The last, located in the *favela* Euclides da Rocha, is described in the chapter on housing. In these centers the staffs of 37 training shops for manual workers taught 777 apprentices in 1967. The Occupational Guidance and Job Placement Service was sought out during 1967 by 6,459 persons, at an average of 43 per day. Of these, 4,490 applied for jobs and 54.6 per cent were successfully placed. This was done through the cooperation of 250 business firms which offered 7,956 job vacancies. The main problem of unplaced job-seekers as well as of the 1,969 who came mainly in search of guidance, was illiteracy, present in 53.5 per cent. Beyond this, many had physical problems. Others, though literate, had no marketable skills. These included minors, many of whom were eventually placed as apprentices in factories and offices.

The fourth service is the *Despensas* ("storerooms" or "pantries") of Providence. Seven of these were operating in 1967 in Campo Grande, Barros Filho, Honorio Gugel, Engenho Novo, Sao Francisco Xavier, Catumbí, and Copacabana; four in conjunction with the Center noted above. Whereas initially they were delivery points for food and clothing, they have gradually been transformed into stimulators of self-help and community organization. Essential items continue to be dispensed, but pieces of clothing made with material obtained at the Centers are sold to the poor at token prices in five Economy Shops. Special activities are conducted for old people and those who are ill, study sessions for families are organized, and direct supervision is given in development projects. The aim is to help individuals and families seeking help "to see and to feel their own situation and to desire to advance beyond it," to awaken in the old and sick "interest in activities compatible with the capacities of each," and in general, "to transform the delivery of material goods into a brotherly encounter" (Banco da Providencia, 1968, p. 4).

The *Carteiras* supplement and expand the work of the services. One provides interest-free loans, most of which are repaid at the rate of 10 per cent monthly. These again offer an opportunity for rehabilitative and counseling interviews. In 1967, 9,488 such interviews were carried out, mostly in the homes. The real problem is not always financial but something which may be resolved with counseling. Occasionally the loan is requested after a responsible family member loses his job. In this case the Employment Section is often successful in finding him new work.

The Education Section gives priority to "abandoned minors, children of parents with tuberculosis, cancer, mental illness, who are unemployed, or those from exceptionally large families" (p. 5). Efforts are directed mainly at obtaining waivers of fees from secondary schools and at placement of children in appropriate schools. Other sections deal with housing, food, and the annual fair. The one most directly concerned with social-psychiatric matters is the Section of Legal Aid and Health. In 1967, with the volunteer collaboration of 10 lawyers, a permanent staff of a social worker, a *despachante* (a person who writes letters and finds his way through the bureaucracy, a combination of public scribe and ombudsman, an expediter), and a receptionist, 351 legal problems were dealt with. A common problem is being discharged from work with no explanation from the employer. As one lawyer said, "The people just don't know their rights."

During the same period two volunteer physicians, each working for two half-days weekly, saw 2,423 patients. They furnished glasses to 286 persons, orthopedic devices in some instances, and arranged the admission of 163 persons to general hospitals and 56 to "asylums." The doctors work in an office in the Banco headquarters lined with floor-to-ceiling shelves filled with free samples of medicine. One of the volunteers, a 76-year-old physician who served in the French army during the first World War, said that the problems encountered at the Banco were more difficult to solve than those of wartime because the complaints were more serious and the resources fewer. Most patients were worried because of unemployment, lack of money to pay rent, and the sickness of one or several family members. The usual presenting symptoms were weakness and fatigue, an exacerbation of a chronic cough, nervousness, or *figado* (liver). This last has the status of a cultural symbol; the liver is considered a delicate organ which may go out of balance from time to time. If one doesn't feel well, or if anything physiological goes wrong, people tend to attribute it to *figado*.

The majority of patients have anemia and other evidence of mild to moderate chronic malnutrition but do not believe the doctor when he tells them about it. They eat a great deal of *farinha* (manioc meal) and *bacalhao* (dried salt cod) and add crude sugar to their coffee, but take almost no vitamins. It is a problem of health education as well as finances.

The health care available in the four *favela* centers is variable. The most consistent and extensive is probably that in the Euclides da Rocha where a nurse—a French nun—has been living for five years. Her office, too, has its walls completely filled by shelves containing free drug samples. She sees from 20 to 25 persons daily, perhaps half of whom are new cases. She is aided by a pediatrician and a general practitioner, each of whom is present half a day a week. A volunteer social worker and psychologist are in the Center every afternoon but are not identified with the health service as such. Their activities with adolescents are described in the chapter on age. The nurse herself, in addition to dealing with diarrhea, fevers, and the usually encountered physical complaints, acts as a general counselor and confidante. Women ask her about their marital problems, difficulties in child rearing, and relations with others. Some of the interpersonal problems about which they want help stem from overcrowding. (For example, a mother, father, and five children living in a one-room shack were joined by a mother, father, and two daughters, making a total of 11 people. According to the nurse the *favelados* behave with her in a child-like, passive, submissive manner.

They do not seem interested in or capable of "any deliberate attempt to orient themselves or discuss their own sense of purpose in life." It is, rather, a dependent search for advice and support. Even their resistance is passive; they may repeatedly agree to some suggestion and then not follow it. Later, after talking with her they may consult the *pai-de-santo* or leader of the Afro-Brazilian cult house (discussed in the chapter on religion) located in the *favela*.

In summary, the sample of poor people seen in the medical

clinics of the Banco de Providencia confirm impressions noted above. Weakness, fatigue, and nervousness are ubiquitous and often attributed to liver malfunction. These are related by professional observers to chronic undiagnosed disease such as tuberculosis or bronchiectasis often associated with crowding and inadequate housing, to dietary anemia (the result as much of poor eating habits as of lack of money), and to constant worry and uncertainty about jobs, housing, clothing, children, and other corollaries of poverty. Moreover, as noted above, they display a passive-dependent and somewhat ambivalent attitude toward the professional helpers who wish to assist them. The efforts of the Banco da Providence in general can be characterized as preventive. The development of self-help groups diminish feelings of powerlessness, reduce social isolation, and eventually provide money for concrete improvement. Emaus, to be discussed in a later chapter, has both curative and preventive aspects.

CHAPTER 2

METHOD OF STUDY:
APPROACH TO THE PATIENTS

DIFFERENT SEGMENTS of the psychiatrically labeled population of Rio de Janeiro are extruded into different hospitals. The majority of regularly employed city dwellers go via outpatient clinics or emergency services to the wards of private hospitals which care for them under contract from the INPS. Some of these who are unaware of their privileges, and the bulk of the unemployed and intermittently employed, are sent to the public mental hospitals, frequently via the emergency services. In time, the most chronic and least capable of caring for themselves are transferred into one of the larger colonies where the psychotic, mentally defective, brain-damaged, and seriously epileptic are warehoused. In these institutions the most aggressive or agitated are tranquilized and sedated; the most amenable have the opportunity to engage in routine types of agricultural or simple construction or craft work; the others live in a milieu which at least keeps them from the sight of the outside world. This general scheme for dealing with the mentally ill is the norm for the Western world, with regional variations in the adequacy of basic amenities such as water, food, shelter, and clothing, and in the humaneness of the attending personnel. A final, and in Rio de Janeiro, very small group receive privately financed care in one of several sanitoria. It is clear, then, that the nature of the patient sample to be studied will depend in part upon the hospital selected as a source of subjects.

33

SOURCES OF THE PATIENT SAMPLE

It seemed desirable for purposes of the present study to have access to people who were becoming hospital patients for the first time in their lives, even though they might have had previous office or clinic contact with psychiatrists. Confining the sample to patients judged in need of hospitalization eliminated most of those whose requests for consultation were a direct reflection of dependency and an expectation that they should receive something from social security for the money deducted from their salaries. It also provided a more easily available population than that in a clinic for diagnostic study prior to a decision as to hospitalization. It was essential that the patients were capable of verbal communication. Finally, it was hoped that family members would be available in order to obtain detailed information about relevant sociocultural variables. With this in mind, three hospitals were chosen as patient sources.

The first was the Pronto Socorro in the Federal Psychiatric Center Pedro II, located in the district of Engenho de Dentro, about 45 minutes by taxi from the center of town. When preliminary work on the project began in the fall of 1964, this was the only such station in the city; another Pronto Socorro associated with the Pinel Hospital went into full operation in 1967 after the data-gathering period for this project was completed. At that time the station at Pedro II was officially designated for the North Zone alone, while the one at Pinel was so designated for the South Zone. Both stations receive patients in the same manner. Most are brought by their families, sometimes on foot or by taxi, often in ambulances operated by the National Service of Mental Disease, and more rarely in police vehicles. Occasional patients, usually repeaters (not included in the present sample) who have already learned where they can find help, come alone. Some are also picked up on the street where they might have had a seizure or exhibited bizarre behavior. This is relatively infrequent, however; in the poorer zones of the city, or in the *favelas,* disturbed behavior which is not clearly destructive does not often result in a call for the police or a doctor.

The Pronto Socorro at Pedro II is staffed by seven 24-hour teams, one for each day, under the direction of a different psychiatrist. Team members include an occasional medical student, nurses, aides, and usually another physician who may not be a psychiatrist. There are eight to 10 people in each. From 20 to 35 patients are seen daily, about half of whom are repeaters. The majority are given drugs and sent home, sometimes with appointments to return to the *ambulatório* associated with the hospitals at the center. From one to six or seven may be admitted as inpatients on any day, and the building can accommodate up to 40 patients in two wards divided according to sex. Usually somewhat more than 50 per cent of the inpatients are readmissions. The limit of residence is 72 hours, and if the patient cannot be discharged at that time he is usually transferred to the 500-bed main hospital of the Center. Most of the patients used for practice in interviewing and recording data were seen here, beginning in October 1964. It soon became apparent that the relatively slow rate of first admissions, and the fact that they arrived at irregular intervals around the clock, would make it difficult to obtain the 300 hoped-for cases in this setting. An added complication stemmed from the emergency nature of the facility and its pressure for immediate treatment. This meant that some first admissions were given drugs and even electroshock within half an hour of their arrival, and were not, therefore, suitable for study. It proved impossible to control this factor despite repeated requests from the interviewers on the spot and the Director of the University Psychiatric Institute. Eventually, a total of 48 cases, or 19 per cent of the final study sample, aside from those seen during the preliminary study period and discarded, were interviewed here.

The Casa de Saude (House of Health) Dr. Eiras is the oldest private psychiatric hospital in Rio de Janeiro. Established in the 1860's in what is now the center of the city, its professional staff includes leaders of the medical community. In the mid-1960's over 1,000 of its 1,200 beds were devoted to patients supported by INPS. Some patients are transferred from the Pronto Socorro; others are sent in after first having been seen in the INPS outpatient clinic, a very few having first consulted private physicians, usually nonpsychiatrists; some come directly for admission without an intermediate stop. Here too, approximately one-half of the patients are readmissions and organic and pharmacological treatment is instituted early, but, the larger number of beds and more leisurely pace made it easier to collect cases for the project. A total of 193, or 76 per cent of the cases, were seen here.

In order to obtain a number of patients of higher socioeconomic status arrangements were made to work at the Sanatorio Botafogo, a private hospital with relatively little INPS support. Objections by relatives, however, and the reluctance of private therapists to make their patients available, limited the cases seen here to 13, or 5 per cent of the final study sample.

In all, 254 of the hoped for total of 300 patients and families were interviewed. All patients were seen within 24 hours and usually within minutes to eight hours of admission to a facility. None had received drugs or electroshock prior to the research interviews. Interviews with families were sometimes delayed until a subsequent visiting day.

THE PROBLEM OF PSYCHIATRIC DIAGNOSIS AND DESCRIPTION—
OFFICIAL DIAGNOSES OF STUDY PATIENTS

An initial question centered about the best methods of describing the patients from a psychiatric-behavioral point of view. A strong argument was advanced in favor of using the diagnoses applied by admitting psychiatrists of the various units, perhaps modified by the project staff. Other reports, however, have shown that the same set of patients might yield evidence favoring a high prevalence of manic-depressive diagnoses in one country and of schizophrenic in another. Aside from this, the inherent deficiencies of existing nomenclatures made it seem unwise to depend upon them for research purposes.

An account of the diagnostic labels, criteria, and frequencies of project patients from the Casa Eiras is presented here to give a more concrete idea of the problem. The Brazilian diagnostic system follows an outline issued by the National Service of Mental Disease. This is shown in Table 15. No classification exists for neurotic depression, and mood disorders must be listed under manic-depressive psychoses. Other items reflecting the "official psychiatry" of the country and its differences from the most widely used United States diagnostic systems are: lack of a category for alcoholism other than a subdivision of exotoxic psychoses; the retention of the term, feeble-mindedness (translated from *débilidade mental*, or mental weakness) rather than a concept such as retardation with connotations of reversibility; limitation of the other oligophrenias to two, without effort at operational definition or subdivision into genetic or cultural determinants; lack of specific categories for seizure behavior including psychomotor epilepsy; lumping together of simple, hebephrenic, and catatonic schizophrenias along with the addition of paraphrenic forms and the omission of the category of paranoid condition; the inclusion of a special category of mixed and associated psychopathies; the separation of psychogenic psychoses into a special category without further subspecification; omission of dissociative reactions; and, aside from psychopathic personality, lack of a system of personality trait and pattern or characterological diagnoses. Some differences between the official Brazilian and the American Psychiatric Association nomenclature have been reduced with the latter's 1968 abandonment of the term "reaction" as a suffix to most diagnoses.

Although the system described above is used as the basis for all official statistical reporting and diagnostic discussions, Table 16, including diagnoses made by 10 psychiatrists in the Casa Eiras staff, indicates that many subvariants are regularly employed by individual physicians. It thus contains several ways of expressing a nonpsychotic depressed state and a number of alternatives for schizophrenia, such as "schizophreniform syndrome," apparently judged preferable to "psychogenic psychosis." Similarly, there appeared to be a need for the category of chronic alcoholism. Other rarely used labels reflect the idosyncratic interests of individual diagnosticians. The Casa Eiras, like many well-established and reputable institutions, has diagnostic criteria formulated by a committee or by interested individuals. While these criteria may be officially publicized or informally circulated, they are not, as is clear from Table 16, uniformly followed. The criteria of three of the hospital's senior psychiatrists for the diagnosis of schizophrenia are noted here as examples of the nosographic thinking of leaders in the field.

The first psychiatrist lists four sets of criteria on the basis of which a diagnosis of schizophrenia might be made or excluded: "(a) autism, ambivalence, or dissociation of thought, (b) exclusion both of identifiable organic factors and a comprehensible network

of psychological factors in the formation of symptoms, (c) the possibility of remissions, (d) exclusion of characterological contents
inclined toward a psychodynamic view of the disorder."

A second psychiatrist lists the following: "(a) extravagant
behavior—typical, (b) cosmic preoccupations, and (c) the fundamental symptoms of Kurt Schneider." He includes "schizophrenic
reactions and developments" under the heading of "psychogenic
psychoses." A "schizophrenic reaction" might occur in an "abnor-
mally developed personality." He observed that the frequency of
hebephrenic schizophrenia is greater in the Casa Eiras than
would be expected from its incidence in the general population
because of the "low socioeconomic level of the patients resulting
in impoverishment of thought and the rarity of structured delusions."

The third psychiatrist rarely diagnoses "schizophrenia," considering it a genetic fault: "The illness arises without comprehensible
psychogenic factors, it is irreversible, and therapy can only slow
down the process; there is always a permanent defect." He prefers
the term "schizophreniform reaction" for behavior which has a
"schizophrenic facade." This is considered a "reactive or regressive" syndrome in which, unlike the true schizophrenias, the patient is capable of establishing good interpersonal relations. It
may also occur "in consequence of certain types of epilepsies." In
spite of this exposition, the third psychiatrist insisted that he
makes these diagnoses "without much conviction, following no
single psychiatric school," and often using his "intuition."

Table 16 shows that the most frequent diagnoses in the Casa
Eiras sample (usually unchanged from the time of admission)
were of some type of schizophrenic behavior. Next in order were
alcoholism (mainly considered as a psychosis), neurosis, and
depressive states, some of which were considered neurotic. Most
diagnoses of "schizophrenia" were made by the first and third
psychiatrist whose criteria are listed above. The third made the
majority of those of "schizophreniform syndrome." It is interesting to note that the majority of these latter diagnoses as well as of
"psychogenic psychoses" were applied to females. Almost half the
patients diagnosed as depressive states were female; the two considered manic-depressive, manic were female.

Alcoholism is the most difficult category to interpret. Excessive
drinking was rarely regarded as a major problem by the project

interviewers, although it was acknowledged by 26 per cent of the entire patient sample. The admitting psychiatrist at Casa Eiras, noting its presence in 23 per cent, listed it as the only diagnosis in 13 per cent of the cases from this hospital (contributing 76 per cent of the project cases). Scrutiny of individual case histories and discussions with interviewers suggest that many whose admission diagnoses were "exotoxic psychosis, alcoholism" were, in fact, chronic schizophrenics or socially impaired neurotics for whom the crisis precipitating hospitalization was associated with an episode of intoxication. A great deal of alcohol, mainly cheap *cachaça* (or variants known generically as *pinga,* i.e., rum or booze), is consumed by the poorer people during *festas* or when a few men get together to talk and sing. Although this pattern may result in repeated intoxication and have social consequences because the money so spent could be used more effectively, it is not regarded as pathological or deviant. It represents, rather, an institutionalized way of behaving congruent with the norms of the lower-class community. The upper-class psychiatrist, however, confronted with an intoxicated patient sent to the hospital because of aggressive, hallucinatory, delusional, or panicky behavior, will often diagnose him as "exotoxic psychosis," and in the large majority of cases the admitting diagnosis to a hospital is the final one. The classical picture of delirium tremens was never encountered by the project psychiatrists at the time of their interview on the day, or within a day after, admission. Whether or not some chronically hallucinating patients might have been diagnosed alcoholic by admitting physicians rather than schizophrenic remains moot. Table 16 lists no patients with combined diagnoses of exotoxic psychosis and schizophrenia, suggesting that the latter might have been subsumed under the former. Only seven patients, just over four per cent of the Casa Eiras study population, were diagnosed as chronically alcoholic, that is, with a history of addiction and repeated acute episodes interfering with life adjustment, a figure more in keeping with the project interview results.

THE DATA-RECORDING INVENTORIES

In order to avoid the problem of diagnosis it was decided to record only behavior. This was broadly defined to embrace everything available to the interviewer. Two inventories were devised, one for recording observations of patient behavior, including patients' subjective reports, the other for recording social and cultural information including material about relatives. Before the data-gathering schedules were constructed, a series of ordinary clinical interviews was observed, tape-recorded, and discussed by project staff. These discussions, along with the author's prior experience in Brazilian psychiatric hospitals and the clinical experience and training of the Brazilian interviewers, psychiatrists, and social workers, provided a base for arriving at interview schedules and sequences. Professors Leme Lopes and Cunha added their own broad experience and suggested items of particular importance for both the patient and family interviews.

Each inventory was presented as a list, in pamphlet form, of alternative responses, with the interviewers required only to encircle appropriate numbers; space was provided for handwritten observations if these seemed pertinent. The inventories were constructed by the author with consultation from the project staff, and then translated into Portuguese.

The Initial Interview Inventory, while encompassing items of past history, dealt primarily with what could be observed immediately at the moment of the interview. It is one of a wide range of rating scales and similar devices developed by various workers in recent years for objective recording of patient behavior (Fleiss, Spitzer, & Burdock, 1965; Spitzer, 1965b). These reflect general agreement that in the absence of an objective system of observing and recording, epidemiological tables based on Kraepelinian nosologies reveal more about prevailing diagnostic biases in various countries or hospitals than about the actual nature of the behavior in question (Brody, 1964b). One such device specifically concerned with the initial psychiatric interview is the Mental Status Schedule developed by Spitzer with the collaboration of Burdock and Hardesty (1964, 1965a). This schedule was a major source of ideas in developing the instrument which was finally used. It includes a series of questions to be asked by the examiner in a sequence designed to provide a natural progression of topics, and offers numerous optional follow-up questions. Its major advantage for cross-cultural research lies in its concern with recording publicly observable items of behavior, including the content of the patients' speech. Using this as a base, and adopting its general approach to the ideas and observations of ordinary clinical interviews, an inventory was constructed to fit the characteristics of the patient population encountered in the Rio de Janeiro hospitals described above. This population combined elements of primitive cultures with those from advanced cultures and elements of belief in Western medicine with experience with Umbanda, Macumba, and Spiritism. With a low level of literacy, subsisting in an economically marginal state, often recently migrant from rural areas, it was to an important degree a culturally excluded population (Brody, 1965). The Initial Interview Inventory, then, while clearly derivative from Spitzer's work, also included primitive and folkloric references couched in general terms, did not require adherence to a predetermined sequence of questions, and contained the flexibility which hopefully would allow it to be useful in a variety of cultural settings. (Brody, 1966). It covered all aspects of interpersonal and conventionally defined psychopathological behavior, including the patient's verbal reports of current and past subjective states and life history events, and the doctor's observations of current behavior.

The first page of the Inventory contained a summary of directions for using it which had been discussed frequently during the training period; its presence was a constant reminder to the interviewer. It clearly stated that the emphasis was to be upon "publicly observable behavior, including verbal reports of subjective states, so that investigators of different cultures and nationalities may know the actual observations upon which diagnostic or etiological conclusions are based." The interviewer was described as having "a set which will enable him to be an open-minded, unbiased observer, sensitive to all aspects of the subject's behavior, whether considered as 'sick' or 'well'." The interview "should be conducted in an open-ended manner, following the general progression: present complaint and illness, relevant aspects of past history, further exploration of mental status during the interview." Finally the interviewer was instructed not to

use the inventory as a guide for a question and answer type of transaction with the subject. In the usual manner of nondirective interviewing he should avoid, during the first phase of the interview, giving directions to or responding to the patient in a way that will significantly distort the data or close off certain avenues of approach. There will, of course, be indications of topics which will require more detailed exploration. Later in the interview it will probably be necessary to return to one or more insufficiently investigated areas and to ask specific questions where information is lacking. It is, further, understood that patients with differing problems and of differing social class will require differing types of behavior on the part of the interviewer. Since any interview involves at least two persons, a section on the interviewer's observations of himself is included. The most effective utilization of this form will require the employment of trained and experienced interviewers. It is estimated that two to three hours of interviewing should provide the necessary information.

In every instance an attempt was made to indicate as clearly as possible that the behavioral event in question was something that the patient *said* or *did* during the interview itself. The margin of interviewer error was reduced by limiting his recording to statements that the behavior in question was or was not present, i.e., a true or false judgement. In many cases the item could be registered by circling a yes or no response. More often, however, a series of mutually exclusive statements or judgments of progressive intensity about the behavior in question was offered with the interviewer expected to circle only the most appropriate.

Three examples from the Inventory are shown in Tables 17, 18, and 19. The overall nature of the Inventory observations is indicated in the tables reporting actual findings in the succeeding chapters. The combined Initial Interview and Sociocultural Inventories included a total of 473 items. Two hundred and fifty-six of these were in the former and 218 in the latter, of which only 96 concerned the patient.

Special attention was paid to recording the effects of the doctor and of the interview situation itself upon the patient. The Inventory provided opportunities for detailed recording of how the patient approached the situation, and changes in his behavior during the interview. Because the interviewer's subjective reactions were themselves considered legitimate data of cultural interest, space was provided for recording the quality of his feelings about the patient. All Initial Interview Inventory interviews were conducted by the project psychiatrist in a private room in the hospital to which the patient had been admitted.

After both inventories were completed, a section concerned with the pathway to the hospital was executed on the basis of answers from relatives (who accompanied 72 per cent of the patients) and other informants (friends, physicians, authorities) as well as the patient. This listed the way in which the patient came, who accompanied him, statements or acts which resulted in his being considered ill, the family's theories about etiology, their expectations and wishes for the future. In addition, a separate series of sheets was used to record the results of a cursory physical examination.

The Sociocultural Inventory had sections for information about the patient, his father, his mother, his siblings, his spouse or mate, and his children. The section dealing with the patient was the most extensive and detailed; the others duplicated parts of it. (Initial analysis of the completed data showed that except for a few items, the only section providing useful material was that concerning the patient himself.) The social worker's method of recording was the same as that employed for the Initial Interview Inventory. These interviews included one or more family members in 85 per cent of the cases. Approximately a third were conducted in the patient's home, making it possible to obtain information from relatives of the 28 per cent of patients who had been brought to the hospital by friends or other nonrelatives.

All the data were transferred to punch-cards and then to magnetic tape, thus permitting rapid production of a large series of frequency tables using sociocultural items as independent, and both behavioral and sociocultural items as dependent, variables. Detailed scrutiny of these tables, and the transformation of their contents into percentages, made it apparent that in some instances many of the variables did not yield differences of even a few percentage points, and that in other instances differences did not occur in a consistent direction. It also became clear that far too many items or subdivisions had been used, frequently resulting in very small numbers of patients in each subcategory. This last reflected a cultural problem as well, for the initial inventories which had been presented to the staff for discussion were greatly broadened by their insistence that important aspects of Brazilian life or of psychopathology should not be omitted.

All ambiguous, nonproductive, or inconsistent categories were excluded from further analysis. These included the cursory physical examination schedules which revealed little unambiguous pathology and a range of interindividual differences too narrow for comparison between social groups. Subitems were combined to produce larger numbers of data points when this could be done without destroying the original meaning. In this way the extensive lists of items were finally condensed and combined to cover the ensuing categories of information.

Within the Sociocultural Inventory the following items were retained: Socioeconomic characteristics included education, occupation, housing, and socioeconomic status mobility. Migratory status was included in its various aspects. Demographic characteristics included color, size of family of origin, number of children, marital status, age, sex, and religion. Childhood influences included various indices of family stability, whether the father had died before the patient was 12, who had been in charge of discipline and how it was accomplished, parental literacy, and paternal occupation. Data on information and social participation included access to and ownership of informational media; relations with friends and neighbors, the clergy, and social welfare workers; and attendance at dances and soccer games. Data on hospitalization and the family included previous contact with psychiatrists, length of present illness, hospital where seen, who accompanied the patient to the hospital, reasons for hospitalization, and the family diagnosis.

Within the Initial Interview Inventory the psychiatric and behavioral characteristics of the patients which could be extracted from the mass of data coalesced around the following topics. One category included items reflecting the presence of tension, anxiety, sensitivity, and frustration. These covered observations of the patient during the interview, the psychiatrists' own reactions, anxiety symptoms including those related to situational factors, and evidence of interference with function, hostility, and impulsivity. Depression, including feelings of guilt comprised another category. Many items subsumed under the category of reality contact referred to a possible break with reality, such as general attitudes of suspicion, paranoid and grandiose beliefs (some of which were presumably delusional), and insistence on the reality of hallucinations and delusions. Somatic problems included a focus, anxious or hypochondriacal, on particular organs and psychophysiological complaints. Sexual problems occupied a separate category. Few items in the category of past psychiatric and developmental history yielded positive results, and these were not always consistent. The major items in the inventories which were retained are shown in the data tables in the following chapters.

CULTURAL SOURCES OF METHODOLOGICAL DIFFICULTY IN INTERVIEWING AND RECORDING

The basic data-gathering situation was the clinical interview of psychiatrist with patient, or social worker with family. Differences in the attitudes of project participants toward interviewing and data recording were apparent from the outset (Brody, 1966). North American investigators are accustomed to working with direct observations, which may conceivably lead to the development of new categories of classification. This means an emphasis on publicly observable behavior. In contrast, the Latin American tradition, more in keeping with that of Europe, classically depends upon first principles, on the basis of which a theoretically consistent scheme of data recording may be organized. Most accepted diagnostic systems are of this variety since the label to be attached to a particular patient is determined not by immediately observable behavior alone. It is determined by a complex set of inferences and deductions about the history leading to the current behavior and its probable future; by the motivational or interpersonal significance of the behavior; by its "functions" for the patient; by its adaptive value or lack thereof; by its possible genetic or biochemical bases; and by its modifiability. A particular problem posed by the use of such diagnostic systems is that the clinician who uses them makes decisions on the basis of culturally implicit but unstated connotations which load the most explicitly stated criteria. This may not impede communication between clinicans who belong to the same culture, but it does make it difficult for scientific messages about patient behavior to be transmitted across cultural boundaries.

Agreement on a standardized system of recording publicly observable behavioral events was further complicated by the nature of the interviewer-patient relationship. There was no question

about the desirability of having the research interviews conducted
by Brazilians, not only because they shared the language with the
patients, but because of nonverbal and other cues which sustain
communication between members of a single culture. The Brazilian psychiatrists, however, wondered if the use of a prearranged
sequence of questions or a predetermined interview structure
might not interfere with their own natural rapport with the patient and with the latter's spontaneity. This question assumes particular importance in a culture in which interpersonal warmth
and expressiveness are so marked a part of dyadic interchange,
and in which any evidence of impersonality is apt to be seen as
coldness, hostility, or, what is worse, indifference. The author's
repeated observations of interviews carried out by young psychiatrists, members of the project staff, and others, did, indeed, suggest a culturally influenced interviewing style—a mixture of benevolent-paternalistic and egalitarian elements. On the one hand,
the lower-class interviewee's perception of the psychiatrist as a
doutor (any upper-class person may be addressed by this title,
"doctor," by any lower-class person), or in some instances a *patrão,*
or patron, a member of the more educated and powerful class, fits
the psychiatrist's own self-perception, thus reinforcing the patient's tendency to respond acquiescently whenever the doctor
seems to have a preference for a certain answer. This last fits the
impression of passive-dependence with some ambivalence, noted
in the preceding chapter. (Acquiesence is also a way of evading a
question—a form of passive aggression.) On the other hand, the
doctor's culturally reinforced sense of status-security, coupled with
the cultural emphasis on respect for the patient's personal dignity
(since this is in part all that a poor man possesses), allows him an
apparent interpersonal openness, a human-to-human encounter
with the patient not ordinarily seen in the United States psychiatric resident. This is an aspect of a value brought to all of Latin
America, perhaps in most marked fashion to its Hispanic areas,
from the Iberian peninsula: all men have a unique inner dignity
(in Spanish, *dignidad de la persona)* which requires respect from
everyone including those at higher social levels. *Machismo,* the institutionalized emphasis on maleness or masculinity, less prominent in Brazil than in other Latin countries, is one aspect of this.

Another related value is that of establishing a mutual support relationship involving reciprocal favors or assistance between lower-and upper-class persons. However attenuated, this tradition imposes another constraint upon the interaction of doctor and lower-class patient.

Continued feedback from the patients, often frightened and confused, depended to a significant degree upon repeated demonstrations of the doctor's affectionate and respectful interest. Under these circumstances it began to seem likely that artificial systematization imposed upon the interviewer by a predetermined schedule could well deprive him of inner cues necessary to sustain his accustomed patterns of interpersonal behavior.

Another problem arose from the patients themselves. Predominantly from the lower class, most were unaccustomed to talking at length about themselves to others, especially to physicians who were from another social world. As noted in the preceding chapter, the usual expectation from a psychiatrist is that he will prescribe medicine and converse only briefly in order to give directions or offer encouragement and sympathy. The patients' ease of communication with educated people was impaired by their own complete or partial illiteracy which was compounded by some self-consciousness and feeling of inferiority and, often, suspiciousness as to why the doctor should be interested in knowing so much about them.

The difficulties were resolved in part by the decision to combine a free-flowing style of interviewing with nondirective elements, and a more structured schedule for recording data, the Initial Interview Inventory. This meant the psychiatrist was to treat the transaction as he would a therapeutically oriented clinical interview, but to make sure that he had acquired the wished-for data by going back to inadequately covered points. The "going back" phase often involved asking specific questions, but by this time the interview had usually been in progress for at least an hour, and a pattern of rapport and information-giving had been established. Since the data-gathering form, the Initial Interview Inventory, was used so often by the psychiatrists, it inevitably exerted an influence on the interview procedure.

THE HISTORY OF THE DATA-GATHERING OPERATION

The first phase was devoted to practice and familiarization with the inventories. Approximately 30 interviews were conducted and the results recorded on the inventory forms and discarded between October 1964 and the spring of 1965. The interviewers were trained by the author through direct observation and analysis of tape-recorded interviews, with special reference to the technique of asking open-ended questions rather than specific, concrete, restrictive ones. The issue of providing the patient with enough freedom and comfort to say what was on his mind was always uppermost. Eventually, the interviews became standardized at between two to two-and-one-half hours each. Repeated observations of the process of transferring clinical notes to the data forms were also carried out. An unforeseen problem in interviewer differences arose when a psychiatrist who began the project was forced by political circumstances to leave the project, and some time elapsed before his replacement was recruited. (Shifts of personnel because of governmental or economic instability are a research hazard in developing nations whose growth involves abrupt shifts of regimes.) No data recorded by the lost psychiatrist were included in the final data, so that more time passed while his replacement was trained until both interviewers' skills were judged to be comparable. At this point, when confronted with the same patient, both arrived at virtually identical ratings of behavior; comparisons of their ratings on a sample of patients matched for age, sex, and education revealed no systematic differences between them.

Less training time was spent with the social workers who interviewed family members accompanying the patients, and when they were unavailable, made home visits. In the very few instances when families were totally unavailable, either at their homes or during visiting hours after admission, the social workers interviewed the patients themselves in order to obtain the desired sociocultural information. There seemed to be less of a social gulf and considerably less of the benevolent-paternalistic style reflected in the social workers' interviewing manner, partly perhaps because of their less elevated status as females and partly because they were not being perceived as *doutors,* members of such separated social worlds. Fortuitous personal and social characteristics also played a part; one social worker, herself a *nordestina* of unobtrusive manner and slightly darker skin than the others, was conspicuously more effective at establishing rapport than any of the other project interviewers. Finally, since almost all their interviews were with family members rather than patients, the social workers did not have to cope with the disturbed outlook and high anxiety which made the doctors' interviews more difficult.

Data gathering on patients progressed on an irregular schedule through every month between April of 1965 and November of 1966. The long period and slow pace were due to the fact that all the project psychiatrists and social workers worked only part-time on this study; all were employed elsewhere in at least one and sometimes two or more positions. They, as well as their patients, were trapped by the rapid inflation and the limited salaries offered by educational and clinical institutions. A psychiatrist and social worker would operate as a team, devoting a day, or more often half a day, to a particular hospital, trying to see each new patient and his family who arrived while they were on the scene. Hospital visits were made every day of the week, except Sunday. Patients were almost never admitted during the night to Casa Eiras or the Sanatorio Botafogo. Those coming to the Pronto Socorro at night were usually not available for study because they were medicated almost immediately.

Data gathering on the social-cultural contexts in which patient behavior occurred was completed between July and September, 1968.

CHAPTER 3

THE CONTEXT OF BEHAVIOR:
METROPOLIS IN A DEVELOPING COUNTRY

"Psychological phenomena and the environments in which they occur are interrelated; they are interdependent" (Barker, 1969, p. 34). The environment or context of behavior is

> *not* a passive probabilistic arena of objects and events . . . the everyday situations within which people live . . . do not provide inhabitants with a limited and fixed array of environmental inputs, but with inputs that vary widely in accordance with the differing motives and cognitions of the inhabitants . . . [and] in such a way that the characteristic behavior patterns of the settings are generated and maintained *in spite of* the greater variety of interior conditions inhabitants bring to settings [p. 35].

Rio de Janeiro, like any behavioral setting with physical boundaries and functional regularities, can be viewed as an environment tending to reinforce or extinguish certain behaviors, one which poses particular problems of adaptation and offers special challenges and opportunities for personal support. It provides a large variety of stimuli to a heterogeneous group of receivers whose own varying perceptions and acts evoke or trigger different environmental inputs for different individuals and for the same individual at different times. An environment itself is produced and modified in part by the people who—along with other animate and inanimate entities and patterns—constitute it. The individuals and the social context, interacting with and modifying each other through self-regulatory feedbacks, maintain a degree of behavioral constancy at the same time that social-technological evolution continues. This chapter presents some aspects of Rio de Janeiro as a changing physico-human context for behavior. It is intended as a background from which to view the data of patient behavior in succeeding chapters, which are organized according to major sociocultural headings such as migration, literacy, or religion.

THE NATIONAL SETTING

The city, more than half of whose inhabitants were born elsewhere in Brazil, is part of a larger national system which can also be viewed as a behavior setting or in a general sense as an ecological-behavioral system. It is one corner of the "golden triangle" containing the bulk of the country's economic, financial, educational, and cultural institutions. The other corners are formed by Belo Horizonte, capital of the State of Minas Gerais, and São Paulo, capital of the State of the same name. Rio de Janeiro and São Paulo, 200 miles apart, are connected by rail, highway, and a *ponte aérea* or aerial bridge, with half-hourly flights throughout the day. In the Paraiba Valley between them, at Volta Redonda, are the largest steel mills in South America. Approximately a fifth of all factories and processing plants in Brazil were located in this subregion in 1968. The per capita income for the Rio-São Paulo region is at least twice that of the country as a whole. The people living here are more apt than elsewhere in Brazil to be caught up in the process of industrialization and in the often conflictful cultural transition from traditional to modern values, attitudes, and practices. Those whose attitudes and activities maintain the rate of change include many who are native to the area, large numbers whose immediate ancestors brought such aspirations with them from Europe, and internal migrants attracted by opportunity and new freedoms. For others, change is imposed upon them and constitutes a source of anxiety.

Another 500 miles down the coast from São Paulo is Pôrto Alegre, one of the most rapidly growing cities in the nation. Pôrto Alegre, capital of the southernmost State of Rio Grande do Sul has little of the African influence of the subtropical North; with its more temperate climate and large immigrant population it is European in manner and appearance.

The official national population according to the 1960 census was 70,967,185; in 1969 the Ministry of the Interior estimated it at 90,000,000. Brazilian leaders and many of their countrymen who are aware of the physical size, population growth (annual rate, three per cent), and undeveloped natural resources of their country, perceive it as the "Land of Tomorrow." Depending upon the definition of its boundaries, Greater or Metropolitan Rio de Janeiro included at least 5,000,000 residents in 1969, an increase of approximately 40 per cent over the 1960 population.

Sheer size is a prominent feature of the Brazilian context. Rio de Janeiro and the area of the "golden triangle" cover only a fraction of the 3,289,440 square miles of national territory. This vast land mass with a 4,600 mile coastline on the Atlantic Ocean occupies nearly half the surface of South America. An awareness of the unfamiliar inner reaches of his country and a semi-humorous contempt for the backwardness of its inhabitants is part of the city dweller's world view.

Most educated Brazilians have been more familiar with Europe and the United States than with the interior or distant coastal points of their own country. Very recently, however, outbursts of newspaper publicity, have reflected growing sensitivity to hints of foreign exploitation or control of the undeveloped territories, par-ticularly the Amazon region, itself a symbol of national hope and aspirations. The fact that Brazil's original colonization was along the coast and up the waterways, and that the old cities were sep-arated by mountain, jungle, and semidesert have contributed to a still-persisting regionalization almost unique in the Western Hemisphere.

Brazil never had a railroad age, and it was only in the late 1960's, stimulated to an important degree by the presence of Bra-silia, that motor roads began to connect the coastal cities with each other and the burgeoning centers of the interior. The air-plane has been the passenger bridge and beast of burden, giving a sense of national unity to the widely separated regions, and even in the late 60's the small-town airport filled with relatives greeting new arrivals or wishing *boa viagem* to those departing was reminis-cent of the bus station of the United States midwest in the 30's and 40's. This regionalization contributes to the behavioral im-pact of new settings upon migrants and allows the persistence and transfer into new areas of traditional beliefs and practices, especially as these involve work and religious observance. Size and regional isolation have contributed to a high degree of physical and cultural diversity, including contrast, among the Brazilians. And yet, as Poppino (1968) has pointed out, after more than four centuries since its colonization the overwhelming majority of Brazilians continue to live near the sea which provides a point of common interest and experience. In 1960, 13 of every 14 resided in the band of states from Maranhão on the North to Rio Grande do Sul in the South, only one of which, Minas Gerais, has no sea-coast. In nearly all the coastal states both the largest cities and the heaviest rural concentrations are within less than 100 miles of the Atlantic—a situation resembling that of the United States at the time of independence.

The past decade has been marked by an increasing tempo of planning for systematic area development. In 1969, the two major agencies developed for this purpose were SUDAM and SUDENE. SUDAM is The Superintendency for Amazon Development. It covers the States and Territories of Maranhão, Pará, Amapá, Amazonas, Northern Mato Grosso, Acre, Rondonia, and Northern Goias. This largely primitive area of about five million square kilometers contains only 6.3 million people and is promoted by the Ministry of the Interior as "one of the world's richest regions" and the potential "breadbasket of the Americas." SUDENE, The Superintendency of Northeast Development, is an autonomous agency of the Ministry of the Interior responsible for the "economic and social development" of the nation's most backward though populous region, the poverty-stricken "polygon of droughts." The area includes Eastern Maranhão, Piaui, Ceará, Rio Grande do Norte, Paraiba, Pernambuco, Alagoas, Sergipe, Bahia, and Northern Minas Gerais. One of the unstated aims of the program has been to provide job opportunities which will stem the tide of migrants toward the large coastal cities of the South.

The tremendous geographical, ethnic, and cultural diversity of Brazil, perpetuated in part by its inadequate transport system, has led to a series of attempts to subdivide it for purposes of analysis. Two such attempts by social scientists are the division of the country into culture areas (Diegues Junior, 1960), and into zones based on physical, ethnic, historical, and cultural patterns (Wagley, 1963). References to the folk types coming from these areas still persist as descriptive reference points in Rio de Janeiro conversation. Many of these come from the Northeast coast (the States of Rio Grande do Norte, Paraiba, Pernambuco, Alagoas, Sergipe, and Bahia), the traditional area of sugar *engenhos* or family-owned plantations with mills, now replaced mainly by large corporation-owned farms with their plants, the *usinas*. These states were the delivery points of the largest number of slaves (who were sent to Salvador do Bahia and Recife in Pernambuco until the opening of the mines of Minas Gerais), they have the largest concentration of blacks and mulattoes, and they are the site of the most viable African cultural heritage in the country. The Bahiano from Bahia is a familiar folk-type for Cariocas who are fond of bahiani food, music, and jokes. Umbanda, the syncretistic Afro-Catholic religion found mainly in Guanabara, owes much of its content and form to the Candomblé established by slaves in Bahia.

Another region described by Wagley is the arid pastoral Northeast inland from the coastal agricultural belt and including large areas of the States of Maranhao, Piaui, Ceará, Pernambuco, Rio Grande do Norte, Sergipe, Alagoas and Bahia. Its limits defined by federal law are those of the *polígono das sêcas* (polygon of droughts), regarded as a disaster area and long subject to special attention. Although the traditional economic activity here before the recent effort at factory building was cattle grazing, it supported less than 10 per cent of the nation's cattle. Its herdsmen, or *vaqueiros*, lead a seminomadic life and share the area with squatters or sharecroppers who practice a primitive agriculture as well as collecting from wild stands. This area is the *sertão* or backlands, the source of so much Brazilian folklore, of primitive folk Catholicism, of periodic messianic movements, and of isolated rebellions. The Nordestino is a familiar type in the metropolis, stunted, thin, and "tan" skinned; according to stereotype he is driven from his land by natural catastrophe yet retains an intense love for the freedom and open horizons it affords. Some of his songs are well known in Rio de Janeiro, including those of the Cangaçeiros, early bandits of the region.

Two other Northeastern stereotypes are frequently mentioned in Rio. One is the Pernambucano, supposedly quick to sing, dance, and drink. Many live in the city, including members of the artistic and intellectual world, and they retain their cultural identity as a source of pride and pleasure. The other is the Cearense; they are known as shrewd peripatetic traders. Their state is one of the poorest in the nation with one of the higest birthrates, but these sharp-eyed natives are proverbially successful dealers, said to extract a profit, however small, from every transaction.

The Eastern Highlands, another of Wagley's regional divisions, includes most of Minas Gerais, the western part of Espirito Santo, and the southern part of Bahia. This area was the scene of several mining booms and is still a major source of gold, precious stones, and industrially important metals, but agriculture and raising stock are its principal economic activities. A region of small towns as well as the planned modern city of Belo Horizonte, it is known for conservatism and hardheadedness and for the continuing strength of family and religious ties. Many Mineiros have achieved national political prominence.

The Amazon Valley constitutes a fourth region which accounts for about 45 per cent of Brazil's total area, but less than five per cent of its people. This is the area of the most static economy and the highest rates of infant mortality, illness, and illiteracy.

South of Rio de Janeiro is São Paulo and its port city of Santos 30 miles distant, which is the nation's most active. São Paulo State's wealth began with coffee, but unlike the sugar *engenhos* of the North with their slaves, the coffee *fazendas* depended upon immigrant tenant farmers or *colonos*. As noted above, much of the character of this area is rooted in its semitemperate climate and its immigrants; the Italian and Slavic influence are especially notable in São Paulo. The state also includes at least a quarter of a million Japanese. Paraná, Santa Catarina with a major German influence, and Rio Grande do Sul in the extreme South have been almost completely uninfluenced by the feudal slave culture of the North. Unimpeded by the classic Brazilian disdain for manual labor, the immigrants rapidly formed a middle class which in time became effective in urban as well as rural areas. The European homesteader also brought with him the tradition of diversified family farms. Some of the story of the early pioneers is told by Erico Verrissimo (1946) in his epic novel, *Of Time and the Wind.*

The great ranches of the Rio Grande do Sul *pampas* have much in common with those of Argentina and Uruguay with which they are contiguous, and there is indeed a strong Hispano-American influence seen in both the behavior and the speech of the people. The typical folk figure is the *gaucho,* the colorful, swaggering cowboy who lives on horseback and rides herd on his cattle (and now sheep). Even the thoroughly urban upper-class resident of Porto Alegre enjoys a direct, free-swinging manner in song, dance, or intellectual debate, and many living in Rio claim this to be their natural privilege as a *gaucho.* The *gaucho* stereotype is that of a person more persistent, productive, and hardworking than his *carioca* counterpart. Intellectuals, politicians, and businessmen from the South are important in national life. This region, however, contributes few lower-class migrants to Rio de Janeiro. In general, it is the North with its feudal heritage and continuing production of migrants which continues to be a problem for the relatively well-to-do South with its cities, strong European influence, mechanized agriculture, and a developing, educated urban middle class.

A final region, identified by Wagley and others, is the West. Still a frontier area much of which remains unexplored, its 22 per cent of the national territory includes Brasilia and just over four per cent of the population. From time to time gold and diamond booms occur, and with them appear new frontier towns in the tradition of the American West. Western Paraná is the site of rapidly developing new coffee farms and much land speculation. These areas do not draw significant migration from Rio de Janeiro although they influence its business, and urban speculators may gamble on land development or own farms in the frontier zones. They are, however, draining off the migratory streams from the Northeast, many of which now seem to be bypassing their traditional coastal destinations as they turn inland to the west, stimulated in part, again, by the existence of Brasilia.

The Bureau of the Census subdivides the country into five "physiographic" regions which have much in common with those described above. While these follow the political boundaries of

Brazil's 23 States, two Territories, and Federal District, they correspond in general to physical-geographic features of the land and to historical patterns of settlement, economics, and culture. Table 20 lists these regions, their component political entities, and their populations as well as that of their capital cities at the time of the 1960 census.

RIO DE JANEIRO CITY AS A BEHAVIORAL SETTING

SKELETON OF THE CITY—STRUCTURAL UNITS

Rio de Janeiro is a city-state. Its political boundaries are those of Guanabara, created by Federal Law Number 3,752 on April 14, 1960, on the site of the former Federal District. Its governor is the senior elected official of the city of Rio de Janeiro. The areas outside of Guanabara which are considered socioeconomically integral with the city are political subdivisions of Rio State. This latter had a population in 1960 almost identical with that of Guanabara dispersed over a considerably larger area. In 1968, after almost 20 years of discussion, arrangements were finally concluded for the construction of a bridge across Guanabara Bay connecting the population centers of the two States. If this becomes reality a true metropolitan region will emerge and new governmental arrangements for the region may be considered.

The city's limits include the natural barriers of the Atlantic Ocean and Guanabara Bay. As a functional socioeconomic unit, it spills out beyond Guanabara into the neighboring State of Rio de Janeiro. Within Guanabara, itself, there exist circumscribed pockets which, despite their proximity to the urban center, can best be described as rural. The following account of the city's structure is presented as a background for the later discussions of social influences on behavior which impinge upon people in their own neighborhoods before they become patients, as well as a description of the social context of which mental health services are a part.

Table 21 presents the most inclusive concept of the urban area. This scheme differentiates between "urban space" (the central section with its districts or *bairros,* suburbs, and peripheral towns, also called suburbs) and the so-called "urban pioneer zone," sometimes known as the *faixa*, or belt. The present city center corresponds approximately to the oldest area of Rio de Janeiro. The central peripheral zone surrounding the main business district is variable in nature, but includes some railroad stations as well as the areas regarded as obsolescent or deteriorated. The urban residential zone includes those of the well-known beaches, mainly to the South, the poorer homes in the North, and Santa Tereza hill.

The suburban zones are identified by railroad lines which serve the neighborhoods composing them. By common consent, most were initially defined as areas reachable only by trains; now many are the sites of light and medium industry as well as the homes of workers employed in the plants. The longest established *bairros suburbanos* which grew up along the rail lines (the E.F.C.B., Estrada de Ferro Central do Brasil, first laid from the center to the most accessible undeveloped areas), have become urban. Their growth was later hastened by the construction of major roads such as the Avenida Brasil. The older subdivisions stretching inland toward Rio State had a combined population of 912,074 in 1960, an increase of about 25 per cent over 1950; informal estimates place the probable 1970 population at almost 1,250,000. All are densely populated with both lower-class and moderately comfortable residences. The subdivisions require 30- to 60-minute train rides each way for the *funcionários* and the poorly paid white and blue collar workers employed in the central city, but they offer more adequate housing at lower cost so that most of the lower middle class are prepared to undergo the discomfort and small expense involved in commuting. In fact, the term "suburbanite" has acquired the informal meaning of a poorly paid but respectable worker, a family man with regular hours who works hard with little hope of advancement.

Meier is the largest center in the suburban zone noted on Table 22 and is equipped to care for all of its population's needs. Madureira, the second largest, is a *boca de sertão* (mouth of the *sertão*), a market for products from rural areas. Each occupies the status of a major town in its census zone, as noted in Table 22. While the stores in these major suburbs carry a wide variety of goods and appliances, they also deal in those especially suited for areas without electrical power. Pedal-driven sewing machines, for example, are displayed along with the latest table models.

The more distant inland areas, occupied mainly by the poorer classes, have ecologically discontinuous residential, industrial, and military sections. These have doubled and tripled in population since 1940 with the coming of new industries and construction of apartment blocks and lower-class *vila* by various social security and union-connected groups.

The peripheral zones listed on Table 2 are all major centers of Rio State. Niteroi, the capital, is a large city in its own right, the site of businesses, factories, and a university with a school of medicine. Sao Gonçala, Duque de Caxias, Sao Joao de Meriti, Nova Iguaçu, and Nilopolis are but five of the other *municípios* or townships (each of which contains one or more urban nuclei) of Rio State. The last four comprise what is known as the *Baixada Fluminense* (the Rio State lowlands), an area which at the time of the 1960 census contained 1.5 million people, many of whom had migrated in the preceding two decades from elsewhere in Brazil. By 1960 an estimated 70 per cent of the inhabitants of Duque de Caxias were *nordestinos*.

Outside of the urban space is the somewhat misleadingly named "urban pioneer belt." This includes new satellite towns and many old ones as well. Petropolis, the former summer home of the Emperor and one of the nation's historical shrines, continues along with Teresopolis as a fashionable weekend retreat for well-to-do Cariocas. During the oppressive humid heat of the summer the entire family may move to this cool mountain town only an hour from the city, while father commutes on weekends. Although the towns in this outer belt are surrounded by agricultural activities, they are not rural in structure or function and their inhabitants share an urban outlook with those who live in the metropolitan centers.

The zones and tracts used by the 1960 census are shown in Table 22. These were defined in part on physiographic features, on traditional fiscal subdivisions, on neighborhoods and districts gradually formed and named by public consensus over the years, and in part by the nature of roads, the presence of parks or city squares and the uniformity of housing in particular areas. Most of the traditionally established districts have also been given status as census tracts and are listed in Table 22. Others, such as Catumbí, have not been used for census purposes. The poorer class residential and business *bairros* of the traditional Zona Norte, include: Andarai, Catumbí, Grajau, Maracaná, Rio Comprido, São Cristovão, Tijúca, and Vila Isabel. Most of these are in the Tijuca Census zone. The well-known residential and hotel districts of the Zona Sul include: Botafogo, Copacabana, Flaméngo, Gavea, Ipanema, Lagoa, Laranjeiras, Leblon and Urca. As seen on Table 22, most of these districts are included in the Guanabara Bay and Seacoast Census Zones.

MORPHOSTRUCTURE OF THE CITY

Like all men, the Carioca is assaulted by and a creature of his physical environment, but the color, the noise, the crowds, and the vistas of the Cidade Maravillhosa are perhaps more inescapable than in most behavioral settings. There is no point from which the blue of the ocean or bay, or the jagged outlines of peaks to the landward are not visible. At night, even when shining through the haze of a raincloud, the illuminated figure of Christ floats atop the Corcovado mountain. The press of people and the sounds of traffic are pervasive and endure far into the night. The constant inflow of vivid, intense, sometimes pleasurable sensory stimulation is an accustomed feature of the environment. This may be assumed, depending upon the fluctuating needs of individuals, to have supportive value, to make silencing mechanisms necessary, and to contribute to the cognitive, affective, and communicative styles of the people.

Yet the city is like a beautiful woman who has aged and is not well. From a distance she is radiant; her contours and color are magnificent. But cracks in Rio's famous mosaic sidewalks are encrusted with dirt, and sidewalks as well as streets are often a wilderness of potholes which become small lakes after periodic downpours. The distant view from Corcovado shimmers with color, but straight down are waste papers and the ubiquitous orange peels. And the *morros* or granite hills which split the city into a series of great basins connected by tunnels, are sprouting with fungoid shacks and hovels, housing at least a fourth of the population. The Carioca lives with antitheses; he knows the beautiful conceals the ugly.

While the beaches, the mountains, the monuments, and the slums are most apparent, they are but a few of the many Rio de Janeiros in which different segments of the population participate. There is the Rio of the port, with its great cranes and ships; the Rio of the business center, including 77 head offices and 635 subsidiary branches of the banking network; the cultural and sporting Rio of libraries, museums, radio and television stations, cinemas, theaters and stadia; the Rio of industry, with its small to middle-sized factories manufacturing a wide variety of products; the Rio of rural pockets away from its center, as well as the sprawling unformed development on the periphery and in the State of Rio de Janeiro. Finally, there is the Rio of government and bureaucracy. Although the capital and the Distrito Federal are now in Brasilia, nearly a third of the federal payroll in 1968 was spent in Rio. For all of its slums and underemployed people, the "marginals" as they are called, the per capita income for Guanabara is about three times the national average. The Carioca usually has more money than other Brazilians, and if he is poor, he is more regularly exposed to the wealth of others.

The city is a prisoner of its topography. Beaches, lakes, hills, and mountains occupy more space than flat ground. Since it cannot expand horizontally with increasing population, it must grow vertically. Since it cannot cross the *morros,* it must tunnel through them for communication, and tolerate the connecting passageways —noisy and redolent of fumes and sweat at the rush hour. A profusion of Volkswagens and other locally produced models is replacing the ancient American cars which formerly dominated the streets. The huge buses which roar at high speeds down the crowded avenue constitute a particular hazard; the Carioca at the throttle of his own tiny car seems called upon to demonstrate that he, too, is a man to be reckoned with, and accidents are frequent. All of this lends credence to the tale of the *Bahiano* who left the city for his home after six months because he had not yet learned how to cross a street.

The contrasts so much a part of Rio de Janeiro are also seen in the proximity of the old and the new. The city's 400-year history is reflected in its many churches, some of which remain oases on busy thoroughfares, dwarfed by nearby office buildings; in the remnants of colonial architecture, much of it now in disrepair in the central section; in the aqueduct; and in the narrow streets of

some districts. Here and there among the rectangular office buildings are examples of the school of architecture led by Oscar Nie-
meyer; Cariocas are pound of the new Ministry of Education and
Health, of the Museum of Modern Art with its formal gardens
designed by Roberto Burle Marx (but no permanent art collection), and of other structures—all symbolically tied to the new
capital of Brasilia, which, while it continues to evoke mixed feelings as a practical venture, is a source of national pride for its
concept and design. Another aspect of the physical scene, and one
not congruent with the Carioca stereotype, is the constant building activity, which is facilitated by the use of reinforced concrete.
The stark gray skeletons of unfinished structures on which work
has stopped for lack of money have become a trademark of the
city.

The limitations of the *espaço urbano Carioca* as city planners call
it, have led to severe crowding. The density of the population, estimated in 1960 as 6,000 per square mile for all of Guanabara
(Poppino, 1968), contributes to the insufficiency of water, electricity, schools and other municipal services, and to congestion on
the sidewalks as well as the streets. Nevertheless, the Brazilian,
even the small-town dweller, is accustomed to this, and he likes
the *movimento* which comes from many people living close together, walking, talking, singing, dancing, and playing their radios. Faced with the relative emptiness of most United States
main streets, especially at night, he feels lonely and isolated. At
the same time, the constant contact with others, while dealt with
by an elaborate system of courtesy, is said by some Brazilian psychiatrists to engender a form of tension which has no solution,
since the longed for isolation is, in itself, distressing.

The most widely known district of the Zona Sul is Copacabana. (As noted in Table 22, more of the Zona Sul is included in
the Guanabara Bay—Southern Border and Seacoast Zones.) In
Copacabana in 1958 there were 4,600 inhabitants per block
(Segadas Soares, 1965) and some observers believe this figure was
doubled in the ensuing ten years. Copacabana's population explosion began in 1945 (Geiger, 1960). By 1965 it had reached
240,347, and informal estimates for 1970 suggest that with increasing high-rise apartments the level may approach the
half-million mark. To this figure there must be added the tourists,
inhabitants of other districts attracted by its stores and entertain-

ment features, hotel workers, maids, and office workers, all in less than four square kilometers.

The rapid growth of this area has stemmed partly from the deterioration of the central section of the city. For 20 years the better stores, movie theaters, night clubs, and restaurants as well as medical and dental offices have been moving into Copacabana. Another reason for increasing density lies in social heterogeneity. Most neighborhoods contain a variety of social classes. Throughout the Zona Sul, mainly along the seacoast, deluxe buildings alternate with homes of the middle class and the proletariat. Those who live in apartment houses mingle in the streets and squares with *favelados* whose shacks are perched on the *morros* looming overhead. In Ipanema, for example, in the Praça General Osorio, around which are several galleries, a theater, and restaurants frequented by the young artistic-intellectual set, white preschoolers accompanied by mothers or maids share the play areas with older black and brown children who have descended alone from the Morro of Cantagálo. At the dead end of a street occupied by apartment buildings, valued because it is near the square and the beach, there is a pump around which the *favelados* gossip and wash clothes before beginning the steep ascent back to the top of the *morro* with their precious water balanced in gallon tins on their heads. The green area between the circular drive around the Roderigues Freitas Lagoon (part of the Zona Sul—lagao district) and the water is used for clothes-washing, outdoor cooking, and impromptu soccer games by residents of the *favela* spilling down from the unoccupied hillside inland from the drive. The *favela* Praia de Pinto, on another shore of the Lagoon, was popularly considered the most noisome and a refuge for criminals before it was burned and razed in 1969. It protruded into Leblon, across the street from a luxury restaurant and a block from its major shopping thoroughfare. With rare exceptions the movement is one-sided; although the *favelados* penetrate freely into the surrounding city, the apartment dwellers almost never enter the slums and speak of them mainly with fear and loathing. (These issues are discussed at greater length in the chapter on housing.)

Construction of one-bedroom apartments for speculative purposes has perhaps reached its peak in Copacabana, putting non-*favela* housing here within the reach of those with few resources. This is reflected in the 1960 census finding that in spite of its high concentration of hotels and shops the relatively small area of Copacabana contained the highest proportion (six per cent) of the city's total of permanent private residences of any census tract. By informal estimate, these proportions will probably remain constant through 1970.

In the Zona Norte (much of which is included in the Tijúca Census Zone shown on Table 22), there are almost no open lots; land is not so expensive as in the South and skyscraper construction not so prevalent. Here are middle-class bungalows, *vila*, which are actually multiple dwellings often grouped around a single courtyard or alleyway, and in most *bairros*, larger and more comfortable residences as well. Apartment houses are becoming more common, especially in Tijúca, the most affluent section of this zone. The more educated and well-to-do people from the Zona Norte and its suburbs, however, continue their gradual movement into the South.

In the center city many of the old buildings serve commercial purposes while at the same time containing much lower-class housing occupied by recent migrants and those who have found lodgings near their places of work. These formerly elaborate dwellings are fragmented into offices, rooming houses, and *casas de comodos*, i.e., pensions for single men, often drifting, who may remain in any one lodging for only a brief period. In its old sections, the center city is also an area where homeless people may find a place to sleep for the night in a doorway or a square, or where they may squat selling small articles or food. The Praça Tiradentes (Place of the Toothpuller), named after a dentist who was one of the fathers of Brazilian independence, is such a place. The streets around it are heavy with the noise of buses and automobiles, and often it is half-ringed with booths selling books or records. Nearby are bars and the closest Rio equivalent of a burlesque show. On a typical night a family from the Northeast, a grandmother, her daughter, and two young children, were squatting at the far corner of a shelter for bus passengers. With a glowing charcoal brazier, they cooked tidbits of regional food, which the pajama-clad children offered for sale to passersby. Two crates covered by a blanket formed a secluded nook in which the children would eventually sleep. Customers were rare, but the passersby were friendly and polite. The family's overall air was not one of desperation or unhappiness, but rather of cheerful acceptance, and they seemed very much at home as the traffic swirled around them. This scene, with variations, is replayed nightly in many sections of the city, especially in the older parts of the center.

MUNICIPAL SERVICES AND THE TELEPHONE

Services taken for granted in more highly developed countries continue to be erratic and idiosyncratic here. Recurrent failures in electric power, water, street and sidewalk repair, gutter and storm sewer functioning, and other aspects of the normally un-noticed infrastructure of urban existence are constantly visible elements of city life.

Perhaps the best illustration concerns the telephone service. Ac-cording to officials of the CTB or Brazilian Telephone Company, even a light shower may be enough to soak underground cables and interfere with the operation of entire exchanges. More serious is the absolute insufficiency of the system. In 1968 there were ap-proximately 62 incorporated municipalities in the country which did not contain a single telephone. Even in the largest metropolitan centers home owners and apartment dwellers considered them-selves lucky if they were so equipped. In Rio de Janeiro approxi-mately 400,000 telephones served a population of between 4.5 and five million. For millions of marginal slum dwellers as well as those in the more stable lower class, the twentieth century practice of person-to-person voice communication across distance simply does not exist. Even well-to-do business and professional people often resign themselves to the need for face-to-face contact (reinforced by traditional cultural practices) which may involve tiring auto-mobile trips through heavy traffic in order to resolve many issues dealt with elsewhere by telephone. The public telephones at Ga-leão, Rio's International Airport, provide a sample both of the mechanical and the human aspects of the situation. There are "good" telephones and "bad" ones—the former requiring shorter waits before the dial tone signals the user to insert a previously purchased slug. It is not uncommon to see a man straddling two phone booths, holding a receiver in each hand, awaiting the arri-val of the tone or cessation of a busy signal from overloaded lines; by and large, telephone users are good-humored as though inured to the minor annoyances of life in their city. Life at close quarters, under the pressures of many minor frustrations, with transactions conducted on a personal basis, may well contribute to ironically humorous styles of relating and a reliance upon traditional forms of courtesy.

As is true for many problems, suggesting a failure in the capacity for collective action at the local level, this has become a matter of federal concern: A National Council of Telecommunications was created in 1962. Active development and implementation of plans were delayed, however, until 1968 when Contel (Conselho Nacional de Telecomunicações) announced a short-term plan aiming at the development of an effective national network within four of five years, to coincide with the establishment of an inter-American network—Rêde Interamericana de Telecomunicações (RIT)—under the auspices of the Organization of American States. In this instance the orientation toward international rather than domestic values, suggested by some observers as characteristic of developing countries, may provide a stimulus for movement. The chief motive appears to be status or "face" in the eyes of others: It has been said that work on the project should be accelerated so that Brazil will not be the cause of a delay in the installation of RIT in other Latin American countries.

In the summer of 1968 the *Jornal do Brasil* (Aug. 4) ran a headline epitomizing a salient attitude: recognition of present problems coupled with faith in the future. The banner spread across the top of a page read, "Brasil is 30 years behind in its communications but the future is encouraging." The article noted that a telegram between New York and Moscow requires a tenth of the time involved in getting a telephone call through from Belém to Porto Alegre. It went on to comment wryly that this situation exists in an era when plans are afoot to employ satellites in an inter-American communications system and to establish color television in Brazil.

CRIME AND POLICE SERVICES

In mid-1968 the Guanabara police force of 30,000 men, consuming 10 per cent of the state budget, was a storm center of controversy. It was described in the press as an army, larger than that of many small Latin countries but unable to guarantee the security of the people. The police had been the target of criticism before, but mainly for brutality as in the much publicized disappearance of a number of beggars whom they had allegedly murdered some years earlier. On this occasion, however, the storm broke after the early morning killing of a series of taxi drivers. Crime then was added to the poorly regulated traffic as a topic of serious discussion. It was pointed out that there occurred daily in 1968 an average of four assaults, three automobile robberies, and one homicide, this last figure compared with a total of 20 homicides for the entire year of 1960 (*Jornal do Brasil,* Aug. 8). Robbery and assaults within the *favelas* are not fully reported to the police. Armed robbery of an upper-class person by a lower-class assailant appears to be still rare. Anecdotal evidence suggests that rape as well as assault and theft are not uncommonly perpetrated by the poor against the poor, within *favelas* or similar areas. Nonetheless, these crimes, regarded by both their victims and the agencies of social control as part of the ordinary context of a dangerous and deprived life, go unreported.

Fear of burglary and house-breaking is so commonly met among the middle class in the absence of actual incidents that it appears to be almost an institutionalized form of anxiety. The source of danger is generally identified as the marginals. The connotations of "marginals" are many. At times it means the underemployed *favelados* who have little to lose and everything to gain, and for whom anyone with property is fair game. Often it refers to a loosely defined "criminal element," sometimes organized, occasionally with money, but always parasitic, ready to prey on the established working class or bourgeoisie. The general lack of confidence in the Guanabara police organization is reflected in the growth of private police forces employing several thousand guards.

SELF-HELP AND COMMUNITY ASSOCIATIONS

Besides the need for adequate protection, other problems such as maintaining the cleanliness of streets, the general upkeep of parks and plazas, obtaining adequate street lighting, water sup-

plies, transport, garbage removal, and the repair of broken street
pavement have stimulated joint action. Most of the associations
are made up of businessmen who contribute fixed amounts to hire
the necessary help. In this case collective action has been effective
to a degree, but it involves relatively few business leaders and
does not include a broad popular base. These associations have
planted trees, developed parking areas, built a tourist center, installed new equipment in police stations, sponsored improvements
in primary schools, established a garbage collection service and
permanent services for sidewalk maintenance.

One hoped-for improved government support of community
services lies in more effective tax collections. Traditionally the
income tax has been regarded as a penalty to be avoided by anyone with intelligence; bribing collectors was one of the accepted
means of dealing with it. New enforcement procedures, however,
and a stiffening attitude by high administrators since the military
government was installed in 1964, have begun to increase collections; the first arrest on tax evasion charges in the nation's history
was made in 1967. The names of delinquent individuals and businesses were publicized, agents' salaries were increased, and they
were awarded a proportion of the fines imposed as a result of
their work. In consequence, tax revenues have more than doubled
since 1965. The tax rates are still much lower than those of the
United States, and while there are many huge family fortunes, no
more than four to five per cent of the population have the income
of at least $150 monthly on which taxes are levied.

DIVERSION

Many diversions may be regarded as among the constant or
recurring patterns of behavior which help to make a behavioral
setting (Barker, 1968). They are bounded by space and time and
are associated with the milieu, all of which are essential to the
behavior. Examples of such milieus are classrooms, stadia, theaters, and doctors' offices. Persons are required or not, attracted or
not, to participate, so that the significance of the milieu for individuals within the same city may be highly variable. Participation in any diversion or behavior pattern is, like all participation,
a function of a mix of socioenvironmental and intrapsychic fac-

tors. Many would say that the chief Carioca amusements are chatting, drinking, singing, and dancing. The salient physical features of the city, however, which most strongly influence its recreational habits are the beaches. These are present as a concept and as a visual stimulus even for those who do not use them. They constitute a playground, easily accessible without cost from most parts of the city, although the ocean requires an hour by train or bus from the deep North Zone and major suburbs such as Meier and Madureira. They provide relief from the oppressive heat and humidity, swimming, sunbathing, fishing, looking, walking and running space for those who spend most of their lives constrained in cramped, noisy, and dirty quarters; they are also the sites of volleyball and soccer games between neighborhood or business-based teams, and meeting places for all of the disparate elements which make up the Carioca population.

Only the still largely undeveloped beaches of Barra da Tijúca are limited to those with private automobiles. For the poorer inhabitants of the South Zone, the beaches of Botafogo and Flamengo on the bay are available. Although the polluted waters of the former make swimming undesirable, many improvements have been made at the latter as well as in the nearby park along the bayshore drive to increase its recreational usefulness. Farther inland, toward the head of Guanabara Bay at the road to Ilha do Governador and the International Airport, another beach, Ramos, has been developed. This is utilized almost exclusively by North Zone inhabitants including those from a number of nearby *favelas*. The precise influence of the beaches on the adaptation of poor and otherwise frustrated people is a matter for conjecture. It can only be said that they are an important part of the life space of the Cariocas, and for many add an extra dimension of pleasure as well as of necessary relief.

The beaches have yet another significance for these people, so many of whom have been accustomed to living or working near the shore or upon the sea. This is revealed in the sweeping nighttime view of Copacabana seen from the top of the Hotel Miramar at the far end of Avenida Atlantica near Arpoador (Harpooner's) Rock. Between the ribbons of light created by cars on the Avenida and the irridescent whitecaps as the breakers rush in lies the darkness of the sand. After a moment, on most nights the observer can see a series of faint yellow points glimmering against the black strip between roadway and water. These are votive candles lit in homage or supplication to Iemanjá, goddess of the waters, and protected against the wind in little scooped out sand hollows. The early morning stroller will often find the burnt candle stubs, sometimes surrounded by square or other ritual markings in the sand. On this or any other beach he will also find from time to time roses, gladioli, or white carnations lying limp or still caught up in the tidal wash, or he may occasionally see the worshippers or supplicants themselves. On particular holidays such as New Year's eve, before January which is the month of Iemanjá, thousands of all colors and social classes, may appear, dressed in white robes. Most of the time, they are dressed conventionally and attract no attention. One such, in the dusk near Arpoador Rock, was a middle-aged soberly dressed white woman who, removing her shoes, walked to within 15 yards of the water; she knelt, scooped a hole in the sand, lit a candle and then stood silently facing the ocean for several minutes before repeating the procedure with another candle. On another occasion, in the gathering darkness on a chilly, windy August evening in Ipanema, a young black woman stood chanting on the sand, then waded into the water until her hem was soaked, deposited a newspaper filled with flowers into the waves before returning to repeat her prayers.

The shared recreational interest which is most ardently discussed among the Cariocas is soccer, or *futebol*. This is truly a national sport, even more so than baseball in the United States, and is played by young men and boys of all social classes, on every type of possible terrain, in the most remote as well as the populated parts of the country. There is no little boy who does not know of Pelé, the Negro national hero who first led his country's team to the world soccer championship in 1958. Even dignified older Carioca professors have been seen standing in the rain in other South American countries hoping for a glimpse of Pelé as their nation's team entered or left a hotel. *Futebol* inspires strong feelings and outbursts; team banners carried by spectators dwarf the pennants of United States football crowds, and the wildly flag-waving, passionately roaring crowd at Maracaná, largest stadium in the world, is almost frightening to the first-time observer. The huge bowl is usually filled to capacity, especially for games between the Flamengo and Fluminense (Niteroi) teams, "Fla" and "Flu" as they are popularly known. Spectators strip to the waist in the hot sun on the top ranks of concrete bleachers where most are seated, movement is intense in the stands as well as on the field, and, as much as physical barriers permit, the watchers are true participants in the action. There is no better description of this vital event than that contained in a special 1968 issue of *Manchete,* the Rio picture magazine. The Maracaná, it states, is ". . . still too small to contain the anguish or ecstasy of the Carioca's greatest passion . . . (he) . . . is an unleashed, howling creature, talking only in screams . . . Rio transforms her football into carnival, the players dancers on the field, the fans revellers in the main stand. Above all things, the Carioca is a frustrated Pelé . . . a demanding and often intolerant show of world champions" (p. 20).

The significance of *futebol* like that of beaches for Carioca life is a matter of conjecture. It is plausible to suggest, however, that while the ever-present beaches provide support, relaxation, and an opportunity for surcease from tension, the preoccupation with *futebol* and the matches themselves constitute an opportunity for abreaction, a periodic displaced outpouring of built-up tension, as well as a focus for distracting attention from the rigors of reality. It is a collective activity as well, in which the suspicious or socially isolated may feel themselves, at least temporarily, part of a group. *Manchete's* comparison with *carnaval* is apt, since preparation and anticipation for this last also offers an ongoing focus of attention which gives meaning to life in addition to its yearly four-day collective frenzy of dancing, drinking, and forgetting.

Carnaval is the most impressive denying, distracting, and substituting collective activity of Rio, concentration on which permits the shutting out of the squalid misery of *favela* life. In one popular song the memory of a *"carnaval* of which there can never be another"* is presented like a fantasy of paradise. This also has meaning for well-educated, well-to-do Brazilians. While many leave their city homes to escape the crowds of *carnaval,* the *favelados,* whose dancing dominates the *carnaval,* influence the cultural life of the country as a whole and particularly of Rio de Janeiro. The response of a group of well-to-do patrons in an upper-class night club, at the climax of a *carnaval* scene when confetti and streamers were being thrown, was complete involvement—flinging streamers with abandon, laughing, moving to the rhythm, singing the words of well-known *carnaval* songs—participating in the renactment of a yearly ritual with its roots in their own childhood experience.

Another diversion immensely popular among Cariocas is movie-going. The newspapers carry intense and lengthy critical cinema columns, and the major theaters are usually filled. On weekends long queues stretch into the streets when the best advertised films are showing. Audiences seem to be of two clearly differentiated types. The newest films in major theaters on the Avenida Nossa Senhora de Copacabana, for example, attract audiences which appear middle class and often resemble United States college students in clothing and age. This is especially true on weekends. Older theaters with lower rates, in which the seats are apt to be wooden rather than upholstered, may—especially in midweek when they have off-duty nights—attract maids, laborers, doormen, and the like. The difference is clearly visible in the clothing and often in the predominantly darker skin color of the patrons. These latter audiences are often noisy, catcalling at the screen and sometimes talking loudly to each other.

Two other aspects of movie-going may be related to cultural patterns. One is the rule concerning age of attendance. No child of 14 or less is permitted to enter a theater after six or seven p.m., even if accompanied by his parents. And a large number of movies, such as *Tom Jones* which had unrestricted viewing in the United States, are not open to people of 18 years or less. With some exceptions the rules are strictly observed by theater managers under pain of fine or license loss. Films may be prohibited on grounds of what is considered either excessive sex or violence. The Brazilian middle class, though less so in urban Rio than in more traditional areas to the North, sharply differentiates between the kind of stimulation permissible in the home surrounded by the family, and the uncontrolled input which may occur in a public setting. The other striking aspect is the number of foreign films, with those from Hollywood predominant. They are shown with the American speech muted and Portuguese subtitles. While the best theaters show currently popular features, in many of the others the standard is the "Class B" Western. Thus the movie-going Carioca is subjected to a steady exposure of North American language and stereotypes. In consequence, he is, perhaps, familiar with many individual American words, but the effect of this regular exposure to strange scenes with no possibility of validation can only be guessed.

For those who can afford it, television also carries a steady stream of canned one- or two-year-old United States programs. In these cases verbal Portuguese is substituted for the American.

The Samba,* along with its newer derivatives such as *bossa nova*, is heard most prominently in Rio de Janeiro and is the most well-known and widespread of all forms of popular music in Brazil. It was derived from the African rhythms, called *batuque*, brought into the country with the slaves; early foreign observers of the dances set to these rhythms were impressed by their frankly sexual motions not seen in the popular dances of Europe. Since then it has undergone changes while preserving much of its basic character to become one of the most authentic expressions of the Brazilian ethos. It is possible to use *samba* to describe the setting, the institutions, the value system, the relationship between the sexes, and race relations in Brazilian life. A recent wish-fulfilling song, for example, concerns the beautiful daughter of a rich lady who fell in love with a black man. Her mother forbade her to see him, so she ran away to live with him high in a hilltop *favela* and became a queen of the *samba*.

In the early 1900's the *samba* was still seen as an expression of marginality related to lower-class status, to life in the suburbs or on the *morro*, in contrast to the urban center, to irresponsible behavior and even to antisocial actions. Nowadays it has a new prestige. This began with Noel Rosa, a composer of more than a hundred minuets, who died in 1937 at the age of 27. He was known for the sense of humor with which he drew a caricature of the Brazilian way of life in his music. He did not leave untouched even LeComte's Positivism, so dominant for decades, with its motto of "Order and Progress" incorporated in the Brazilian flag. His *samba* "Positivism" began by stating that, "Truth, my love, lives in a well," and went on to explain how the unhappy end of a romance was due to the failure to obey LeComte's law.

---

*This section on The Samba was written by Dr. Manoel Wilson Penna.

The *samba* since Rosa reflects a pervasive Brazilian mood as well as an attitude toward life; there is hardly a well-known *samba* which does not have a touch of sadness. As the words of one of them go, *samba* is "to cry out of joy, is to cry out of nostalgia, within a melody." The rhythm and the melody can be light, fast, and gay, the words can be humorous and describe tragedy almost as a joke, but the sadness is still there. One of its most important elements is fatalism, a recognition of man's powerlessness in the face of life; submissiveness without despair. This may be described in terms of a certain passivity, even a rather weak acceptance of one's place in life. The anguish or rebellion, if there is any, is submerged and shunted aside by music and dance or expressed in disguise by clever sayings and jokes. This mood may be related to the actual powerlessness of the bulk of the population. It can also be related to other characteristic features of Brazilian life, such as the forms of religious expression. If Brazilians have no expectations of bettering their real lives, they turn to the supernatural world, seeking strength and courage.

Along with the mood of sadness and passivity, the *samba* reflects defensive attitudes: cynicism, a disbelief in social institutions, and a wariness of other people's motivations—especially those of public officials. In the 1960's a group of young composers in their teens and early twenties brought the *samba* fresh vitality. A new category was created, the *samba de protesto,* which harshly criticizes Brazilian life and institutions. Years ago there was a *samba* about the *morro,* a poetic idealization which said that although people lived in slums atop the *morros* they were happy because they could hear the birds singing and lived closer to Heaven. Now a *samba* about the *morro* says: "Ugly, it is not pretty/the *morro* exists but asks to be extinguished/It sings but its song is sad/Because it has only sadness to sing." Brazilians feel themselves prisoners of the "wheel of life." *Roda Vida* (Life Wheel) by Chico Buarque de Holander, 23 years old, describes the helpless feeling of a man who finds that the larger world is in actual control of his life. The first lines state: "There are days when one feels/As if one has departed or died/One has stopped all of a sudden/Or it was the world that grew up/One wants to have an active voice/And his destiny command/But here comes the life wheel/And carried the destiny away."

EATING AS A DIVERSION

With increased crowding and business activity as economic life has become more intense, a new breed of restaurant has appeared. Entitled, with the Brazilian fondness for incorporating and modifying North American words, *lanchonetes,* these quick-lunch establishments, so out of tune with the siesta tradition, offer anything from a pastry to a complete meal, eaten standing at a counter or seated on a stool. Some function mainly as coffee bars where the Carioca gulps his *cafezinho* instead of sipping it at a sidewalk cafe. For most, however, the lunch break continues to be longer and more substantially filled than in the United States. Cheap restaurants have "commercial plates" heaped with rice, beans, and stew at a cost possible for most minor clerks, salesmen, and skilled manual workers. It is more customary than in the United States for institutions and some businesses to supply their employees with bulky noontime meals at low cost. And even the working man with his food in a paper bag is apt to make more of a time-consuming ceremony of eating and drinking. All, including the *favela* dwellers, appreciate the low-alcohol Brazilian beer, usually available in draft as the familiar *chope,* and consumed in quantity, especially during the hottest months.

In general, food continues to be a source of pleasure and an occasion for ceremony. Adult Cariocas originating elsewhere in the country characteristically continue to have a strong interest in the regional food of their early lives. To those who can afford it, and many who cannot, it is important to have several types of dishes on the table as a traditional reflection of the capacity to be hospitable and openhanded. Traditional foods from the era when refrigeration was not available continue to be prominent. As noted in the preceding chapter, the poor inhabitants of this seacoast city still eat *farinha* from the Northeast and *bacalhau,* dried cod from the Portugal of their ancestors. As one middle-class housewife has put it, "I don't feel that it is a meal unless both rice and beans are on the table."

THE SENSE OF BEING A CARIOCA—TYPICAL AND STEREOTYPICAL STATEMENTS

It is hard to find a "real" Carioca in the sense of someone actually born in the city. However, those who move into it soon begin to "feel like a Carioca." The image is that of a persom who knows he lives in the old capital and the present cultural center. "To be a Carioca is to be in the center of Brazil, which is like being in the center of the universe," they say. "Every Brazilian intellectual, no matter where he lives, feels an obligation to come to Rio at least once a year. This is the world of the arts and letters. He used to come just to visit the bookstores, which were almost like salons where he would go to meet his friends, others like him, and to talk, to find out what was going on." For people in the lower class, "It is where there are the best performers and movies . . . you can go to a radio station or watch television and see the personalities." Or, "To be Carioca is to go to the beach and to be a *futebol* fan." The Carioca stereotype—the relation of which to reality is undetermined—is someone who is good-humored, easygoing and irresponsible, who would rather sing and dance than work. Yet, it is beter if he has accomplished something, preferably of an artistic or literary nature, if he has become a *personalidade*, although without too much effort. In this last sense Noel Rosa was a prototypical figure. He dropped out of the second year of medical school to become the leading composer of the 1930's *samba*. He wrote music on the streetcars or in a taxi on the way to the recording studios and spent much of his time chatting, drinking, and singing. "He was an ideal Carioca type from an era when Rio was not yet a true metropolis."

Another frequently invoked characteristic of the Carioca is his fondness for *jeito* or, in diminutive form, *jeitinho*. This has many translations ranging from manner, skill, knack or talent, to diplomacy. To *dar um jeito* is to find a way to manage, or to find a solution. *Falta* or lack of *jeito* is the equivalent of clumsiness. The main point is that faced with problems and frustrations, the *jeitoso* Carioca will, somehow, find a "way" to achieve his aims which bypasses the irksome or insurmountable obstacles, authorities, or objections which impede him. The *jeito* most often involves a skillful manipulation of interpersonal relations and thus requires contact with some member of the family, however distant, or a friend who has a friend highly enough placed to "fix" the problem. This may be understood simultaneously as reflecting a reluctance to work needlessly, a necessary adaptation to a difficult milieu, and admiration for adroitness in human affairs. Perhaps a certain cynicism is also involved, a pervading sense that things are never what they seem to be at first glance, which may be reinforced by the daily contrasts between beauty and squalor. To this is often added a conviction that no one will do anything for anyone else unless some clear personal gain accrues from the seeming altruism or unless the one helped is a member of the family. This is reminiscent of failures in the capacity to engage in collective action noted among the poor of South Italy (Banfield, 1958) and the United States (Harrington, 1962), and suggests the influence of early experience and current pressures making it impossible to see individual gain as stemming from collective action (Brody, 1965). Interpersonal transactions often involve a clear sense of the building of a system of mutual obligations in which a favor done is insurance for reciprocal help in case of later need. The philosophy of *jeito* may be regarded as a special variant of survival behavior in personalistic societies in which an automatically functioning administrative system cannot be assumed. In such situations promotion and success have necessarily been more dependent upon relationships between individuals than upon impersonally judged merit.

Another cultural factor contributing to the *jeito* philosophy is the lack of social reward for responsible hard work. This again is a function of an unstable social-political-economic system which makes long-range individual planning enormously difficult. Hard, consistent work aimed at the system rather than for the individual may produce desirable consequences, but is not uniformly regarded as a virtue in itself; it may even cause a person to be viewed as an unimaginative drudge, although it can be much appreciated by supervisors and colleagues. To this is added the regularly rising cost of living and the periodic devaluation of the *cruzeiro* which make it maladaptive to save money. Bank accounts may be halved in buying power over a space of months. Among those with means, this contributes to a speculative fever, and among the poor, to continued purchases of lottery tickets and gambling. For almost everyone, there is a prevalent attitude of buy now because everything will cost morè later on. One way out for those who can afford it is to buy an apartment which can be occupied while payments are made and, in view of the housing shortage is almost sure to become more valuable. Another is an

automobile. Although expanding national production may decrease its investment qualities, it is still possible to dispose of a
well-kept car after several years for close to its original cost. For
the *favelado* and the large masses of the poor, the "investment"
may be only the temporary pleasure and anesthesia found in a
bottle of *cachaça* or sugarcane rum. Or it is the costume which he
and members of his samba dancing group *(escolha de samba,* or, literally, samba school) will wear at *carnaval.*

Continuing inflation, which contributes to a certain fatalistic or
escapist attitude, also forces those with middle-class tastes and
without special *jeito* or connections—especially in the professional
class—to work long hours and hold several jobs in order to preserve their economic status quo. The long hours, however, are
accompanied by fatigue and reduced efficiency, and the many
jobs often prevent the career investment which motivates individuals to build effective institutions. Instead, the insecurity of
tying a career to an institution, coupled with the personalistic
Latin tradition, combine to support the development of *med-
alhoes. Medalhão* or, literally translated, medallion, means "big
shot" to the Brazilian. This is a man for whom the attainment of
a position of power and prominence is an end in itself rather than
the means to a socially useful goal. *Medalhões* in university administrations are the target of much student unrest, for they are felt
to maintain the status quo in order to avoid change which will
endanger their own prerogatives. The achievement of *medalhão*
status requires careful preparation of several bases or spring-
boards from which a man might move upward, should one or
another prove unreliable or evanescent. This means that he cannot be too thoroughly involved with any of them. Some of the
most successful are astonishingly versatile, but their relative lack
of interest in building stable institutions which may outlast them
(without perpetuating their names) deprives the social structure
of some of their most fundamental contributions. This is especially true as regards the hard, often unrewarding work of social
and community development. The true *medalhão* in the stereotyped sense of the expression must blind himself to the poverty
and institutional weaknesses of his society in order to devote his
attention to larger theoretical, intellectual, artistic, or political
issues with proven public relations value. The historical, cultural,

and physical environments combine to produce the Carioca *medalhão* as much as they do the unemployed laborer.

RESPONSE TO STRESS—THE FLOODS OF RIO

The way in which a community, viewed both in terms of individuals and of organization, responds to natural disaster indicates something about the people and the social structure. The most characteristic recurring disasters which affect Rio de Janeiro and the Cariocas are floods. These occur mainly in the hottest months of the year, December and January, although torrential rains are not uncommon at other times. Each such event is characterized by heavy loss of life, especially among the shanty dwellers. Each is characterized, also, by public outcries for more adequate construction and preventive planning. Once the event passes, however, it assumes a dreamlike quality, and the memory of it becomes submerged in the hot torpor induced by sun and sky.

The author was present during the most massive and death-dealing floods in Rio's history, beginning on the evening of Monday, January 10, 1966. With intermittent pauses the rain fell almost continuously for approximately 85 hours. Streets soon filled with surging yellow-brown water rushing down the steep slopes to combine their streams into rivers and lakes. Sewers were rapidly taxed beyond capacity. Water spouted from manholes. Concrete and asphalt surfaced roads collapsed. Huge boulders were loosened from precipitous cliffs. As the earthy superstructures of the *morros* slid and moved they cast down the shanties, boulders, and people adhering to them, raining destruction on those below.

By midday on Wednesday the force of the rain had slackened sufficiently so that some communications were reestablished and the paralyzed transport system had begun to function again, although only partially. President Castelo Branco announced on the radio that government workers who wished to do so could report to work, but that those who did not appear would not be penalized. People were beginning to reappear on the streets, and stock of the damage was being taken. Several hundred were known dead; major roads and bridges were closed; two tunnels were blocked by sliding earth and water; most telephone lines were out; people were isolated by washed-out roads; stores and homes were ruined. Even major streets were covered with mud and stones. Gulches four or five feet deep had been carved in the sand where water from the street had poured across the beach into the roaring ocean. The corpse of a large man was visible there, his body and face covered with a sodden blue blanket, his black ankles and long feet extending out from under the cover toward the sea. Under glistening umbrellas, a group of about 30 spectators silently surrounding him changed in composition as people came and went, whispering to each other, but making no move toward the body. Boy Scouts in blue, short-trousered uniforms assisted with the traffic; occasional workers, barefoot and shirtless, shoveled in a desultory way at the debris on the streets; groups of adolescents, some almost in a holiday mood, stopped cars and asked for money, from 10 to 100 *cruzeiros*, "to help the *flagelados*," the victims. Laters, friends advised us not to give them money because there was no assurance that it would find its way to the *flagelados*.

The *favelados* who were most severely hurt by the storm began to evolve their own theories about what had happened. The most frequently encountered idea was that the cloudburst was a punishment, that God was showing his anger because human beings were trying to fly to the moon. Zilda, a short grey-eyed woman of about 40 with an etched face which would have looked at home in Bavaria, said that this, and possibly "other spatial events" had incurred the wrath of God. When one wondered why such punishment should have been visited on the Brazilians who, after all, had no astronauts, she said only that the Brazilian government was probably getting ready to try.

A refugee from a nearby *favela*, Zilda was housed temporarily with 180 others in the Centro Academico Carlos Chagas, a building in the Medical School complex of the Federal University of Rio de Janeiro. The group was predominantly mulatto with a sprinkling of black-skinned Negroes. Women and children gathered quietly around rolled-up mattresses and bedding. Few men were in evidence, for they were out searching for belongings, trying to repair their shacks, or helping with general clean-up operations. The people in charge exhibited the food preparation

with some pride, observing that the refugees were probably receiving more and tastier food than that to which they were ordinarily accustomed. A colleague commented on the cheerfulness
and loud good humor exhibited during mealtime, saying that he
felt the *favelados* of Rio to be not so emotionally isolated from
each other as those of São Paulo, where the climate was cooler.

That night, the 13th, television coverage from Guanabara Pal-
ace, headquarters of the local government which was serving as a
nerve center for rehabilitation operations, revealed complete bed-
lam. Announcers, including some modishly dressed young women
upon whom the cameras dwelt repeatedly, sent out frantically
uncoordinated, undirected appeals for "medical teams," for
equipment, for bedding, and said that there was "absolutely no
food to distribute" to the refugees. They listed schools that were
being opened to provide sleeping places, and interspersed their
appeals with announcements about the continuing danger of the
flood sequelae. One *favela* on top of a hill overlooking Botafogo
was being evacuated because of the possibility of further land-
slides. Military helicopters and engineers were also being pressed
into service in an effort to discover where further slides could be
expected. The camera moved to a group of laughing *favelado* children, three little Negroes of perhaps eight or 10 years, dressed in
donated clothing. The Brazilians in the room, all Cariocas, kept
up a running fire of comment: "This is a crisis—but the plight of
the *favelados* is never good . . . This is just another time when it is
temporarily brought to public attention. . . . And the *favelados*—
except for those who have lost members of their families—they
actually enjoy the attention. . . . It gives them a sense of identity
which they don't normally have. . . . Look at those kids—that's
probably the best clothing they've ever owned. . . . When the crisis
is over they'll go back to hillsides and build their *barracos* again—
and they will be forgotten again. . . . Their two square meals a
day are better than they ever have ordinarily—many of them prefer their present temporary quarters in schools and public buildings
to their *barracos*—many would like to be *malandros* (operators who
live by their wits) if they could." The talk turned to the use of
the money which had been collected by people on the streets and
by the government offices: "All those millions of *cruzeiros*—come to
about $10,000. . . . How much will actually find its way into

supplies which will be of real use to the *favelados*—how much will be pocketed by various subofficials?" Perhaps this was one reason why the televised appeals were not for money but for supplies.

Other collecting points were being set up throughout the city, with neighborhood schools, military installations, and even warehouses receiving their contingents. By Thursday, January 14th it was estimated that 120,000 people were homeless. About 700 had been treated for fractures and concussions, and 170 dead had come to autopsy. There were no psychiatric casualties and no evidence of mass panic. Rather, observers, including the newspapers, commented on the unusual "solidarity," comradeship, and fortitude exhibited by the people. Perhaps the major emotional casualties were the children. The police had by this time picked up an estimated 500 youngsters between the ages of two and 10 wandering alone through the city. In at least two instances mothers gave their young children to bystanders, leaving no identification at all. A cynical onlooker suggested that they had been waiting for an opportunity to give up the responsibility of child rearing.

By weeks's end a typhoid scare increased in intensity. Nurses were inoculating dwellers from the *favela* of Sereno in the Grajau Tennis Club, where there were now housed 60 *flagelado* families. In a post installed in the *favela* of Mangueira, 2,000 persons were inoculated in two days. The *favela* of Rocinha in the Gavea section was threatened not only by typhoid but by physical destruction. Towering high above the *favela*, separated from it by several hundred feet of sheer cliff, balanced a huge boulder perhaps 20 by 30 feet in size. It showed all the signs of being about to fall with the next downpour. The government radio had been sending repeated warnings to the Rocinha population, many of whom had transistor radios, to vacate the area, but only a few had done so. A black-skinned woman of perhaps 50, wearing a wide, soiled, dark red skirt and a bandanna around her hair was asked if she was going to move. She shook her head, " . . . God will find a way to keep the boulder from falling." This response, heard repeatedly in Rocinha, contrasted sharply with the attitude of the administrators of the Sanatorio Botafogo. An apparently unstable rock was perched on the *morro* above it, too, but lacking the *favela-*

do's faith in God, the doctors had evacuated the patients from the wards closest to the hillside.

The aftermath of the flood brought much discussion by those with social power or status. An intellectual of European birth, who had lived in Rio de Janeiro for 25 years was impressed by the lack of complaints among the displaced people who, instead, expressed tremendous admiration at the constant work of the "nice ladies," the upper-class women who were busy providing them with clean sheets, bedding, food, and clothing in a nearby school where they were sheltered. This, he thought, fitted a mutually accepted value system. It is not uncommon for an upper-class woman to assume responsibility for clothing and schooling the children of an employee. Many such women have at least one lower-class godchild. Several of the *flagelados* told him the food was better than that to which they were accustomed, and that they did not ordinarily sleep on sheets. There was no sign of any wish to exchange their positions of passive dependency for something else.

The newspapers and the government publicized the fact that the Villa Kennedy was not affected by the storm. This was a group of houses built with Alliance for Progress funds to shelter dwellers from another *favela* who had objected violently to moving, but finally did so. News of its safety and absolute lack of flood damage was intended to entice other *favela* communities to move. They did not succeed, however, and by 1967 little change had occurred. The people did not want to leave their shacks, close to their work as maids, handymen, or peddlers. A home in the suburban areas, such as the Villa Kennedy, where other public housing would be built, would require long travel by unreliable transportation back to the city. Furthermore, the *favelados* liked the individuality of their *barracos* and the feelings of ownership, however illusory, which these afforded. In spite of quarrels and suspicious isolation, some friendship networks had developed. These were also considered valuable and an important reason for not moving.

The most striking government statement, because of its timing hard on the heels of the well-publicized typhoid scare, was an urgent announcement that Rio was not after all threatened by an epidemic. This was attributed to the fear that much needed foreign tourism would be curtailed at the time of *carnaval*. The column by Herbert Zeacheche in the *Brazil Herald* (1966) noted,

> The Guanabara state authorities are faced with a cruel dilemma. Shall they spend 14 hundred million *cruzeiros* for *carnaval* street decoration as scheduled, or use the money for flood relief. Either solution will be unpopular and is likely to touch off furious criticism. As a first reaction, groups of slum dwellers who were the hardest hit by the flood calamity protested yesterday. *Carnaval* concerns the *favelados,* and they don't wish their big festival to be restricted or spoiled. Not even for their own benefit.

Ultima Hora noted editorially, how the calamity demonstrated "the social problem of our city." It discussed ". . . the influence of natural factors in this great city surrounded by mountains . . . the importance of the force of the waters which have affected certain structures of more or less solid construction . . . the need for improving the system of water run-off and supply . . . the need for reforestation to stop erosion and for rigorous vigilance about the nature of new construction and anti-flood measures." However, the editorial went on to say

> . . . the real social problem of Rio emerges in all its terrible expression in the apparently poetic situation of the *favelas*. Those who are called *favelados* were those who were most affected by the tragedy, especially since they live in subhuman conditions and are incredibly vulnerable. For them it is more than a technical problem to resolve. Exactly where they are isn't important. The fact is that we always have our places without price. The most unhealthy, the most inaccessible, subject to all kinds of dangers . . .

This general attitude was supported by colleagues who described the white, middle-class group, as completely "detached" from the plight of the *favelados,* with little more concern for them than the traditional white North American southerner for the rural Negro field hand. The failure to take preventive measures against floods and rockfalls was considered due to the low regard in which the life of the *favelado* is held. Others said that it was part of a general inertia and reluctance of the decision makers and holders of national wealth to commit themselves to a program of social services aimed at a noncontributing population.

In summary, the catastrophe was in large measure a consequence of the human contributions to the environment and the responses to it reflected in the attitudes of those at the opposite poles of the social class structure. The consequences of heavy and predictably recurring rains stemmed from overcrowding, an inadequate base of municipal services, massive immigration from the country, and the host of factors leading the poor to colonize the precarious *morros*. The failure to engage in systematic preventive efforts stemmed from the relative detachment from the powerless victims from those with social power, and the passive dependency of the victims themselves, ready to trust in the power-holders or the supernatural; they had little experience leading them to believe that immediate sacrifice, effort, or collective demands rather than filial dependency upon the power-holders might lead to long-term gain.

CHAPTER 4

MIGRANTS BECOME PATIENTS—COUNTRYMEN IN THE CITY

THIS CHAPTER will describe the migratory process as idea and fact, as part of the Brazilian context of behavior. It will indicate the prevalence of migrants in Rio de Janeiro, and the nature of facilities and activities aimed at them. These provide support for new arrivals, most typically those coming alone and without relatives who have preceded them. They constitute alternatives to the clinic or mental hospital and are thus significant elements in the case-finding or patient-identifying process. With these considerations in mind, the patient population will be described in terms of its migratory characteristics. Patients who are recent migrants, i.e., those coming to the city within five years of hospitalization, and the settled population, i.e., natives plus those who arrived more than five years prior to hospitalization, will be compared. Comparisons will focus on social and psychiatric characteristics of the two subpopulations in an attempt to delineate the role of migration, its motives and corollaries, in the process leading to mental hospitalization and in the production of symptom patterns.

MIGRATION AS PART OF THE BEHAVIORAL SETTING

MIGRATORY PUSH, PULL, AND PROCESS

Actual and potential geographic mobility is a prominent aspect of social behavior in Brazil. The physical environment has made migration necessary for survival in some instances; the awareness of others moving, of a continuing frontier and unknown cities with beckoning opportunities, combined with limited opportunities at home make relocation an always imaginable solution to life difficulties. Recurrent drought and famine, disease and inadequate health facilities, stagnant and marginal small-town economies, and lack of schools for their children have pushed rural Brazilians out of remote homesites and provincial towns and villages toward the large cities. Similarly, they have been pulled by the promise of jobs in new industry, the lure of lights and *movimento* in metropolitan centers, and opportunities for educational and personal advancement. Brandão Lopes (1961) described the inhabitants of the semi-arid Northeast as having a "permanent readiness to move and to seek better living conditions elsewhere." Among the single young men in their late teens or early twenties "predisposed to move, a bad crop or even a mere sign that it is not likely to rain encourages [them] . . . to leave home to try their fortune . . ." (p.237). Another important motive, emphasized by Souza de Andrade (1952), is the desire for new experience. The city's freedom for the young and unmarried, previously confined by the strictures of traditional small towns or the isolation of the country, is an important attraction.

The largest movements have been from North to South and from the interior eastward toward the Atlantic Ocean. Their sources are in the dry *sertão* or backlands and isolated villages of the North and Northeast, the eastern states of Bahia, Espirito Santo, and Rio de Janeiro, and the hills and valleys of Minas Gerais to the west. Each of the major coastal cities north of Rio de Janeiro—Belém, Fortaleza, Recife, Salvador—has its slums, final termini for refugees and seekers from the interior. But the most massive movements, over thousands of miles of trail and dirt roads, have been toward São Paulo. Some migrants come directly to the city hoping to work in the new factories. Often the first step has been to the huge coffee *fazendas* and other farms, many of them in the process of industrialization. It is from these that the next move to the city is made. A farm laborer's perception of the process is described by Pereira (1965). During the course of a dozen years he had worked on several *fazendas:* " . . . I earned little . . . there were no amusements, no *futebol,* no sanitary facilities, the worst hygienic conditions. People would move to another *fazenda* hoping for better but the situation continued the same. I had heard people speak of the city and I didn't want to continue my life in the country . . . Friends who had come to São Paulo said that it was good there, jobs, amusements, dances, girls . . ." (p.154). This man, like many, made his move to São Paulo city when he was married, and then, having obtained work and saved some money, brought his family in from the countryside.

Among those who began the journey with São Paulo in mind are some of the migrants who make up almost one-half the population of Rio de Janeiro. Rio de Janeiro is 200 miles closer to the homes of those who started from the North. Its intermediate position constitutes a powerful attraction; it also has bluer skies and a warmer sun than the often gray and misty São Paulo. A man from Belém, three degrees from the Equator where at midday "one must remind himself that elsewhere in the world people are moving and working" said to the author, "Our idea of Paradise is to live in Rio." Many migrants also respond directly to the economic opportunities around Guanabara Bay including shores on both the Guanabara and Rio State sides. Here, especially since the middle nineteen-fifties, the development of small industry and agriculture has accelerated. Migrants from Minas Gerais, Espirito Santo, and the interior of Rio State often find that Guanabara and greater Rio de Janeiro represent known quantities, the possibility of closer ties with relatives left behind, and a more familiar and traditional atmosphere than frighteningly busy São Paulo.

GENERAL RESIDENTIAL INSTABILITY

The major migrations to the two largest metropolitan areas of Rio and São Paulo have occurred in a context of general residential instability, fueled, as Brandão Lopes (1961) put it, by a "permanent readiness to move." Those least burdened with personal goods have been more attached to a region, a cultural area that is part of their identity, than to a particular house or village or neighborhood. This identity is not lost and may in time draw them back to the point of origin (where a relative may still hold a small piece of land), but it does not inhibit changes in location. The seasonal and circular journeys of farm laborers have been traditional, especially in the Northeast, and they continue. In the dry months thousands of men from the interior work in the coastal sugar cane fields. Yet the large majority do not lose their attachments to their inhospitable homeland and only await the opportunity to return. As de Carli (1940, in Smith, 1963) described it: "They remain three or four months, until the evening in which, crazy with happiness, they see in the direction of the *sertão* the distant reflections of the lightning cutting the skies . . . In an instant the *sertanejo* disappears. He has returned to the land which is so ungrateful to him and so harsh" (p. 163).

Limeira Tejo (1937, in Smith, 1963) similarly regarded the "immense individual liberty" giving rise to people "undisciplined, without submission to work" as fundamental to the seasonal workers' return to an area offering so little in the way of realistic support. These descriptions may be regarded by present-day observers as romanticized, but they indicate the nature of the conflict in which the Nordestino, and the potentially migrant rural Brazilian in general, are caught. On the one hand, his homeland signifies freedom from the discipline of routine work and responsibility to an immediately directive boss. On the other hand, it signifies poverty, chronic fatigue, early death, and lack of opportunity for advancement. The consequences are a restless circularity within nearby areas and a constant extrusion of individuals and families to more distant places, where the gradual sinking of social and economic roots must compete with recurrent nostalgia for idealized elements of the past.

Harris (1956), close to 20 years ago, noted that at least 30 per cent of the adult males of two farming communities in the Eastern Highlands of Bahia were working or had worked in the States of São Paulo or Paraná. About 80 per cent of these émigrés, mainly young unmarried men, could be expected to return within two or three years. As he put it, they returned in the status of heroes: "Few actually manage to save much money, but the experience and the foreign mannerisms are considered to be great assets." Among the inhabitants of the principal small town in the area, the movement was just as intense but with considerably less likelihood of return. This was because the majority of town émigrés were unconnected with agriculture: "The city dweller is evidently more successful in cutting off home ties than the villager who has a piece of land, however small, which belongs to him, and which may be augmented someday when he inherits from his father" (pp. 90-93).

Backward forms of agriculture and the nature of the country itself still contribute to residential instability in certain areas. The historically stereotyped "notorious . . . nomadic or migratory habits" of the "rural Brazilian of the lower classes" have been discussed in detail by T. Lynn Smith (pp. 144-148) who described how life conditions in the North and Northeast militated against the development of items and institutions binding men to a piece of land. The residential instability of these peasant families was so impressive to professional observers in the nineteen-twenties and thirties that an *instincto migratorio* was once postulated as the motivating force behind it.

The opening of new frontier areas has often converted aimless movement into directed migration; newly available agricultural and mining areas continue to inspire entire families to long overland treks. In the late 1960's, workers and families flowed toward the Territory of Amapá in the extreme North, drawn by industry surrounding manganese deposits and intermittent reports of discoveries of gold and oil. Heavy migrations continue into Goias, home of the new Federal District on the *altoplano,* the high, dry plateau of limitless horizons. With the building of Brasilia the long dreamed of "March to the West" has become a reality. New "pioneer" zones are in a constant process of development. These include parts of Matto Grosso and of central Maranhao, a·potential farming area which attracted large numbers of settlers from the Northeastern drought in 1958. The coffee of Paraná is a major boom attracting both migrants and city investors. Connected with Paraguay by a new major bridge, Paraná is the main link for trade between that country and the rest of Brazil. It is rich in electrical power, already one of the nation's main breadbaskets, and the site of the largest paper industry in South America. Its population growth, largely through migration, has been explosive; Curitiba, the capital, will soon have one million inhabitants.

THE PULL OF NEW INDUSTRY

This factor can be viewed in terms of two interrelated elements. One is the rapid movement toward industrialization which has created demands for a new labor force of both factory and construction workers, especially in the large centers of São Paulo and Rio de Janeiro. For many, the opportunities of industrialization imply a new level of personal freedom. Pereira (1965) documented this in his case histories of mobile workers coming into urban factories for the first time. In the words of an 18-year-old mechanic whose early work experience included sharecropping with his father and, when he was 12-years-old, helping a butcher in a small interior town of São Paulo, "He who works on the *roca* [the land] has no minimum salary, no social security, no protection." A Northeast migrant who still had a small holding in Ceará said, "The worker on the land isn't an employee, he is a slave." The complaint that the rural worker " . . . doesn't have rights with the owner" (p. 47) is a constant theme in these case histories. These men include many of those described poetically by Tejo as free, even though they might be sharecroppers in debt to an absentee landlord. They also include sugarcane workers and others bound to a particular *fazenda* or plantation, working under the supervision of overseers and totally dependent upon a company store. The second element is the opening, emphasized by Hutchinson (1963), of an entirely new avenue to a social promotion in contrast to upward mobility in a static structure. Knowledge of these new possibilities for increased status in developing industry has apparently stimulated the migration of both skilled manual and nonmanual workers. It is this group within the new industries which contains the heaviest concentrations of migrants: " . . . the expansion of industry has played a crucial part in throwing open new status positions, which the migrants have been particularly ready to claim for themselves" (p. 48). Migrants from the lowest occupational class, however, including mainly unskilled manual workers from rural areas, were least likely to move upward from the status of their fathers, for they lacked training and basic education. Failures of upward mobility among the unskilled rural migrants may also be associated with lack of consistent ambition and with certain attitudes toward work. (This will be discussed further in the chapter on occupation.)

One-third of Pereira's cases came to São Paulo industries from the Northeastern region, the rest from the interior of São Paulo State and neighboring areas such as Minas Gerais. Most had migrated in family groups. Their customary work relationships were dominated by traditional norms rather than by impersonal and rational standards. Previously accustomed to home industries or farming, factory work meant their family was separated, their sense of cohesion and meaning lost. They frequently thought of employment as merely a way of accumulating enough money to permit them to return and buy some land or to begin an independent craft or business in a town or village. A central goal for many was to start life anew working for themselves and not for "others."

Migrants from small towns and the country bring with them values and work habits which sometimes impair adjustment to the industrial environment. Harris (1956) repeatedly encountered failures in the ability to act collectively, and evidence of the high individualization of work patterns and achievement. Most marked among villagers, this individuality was also present to a striking degree in town. The low value placed upon communal conformity, or working together (with its necessary sacrifice of some individual "sovereignty") to achieve a common aim, was revealed in such disparate ways as indifference toward the community's patron saint and a proliferation of personal patron saints, a proliferation of stores and workshops, resistance to business mergers, and in political schisms. Such values seem prone to engender conflict when the migrant is placed in work situations requiring cooperative effort with others. Another value which has prevented the use of individual funds for local development is the townspeoples' disdain for anything related to agriculture. As Harris noted, "From the viewpoint of the townsman the man who is willing to spend all day under a hot sun hoeing up the soil is *de facto* deficient in civilized qualities" (p. 94). The townspeople "despise the work of the peasant and see in him the destroyer rather than the creator of civilization. . . . When fortune comes, they desert the interior and take their skills and money to the coast" (p. 288).

THE PULL OF NEW TRANSPORT FACILITIES AND MASS MEDIA

Migration has also been encouraged by the development of communications, including roads. This development was greatly stimulated by the creation of Brasilia as the national capital. New roads have made low-priced transport by truck over long distances available to people who formerly had only the choice between expensive air travel or the slow tedious movement via foot, wagon, boat, or irregular train service. Even now, especially in the western interior, ox-drawn wagons are not an unusual alternative to travel by foot. In Amazonia, motor launches pulling strings of native canoes and similar craft, the "river-horses" with produce for market, also transport groups of people down-river toward Belém, where they may start the long voyage south. The important word-of-mouth transmission of news about new localities, now amplified by telephone and telegraph, is vastly facilitated by the developing highway system. Entrepreneurial highway truckers stimulate new wishes in the populace and business for themselves, and their passengers carry messages and invitations to relatives and friends. Thus the concept as well as the fact of internal migration as a means of resolving problems and fulfilling wishes becomes increasingly significant as part of the context of individual behavior. For those with more ample funds, intercity bus service has achieved an adequate level of comfort on the main runs. Brasilia's central bus station is one of the busiest points in the city, its importance underlined by its location in a complex of shops including an always-open drug store. The Rio-Brasilia-Belém highway, which has at times been called (after the president who brought Brasilia from the drawing boards into actuality) Kubitchek's Folly, runs 2,100 miles along a North-South axis. Mainly dirt and with little as yet in the way of roadside facilities, it is in regular use throughout the year, except for periodic washouts in the rainy season. The Brasilia–Belém section of the road, still under the supervision of Army engineers, represents an initial step toward conquering the vast green expanse of jungle and forest which has divided tropical inland Brazil into isolated centers reachable only by air or boat. Major trunk roads have been finished, or are still in construction, between deep interior Pôrto Velho and Rio Branco, and between Pôrto Velho and Manaus, the city 1,000 miles up the Amazon created by the rubber boom of the early twentieth century.

The mass media, too, exert an increasing impact among formerly isolated peoples, and with the wider dissemination of transistor radios even the barrier of illiteracy can be surmounted. Such organizations as The Catholic League, The Peasant League, and The Union of Agrarian workers, while aiming at change within the rural areas, have also contributed impact to the migratory impulse through their educational programs.

INTERNAL MIGRATION AND URBAN GROWTH

Between 1940 and 1950, according to estimates by Smith (1963) almost 393,000 migrants came into Rio de Janeiro, the then Distrito Federal. This movement accounted for 68 per cent of the total city growth during that period. The largest number (30 per cent) of internal migrants came from the neighboring state of Rio de Janeiro, with 24 per cent from Minas Gerais. A preponderance was female with a sex ratio (number of males per 100 females) of 86.5 for the entire migrant population and 76 and 78 for Minas Gerais and Rio State respectively (p. 149). Informal observation suggests that adult sons may be left behind to hold on to property or may remain as a matter of personal independence. Thus, migrating families may include disproportionate numbers of female relatives of all ages, including those with dead or absent husbands, as well as unmarried daughters.

A description of one subsample of female migrants is provided by Bosco's (1965) study of 79 who were seen at the São Paulo State Department of Immigration and Colonization. They came from the Northeast, Bahia, and Minas Gerais. All were married and had had as many children as possible for their ages, but with few survivals; one woman had borne 17 children of which one had survived, another had 15 with six surviving, and so on. It was a malnourished group for whom dietary staples were coffee, beans, rice, *farinha*, and occasionally the traditional dried meat of the pioneer. Seventy-one per cent were between the ages of 19 and 31, and of the remainder, none was over 55. Fifty-one per cent were white, 37 per cent brown, and 12 per cent black. These figures are more representative of the rural than the Rio population with proportionally fewer whites and more browns. Seventy-one per cent had helped their husbands with agricultural labor, while the rest confined themselves to household duties. Eighty-six per cent were illiterate. Because most of them lacked documents, only four per cent were entitled to vote.

The July 1, 1950 census data showed approximately 40 per cent of the 2,377,451 official inhabitants of the Federal District, later to become Guanabara State encompassing all of Rio de Janeiro City and most of the metropolitan area, were internal migrants, mainly of rural origin. Since the middle 1950's, according to Beyer (1967), the urban growth rate in Brazil has been approximately four times that of the rural.

In 1960, the time of the last available census figures, 45 per cent of all Brazilians lived in cities; 92 per cent of the Guanabara population was native Brazilian, with the remainder of foreign birth. The proportion of those born elsewhere in Brazil remained constant at 40 per cent with a sex ratio of 83. Of the total internal migrant group, 24 per cent (approximately 10 per cent of the total population) had lived in Guanabara for five years or less, 19 per cent (approximately eight per cent of the total population) between six and 10 years, and 56 per cent (approximately 22 per cent of the total population) for 11 years or more. Within the *favelas* the proportion of males was higher with a sex ratio of 95. The percentage of *favela* dwellers who had been in the city for five years or less was 28; between six and 10 years, 25; and 11 years or more, 45.

Nonmedical Support Facilities for Migrants

The facilities and activities described in this section offer support and sometimes temporary shelter for some migrants who might otherwise come voluntarily or involuntarily to hospitals or clinics. They are thus essential components of the social system preventing or determining the transformation of a migrant into a psychiatric case. Those who became cases, i.e., data for the present study, were those whose disturbances were too intense or socially obvious to permit their alleviation in a nonmedical faculty, or those with families whose care made use of the nonmedical facility unnecessary, but who later decided that medical care was required and brought the disturbed person to a hospital.

ALBUERGUE JOAO XXIII.

This "shelter" or "inn" is the only center administered by the

Guanabara government for the care of homeless people. It is aimed particularly at migrants. Established in 1934, it was first known as the Shelter of Good Will. After the death of Pope John XXIII it was given his name. Other changes have taken place. The old square on which it is located is near the docks in a deteriorating section of the city called Saude (the Portuguese word for health). It was formerly called Praça Harmonia. Now, named after a military man, it is known as the Praça Coronel Asunção.

The building, seen from the worn brick street on the other side of the square, projects itself as a gloomy gray fortress. Its depressing severity is relieved on appropriate holidays by strings of small gray paper pennants. The wall is interrupted by a small doorway opening onto a main courtyard, about 60 by 35 feet, paved in gray concrete. Two concrete benches on either side of the area flank a potted palm.

On a typical morning three men sat together on a bench. One was black, two were tan. All were unshaven, scruffy-looking, wearing worn rubber sandals and dirty, shabby clothing. They were unobtrusive, thin, passive and gently slouched, and seemed in no hurry to move. Like the other 300 people who had slept at the shelter the previous night, they had been photographed, fingerprinted, and inoculated. Usually men are given breakfast and are expected to spend the day looking for jobs before returning for the evening meal. A few remain during the day to work in the dining room, kitchen, laundry or at general menial tasks. For this they receive lunch and a small wage. Women are not required to leave during the day. Many of the women are accompanied by young children. Of 12 women lined up for a screening procedure, most were brown and young, three were pregnant, and two were elderly. A young white woman, cleaner and better dressed than the others, said that she was not a migrant but had been living with her mother. Then she had an illegitimate baby and her irate mother had put her out. Now, during the 15 days permitted at the Albuergue, she hoped to be able to find a home for her baby.

The courtyard is surrounded by a red-tiled walk, slick with age and assiduous washing, separated from it by a concrete railing. On one side small offices open onto the walk. A record room contains cards bearing the photographs and other notes. A brief admission note about each person is entered in a log book. One typical note in its entirety stated: "He came from the State of Rio where he had lived alone. He came here to look for a job." The clerk in charge said that he thought more people came from Minas Gerais than any other locality. Another office opening onto the courtyard is a dispensary. The Albuergue functions, as does the Pronto Socorro Psiquiatrica, as a general public health registration point. A part-time physician gives each person a cursory physical examination and vaccinations for smallpox and typhoid fever, and a portable X-ray is taken. Those with active tuberculosis are not admitted but sent to a hospital. The one or two psychiatrically disturbed people who appear each week are taken to the Pronto Socorro in Engenho de Dentro which sometimes does not accept them because they are not considered acutely ill. The usual practice then is to arrange for the sick person to be sent back to his home city if this is feasible. About once a week someone already in residence at the Albuergue develops apparently psychotic behavior. The doctor believes these to be previously ill people relapsing from a state of remission. They can usually be placed in the Pronto Socorro but the Albuergue staff is reluctant to take them back after the acute phase has passed, especially if they have been aggressive.

Upstairs dormitories accommodate up to 400 people. Each person reports in after dinner, puts his clothing in a locker, is issued pajamas and bed clothing, and goes through the shower. After this he enters the dormitory and lowers a canvas cot which is bolted against the wall during the day. No one is permitted to leave the dormitory until morning. In addition to work areas, the Albuergue contains a nursery with 22 bassinets. Only a few of these are occupied as a rule. The walls are decorated with large poster pictures of plump, rosy, blond, blue-eyed youngsters enjoying Nestlé dairy products.

Statistics for the population flow through the Albuergue are shown in Table 23. They indicate the nature of those in need of immediate help, nine out of 10 of whom have moved into Rio de Janeiro within five years. This is a markedly deprived population which, like those who became patients, may be regarded as fallout from the migratory stream. Almost two-thirds are male, and at least three-fourths of the total are without legal spouses; as a group they lack the family support which both keeps migrants out of nonmedical support facilities and is involved in their admission to mental hospitals. Approximately three-fourths are illiterate or partly literate. Whites are in a clear minority, browns are most heavily represented, with blacks intermediate.

They come on their own, having heard of the place by word-of-mouth, although occasionally someone who knows the Albuergue will telephone about a family in need of help and a minibus will be sent to bring them in. Typically, such families appearing lost and without resources will be identified at the Rodaviaria, the main bus station in the Sao Cristovão district, which is the terminal point for travellers coming from the Northeast into Rio de Janeiro. Others may be found sleeping in the street. A favored spot, sheltered from the rain by a continuous arcade protecting the sidewalk and not far from the decaying districts of Saude and Praça Onze where cheap lodgings may be found, is on the Avenida Getulio Vargas across from the old church of Candelária. An occasional homeless man sleeps at the entrance of the church itself. Even at the height of business hours on the crowded Avenida Rio Branco one may encounter a few straggly-haired women squatting in a doorstep with one or two young children holding out their hands for alms. Their stories are vague in detail but consistent in content. They have been living in a small town or hamlet in the State of Rio, in São Paulo or in Minas—more rarely in the distant Northeast. The husband died or disappeared; there was nothing to eat, no job, and no place to go, so they came to Rio. Or the man had accompanied them to the big city, and then had disappeared or become ill. Now they wanted money to go back, or to support themselves and their children until a job or a place to stay could be found; or they were looking for the "mayor's office" having "heard" that it might offer help, or for the Albuergue Joao XXIII, or the Society for the Protection of Northeasterners, or some other place which might offer at least temporary assistance.

Perhaps 40 per cent of any single night's residents at the Albuergue are repeaters. After the allowed 15-day period has elapsed clients may not return for six months. A number of these are always waiting at the door on the first day of the seventh month. So long as there is room, all applicants are accepted except for those who are clearly sick or unmanageable. Social service is limited, but upon request every effort is made to help the clients find jobs and the mothers to find day-care facilities for their babies so that they may work. Considerable effort goes into obtaining airplane or bus tickets to return individuals or families to their points of origin. Some of these are referred to the Association for the Protection of Northeasterners (described below). The Aluergue's director, a physician, believes there is more circular migration of people who become disillusioned, unsuccessful, or lonely than is generally recognized. Some make the round trip several times, with sojourns in the Albuergue on each occasion.

ASSOCIAÇAO DE PROTEÇAO NORDESTINO

The Association for the Protection of Northeasterners is fittingly located on the Rua Ceará, named after one of the Northeastern states which has contributed high percentages of its people to the migratory streams. This facility is located in the North Zone, not far from the Maracaná soccer stadium, the Rodaviaria bus terminal, and the Campo São Cristovão. In this last, a vast old square surrounding a recently erected commercial exhibition hall, a street fair where Northeastern migrants meet each other and sell food, purchased or homemade articles, is held each Sunday morning.

Rua Ceará is a long street, paved with irregularly contoured bricks. It is faced by small stores and repair shops, with apartments and rented rooms on the second floors of the low buildings. Once on the street, no one can miss the Association. A two-foot-high banner announces its presence across 10 feet of the building front and states that it is registered as a public utility. The office is on an open porch which can be closed off against rain. In front is a small courtyard. Several people, mainly women and children, are usually waiting for food distribution. Sometimes the distribution of food and clothing is not scheduled until several days later, but they nonetheless remain.

The walls of the office area are covered by two paintings of drought refugees in the Northeast and several large photographs of long lines of people receiving food and clothing. Each photograph prominently features the Association's president who may have political aspirations. According to the secretary-treasurer, by 1968 the Association, which was founded six years earlier, had cared for 80,000 families or approximately a half million people who learned of the service partly because of newspaper and television publicity but mainly by word-of-mouth. The Association distributed food—much from the Alliance for Progress and private North American sources and some from the Brazilian federal government—and used clothing to about 500 families including from four to 20 children each week. Its most spectacular activity, however, was returning migrants to their homes in the Northeast. Through the Brazilian air force, it arranged for a plane to leave Rio de Janeiro each Friday, stopping at all the major cities on the coastal route North. Passengers disembark at Salvador, Recife, Terezinha, Fortaleza, Natal, and Belém do Pará and from there make their way back to their former homes in the interior. The secretary estimated that 10 to 15 per cent of those who come to Rio from the Northeast try to get back, and in most instances this is a permanent return. There are even a few Indians from Amazonaus who have found their way to the Association in search of transportation. Most of the people who ask for food or wish to return are husbandless women with children; some are accompanied by grandchildren.

Association officials have also written to mayors asking that jobs might be arranged for people who are returning. They have found several physicians willing to volunteer time to give medical aid to people who come for help. Two volunteer social workers do what they can to solve problems. Support for the Association is uneven, however, and in August, 1968 they were two months behind in their rent. A group of Associates pays a certain amount each month and systematically canvasses large businesses, particularly in the United States, for help. Their success with Brazilian businessmen and government agencies has been limited except for the contribution of the Air Force plane.

THE FEIRA NORDESTINA

This Northeastern Fair resembles other street markets or fairs, which, with their colorful vegetables and fruits, meats and dried fish, appear each weekday morning in different city neighborhoods. The crowds are not the usual housewives, however. Among the customers and venders are large numbers of the poor, thin, dark, and sallow-skinned people identified as Nordestinos. Many have come down from nearby slum areas. Three or four are beggars. Others cluster around a man singing in a hoarse voice as he laboriously squeezes a cracked accordian. Seven young men, staring intently into space and dripping sweat, beat out a frantic rhythm on percussion instruments. An elderly man with tan skin and a gray stubble, hollow eyes shaded by a large felt hat, gives a piece of bread to a curiously flabby young woman sitting on a bench under a tree. She is pale, and upon closer inspection, blind.

A large section of the Fair is devoted to cheap manufactured goods: shoes, plastic satchels, dresses, and sport shirts. There are also booths near which trucks bearing Pernambuco and Bahia license plates are parked, where Northeastern food, mixtures of rice and beans and sometimes fish or dried meat are prepared. The cooking is done over small charcoal and scrap-wood fires built in discarded tins or grates. The food smells good, is cheap, and is eaten hungrily. The Fair, like the Albuergue and the Association, provides a measure of support and social contact for those who might otherwise become so lonely, depressed, or out of touch with reality that hospitalization is required.

ASSOCIAÇAO DE NORDESTINOS DE ITUIUTABA

It was only in the late 1960's that the migrants, discovering themselves as a special group, began to experiment with self-determination. Accepting the charity of Joao XXIII and the Proteçao Nordestino continues in the tradition of passively receiving and moving in the direction of least resistance. Banding together with specific aims requiring aggressive action is a step toward a totally different tradition. The Association of Ituiutaba in the Zone of Pontal covering eighteen *municipios* in Minas Gerais was the subject of a newspaper feature story by Pinto and Contreras in July of 1969 and suggests the direction which similar organizations might take. It was formed with the dual purposes of putting an end to the "slave labor" conditions imposed upon migrants by landowners and promoting the integration of Northeasterners into the local society. Denunciations received by the Association are forwarded to local courts which warn the accused plantation owners and provide legal aid for the plaintiffs. The most common complaint refers to the confiscation of their peons' (The Portuguese word, infrequently encountered in Brazil, is *peões*), boots, suitcases, and clothing, and threats of physical force to prevent their flight. This occurs during the first months after arrival on a *fazenda* when the migrants, who may best be described as sharecroppers, must pay off their contracted obligation by working for the owner. Their day begins at five in the morning with coffee, sometimes accompanied by manioc meal; the food supplied by the owner does not include bread. Then there is a tedious walk to the place of work, followed by long hours of weeding, hoeing, digging, and sowing before the midday meal of rice, beans, meat, and hard brown sugar. This last is the sole item which never fails in times of a poor harvest. On most days they are back in their huts by seven in the evening. If all goes well, after three or four months the basic obligation is paid as are sums for food and the use of tools. Then the workers may begin to collect the equivalent of about 75 cents each afternoon. Their first act upon "being liberated" tends to be a trip to the nearest town or village to buy a transistor radio. The hunger for objects is impressive and the image of the Northeasterner in the eyes of the townsmen is that of a "spendthrift" or "squanderer." As a storekeeper of Ituiutaba said, "They buy everything and don't worry about going back to the *fazenda* without a cent. They don't bargain or ask for price reductions and they decide what they want as quickly as possible." Most of the migrants in the Zona do Pontal come with wives and children to whom they are much attached, an attachment which is said to account for their willingness to "suffer the worst consequences" and to show a "submissiveness which at times is subhuman" (p. 32). Single men who come without such attachments, especially those in *fazendas* far from any town, often succumb to nostalgia for the Northeast and soon attempt to leave. The Association usually tries to help arrange transportation back to their home areas. These account for no more than 10 per cent of the migrants, however, and of those who remain, many begin small trading operations as soon as they begin to receive money. The Association presently includes several Nordestinos who have become small shopkeepers and even owners of gasoline stations who

now help the less fortunate and the new arrivals. Formerly, anything that went wrong in the community was blamed on the Northeasterners; they were regarded as uniformly uneducated and illiterate. The Association attempts to combat these attitudes and
urges its 2,000 members, as well as the rest of the approximately
100,000 migrants in the region, to send their children to school
and to learn what they can themselves. Now, they say, it is rare to
find one who cannot read and write. What is perhaps most
impressive, the last president of the Ituiutaba Rotary Club was a
Northeasterner.

THE PATIENT SAMPLE

Migratory characteristics of the patient sample are summarized
in Tables 24 and 25. Only 45 per cent of the 254 patients had
been born within Greater Rio de Janeiro. Of the 55 per cent originating elsewhere, most were born and reared in rural or provincial settings and had moved into Rio within 10 years preceding
their hospitalization. Of these, a few had lived in cities with populations of 70,000 or more prior to their move to Rio de Janeiro,
and in some instances the city sojourn had been a temporary stop
en route from the interior. A man from rural Pará, for example,
had stayed with relatives in Belém for three years before pushing
on to Rio. In another instance, a rural family from the Northeast
had moved to a suburb of São Paulo and then come back north to
Rio.

The proportion of relatively recent arrivals within the group of
migrated psychiatric patients was more than twice the 30 per cent
reported by Hutchinson (1963) as within the total migrant population of the city. This was in spite of the increase in psychiatric
facilities in the native regions of potential migrants since 1960.
These figures suggest that the first years after arriving in a metropolis constitute the period of greatest risk of hospitalization for
migrants.

Not all those born in the metropolitan or Greater Rio area
came from the city proper. Eight, approximately three per cent,
of the total patient group who came to the city for the specific
purpose of obtaining psychiatric treatment, lived in other townships such as Petropolis, regarded by local planners as part of

Greater Rio. Another 10 per cent came from hamlets and rural pockets within the metropolitan area. The remaining figure of 32 per cent born within the city proper is close to that of 39 per cent of the total 1959–1960 population reported by Hutchinson (1963) as native born.

In contrast to Hutchinson's specialized research effort, however, census figures for 1960 report 52 per cent of the inhabitants at large as Guanabara-born and 40 per cent as internal migrants, with the remaining eight per cent from abroad. If these data are accurate, it would appear that the patient sample (which includes only four persons coming from abroad) contains approximately 15 per cent more internal migrants than the population at large. But these figures are contaminated by an additional 10 patients, approximately four per cent of the total patient population and seven per cent of all migrants, brought to Rio from other areas for the express purpose of hospitalization. Thus, while the data are suggestive, they are not sufficient to conclude that internal migrants are overrepresented in the mental hospital sample.

Twenty-eight per cent of all the patients (designated from now on as "recently migrant") were born outside of greater Rio de Janeiro and had arrived within the five years preceding hospitalization. This includes the 10 brought by family members who had already identified them as needing psychiatric help. The data on this last group, not truly migrant because their homes remained in their points of origin outside of Rio, dilute the comparative findings concerning recently migrant and settled patients; they were included nonetheless because in every instance a home base was established in Rio, either by a parent or spouse moving with the patient or with a relative already living there. (All these patients had at least one resident relative who provided a point of contact in the city.) Furthermore, upon undertaking the trip, all had accepted the possibility of outpatient care and were prepared to live in Rio de Janeiro to obtain this kind of treatment if hospitalization was not required by the doctors. Even without these individuals, the proportion of recently migrant members within the study group is almost three times that in the general Rio population. It is, however, similar to that among *favela* dwellers, so that there is an overrepresentation of recent (five year) arrivals into Rio in both the patient sample and in the *favelas*. Almost a quarter of these recently migrant patients had been in Rio one year or less, and most had arrived as adults.

The 72 per cent of all the patients who had lived in Greater Rio de Janeiro for more than five years preceding their hospitalization are designated from here on as "settled." (While the majority are natives of the area, 38 per cent are migrant.) Their other mobility characteristics are summarized on Table 25.

These figures suggest considerable differences between recently migrant and settled patients in terms of their integration into the urban community, as well as a comparatively high continuing influence of non-Rio (mainly rural) origins on the former. It is with this in mind that the following comparisons deal largely with the recently migrant versus the settled segments of the patient group rather than with the native of Rio de Janeiro versus those coming from elsewhere. Put another way, the major comparisons will be between relatively recent migrants (who arrived within five years) on the one hand and a mixed group of more established migrants plus natives (settled) on the other. This should maximize differences associated with the motivations for and immediate consequences of the move and at the same time reduce the problems of interpretation due to the mixture of urban and rural environmental influences among migrants living in Rio de Janeiro for varying periods. Unless comparisons of the migrant and native groups reveal significant differences they will not, as a rule, be reported.

One index of community integration is the hospital to which the psychiatrically disturbed person goes. While 38 per cent of the recently migrant had been seen in the Pronto Socorro, this was true for only 11 per cent of the settled patients. Conversely, 82 per cent of the settled, in contrast to 56 per cent of the recently migrant, were patients in the Casa Eiras. Similar proportions were residents in the Sanatorio Botafogo. In other words, proportionally more of the recently migrant came to the Pronto Socorro which requires no social security coverage and usually no previous clinic consultation. This was true even though patients brought directly from other cities for psychiatric care were generally taken to the Casa Eiras because the family head was covered by INPS. This last group, more educated and affluent than the other recently migrant, dilutes the expected differences between recently migrant and settled patients.

The most encompassing difference between the recently migrant and the settled groups is the rural-provincial origin of the former. Further, migrant members of the settled group have had a longer period of acculturation and an opportunity to acquire the values and cognitive and affective styles of the city dwellers. Migrants among the settled for whom the move was traumatic have had time to recuperate, and the socially isolated have had an opportunity to find new friends. It is assumed that the recently migrant will include most of those who, moving themselves to the city (in contrast to those brought by relatives) because of emotional or interpersonal problems or a deliberate search for psychiatric help, will have entered the hospital as part of the relocating process itself.

SOCIAL CHARACTERISTICS

The following material is intended to differentiate the recently migrant from the settled, and in some instances the native from the migrant patients, on social grounds. The social data will provide some insights into the motives behind the migratory move and the nature of the migrant's experience in the host community. They will also make it possible to more adequately understand the psychiatric-behavioral differences between recently migrant and settled patients in terms of social factors as well as the experience of relocation itself.

DEMOGRAPHIC FEATURES

The age at arrival of migrants who became patients resembles that of the migrant nonpatient population at large. According to Hutchinson's (1963) estimate, 45 per cent of all migrants coming into Rio de Janeiro during 1959–1960 were aged 19 or under. Thirty per cent of the migrants in the patient population had arrived by age 18 or less, with an additional 18 per cent between the ages of 18 and 21. There were no statistically significant age, sex, or color differences between the migrant and native or between the recently migrant and settled groups. There were no

major differences in marital status between the recently migrant
and settled patients, but proportionally more migrants than natives (74 per cent versus 49 per cent) had spouses or companionate mates. The fact that more migrants, similar in age to natives, have a permanent mate may reflect the process of selection
to become a patient. Unattached migrants who become mentally
disturbed are less likely than those with families to be referred for
psychiatric care and more likely to remain anonymous or to be
picked up by the Beggars Service, Joa XXIII, other general social
welfare agencies, or the police.

Twenty-nine per cent of the recently migrant as compared with
21 per cent of the settled had produced families with four or more
children. Fourteen per cent of the recently migrant and seven per
cent of the settled bore children of different color than themselves. Thirteen per cent of the recently migrant versus four per
cent of the settled described their marriages as "common-law" or
companionate. These differences, none of statistical significance,
are consistent with rural-urban differences in the population at
large.

A 28-year-old brown domestic worker is an instance of a
recently migrant with a common-law marriage. She lives with her
consensual mate in a rented shack or *barraco* without electricity or
water in a suburban *favela*; it was her *amigado* who brought her to
the Pronto Socorro. She was born and reared in Paratí in Rio
State where she completed two years of school; "I always had
trouble learning." Her father, a ship's cook, died of heart disease
when she was 10 but her mother, a laundress, still lives in Paratí
at age 60, and continues to work in spite of "heart disease and a
fallen womb." The patient has been financially independent since
the age of 14, "when I first became a mother." The family moved
into the area in search of jobs five months before coming to the
Pronto Socorro. She is friendly with some neighbors, but the one
next door "cannot stand me and wants to see me destroyed." She
says that social workers have hurt her and have no sympathy or
understanding for poor people. Before she was married she frequently went to *futebol*, the movies, the beach, and dances. Now
she has no time, money, or energy for anything "but survival."
Her mate classifies her acute paranoid syndrome as "a nervous
illness" and believes hospitalization to be necessary.

SOCIOECONOMIC INDICATORS

Clear-cut differences are apparent between groups in level of educational attainment. As seen in Table 26, proportionally more of the recently migrant than the settled were totally without schooling, and fewer had progressed beyond the primary level. Few members of either group had reached the university level. Educational differences are most marked between migrants and natives reflecting the latter's greater exposure to urban school facilities. A similar picture, as indicated in Table 26, exists with respect to literacy. While the origins of these differences appear to lie in the rural childhoods of the recently migrant, they have special consequences for people in the initial phases of enculturation into a new environment. The ability to read, less important in familiar and rural settings, becomes increasingly necessary in the strange city where survival requires more massive and rapid information processing; it is also essential for employment beyond the unskilled manual level.

Forty-four per cent of all migrants changed their type of work in consequence of the move, although it continued as a rule to be manual and unskilled. The occupational distribution within the recently migrant and settled groups is shown in Table 27. For this population of temporary psychiatric dropouts from the labor force, consisting mainly of manual workers, the only significant difference between groups is at the lowest occupational level. This is consistent with rural-urban differences in the population as a whole, based on opportunities for education and the acquisition of occupational skills. Migrants who have lived in the city for several years have had the opportunity to acquire added skills and social competence, increasing the likelihood of their upward occupational mobility.

Unskilled manual workers in the nonpatient population at large appear to have been moving actively into skilled manual jobs which promise further upward mobility. Within the patient group, however, a significantly smaller proportion of migrants than natives (seven per cent versus 20 per cent) continues to be found in supervisory or small proprietor's positions. In this population, migrant status is clearly associated with low occupational status; those with the support of family, previous position and education, grown up in the city, familiar with its ways, and exposed early to its opportunities are the most economically effective. Those reared in rural areas, with little education, accustomed only to the available unskilled work, have not caught up to the occupational level of even their urban psychiatric patient counterparts. In this respect they resemble the migrant population at large in which Hutchinson, as noted above, pointed out that the lowest class individuals are least likely to be upwardly mobile.

HOUSING AND AREAS OF RESIDENCE

Indications of the quality and density of housing are listed in Table 28. The recent migrants had less adequate housing than the settled and in keeping with this, had less privacy.

The nature and location of living areas are listed in Table 29. Proportionately more of the settled lived in the comparatively stable working-class suburbs and other areas peripheral to the center city. (The limits of the "industrial zone" are difficult to define, insofar as small factories are found throughout areas known both as suburban and peripheral urban.) The recently migrant were most frequently found in the nonresidential, including central urban, areas, where cheap, inadequate, and often transitory housing is readily available. Such housing is located not only in *favelas* but in older districts of the city, including Saude, Lapa, Praça Onze, and others inland from the major ocean-going freight and passenger docks at Praça Maua and at Praça Quinze, the point of embarkation for the Niteroi ferry. A somewhat higher but not statistically significant proportion of recently migrant as compared to settled persons resides in small-town environments in or near the Greater Rio boundaries. Migrants, upon arriving in the new area, often settle first in such peripheral sections which resemble their former homesites more than the city proper.

In summary, the greatest concentration of recently migrant as compared with settled persons who become patients was in the nonresidential areas of the center city, followed by sections at the periphery of Greater Rio de Janeiro. More of the recently migrant than the settled lived in substandard and overcrowded quarters. These differences in quality and density of housing do not

appear, however, when the group is divided according to migration per se. With time, inequities in housing resulting from relocation are evidently erased, suggesting that for this population, the
housing deficits associated with migrant status were not continuously significant among the factors associated with mental hospital admission. If housing was important, it was as part of the
complex of factors operant within the first five years after arrival,
i.e., as a concomitant of recent mobility rather than of migration
as such.

MOTIVATION TO MOVE AND ACCEPTANCE OF SOCIOECONOMIC STATUS

There were differences between the recently migrant and the
settled in respect to SES acceptance as indicated in Table 30.
Although the recently migrant rank lower in all socioeconomic
indices, more of them than the settled felt they had improved
their socioeconomic position during the preceding year. At the
same time, a few more of the recent arrivals, perhaps under the
influence of wishes which had motivated their move, described
themselves as aware of a discrepancy between aspiration and
achievement. Approximately 30 per cent of each group estimated
their position as worse than in the past year.

Some differences between the recently migrant and settled in
motivation for the move to Rio are probably associated with the
fact that the study population is composed of psychiatric patients.
Thus, it is plausible to expect that more of the recently migrant
would have decided to migrate because of emotionally conflictful
motives. The settled, including those who were not migrants at all
or whose psychiatric difficulties presumably arose after they had
become reestablished in their new location, would not be expected to have been so importantly motivated to move because of
emotional factors. Table 31 shows that proportionately more of
the recently migrant than the settled migrant had in fact moved
for reasons categorized as personal-emotional. The reasons given
were to join or escape families, search for adventure or escape
from boredom. Some of the recently migrant and the settled migrant whose moves were associated with their psychiatric illness
described their reasons in terms of interpersonal problems involving marital or other family relations, or in terms of symptoms
such as weakness or fatigue interfering with adaptation or work.

In most cases, however, there was a clear recognition by patients or families that mental illness requiring medical help was available only in Rio. The following are examples of two such situations.

A 46-year-old white married man with six years of schooling, a ticket clerk in a bus station unemployed for six months because of drinking problems, was brought to Casa Eiras by a cousin. Born in a central urban area of Nova Friburgo, a small town in Rio State, he had migrated to the city, along with two male cousins, when he was 18. The reasons were mixed: to find work, and also adventure and "see the world." He had various jobs before becoming a clerk. After a number of temporary liaisons he lived in a consensual arrangement for 10 years with a woman (whom he now describes as a "prostitute") and her three children. They had a small house in a peripheral urban zone of the city which had electricity but no water. Four years before hospitalization they underwent a civil marriage, but three years later were separated because of intensifying arguments, apparently fueled by alcohol. He has no idea of her whereabouts or that of the children. Upon losing his job the patient returned to his father's home in Nova Friburgo. After consultation with his father, a 72-year-old retired weaver, and four brothers still in Nova Friburgo, he agreed to seek hospitalization. He returned to Rio two weeks before admission, staying at his cousin's home in suburban Madureira. He had hoped to delay hospitalization, but the cousin brought him to Casa Eiras after discovering that he had "stolen" a liter of alcohol.

A 22-year-old white unmarried student who had finished one year of normal school was accompanied to Casa Eiras by his mother and a cousin. The family, including four siblings, lives in a residential quarter of the central urban area of a medium-sized city in São Paulo State where the father, a university graduate, is principal of a secondary school. The patient was brought by bus to Rio with his parents for the purpose of outpatient treatment or hospital admission following several months of increasing tension, withdrawal, and "estranged" behavior culminating, three days before the trip to Rio, in a drinking bout and threats of suicide. The family has also been concerned in the past about his "effeminate" friends and lack of interest in females. His father has already returned to São Paulo, but his mother will remain for an indefinite period at the home of her sister who lives in a residential neighborhood not far from the hospital.

Fifty per cent of all migrants gave lack of jobs as the primary reason for moving. This was true to a significantly greater degree for the settled than the recently migrant. As we have seen, 44 per cent of all migrants changed their jobs in consequence of the move but remained in the manual workers category. The low overall proportion of achievement/aspiration discrepancy responses (encountered in only 20 per cent of the entire patient group) is consistent with the resigned attitudes generally attributed to deprived and mobility-blocked lower-class Brazilians. It may be plausible to attribute the slightly greater proportion of achievement/aspiration discrepancy responses among the recently migrant to psychological tension not necessarily related to economic or job dissatisfaction. Even among those giving lack of a job as the primary reason for moving, other factors not related to conventionally defined achievement may be more important in determining a subjective estimate of the current success, failure, or achievement. Approximately a third of the 50 per cent of the total migrants who gave economic or job-related reasons for their move, volunteered the presence of other reasons as well. A typically encountered example was a young man from rural Minas Gerais who, coming to Rio to find work, mentioned that he wished to escape "exploitation" by his father whom he assisted as an apprentice shoemaker. A man in his forties who had come from Recife 17 years earlier, gave the search for a job as a primary reason, but also noted that he was looking for adventure and wanted "to see Rio de Janeiro." In other instances, a personal-emotional reason was given first and then followed by an occupational one. A young woman in her twenties, for example, a housewife at the time of hospital admission, had come from Pernambuco a few years earlier because she "did not get along with" her stepfather. "Beyond this," she added, she "wanted to find a job." In still other cases the primary motive for leaving might have been obscured by rationalizations; an office clerk in his forties said that he had come from Fortaleza 18 years earlier in order to study medicine. He had been, he said, forced to give up his schooling and support his mother, who moved to live with him in Rio after his father died.

These data support the assumption that in this population of psychiatric patients the conventional economic or job-related reasons for moving may be related to a number of other emotionally relevant factors. They indicate that those migrants hospitalized within five years of relocation were motivated to move for personal-emotional-psychiatric reasons to a significantly greater degree than were those who did not become patients until more than five years after arriving in Rio. Almost two-thirds of the recently migrant patients had left their homes and come to Rio because of personal (as contrasted to economic) dissatisfaction, emotional tension, or because of psychiatric illness recognized by them or their families.

ORIGINS

As indicated in Table 31, 83 per cent of all migrants came from rural or small-town settings, predominantly the former. The traditional Northeast sources (Ceará, Maranhão, Paraiba, Pernambuco, Piaui, Rio Grande de Norte) supplied 39 per cent of the migrants, with the majority coming from the Eastern states (Bahia, Espirito Santo, Minas Gerais, Rio State, Sergipe); a few individuals came from the South and West. Equal proportions of the recently migrant and the settled migrant are rural and provincial in origin.

SOCIAL SUPPORT FROM RELATIVES AND FRIENDS

Similar proportions of the recently migrant and settled had lived in long-term relationships with spouses or mates prior to hospitalization. More migrants than natives, however, as noted above, had consistent mates, and these were presumably a source of support rather than strain. This difference was considered a possible consequence of the selection process to become a patient since unmarried, socially isolated migrants appear more apt to continue as floaters, or to be temporarily picked up in nonmedical facilities, than to be referred for psychiatric assistance.

One index of the migrant's vulnerability to stress, including both personal predispositional and situational factors is the group with which he travels. The presence of a family group protects him from loneliness and mishaps along the way and also indicates his capacity to relate to others. For most of the sample the act of migration was accomplished with relatives. Table 32 shows that significantly more of the recent than the settled migrants had come with conjugal family members; more of the latter had come with parents, siblings, or others of their families of origin. Since the recently migrant and settled migrant groups are of similar age, with most concentrated between the ages of 21 and 40, this may be a matter of age on arrival, i.e., the settled, migrant patients came when they were younger; 40 per cent of the settled migrants versus 15 per cent of the recent migrants did, in fact, arrive before age 18. The recent migrants thus include proportionately more who were adults during migration. Coming alone, they had to depend on themselves; coming with spouses and children, they were more responsible for the care of others than the settled migrants. They had less support from older family members and an extended kinship group and carried more individual responsibility for decision making during geographical relocation.

As shown in Table 32, 30 per cent of the total migrants in the patient sample had come to Rio alone. This is close to Hutchinson's (1963) finding of 36 per cent of all migrants (57 per cent of the men and 15 per cent of the women) entering Rio de Janeiro alone in 1959–1960. A solitary transition between the old and new environments thus need not differentiate the psychiatrically vulnerable from the stable populations. The fact that proportionately, more of the recent in comparison to the settled migrants traveled alone is, however, compatible with the proposition that the first years after migration are those at highest risk of mental hospitalization; it is in this period that individuals motivated to move for personal-emotional factors or traveling without support for other reasons are most apt to decompensate.

Table 32 presents additional material about the supporting network of relatives, friends, and neighbors. Ninety-two per cent of all respondents had relatives in the city aside from nuclear family members, and there were no differences in this respect according to migratory status. As will be shown below (in the chapter on housing), only four per cent of the total patient group lived alone and just a few more of the recently migrant than the settled (nine per cent versus one per cent) lived with people to whom they were not related. Most of the migrants who traveled alone had evidently been preceded or were soon followed by other relatives. In the majority of instances, however, members of extended families did not live close to each other, and significantly fewer of the recently migrant individuals had such family members in the same district or nearby. While the lack of family support was filled to some degree by friends regarded as sufficiently "close" so that the subjects "could talk" with them, differences also existed in this respect between the recently migrant and the settled. As shown in Table 32 half of all the migrants, including significantly more of the settled than the recent, had such friends. This seems to mark a departure from the historically embracing nature of the Brazilian family which traditionally did not permit personal problems or feelings to be shared with others than relatives.

About a quarter of all migrants, including significantly more of the settled than the recently migrant, said that they "knew nothing" about their near neighbors. It seems likely that the recently migrant had greater needs in terms of becoming established while the settled were more self-sufficient. The greater lack of knowledge of the settled than the recently migrant about their neighbors (which still left 75 per cent who did know about them) may have been owing largely to (perhaps protective) indifference. This is suggested by the larger proportion of the recently migrant who reported hostile relationships with close neighbors. Since outsiders must generally earn their acceptance into a new group, it is probable that the more recent arrivals encountered more hostility and reacted in kind.

In summary, a number of social-support-related factors appear to contribute to a higher risk of mental hospitalization among recent than settled migrants into Rio de Janeiro. Among these are (1) the pressure of unshared family responsibilities, (2) the lack of social support for solitary travellers, (3) lack of social support from extended family members and close friends during the first years after arrival; and, (4) more hostile relations with neighbors during the first years after arrival.

SOCIAL SUPPORT FROM RELIGIOUS, WELFARE, AND OTHER GROUPS

Table 32 shows significantly higher proportions of the recently migrant than the settled reporting contact with and friendly feelings toward the clergy. This may reflect a perception of the socially helping role of priests, in contrast to a historically rooted anticlericalism, as well as the rural Brazilian's traditional respect for the ideal of the religious devotee. Interview data also indicate that for many of the patients social services obtained through the Banco da Providencia are clearly identified as a form of religious support. The differences in actual religious participation, however, reported by the recently migrant and settled groups are slight. As noted in Table 33 most of the patients describe themselves as Catholic and there are no Jews among them. A very few more of the settled than the recently migrant admit to belonging to Spiritist, Afro-Brazilian or other groups; similar proportions admit to such participation in addition to their primary religion. In view of the reluctance of most people to admit such affiliations, it may be assumed that some of those denying any religious membership also attend Spiritist, Umbanda, or other Afro-Brazilian cult centers.

The possibility that individuals recently arrived from rural areas tend to be more traditional in their religious observance (as suggested by the smaller proportion belonging to African or Spiritist groups) is supported by their more regular attendance at church services; 35 per cent of the recently migrant versus 20 per cent of settled attended at least once monthly. Religious practice is an important form of institutional participation permitting some carryover from the old to the new milieu. Fourteen per cent of the settled versus 6 per cent of the recently migrant population acknowledged a change in principal religious affiliation around age 18. For this small fraction of the patient population, loosening of traditional religious ties as part of the acculturative process seems to have taken place along with greater readiness to use nontraditional sources of support. Rio de Janeiro is thought to contain a higher concentration of Macumba, Umbanda, and other Afro-Brazilian cult variants than most of the rural hamlets and *fazendas* from which the majority of migrants come, and the relative anonymity provided by the vast metropolitan area permits greater freedom of choice and experimentation in religious as well as other matters.

The people most in need of social assistance seem least able to find it. Table 32 shows that more of the settled than the recently migrant report contact, friendly feelings, and frequent use of social welfare workers and services. It appears more difficult for recent migrants to successfully seek help from the welfare institutional structure of the city than from individual priests who represent some continuity with the old environment. Social worker's attitudes, conditioned by middle-class backgrounds and by a self-conscious professionalism, impair communication with poor, uneducated, rural migrants, especially those recent arrivals who have not had time to become fully oriented to their new surroundings.

Organizational membership was extremely limited for the entire population, nor did the fact of membership mean active participation. Thus, while 11 per cent of the recently migrant and 20 per cent of the settled reported membership in trade unions or occupational organizations, only a few individuals in each category attended meetings. Similarly, 7 per cent of the recently migrant and 16 per cent of the settled reported sports or social club membership, but only three and six per cent respectively were active participants.

In summary, recently migrant in contrast to settled patients were less able to relate to and gain support from welfare workers and secular organizations and related more significantly to religious figures and groups.

PARTICIPATION IN THE INFORMATION AND ACTIVITY NETWORK

There were no statistically significant differences between the recently migrant and the settled in participation in the national spectator sport of soccer or in beach-going. Apparently these activities claim those who are interested within the five-year criterion period because they require neither special talents nor the acquisition of unavailable skills. More of the recently migrant, however, did attend dances and did so more frequently than the settled. Whether this reflects a continuing influence of rural life, a greater propensity to activity among the recently migrant, or the increasing age, conservatism, and reluctance of the settled to have close physical contact outside the family circle is uncertain. A number of patients commented that their attendance at dances had declined since marriage.

Adaptation to a new environment requires a continuing flow of information which may not all be available by word of mouth. Thus the question arises of how recent arrivals are attached to the general information network. Table 34 shows that the major informational source is the radio, usually the transitor. For approximately a third of the settled, and even more of those arrived within five years, this continues as the only informational medium. There are statistically significant differences between the settled and the recently migrant only in the ownership of television sets and one or more books; considerably higher proportions of the former than the latter claim such possessions. Slightly more of the settled claim regular exposure to the various media, and there are no differences in attendance at the movies. The cinema provides an important source of stimulation and amusement to newcomers as well as to settled inhabitants of the city. Since many of the films shown in the least expensive theaters are grade-B United States westerns it is doubtful whether they supply information useful to the enculturative process. In general the settled, whether native or migrant, have greater access to information than the recently migrant.

CHILDHOOD INFLUENCES

Table 35 shows a series of consistent though small and not uniformly significant differences between the recently migrant and settled patients. More of the former lost their fathers prior to age 12, fewer (possibly in consequence) had siblings by both parents, more earned money prior to age 14, and more were financially independent by that age. More also, as might be expected in less stable and secure circumstances requiring early work for money, reported being disciplined mainly by beatings. The mother was the main source of discipline for significantly fewer of these recently migrant patients, primarily of deprived rural origin. The mother's greater control among the settled may be regarded as a concomitant of urban life where the father is absent from the family during the working day. The early financial independence reflects general rural-urban differentials. Thus, Hutchinson (1963) estimated that of the entire Rio de Janeiro population in 1959–1960, 15 per cent of the farm-born versus eight per cent of the urban-born males, and eight per cent of the farm-born versus three per cent of the urban-born females had worked for money prior to age 10.

The fathers of the recently migrant group, as indicated in Table 36, were more often illiterate than those of the settled. Data for education included such large proportions of indeterminate responses that they were not tested for significance; 32 per cent of fathers of the recently migrant compared to 17 per cent of fathers of settled were reported to have never attended school at all. The unavailability of rural schools suggests that these are minimal figures. Data for the mothers, who were generally less educated and literate than the fathers, showed similar differences.

There were no marked differences in paternal occupation between the recently migrant and settled. This is evidently due to the pooling of data from natives and migrants within the settled group. As shown in Table 36, differences do exist according to migratory status per se, with more fathers of migrants than native, in the unskilled manual Class VI and more fathers of native, in the skilled manual Class V. This follows the distribution for the nation at large, reflecting the nature of occupations available in rural and small town areas. In Hutchinson's (1963) 1959–1960 sample of the inhabitants of six Brazilian cities, including Rio de Janeiro, the following proportions were found to engage in Class VI occupations: farm-born fathers, 67 per cent; small-town-born fathers 50 per cent; city-born fathers 22 per cent. This is comparable to the more than half of the fathers of all the migrant patients in the present study, some of whom had lived in small-town and urban environments, who were unskilled manual workers and in contrast to the smaller percentages who were in skilled manual or clerical nonmanual occupations. Among the natives' fathers the situation is reversed. Within this group the remainder are more evenly spread throughout all the nonmanual categories.

In summary, the recently migrant appear to come from more personally and economically deprived backgrounds than the settled, including migrant and native. They could depend less securely upon parents for support and for information useful for adaptation in the city or upward occupational mobility.

HOSPITALIZATION AND FAMILY DIAGNOSIS

As shown in Table 37 more natives than migrants in this sample of first mental hospital admissions had had previous contact with psychiatrists. This finding, while not statistically significant, undoubtedly reflects the greater concentration of outpatient facilities in Rio de Janeiro, especially those sponsored by the social security system. It may also reflect a greater tolerance for psychiatric symptomatology in rural areas and in undemanding agricultural occupations. Economic reasons, i.e., failure to work, occur slightly but significantly more often among the recently migrant as precipitants of hospitalization. This suggests the difficulty recently arrived families have in supporting noncontributing members. It also suggests a relatively greater tolerance within this group for deviant behavior so long as it does not interfere with adaptation.

Anxiety, depression, suicidal thoughts and attempts were more frequent precipitants of hospitalization among the settled than the recently migrant and the most frequent among the natives. The impact of tense, depressed, or suicidal behavior appears greatest upon native families who are less preoccupied with reality problems than families who have been geographically relocated. That this indeed represents a difference in family or community response rather than in patient behavior is indicated by the fact that among the patients themselves (see Table 42) relatively more of the recent migrants than the settled exhibited depressive symptoms. Regardless of the actual symptomatology exhibited by recently migrant patients, dislocated families under stress sought medical help when a member showed his disturbance by not working; stable, native families under less environmental stress responded to the member's primary expression of tension or personal discomfort by seeking medical help.

As shown in Table 38, the majority of both recently migrant and settled families believed life stress to be the major underlying cause of disturbance in the hospitalized member. Twice the proportion of the recently migrant than the settled families described the disturbed behavior as a response to persecution of some kind—harrassment by spouse, other relatives, employer, neighbors, or the police, and occasionally religious figures including both priests and cult leaders. It seems likely that this etiological theory was at least a partial reflection of reality stresses to which the new arrivals were required to adapt. It may also reflect a general tendency to externalize or to look for the causes of personal events in outside sources, more prominent in rural areas isolated from sources of information and lagging in the process of modernization. An example of family diagnosis is seen in the following case.

A 41-year-old white married woman with two years of schooling, employed as a servant in the justice ministry, was brought to Casa Eiras by a married sister. She was born in Teresopolis, approximately one hour away from the city, and lived there with her parents and three siblings until her father deserted the family when she was 15. At that time she went to live with a prominent family as a live-in domestic, moving with them to Rio de Janeiro when she was 18. Unlike some natives of Teresopolis, she felt the city to be a strange place and still regards herself as a migrant who has never truly become a Carioca. She now lives with her husband and 10-year-old daughter in a *vila* on the Ilha Governador with electricity but no water. It is one supplied by the justice department to its employees. Until the present illness she has always been friendly and outgoing, although shy with strangers; in recent months she has become paranoid and depressed. The patient's sister and brother in law believe her to be mentally ill and probably in need of hospitalization. They feel, however, that her husband persecutes her and has driven her to attempt suicide, and that separation from her husband may be more important for her recovery than hospital care.

Table 38 shows that in addition to indicating their opinions as to the underlying causes of emotional disturbance, families made diagnoses of physical or mental illness or strange behavior. There were no significant differences in family diagnosis according to migratory status.

Psychiatric and Behavioral Characteristics

As indicated above, the recently migrant are differentiated from the settled patients by a number of social factors in addition to their recent arrival and rural origins. The most prominent so-

cial differences among the recently migrant consistent with their
recently rural background include lower levels of education and
literacy, less literate parents, lower occupational status (mainly
unskilled manual), and more friendly contact with religious
figures and groups. The recently migrant in comparison with the
settled had more job changes, more temporary unemployment,
less adequate housing in less stable neighborhoods, more aspiration-achievement discrepancy, fewer extended family members in
the neighborhood, less friendly contact with social agencies and
workers, less organizational membership, and less available and
regular information about the society. More migrated because of
illness or personal-emotional reasons, more moved as responsible
adults with dependent families, and more migrated alone rather
than as part of a group. Families of the recently migrant more
often precipitated hospitalization because of the patient's inability
to work, and more often regarded the patient's disturbed behavior
as a consequence of persecution. Settled families more often recommended hospitalization because of tense, depressed, or suicidal behavior. It is in the context of these social differences between recently migrant and settled families and their patient
members that the following psychiatric-behavioral differences
should be viewed.

TENSION, ANXIETY, SENSITIVITY, AND FRUSTRATION

Interview behavior, as noted in Table 39, differed markedly
according to migratory status. The settled patients were generally
more easily understood, more cooperative, more comfortable than
the recently migrant. More of the latter requested direct help, a
few more were hypervigilant and distractible, and expressed
unsatisfied dependent wishes. More of the recently migrant
showed a decrease in tension during the interview (perhaps because of initially high levels). These behaviors are those commonly reported for countrymen in the city. Their caution, apprehension, and defensiveness reflect both the continuing cognitive
style of the rural inhabitant suspicious of strangers and the impact of a new environment. Along with the clearer evidence of
dependent expectations they reflect, too, the ambivalent passivity

of the sharecropper or farm worker, or the economically precarious urban poor in relation to the *patrão*, or the rich man who
may be able to help, in this case the doctor.

Similarly, the psychiatrists, maintaining a pattern of mutually
supporting interaction, expressed themselves as feeling more interested, empathic, cheerful with, and liked by the settled. In contrast, they more often felt remote from, apprehensive of, or hostile
toward the recently migrant. In this way they were responding to
the suspicious apprehension of relatively new arrivals in a still
strange environment, to features characteristic of rural people
from other parts of the country; and to socioeconomic class-linked
behavior. The tension of recently migrant patients, as well as
their needs for concrete assistance, might plausibly be linked with
anticipatory and defensive needs emanating from having had to
cope with the hostility of strangers and the problems of becoming
reestablished in unfamiliar surroundings. These factors probably
contributed to some uncertainty in the role relationship between
subject and interviewer. (While the doctors, as noted in later
chapters, were less comfortable and empathic with the illiterate
and undereducated, they were more comfortable with blacks than
browns—presumably because of the persisting institutionalized
roles of white and black with still functional styles of communication between them.)

As indicated in Table 40, a few more of the recently migrant
expressed situation-linked and probably realistic anxiety about
jobs (not statistically significant) and family. More also complained of discrete anxiety attacks. While significant differences
were found regarding organ anxiety and fear of disease in the
stomach and head, the somatic focus of anxiety frequent in medically unsophisticated and partly educated people was not accompanied by relative freedom from depression. Depression, anxious
tension, situational apprehensiveness, and somatic concern were
all present as part of the same constellation of symptoms. The
ubiquitous presence of chronic though not obvious physical malfunction, greater in rural than urban populations, makes it impossible in this group to rely solely upon psychodynamic explanations of somatic concern.

Interference with function, aside from communication in the

interview, was reflected mainly in thought processes. More of the recently migrant complained of impaired mental efficiency and capacity to concentrate and think clearly. Difficulties in concentration and thinking may only reflect the greater anxiety and tension of the recently migrant, but such processes are presumably most vulnerable to anxiety-induced disruption when they are not highly refined by education and practice or used as major agents for adaptation. The requirements of survival in the intellectually less demanding rural environment may be assumed to produce a different pattern of cognitive activity in the service of adaptive needs than the conditions of the urban context.

As Table 41 indicates more of the recently migrant reported that they felt uncomfortable with others and that others did not think well of them. This is consistent with the familial concern with persecution and the sensitivity and caution of the recent arrival. No differences between recently migrant and settled were recorded in either the positive expression or denial of feelings of anger or rage.

DEPRESSION

Indications of depressed mood or feelings of inadequacy and guilt, as indicated in Table 42 were more frequently reported for the recently migrant than the settled. The trend is uniform for all of the usual indices of depression except suicidal thoughts, although only feelings of sadness, loneliness, of being slow, and of parental guilt were statistically significant. Sucidal ideas were expressed during interviews by neither the recently migrant nor the settled. Their occurrence prior to admission suggests that they reflected less a true expression of an inner wish for oblivion than a socially acceptable cry for help aimed at relatives.

Feelings of sadness, loneliness, inadequacy, and inferiority might be expected in people who have left their homes and who, while carrying family responsibilities, are still in the process of finding new roots and becoming accustomed to a strange environment. Nostalgia for home, even for the arid Northeastern "polygon of droughts," was expressed by most of the migrants even as they referred to their past hardships. Some of this is condensed into the word *saudade,* a not thoroughly translatable amalgam of yearning for persons, places, past times, and states of being. The still intense regionalism of Brazilians, who after years in Rio de Janeiro continue to identify themselves as "Gauchos," "Paulistas," or "Pernambucanos," suggests the degree to which native soil contributes to identity formation. This was seen most clearly in patients who repeatedly expressed their wish for the cooking of their home regions. Whether it is legitimate, however, to tie the occurrence of reality-based mood changes to the appearance of clinically depressive symptoms is uncertain. Similarly, the guilt feelings expressed to a slightly greater degree by the recently migrant may be realistically associated with unfilled promises made at the time of the decision to migrate or unfilled responsibilities toward family members who were left behind.

THE BREAK WITH REALITY

It is difficult to determine in these patients whether or not feelings of being persecuted or maltreated reflect a delusional system, an irrational paranoid attitude, or a culturally reinforced response to the real hostility of strangers and stressful life circumstances. The differences between the recently migrant and settled shown in Table 43 are not large, but they are consistent and statistically significant. More of the former feel badly treated, stared at or talked about, persecuted or harassed, or regarded as inferior by others. They feel that others are not trustworthy, and more are plagued by feelings of jealousy. Approximately half the recently migrant, almost twice the proportion of settled, exhibit some evidence of possibly compensatory grandiosity, saying that they feel especially emulated or loved by certain others. These statements, generally occurring in a constellation of paranoid expressions, appear to be delusional. The recently migrant-settled differences in this respect resemble those between general public and private hospital admissions as noted in Chapter I, with more of the former labeled manic (grandiose and euphoric); there are no differences, however, between the two groups in elated or manic behavior. Symptoms which seem most likely to be delusional and associated with a clear-cut paranoid psychotic process are feelings that others control one's thoughts and actions and know one's inner thoughts and feelings. These occurred in somewhat over a third of the recently migrant and in a smaller number of the settled.

Table 44 lists the occurrence of hallucinatory phenomena, supporting the impression that more of the recently migrant than the settled were unequivocally psychotic. Not only did more report auditory and visual hallucinations, but the phenomena were more ego-syntonic and meaningful for them: More recent migrants insisted on the reality of, and planned their actions on the basis of, these experiences. Congruent with these findings were the larger proportions of the recently migrant who misinterpreted or attributed special meaning to sensory stimuli as well as to written and verbal communications. The only clue to a specific cultural determinant of hallucinations was the finding that more (though a very small absolute proportion) of the recently migrant hallucinated religious, folkloric, or ghostly figures.

As might be expected, the higher incidence of impaired reality testing was associated with disorientation in time or place in more of the recently migrant than the settled. Table 45 shows that temporal disorientation (day, month, or year), generally transitory in nature, occurred in a fifth of the recently migrant and less than 10 per cent of the settled.

SOMATIC PROBLEMS

As noted elsewhere, anxiety about organ function and a tendency to concentrate attention on body parts seems more characteristic of less literate and less educated people. More of the recently migrant did report anxiety about bodily function or integrity. Only a very few more, however, had specific complaints about body function. Fatigue and weakness, present in more than half of both groups, may be part of a depressive picture. As suggested above, however, data on the general health of lower-class, particularly rural, Brazilians suggest that these complaints may also be a function of overwork, undernutrition, and chronic though not incapacitating illness. The feeling of something strange inside the body, a complaint of delusional quality, may be classed along with other psychotic symptoms.

The major finding in this area, as indicated in Table 46, was that relatively more of the settled complained of psychophysiological complaints, psychological reflections of actual organ dysfunction, such as awareness of rapid heart beat and a feeling of shortness of breath. Similar reports (Langner & Michael, 1963; Hollingshead & Redlich, 1958) have been made about other groups, suggesting that such complaints accompany greater socioeconomic security associated with less possibility of direct expression of feelings and need for action. These findings are more impressive in this group of generally lower-class subjects where it might be expected that the concomitants of poor physical status would diminish the recently migrant-settled difference.

In contrast to the groups divided on the basis of color, education, or literacy (described in later chapters), there were no significant differences in sexual function associated with migratory status; a few more of the recently migrant than the settled, however, regarded their current pattern of sexual functioning as being associated with their psychiatric illness.

PAST PERSONAL HISTORY

The questions in this category yielded no statistically significant differences between the recently migrant and the settled groups. When both groups are composed of psychiatric patients, differentiation on the basis of mobility does not reveal differences in earlier, possibly traumatic, experience which might contribute to later psychiatric breakdown.

DISCUSSION

Migration provides a set of concrete operations for the study of adaptation and mental illness in relation to social change. A shift in residence involves not only new places, but new faces and new norms. It implies the crossing of social system boundaries, whether the systems are defined in terms of national entities, regional subcultures, or immediate friendship and kinship networks. The migrant leaves his social system of origin impelled by push factors such as disease, hunger, lack of jobs, schools for his children, and stressful personal relationships and obligations. He is pulled by the lure of novelty, excitement, and the promise of need fulfillment not supplied in his point of origin. Beyond this he may have private or internal motives which have little apparent connection with environmental circumstances. Some migrants are risk-takers, others are geographic escapers who deal with personal conflict by physical flight. For some, migration occurs at a point in a personal trajectory of social change when a combination of individual and environmental factors conspire to make geographic relocation an inevitable next step (Brody, 1970). Although a considerable literature (Sanua, 1970) suggests that migration may at times be correlated with increased mental illness and hospital admission rates, why or how the impact of migration on psychiatric disturbance varies between groups and social contexts remains unclear.

The present study cannot answer the general question of whether migratory experience influences the incidence and nature of mental illness in the population at large. Concerned with a population of already hospitalized patients, it attempts to clarify the relationship between migration from other parts of Brazil into Rio de Janeiro on the one hand, and the nature of psychiatric symptomatology and the process of mental hospitalization on the other. It is concerned with the personal and the sociocultural characteristics of migrants and the ways in which these characteristics promote or impair adaptation to Rio de Janeiro life. The personal characteristics reflected in motives for leaving home and searching for new solutions in the city have contributed to their apparent vulnerability to psychiatric breakdown in a significant proportion of migrants. Their migratory behavior can not be regarded as purely symptomatic, however, since it occurred in a national context in which geographic relocation is an accepted form of problem solving. Almost all the migrants in this study overcame major obstacles in order to relocate themselves or their families in pursuit of widely accepted socioeconomic or personal goals. Beyond this, more migrant than native patients had achieved a stable marital relationship so that they may be regarded in some sense as at a lower risk for mental hospitalization than natives.

Problems in adaptation to the new Rio de Janeiro environment are regarded as central to developing the disturbed thinking, feeling, and acting which lead to a migrant's being labeled a "patient" and admitted to a mental hospital. These problems occur despite a series of ameliorating and supportive circumstances: the move to Rio was voluntary; over one-half the Rio population is non-native; migrant associations and social agencies are increasingly available as helpers; and some communication with family members is usually maintained. Nonetheless, the migrant is more alone, and his capacities and opportunities for emotionally meaningful communication are less than those of the native. Those who become mental patients have not become integrated into the new social structure. The friendship and institutional network, including the work structure of the new environment, remains closed to them. For them, the stresses of the new urban context and the loss of support following departure from the home community appear more important determinants of mental hospitalization than earlier predispositions of the sort reflected in prior failures to marry or to achieve in other ways. In contrast, natives who in the apparent absence of the kind of stress associated with migration, become patients, may constitute a group psychologically more vulnerable on the basis of early predispositions than migrants, except for those few who migrated specifically seeking medical help.

The recent migrants, i.e., those hospitalized within five years of their arrival in Rio de Janeiro, are assumed to be most vulnerable to decompensation in the face of adaptive demands and least capable of developing viable connections with the new community. In some instances the failure of migration to solve their problems has also contributed to their decompensation. In contrast, the settled migrants, i.e., those hospitalized more than five years after arrival in Rio de Janeiro, are assumed to have dealt more or less successfully with the loss of old supports and the immediate stresses of entry into the new environment. Their psychiatric disorders, like those of the natives, are probably more a function of early predisposition and chronic stress than of acute aspects of the migratory process, i.e., of a social system boundary crossing itself.

The available literature supports the assumption of highest psychiatric vulnerability in the early postmigratory period. Thus, Hunt and Butler (1970) found the largest proportion of lowest social class anomics to be recent migrants into Los Angeles. This was associated with disruption of their participation in the informal social structure as contrasted with the formal and work structure. Malzberg and Lee (1956) found the rate of admission for United States migrants into New York State, after corrections for age and sex, to be significantly highest within the first five years after their arrival. Wilson, Saver, and Lackenbruch (1965), reporting more than twice the mental illness rates among migrants than natives in Los Angeles County, found the rate highest within the first year after changing residence. Similar findings have been reported for international migrants. Hemsi (1967), who recorded a considerably higher psychiatric first admission rate for West Indians than natives in two London boroughs, noted that 25 per cent of the West Indian patients were ill on arrival or within three months thereafter. This compares with the seven per cent psychiatric hospitalization rate prior to their migration reported by Gordon (1965) for a group of West Indian patients in London. He concluded that environmental factors contributed to their illness. The possible role of hostility to the new environment in adaptive failure is suggested by Richardson's (1957) study of manual workers immigrated into Australia. Those with the greatest difficulties of adjustment tended to feel strongly identified with the social order in Britain so that Australia became a scapegoat for all difficulties, real or imagined. The satisfied immigrants came with a greater readiness to change their behavior to fit Australian conditions. Krupinsky, Schaechter, and Cade (1965), also in Australia, attributed what they felt to be a high incidence of schizophrenia to the migration of unstable single men breaking down during the first year of the struggle for socioeconomic survival.

In the present study more of the recent than the settled migrants came with adult responsibilities for their own conjugal families. Proportionally more also traveled alone, adding to the responsible and highly taxed segment of this group another segment vulnerable because of antecedent circumstances as well as lack of support during transition. Finally, more of the recent migrants were vulnerable, having moved for clearly identified personal-emotional or psychiatric reasons.

Specific obstacles to integration of the predominantly lower-class recent migrants into the social structure of their new environment are their inadequate and poorly located housing, their exclusion from the cultural mainstream owing to lack of education and literacy, and their rural origins, which influence their attitudes toward others and produce habitual cognitive and affective styles not appropriate to the complex adaptive demands of the urban setting. The effects of inadequate or distorted information about the new setting, resulting in a state of relative perceptual deprivation, are intensified by their comparative isolation from friends and relatives and inability to gain needed support from social agencies. Proportionately more are in the unskilled manual category; though many have changed jobs upon arrival, most have done so without upward mobility and, more than the settled, suffered from temporary unemployment in the year preceding hospitalization. These findings are generally compatible with Hutchinson's (1963), which indicate that lower-class migrants into Brazilian cities are least likely to achieve upward occupational mobility. They also fit those of Lipset and Bendix (1959, in Hunt and Butler, 1970), who found that lower-class migrants into United States metropolitan areas most often took low-status jobs, while lower-class natives were more often successful in moving up the occupational scale. Migrant patients in the present sample, regardless of recency of arrival, were less likely than natives to be in supervisory positions. Though access to the opportunity structure of the city is restricted both by poverty and by unfamiliarity with the new setting, their level of achievement-aspiration discrepancy is low, in keeping with the generally resigned attitude of the Brazilian lower class. This is compatible with Parker and Kleiner's (1966) finding that among migrant Negroes into Philadelphia such discrepancy is more often found in the better educated second generation, whose occupational achievement is not commensurate with their education. The slightly greater frequency of achievement-aspiration discrepancy among the recently migrant than the settled seems more plausibly attributed to the psychological tensions motivating or consequent to geographical relocation than to frustrated occupational ambition as such.

Feelings of loss and sadness were prominent in the recently migrant patients. These stemmed in part from certain occupational consequences of migration. Traditionally, these rural families worked together. Everyone was a contributing member of the family economic unit, in the fields or in home crafts. In the city, however, adults work in factories or other jobs. Not only do they lose an important area of shared concern and activity, they also suffer a degree of alienation from the products of their labor. These losses are added to loss of familiar persons and places in their former home. Associated with them are the guilts from unfilled responsibilities to family members left behind, and the feelings of inadequacy stemming from uneven competition with already experienced city dwellers.

Suspiciousness and distrust of the unknown were characteristics brought from the rural environment and intensified in the strange city context. Paranoid tendencies have been identified by many observers as prominent in migrants who become psychiatric patients. Gordon (1965), for example, found a marked excess of paranoid tendencies in schizophrenic and schizo-affective West Indian patients in England in comparison with native-born patients. A similar difference in respect to paranoid illnesses was also reported by Tewfik and Okasha (1965). Listwan (1959) found that twice as many immigrants as native-born were paranoid in a sample of first admissions to the Sydney Hospital psychiatric outpatient department. Schaechter (1962) regarded the large percentage of non-British female immigrants diagnosed paranoid schizophrenic as reflecting difficulties of assimilation into Australia. The observations of a number of other authors, all indicating a predominance of paranoid features among both internal migrants and immigrants as compared with residentially stable patients, have been reviewed by Sanua (1970). In many instances, especially for refugees and others crossing national boundaries, the reality problems associated with geographical relocation appear to have been more severe than for internal migrants into Rio de Janeiro. Perhaps this is why major differences in paranoid behavior were not found in relation to migrant status in general in the present sample, but were found specifically in relation to the recency of migration.

Little education and a high incidence of illiteracy, more characteristic of rural than urban inhabitants, contribute to a relative lack of information with a need to fill in the gaps; people and situations are threatening when they are only partly known. The illiterate or partly literate migrant is more lost than the similarly handicapped native—he can neither extend his symbolic horizons nor see himself in the diverse pattern of reference groups in the host society. Without education and literacy upward mobility within the new social system is impossible, so that his powerlessness and low self-esteem are further emphasized. The hard manual labor, unsanitary living conditions, and associated illnesses of the poor and unskilled contribute to fatigue, body concern, and depression. Depression is further compounded by a sense of hopelessness, voiced by many during their interviews. This stems not only from lack of skills for city living but from daily exposure to goods and privileges which they knew only abstractly before migrating. Low motivation for upward mobility is associated with an awareness, however dim, of being denied access to what is desired. Failure to participate in existing social structures may be as much a consequence of this factor as of lack of knowledge and fear and suspicion of strangers.

It is fair to assume that of all the Rio de Janeiro inhabitants with demonstrable psychiatric difficulties, a considerable proportion never become patients. Adaptive failures of recent migrants, when they are not clearly identified as psychiatric casualties (although they may, for example, be alcoholic) are often handled by agencies dealing mainly with men who are separated from families, or with smaller numbers of women, most of whom do not have husbands or other relatives to help care for them or their dependent children. Unable to survive without assistance, these people may have come in contact with rehabilitation or sheltering rather than with medical-psychiatric components of the social control system, either by accident or in consequence of continuing adaptive capacity. Potential patients whose communicative and reality-testing abilities are not greatly impaired are thus drained off, leaving a more obviously sick group to the mental hospital. It is not until a resident of one of these sheltering agencies becomes markedly agitated that he too is transferred to the mental hospital. In order to enter the patient role, a recently migrant person without a family must be more floridly disturbed and socially impaired than one who is settled.

For more than three-fourths of both the recently migrant and settled patients, family attitudes were the chief determinants of entrance into the status and role of patient. This supports the idea

that the unattached or socially isolated person, whose behavior is
not constantly monitored by people living at close quarters with
him, must be more disturbed than the attached before hospital
admission, and suggests that the recently migrant family may
have been more tolerant than the settled of deviant behavior up
to the point of economic impairment. A clear separation appears
between the psychiatric characteristics of the patients and the
reasons given by their families for bringing them to the hospital.
While the recently migrant are more depressed, anxious, paranoid, deluded, and hallucinated than the settled, their families do
not more often list frankly disturbed behavior as a reason for
admission. Conversely, while fewer of the settled patients are depressed, their families more frequently list depression, anxiety,
and suicidal attempts as reason for hospital admission. Settled
families seem to have a lower threshold of response to disturbed
behavior than the recently migrant families and to be more inclined to utilize psychiatric facilities to deal with such disturbance.
Another factor contributing to differential tolerance is suggested
by the family diagnosis of "reaction to persecution," offered by
twice as many recently migrant as settled families. A rational explanation of this sort, based on shared perceptions of strangers
and the new environment might reduce the likelihood of a sick
member's extrusion by the family into a hospital until his disturbed
behavior begins to interfere with its survival as a socioeconomic
unit. If such differences in family tolerance do in fact exist, they
would account for at least part of the greater frequency of anxiety-
produced functional impairment and impaired reality testing
among the recently migrant who finally become patients.

CHAPTER 5

SKIN COLOR, SOCIAL STATUS
AND PATIENT BEHAVIOR

COLOR AND BEHAVIOR IN THE UNITED STATES

THE COLOR of a man's skin, the contour of his features, the quality of his hair are physical facts having sociological significance. Together they convey a host of messages to members of a pluralistic, multiracial society. Moreover, they are psychologically important; from the onset of self-awareness they are part of his self-concept, his sense of personal identity. The attitudes of others, including members of his family, reinforce their significance. United States parents with children of different hues report attitudes which vary with the lightness or darkness of a child's skin, attitudes of which the child himself is soon aware. The relationship between society and culture and the personality of United States Negroes, especially in the semirural "black belt" of the South prior to World War II, has been amply documented by Dollard (1937) and others. In the middle-class Negro communities of northern cities such as Chicago, Davis, and Havighurst (1946) and others found that white bourgeois standards of child-rearing were adopted with exceptional vigor as part of the upward reach. Some evidence has been accumulated about the impact of social transition on personality and behavior, but the relationship between caste, class, and color on the one hand, and the occurrence and nature of mental illness on the other, is less clear.

Studies of Negro mothers and sons living in the southern border city of Baltimore in the early 1960's, utilizing play techniques with puppets of different colors, demonstrated that the child is sensitive to Negro-white differences at an early age. Six- to 10-year-old Negro boy subjects showed significant conflicts involving anxiety or guilt-laden wishes to be white rather than Negro (Brody, 1963). On the basis of interview and play data, several trends were identified as basic to their ambivalence about identity. One was the reality-oriented wish to be the more powerful white and abandon the less rewarding Negro identity. Another was an identification with the aggressor as a way of dealing with the powerful and feared white world, particularly as perceived through parental attitudes and feelings. A third was a tendency to deal with hostile feelings toward the white world, usually mediated through the parental relationship and stimulated by the mother's contradictory messages about skin color, by turning them against the self. Self-hatred was therefore, a frequent characteristic of their ambivalence. It was also inferred that hostility apparently directed toward a symbol of the white world, i.e., the puppet, or more abstractly "skin color," was at a more fundamental level aimed against the parent, who was perceived by the child as responsible for his uncertainty about himself.

A study using identical techniques with a similar group of white boys and their mothers (Brody, 1964a) demonstrated the way in which the social psychological atmosphere of childhood produced the complementary situation. The white boys' perceptions of Negroes, as revealed by puppet-play techniques, were ambivalent and conflictful, with the latter representing inferior, dangerous, unacceptable, or otherwise anxiety- or guilt-laden elements in themselves. In other words, the "white identity" of a child raised in an atmosphere of racial tension contains within it partly conscious fragments of "Negro identity" to the degree that the entity, black, as learned from the surrounding culture and personal experience, becomes associated with independently originated fears and conflicts.

White mothers, as did the Negro, gave mixed messages to their sons. Both consciously tried to instill egalitarian attitudes in their children, but, without being aware of it, conveyed in a variety of ways their deeply felt hidden hostility toward, and distrust and fear of members of the other group. Negro mothers differed from white mothers in that they verbally denied the real significance of color in their own lives while simultaneously displaying acute sensitivity to any issue concerning race in general.

Another series of studies concerned adult black mental hospital patients and their families. One psychotherapeutic study of a group of 10 young male schizophrenics (Brody, 1961) showed the following characteristics not encountered to the same degree in similarly diagnosed whites of similar social status: (1) Essentially matriarchal families with aggressive, central mothers and passive absent or remote fathers, (2) important, apparently substitutive relationships, with slightly older or more successful male peers (including siblings and cousins) and a tendency to disruption of these relationships before the psychotic breaks, (3) psychoses with prominent elements of confusion and somatic concern, and a paranoid attitude, but poorly organized or absent delusions; and, (4) a tendency to overt homosexual concern or a past history of homosexual interest or activity. Beyond this, lower-class Negro families of nonpatients as well as patients appeared to share features which might plausibly be considered to be productive of schizophrenic behavior. These include problems in forming a satisfactory identification with a father figure, the need to resolve anxiety induced conflicting identifications with white and black authority figures, and a variety of social factors promoting the use of defensive techniques, such as denial, which impair the ability to evaluate and act upon reality. (With these factors in mind one wondered why all Negro males did not become schizophrenic.) Along the same lines, an interesting difference between a black schizophrenic patient group and a black nonschizophrenic control group has been shown by Rorschach and other psychological testing (Goldenberg, 1953). Those who were schizophrenic showed more overt hostility against Negroes—interpreted as caused by the acquisition of white attitudes—and a greater tendency to identify with whites than did the nonschizophrenic group. In contrast, the nonschizophrenic group showed a "greater tendency to accept their own group membership and exhibited more" conscious fantasied retaliation against whites (p. 76).

An additional study made of a sample of 43 black patients and their families, including home visits, produced similar findings and yielded further clues regarding protective factors built into the culture (Derbyshire, Brody & Schleifer, 1963). That is, during the socialization of their children, all the parents (most frequently the single parent—the mother) made extensive use of female relatives residing outside of the immediate household; the children were encouraged to extend their emotional investment beyond household boundaries. This apparently helped to protect them against some of the stresses, such as illness, separation, and death, which are normally considered to be disorganizing. Nonetheless, while female children had opportunities for additional identifications, the boys remained without adequate same-sex role-models.

Finally, additional studies examined factors leading to the identification of disturbed Negro men as mentally ill and their admission to mental hospitals (Brody, Derbyshire, & Scheifer, 1967). Nonwhites, according to official statistics, have a markedly greater risk of public mental hospitalization in Maryland than whites, and nonwhite males are particularly vulnerable. These figures reflect in part the higher public hospitalization rates for urban than for rural dwellers and for those of low socioeconomic status, since most Maryland Negroes live in Baltimore and are of lower socioeconomic status. The study data, however, indicate that current rates of mental hospital admissions do not, as one might suspect, overrepresent the disturbed Negro population, but rather the contrary. That is, social factors have conspired to reduce rather than increase Negroes' use of public mental health facilities. Great delays in identification of disturbed behavior as due to mental illness occurred for two major reasons. One is the attitudes of the police, which produce a pattern of repeated arrest and incarceration in jails, sometimes over several years, before mental illness is recognized. The other is the families' failure to recognize mental illness. They attribute the deviant behavior to reality aspects of the environment or regard it as adaptive rather than sick. In most instances, therefore, hospitalization was not initiated by lower-class Negro families unless the patient engaged in uncontrollably violent behavior or because his failure to work became an intolerable economic burden. An examination of symptoms suggested that in urban Baltimore it has usually been necessary for a Negro to be sicker or more dramatically disturbed than a comparable white person in order to receive hospital care.

In the harshly drawn segregationist atmosphere of the United

States before the second World War, individual behavior in general reflected the accommodation of a minority group with a less viable culture to a dominant majority with a functional and deeply rooted culture. For those defined as white, discriminatory actions and percepts were habitual; automatic discriminations avoided energy-consuming decisions and the anxiety associated with reconciling incompatible standards and viewpoints. The persisting force stemming from unconscious conflict was revealed mainly in the vigor and tenacity of racial prejudice and its sometimes bizarre reflections in suspicion, lynching, and sexual mutilation.

During World War II and after, with an acceleration following the Supreme Court's school desegregation decision of 1954, Negroes began to acquire the information, expectations, and political and economic power necessary for a transformation of self-concept and social role. Explosions of destructive action, especially during the "long hot summers" of the nineteen-sixties, have been interpreted by some as eruptions of pent-up rage against the oppressors and those who symbolize them. They may also represent a convulsive communication on the part of those for whom other channels have been blocked—a cry for help as well as of self-assertion.

Progress has been made toward the development of a positive identity, toward understanding that the group must share more than a common state of misery or of hatred of whites. Attempts at cultural revitalization through establishing social and historical links with Africa and in the concepts of "soul" and "brother" are reflections of this. All, like the more poetic "Negritude" of Leopold Senghor of Senegal, are aimed at emphasizing what is unique, valuable, and viable about being black. Nonetheless, many observers have regarded the use of physical violence and other visible manifestations of power to frighten or manipulate the white majority as the most significant elements in the production of a new identity.

COLOR AND BEHAVIOR IN BRAZIL

How does the Brazilian situation compare with that of the United States? Is there a relationship between color (as distinct from economic status) and behavior, normal or deviant, for Brazilian patients?

Perhaps the first point of difference is that the turbulent era of transition upon which the United States is now embarked reverberates in a still distant way upon the Brazilian scene. Thus, neither the racial violence nor the "black is beautiful" mystique, classic aspects of the personal and cultural transformation of Negroes in the United States, have real meaning in Brazil. Florestan Fernandes (1965), denying an uncompromising division between black and white in Brazil, has noted the distinctions made by black people themselves between Negroes who are "disorderly", or *malandro* (a rascal, bum, or thief) on the one hand and those who are "orderly" or "elite" on the other. He finds a general condemnation of the idea that "we are all the same, Negroes." At the same time, no such distinctions are made between the white "elite" and "rascals" (p. 139).

Oracy Nogueira (1955) has described racial prejudice in Brazil as being related to appearance and not to origin, as in the United States. This is not to say that Brazilians are not color conscious, but rather that they are much more sensitive than North Americans to fine variations in the appearance of hair and skin. The distinctions reported by Marvin Harris (1956) for the inhabitants of a small town in the interior of Bahia in the early 1950's reflect the classification style of the country as a whole. These distinctions, similar to those encountered elsewhere in Brazil, include the *moreno* ". . . wavy hair with the skin coloring of a heavily sunburnt white . . .," the *mulatto,* darker with "crisp, curly hair," the *chulo* ". . . with crisp, rolled hair and his skin is the color of burnt sugar or tobacco," the *creolo,* with . . . "fine wavy hair . . . almost as dark as the *chulo,* but has smoother skin," and the *cabo verde* who "has very straight hair and is the color of the Negro" (pp. 96–146). Brazilians also have special names for racial intermixtures which are used with variable frequency in different parts of the country, such as *caboclo* (Indian-white), originally applied to domesticated Indians, *cafuso* (Indian-Negro), and others. Van den Berghe (1967), who has listed 20 special color-linked labels, regards "this very consciousness of, and concern for, physical appearance" as having "paradoxically militated against the drawing of precise color lines between distinct groups (p. 71)."

Brazilians then, do perceive each other in terms of a *gestalt* in which color is an important element but they are not totally blinded to physical reality by the symbolic significance of a label. The kind of reality testing which allows a North American to refer to a light brown-skinned blue-eyed child of the economic middle class as "Negro" is not present there. This is partly owing to the existence of the large mixed *mestiço* or mulatto population which, while often lumped together with those who are black, is widely regarded as a distinct subgrouping. In the summer of 1968, for example, a popular musical show was entitled *"Nem Todo Crioulo e Doido!"* or "Not all Mulattoes (creoles) are Crazy!"

The historical roots of racial interpenetration in Brazil are varied and have been reviewed in detail elsewhere. The most familiar accounts are the romantic versions of Gilberto Freyre (1964). He writes of the white attitudes toward dark-skinned people, an attitude still influenced by a heritage of 800 years of Moorish occupation. Portugal was one of the last parts of the Iberian peninsula so occupied; thus for centuries a light-skinned person who married a dark one moved up the social scale. It was during those years that the daughter of the black prince became the "symbol of sexual enchantment" for the white Portuguese peasant. The linkage of nonwhite skin and sexual desirability was reinforced during the "procreative frenzy," as Freyre put it, of the first Portuguese explorers who brought no women of their own to the new world. They initially mated with Brazilian Indians, then with black slaves, and later with the resultant people of mixed blood. The institutionalized attitudes of the white men toward their female companions is contained in a saying quoted by Freyre, "A white woman for marriage, a *mulata* for a mistress and a Negress for work" (pp. 278–403). The *mulata* girl, rather than the black, is celebrated as the passionate lover and mistress of the *senhore de engenho* or plantation owner. It is the *"Moreninha* of Itapuan,"* the "tan-skinned" girl of the storied Bahian beach, who is the central figure in the song made popular by Dorival Caymmi.

The cultural superiority of many Africans transported as slaves to Brazil was also important to the early Brazilian perception of color as linked to greater rather than less status and influence; in 1835 more of them than their masters in Bahia could read and write. As Freyre and others have indicated, the impact upon the whites of their early relationships with a black *mucama* or milk mother was extended by her capacity to use her intelligence and cultural knowledge in order to perpetuate her own dominance. Sometimes this knowledge related to love charms or healing herbs or incantations, and sometimes to traditional or superstitious sources of wisdom enabling her to foretell the future or to offer advice in moments of crisis. Even today (as described in the chapter on religion) countless Brazilians invoke the wisdom of the "spirits of the old black ones," the *pretos velhos,* as they "come down" and are "incorporated" by practitioners of various therapeutically oriented religious cults. In this way a certain real power occasionally comes into the hands of the nonwhite household maid who may be the referral link between her master or mistress and a center in which the desired help may be found.

The early attitudes toward dark-skinned women and their derivatives persist, though in diminishing form. It is still possible to hear an educated white man, even in southernmost Brazil where there is the most overt discrimination, refer to his white wife or mistress as *minha negrinha* (my little Negress). The possible interest of white Brazilian women in mulatto or black men remains undocumented.

In contrast to Freyre's emphasis on the interbreeding of blacks and whites on the colonial plantations of the North, Florestan Fernandes (1969) sees the historical origins of present-day relations between white and nonwhite Brazilians in the inability of former slaves to compete with a more able and aggressive white labor force. This included natives, but more especially immigrants from Europe accustomed to a free labor market with its economic and social implications. Unlike Freyre's, Fernandes' observations deal more with the cooler, less colonial and feudal South, particularly São Paulo State. The competitive social order and the consolidation of the class system in São Paulo revolved, he believes, around the dominant figures of the plantation owner and immigrant almost to the complete exclusion of the formerly enslaved rural Negro or mulatto whose difficulties were enormously increased by rapid urbanization. Reasons for exclusion, in his view, included many personal factors: work for the Negro and mulatto, in contrast to the immigrant, was "an end in itself—as though in it and through it they might assert their dignity and freedom as human beings" (p. 12); in contractual relationships Negroes and mulattoes "behaved as if their basic human rights were at stake—that is to say, as if they were selling themselves . . ." (p. 13). The swift development of a competitive social order in São Paulo diminished their opportunity to learn new ways of doing things, and their employability remained impaired because of "refusal to perform certain tasks and services; unreliability in reporting for work; the fascination for occupations that seemingly or actually conferred status; the tendency to alternate between periods of regular work and more or less prolonged phases of idleness; the aggressive reaction to direct control and organized supervision; [and] the lack of incentives for competition with colleagues or for making salaried work a source of economic independence . . ." (p. 13). All these factors contributed to the nonwhites' inability to adopt the urban life style: " . . . they lived in the city without being of it" (p. 74). Excluded from jobs for which they had no training, they turned to what was available; the poorly paid, the health-endangering, the menial. The economic, social, and cultural deprivation which resulted often made it seem to the young that crime and vice offered "the best perspectives for a career" (p. 79).

Fernandes writes at length about the influence of this limited opportunity, with its corollaries in overcrowded housing and disorganized families, upon the early initiation, polymorphous nature, and promiscuity of sexual relationships. "These may be understood by us as the major source of available pleasure and base of interpersonal transactions." He concludes: "Sex came to be the source, par excellence, of the intensification and revitalization of the factors of social anomie among Negroes and mulattoes" (p. 84). Central to this was not the breakdown of the family as a social institution, but rather its failure to become organized as such after the release from slavery. He describes the incomplete family with its tendency to abandon its unwanted children, its sick and its old, and its later organization around the woman which led to a further demoralizing of the man. Drinking, especially among the men, became an accepted way to "pass the time," to gain membership in cliques, to entertain friends, and to gain personal prestige. The cliques, developing interests around " . . . the samba, gambling, vagrancy, and sex . . . provided channels for the expression of . . . needs that had been suffocated by society" (pp. 94–96). This set of interrelated circumstances inevitably led to increased prejudices and repressive measures among the whites, and thus a classic vicious cycle, beginning with the residual perceptions of the slaves as unreliable, dirty, and dangerous, was reinforced.

Fernandes provides the most thorough and detailed documentation of antiblack prejudice in Brazilian social science literature, labeling the official racial ideology deceptive. He specifically notes the misleading tendency to equate color prejudice with class prejudice: "Even the Afonso Arinos Law (1950) which includes among 'legal offenses all practices resulting from race or color prejudice' stresses that it is aimed at 'a change in the racist attitude that prevails among us, especially in the country's upper social and government spheres' " (p. 406). As delineated by Fernandes, this attitude pervades all levels of the social structure. Its perception by the targets, however, the nonwhites themselves, appears to vary with urbanization. The rural worker, while describing in minute detail the color-based rejection to which he is subjected, is apt to deny that it represents prejudice and to understand it in specifically interpersonal and familial terms. Those in the metropolitan centers, more aware and involved, have come to see the overall nature of the problem. The developing nature of awareness can be seen in the rural migrant who, as he comes to know the city, gradually learns " . . . to shield himself from the concealed or obvious expressions of color prejudice." However, " . . . the same problems are posed anew with each generation, as though the experiences amassed collectively were useless" (p. 429).

Aside from the rurally based poor, Fernandes does indicate a gradual increase in upward social mobility among nonwhites in São Paulo (generally considered to have more urbanized Negroes than Rio de Janeiro) after 1930. "Some stimuli which functioned in the past are still present: . . . the socializing influence of the white family and white paternalism . . ." (p. 270). These are of diminishing importance, however. White paternalism in particular is less acceptable to both whites and blacks, and the most important factors in "the modernization of the Negro's cultural outlook [are] linked to the psychosocial effects of his gradual absorption of models taken from society for the organization of behavior, personality and social institutions . . ." (p. 272). In this small but increasing segment of the nonwhite population, modernization and urbanization are accompanied by greater self-awareness as members of a group which may be able, deliberately, to do something to help itself. Sociopolitical groups, which arise from time to time, such as the Frente Negro Brasileira, have not yet achieved significant power or even national representation. They and other "claims movements," as Fernandes describes them, do, however, indicate the gradual progress of the Brazilian nonwhite in " . . . freeing himself from the moral pressures of the traditional world and consciously adopting the moral climate of the competitive social order" (p. 289).

In present-day Rio de Janeiro it is clear that as one moves down the social hierarchy the number of racially mixed or otherwise nonwhite individuals increases. This inevitably contributes to an automatic dominant-subordinate relationship between the majority of whites and nonwhites. The relationship frequently has a touch of the *patrão* quality in which the white assumes to some degree the role of benevolent master while the black, in return for submission, expects both concrete and emotional support. This is intensified when the black person is a child or female and is most easily seen on the street as beggars, rarely adult males, come through cafes or restaurants open to the sidewalk. The almost exclusively white customers may be annoyed, but they usually smile and offer food from their plates or a small bill which sometimes seems to have been saved for just such an occasion. One warm evening, for example, a middle-aged woman darted across the street to a restaurant on the Praça General Osorio in Ipanema. She carried a shiny metal container which she presented to a diner, a well-dressed young white woman, who with little hesitation scooped a large part of her meal into it. The beggar then went back across the street into the park where she shared her food with two children who had been waiting in the shadows. Youngsters of varying hue, between about six and 12 years old, often offer candies for sale or, even if the customer wears sandals, may suggest a shoeshine. They are frequently successful, even though many of those who are approached know that they are being sent out by adults who collect their gleanings; some children are rented by adults for the purpose. While the *favelas* contain many poverty-stricken whites, white beggars are rarely seen making the evening rounds.

Color is only one of the criteria by which people are placed in the social hierarchy. According to a well-known saying, "money whitens the skin." The same could also be said for education, occupation, good manners, and good social connections. Marvin Harris (1956) provided some important insights into this aspect of the race-class interrelationship in his study of a small mountain town in the interior of Bahia. The gross association between color and class was incorporated into the daily language of the towns-people who referred interchangeably to "the whites" or "the rich" (*brancos-ricos*) and "the Negroes" or "the poor" (*prêtos-pobres*). However, the elite and the lowest or marginal classes were easily distinguishable on the basis of economic, educational, and occupa-tional criteria. It was within the middle class, as it was divided into upper and lower strata, that the decisive factor was likely to be color, with the darkest individuals at the bottom. As Harris noted, the general principle involved is the stable and tenacious belief that some people are better than others and that the best deserve and get the best. Thus, the more Negroes that money actually does "whiten," the more money is required for the whit-ening to take place, and the more important color itself becomes as a criterion for admission to social participation. "Among the townspeople, the superiority of the white man over the Negro is generally considered to be a scientific fact" (p. 114), a viewpoint stated in one of the school textbooks and shared by the teachers, all of whom are white females. A series of photographs of indi-viduals of differing racial types produced consistent results among the townspeople when they were asked to rate the pictures ac-cording to intelligence, beauty, wealth, religious devotion, and honesty; blacks were rated at the low extreme, mulattoes in an intermediate position, and whites at the top of the scale. While the Negro respondent tries to ". . . cling to his dignity and attain worthiness . . . everybody believes it is better to be white" (p. 115). Stories about the Negro's inferiority, unattractiveness, un-trustworthiness, and innately subservient character were wide-spread, although commonly repeated in a semihumorous rather than a bitter vein. The stories heard by Harris in Bahia have their counterparts in folklore and derogatory sayings throughout

the country. Even teachers' college students in São Paulo studied
by Bastide and Van den Berghe (1959) accepted the majority of
anti-Negro stereotypes as they appeared on a checklist.

It is still difficult for black-skinned people to be admitted to
some of Rio's best hotels and to certain small-town restaurants
and hotels, but rather than being bluntly turned away they are
given excuses about the unavailability of space. A friend, living in
an upper-class apartment building in Leblon, told me in the summer of 1968 that his doorman came to him expecting congratula-
tions because he had turned away a Negro—obviously with the
requisite financial capability—who was inquiring about an empty
apartment in the building. The doorman told him that the apartment had been rented. In that same summer, a young
dark-skinned friend from the Northeast, an artist already gaining
a local reputation, politely declined an invitation to accompany
me to dinner in a leading Rio club, saying that because he was
my guest he might be admitted, but that it was sure to be an
uncomfortable situation.

These personal anecdotes and observations support the Fernandes data accumulated several years earlier, as well as Van den
Berghe's (1967) contention that "an appreciable amount of dis-
tinctly racial prejudice and discrimination exists in modern Brazil" (p. 60). He believes that prejudice is inherent in the Brazilian
system of race relations which has moved away from the paternalistic type developed on the plantations toward an essentially
competitive model. The face-to-face global relationships of the
plantation are gradually being replaced by impersonal segmental
contacts in large cities; such social distance mechanisms as etiquette are being replaced by de facto residential segregation. He
buttresses his argument by references to his own work with Bastide and the observations of Wagley and others. In the southern
cities, for example, whites consider the "new" generation of
Negroes, in contrast to the "old," "arrogant, aggressive, immoral,
sexually perverse, physically unattractive, and superstitious. . . .
Mulattoes, who have been socially more mobile than Negroes are
held to be pretentious, arrogant, unreliable, boastful, 'cheeky,'
jealous of the whites and social climbers" (p. 72). Interracial con-
cubinage is less and less common, and intermarriage between
people of markedly differing color and physiognomy is very rare

and socially disapproved. Willems (1949) and Pierson (1942) reported extensive racial segregation in São Paulo City and State, although this was at least in part due to socioeconomic factors.

The literature on Brazil as a whole, and informal participant-observation of the life of Rio de Janeiro, present some seeming paradoxes as to the social role, sense of identity, and burden of prejudice borne by brown-and black-skinned Cariocas. Some of these may be illuminated by reference to the one unambiguous feature of the race-class situation alluded to above: the direct relationship for the masses of people between dark skin color, low economic status, and separation from the sources of societal power. All published comparisons, based largely on data from the Instituto Brasileiro de Geographia Estatistica (1967), agree on this point. In the late 1960's black Brazilians were in the main illiterate or only partly literate and scarcely represented in the school system after the beginning elementary years; they were to an overwhelming degree employees of the least skilled variety; they were only rarely supervisors and even more rarely employers; they were almost totally unrepresented in the government, in the officer class of the armed services, and with a handful of exceptions, in the professional classes of the country. The majority of them lived in substandard housing. It seems fair to infer on the basis of data from the neighborhoods and cities in which they live that their life expectancy is shorter and their morbidity from malnutrition and disease higher than that of brown or white Brazilians. There is no reason to expect significant changes in the 1970's.

The browns are closer the the blacks than the whites, but nonetheless occupy an intermediate socioeconomic position. (Since no patients in this project were so classified, we will not be concerned with the relatively small group of "yellows"—namely Japanese—noted in census data, or with Brazilian Indians who do not receive separate listing in the census, but are classified as *pardo,* or brown.) This is the uncompromising context in which our psychiatric data concerning black and brown patients must be viewed. It is one of *economic, educational,* and *health deprivation.* It is a context in which the presence of superficial good will and interracial friendliness is negated by overwhelming structural obstacles to upward social mobility for the darkest-skinned and lowest-class citizens. These are facts which must be considered in any social, psychological, or political comparison between Negroes in Brazil and in the United States.

THE SAMPLE

The patient sample in terms of color is representative of the Guanabara population as a whole. Sixty-four per cent of the patients were described as white, 24 per cent as brown, and 12 per cent as black. These figures compare with 1960 census data for Guanabara of 70 per cent white, 18 per cent brown[1] and 12 per cent black. These latter are virtually identical with those recorded for 1950. The color distribution for the Guanabara *favela* population, however, according to the 1960 census, shows a much heavier weighting of browns and blacks: 39 per cent white, 34 per cent brown, 27 per cent black. Thus, our sample is considerably lighter-skinned than the *favela* population in general. (There is no significant difference between the *favela* and general population according to sex.)

The interviewers were asked to record facial characteristics as well as skin color. Of the patients described as white, one per cent (two individuals) were regarded as having mixed Caucasoid and Indian features. Of those called brown, 17 per cent were described by the interviewers as having Caucasoid features, seven per cent Negroid features, seven per cent mixed Negroid and Indian features, three per cent Caucasoid-Indian, and two per cent Indian. The remaining 64 per cent were listed as having mixed Caucasoid-Negro features. For this group of "browns" there was evidently some ambiguity of definition in the eyes of the interviewer. The Negro group, like the white, was unequivocal. One individual was described as having mixed Negro-Indian features. About the others there was no question of racial mixture.

SOCIAL CHARACTERISTICS

Brief case reports in the other chapters deal mainly with white

[1] Official data for brown, *pardos,* include all those describing themselves as Indian and estimated by census takers as brown. The criterion is skin color, not a concept of race. Many observers feel that most data are overweighted on the side of "white" because of interviewers' reluctance to classify educated or well-off people as dark.

and brown patients. The following examples, chosen at random, illustrate some of the similarities and differences between the black male patients in this series.

A 36-year-old stevedore, formerly a "rice peeler," with only one year's schooling but literate, was brought to Casa Eiras by his 33-year-old wife of 15 years. He was born and reared on a *fazenda* near Itaperuna in Rio State, and has one dead and three living siblings. When he was 11 his mother abandoned the family because she was mistreated by her husband, a farm laborer, who, since he "wore a black mantle and was very bad," was considered a "witch." At that point the family broke up and the children were reared by a series of friends and relatives also residing on the *fazenda*. At 21 he married a fellow agricultural worker (in a civil ceremony) and they migrated to Sao Paulo City. After five months they had been unable to find work and did not like the climate so they came back to Greater Rio, not too far from their point of origin. Now they and their four children live in a house with one sleeping room and a kitchen, but neither electricity nor water, in a rural area near the border of Guanabara and Rio State. They use a kerosene lamp and a nearby well, and excrete in the woods. It requires almost two hours for the patient to get from home to his job at the port. The family has some relatives in the city whom they occasionally visit. The patient says he has intimate friends, but that they are all white, since he does not consider himself a Negro. His wife says also that he "dislikes Negroes," adding that his friends are really "counterfeit friends who envy him." He has no formal religious affiliation and, according to his wife, "jeers at priests because they wear skirts." In the past year he has been drinking more and more beer, and now two bottles are enough to get him drunk. He has become increasingly quarrelsome. Recently he had a disagreement with a neighbor, who he says called him a "fairy" and "tried to steal a halfmeter" of his land. He has been fighting with his cronies and on the street, apparently while drinking, although he has not always been obviously drunk. Because of these behaviors he has been arrested twice. He has no diversions aside from listening to a transistor radio and occasionally "looking at the sport paper." His wife regards his behavior as the result of his being "possessed by the devil because a 'macumba' has been cast on him." Nevertheless, she believes that hospitalization is necessary "to see whether the doctors find out something in his head or whether it is only 'macumba'." The wife has had three years of school but speaks in a semi-literate manner. She says that she is nervous, complains of sharp and sudden pains in the neck, the "feeling of being hanged," tingling sensations in her fingertips, and is so chronically tired that a few months ago she gave up taking in washing. She is a member of an Umbanda center, but her husband does not allow her to attend regularly, saying that she "goes to 'macumba' to look for men."

A depressed 41-year-old unskilled stone worker in the gardens surrounding a local factory came to Casa Eiras accompanied by his 17-year-old son. His 36-year-old wife of 18 years (civil ceremony) and his children were interviewed during a home visit. The patient was born on a *fazenda* in Barra do Pirai in Rio State. Although he has had no schooling, he is literate and reads newspapers and listens to the radio. He ran away to Rio, unaccompanied, at age 14, because his father, a mule-driver, mistreated him, and he has been self-supporting ever since. He had no relatives in the city, so he moved away after a few years and has lived in several semirural areas of Rio State, including Campos, where he met his wife. They moved back to the city, in the *favela* of Parque União in the peripheral urban zone of Bonsucesso, four years ago and hence are listed as recently migrant rather than settled. He lives in a *barraco* still under construction, which he is gradually turning into a "house." So far, his *barraco* has two rooms and a kitchen but neither water nor electricity. The patient, his wife and eight-month-old baby sleep in one room, while their other eight children share the other. Much of the patient's life has been organized around his Protestantism, and he has been a member, *crente*, of the Assembléia de Deus since age 16. (Both parents were Catholic.) He attended services at least weekly and frequently went to other meetings at the church until his present illness. He gave to the fund for the poor, and, as a teetotaler with no other outside activity, was "beloved" by his neighbors as an exemplary character in the *favela*. His family now regard him as mentally ill and in need of hospitalization. His wife, unschooled and illiterate, complains of feeling nervous, and "shaking inside with tremors" in her body. Her time is fully occupied with the care of her family, but three years ago she joined her husband's church, abandoning her lifelong Catholicism, and since then has attended services.

A 31-year-old clerk for the suburban railroad line, a fourth grade graduate, was brought to Casa Eiras by his 28-year-old brown wife (civil ceremony) of eight years. He was one of eight children born in the central urban section of Rio City. His father was very bad-tempered and beat the children severely, so it was a relief when he deserted the family when the patient was 15. At present, the patient and his wife and two children live in a house with essential services in a semirural neighborhood in Nilopolis in Rio State. They had owned a radio and television set, but these were sold a few months earlier to pay for gambling debts. In the past two years he has become a compulsive card player and has lost considerable amounts of money. Although he is a Catholic he has also, according to his wife, become "obsessive about macumba." He has always been outgoing and cheerful, a movie-goer and member of an *escolha da samba*, but these traits have become much more marked and mixed with aggressiveness and assertiveness. He has become hostile to mulattoes, speaks of his wish to move to the United States because "things are better for poor people there," and has incurred his wife's resentment by exhibiting his mistress with whom he has had two children. On one recent occasion he was placed in jail for "defending" his brother; admission was precipitated by his striking his daughter for fancied misbehavior, an act totally out of character for him in the past. He drinks more than he used to, but alcoholism is not considered a problem. The patient still has occasional contact with his father, now 57, a factory machinist who lends money on the side. His father, a Catholic, regularly attends macumba sessions. His mother is a domestic worker who lives separately. She is 47 and a heavy drinker who is often irritable, nervous, and profane. She too is a Catholic and attends an Umbanda center as a regular devotee but not a member. The patient's siblings are described by his wife as irritable and "ready to attack over trifles." She herself, a fourth grade graduate, is a full-time housewife. Her daughters are aged two and five, and the oldest is markedly aggressive toward her playmates and screams and cries when her mother does not give her what she wants.

A 46-year-old unschooled, illiterate, skilled railroad construction worker, born in rural Duas Barras in Rio State, had been responsible for himself since the death of his mother when he was 10. For several years he lived in Nova Friburgo while the railroad line was being built there and four months before admission to Casa Eiras was transferred to Rio. He now occupies an old house owned by the railroad workers' union in the industrial zone, 10 minutes from the city center. In addition to himself there live in two rooms and a kitchen, his common-law wife, *amigada,* their four children, and two children she had had with a former mate. The patient has no other relatives in the city aside from a 21-year-old son in the army (by a former mate now dead) and a brother-in-law with whom he is not close. He is socially isolated, his sole recreation being the *futebol* matches which he attends alone every week. He has always been a moderately heavy drinker and since coming to Rio has increased his intake to "half a bottle of *cachaça*" a day. His increased aggressiveness, culminating in physical assaults against his immediate family, is attributed by them to mental illness caused by alcoholism. An indifferent Catholic, he admits to no macumba or umbanda participation but has made at least two visits to the house of a *rezadeiro,* a fortune teller or sorcerer.

A 34-year-old unschooled, partly literate, unskilled factory worker was born in suburban Campo Grande where he still lives with his 30-year-old brown wife (civil ceremony) of 15 years and their two daughters in a house with electricity and water. His parents separated when he was two years old, and he was reared by his paternal grandparents who, he said, treated him with great kindness. He was self-supporting after age 14. He leads a life or relative social isolation in spite of several older brothers and sisters in the same area, and attends no amusements. He has always been a moderately heavy drinker, and his wife who accompanied him to the Casa Eiras said that his drinking had increased in recent months. She doesn't know how to explain his progressive withdrawal and bizarre behavior, but believes that drinking may have something to do with it. One sister has been hospitalized and was given electroshock treatments. Several members of his family have had "alcoholic problems."

A 38-year-old railroad mechanic with two years of school,

was accompanied to the Casa Eiras by his 25-year-old wife (civil ceremony) of five years (they had lived together for a year prior to marriage). He had been born and reared by his mother—never knowing the identity of his father—on a *fazenda* in Rio State. He became self-supporting at 18, and at 25 migrated alone, looking for work, to Sao Joao de Meriti which is in Rio State and within Greater Rio de Janeiro. With his wife and four children, he occupies a house without electricity or water, in a rural area. During the past two years he has been drinking heavily and was twice arrested for shooting a gun into the air. He has become hostile to his neighbors and accused one of "having his eye on" his wife. In spite of increasing suspiciousness and aggressiveness, he has continued to have a few intimate friends whom his wife considers bad influences. Hospitalization was precipitated when he began to threaten members of his family. His wife considers him mentally ill because of too much drinking. She herself has become very nervous and easily upset since his personality began to change.

A 45-year-old foreman of railroad line workers with two years of schooling, was accompanied to Casa Eiras by his nephew and his oldest son, age 18. One of seven children, he was born in a small town in Minas Gerais and reared by both parents (his father was a partly literate agricultural laborer and *biscateiro*) until he went to work for the railroad at the age of 18. At 27 he was married to a worker in a textile factory with both civil and religious ceremonies. She has not worked outside the home since marriage and now at age 41, is described as "very authoritarian." Two years later he was transferred by the railroad to Rio de Janeiro. For the past 13 years they have lived in a house with essential services and several rooms in Pavuna in suburban Anchiete. His family includes, besides his wife and son, a daughter aged 15 and his mother-in-law. About four years ago they acquired a television set. The patient is characterized by the informants as a *farista,* someone who likes to drink and make merry. He has always been a moderately heavy, regular drinker although somewhat less so since suffering an accident two years earlier. Nonetheless, drinking may have contributed to a worsening of his economic position in the past year. He himself feels that he has been unjustly deprived of well-deserved salary raises. When he was 25, he was arrested for having "deflowered" a minor, possibly under the influence of alcohol. An indifferent Catholic, he has frequently visited a *terreiro de Umbanda* during the past 18 months. In recent months he has been increasingly irritable, prone to insomnia, preoccupied, argumentative, and physically assaultive. His family and friends have found him "insupportable." They decided to seek psychiatric advice after he twice tried to attack his daughter; she is described as "nervous because of her father's constant threats to beat her." The family considers his behavior "strange" but not reflecting a mental illness: "He is nervous because of too much drinking, he is not crazy." They want him kept in the hospital "long enough so that he will become good again." His mother, unschooled and illiterate, still lives at age 70 in Minas Gerais. She has never worked regularly, is described as "very calm" and, as a devoted Catholic, attending mass several times weekly. One brother has been a patient in Casa Eiras and another died of "acute alcoholism."

DEMOGRAPHIC CHARACTERISTICS

As noted earlier, the color distribution of the sample was 64 per cent white, 24 per cent brown, and 12 per cent black. The age distribution for the three color groups was comparable. The only differences were proportionately fewer (though not statistically significant) blacks in the lower age range between 15 and 25 years: brown 39 per cent; white 36 per cent; black 28 per cent.

Seventy-eight per cent of the blacks were male, in contrast to 65 per cent of the whites and 60 per cent of the browns. This masculine weighting may contribute to the proportionately more frequent occurrence of physically assaultive and drinking behavior among the blacks. While blacks are clearly most different from whites in SES, major psychiatric differences according to color do not involve blacks. Major psychiatric differences do occur between browns and whites, who are not significantly different in their sexual representation in this sample.

RESIDENTIAL STABILITY

As shown in Table 47, differences in respect to housing stability and recent mobility according to color are not statistically significant. (This was true although the majority of those coming from out of town expressly for treatment were white.) More browns than whites or blacks, however, had been born outside of Greater Rio de Janeiro and were classed as migrant.

MARITAL STATUS

A major indicator of conventional participation in a society is marriage, or the maintenance of a consistent relationship with a mate. As indicated in Table 48, slightly less than half the whites had had both civil and religious marriage ceremonies, almost double the number for browns and blacks; while the blacks in particular had had marriages with civil ceremonies alone. Omission of the religious ceremony, as indicated in Chapter IX, often suggests a reduction of the traditional premium on virginity. A total of 64 per cent of whites, 54 per cent of blacks and 46 per cent of browns reported legal marriages, the majority of which among the whites and roughly half among the nonwhites were given additional status by the church. These figures suggest not only that more whites have the economic means and values to conform to cultural ideals, but that the browns rather than the blacks are the least stable in this respect. The difference is due mainly to the larger number of browns reporting that they had had no consistent mate. As might be expected, a few more of their children had skin colors different from their own.

CHILDHOOD FAMILY STRUCTURE

The marital and parental behavior of adults may often be illuminated by reviewing their own childhood experiences with parent figures. Table 49 suggests that family stability was greatest during the childhood of the whites; more whites than browns or blacks report siblings by both natural parents—an indication that the two parents had lived together for a period of time. Statements that the childhood home was not "broken" follow a similar pattern. Similarly, more blacks than either browns or whites reported early financial independence, and, to a statistically significant degree, early parental death, disappearance, or separation. The significance of differences between browns and blacks in respect to childhood family stability is less clear, however, than those between whites and nonwhites. Comparable numbers in these two categories said that they had been reared by parent figures of both sexes, but more of the browns were reared by individuals who were not relatives, and more were dependent during developmental years on groups or series of people. The total percentages are small but considerably higher than those for whites and blacks. This may have contributed to early problems in learning how to relate securely to others and to the relatively greater marital instability of browns in this sample.

LITERACY, EDUCATION, OCCUPATION, AND MIGRATION

Blacks have low status according to all socioeconomic indicators. Table 50 shows them to be uniformly less educated and less literate than whites. Browns, who tend to occupy an intermediate position, are usually closer to the status of blacks. The educational figures for this sample of patients resemble those for other population samples (which will be discussed in the following chapter).

Table 51 reveals a similar picture for occupation. Blacks and browns predominate in the least skilled, least remunerative class of manual workers and are barely represented (in the person of a few browns) in the top three classes of professionals, proprietors, and large and small administrators. In classes IV and V, which taken together represent about 40 per cent of the total sample, the three color groups are roughly equivalent. The chapter on occupation and industrialization has a detailed discussion of these issues.

Table 52 indicates that there has been little change in these respects between the present and the parental generations. Browns and blacks appear to suffer from blocked upward mobility between and within generations. Literacy figures reveal the same break between white on the one hand and nonwhite on the other for both the fathers and mothers of our patients. Among the fathers, a larger proportion of blacks and a smaller proportion of whites, with browns intermediate, worked at class VI occupations.

More whites and browns than blacks, as revealed in Table 53, regarded their socioeconomic status as better than that of their fathers; more blacks regarded their status as worse. Proportionally fewer blacks also believed their status to have improved, and more to have worsened, during the year preceding hospital admission. These differences fit the general observation made in the United States that for those who are socially visible targets of discrimination, the least educated, and at the bottom of the economic ladder, upward mobility is most difficult. They also suggest that the gradual increase of psychiatric impairment culminating in eventual hospitalization, resulted in maximal economic impairment precluding upward mobility in these socially vulnerable people. That is, the final SES of blacks en route to becoming patients represents a summation of social and psychiatric deficits.

Table 54 shows that proportionately more of the blacks—although the absolute number was small—had moved to the city from plantations, even though, as we have seen, proportionately more brown patients were born outside of Rio de Janeiro. Thus, proportionately more blacks than browns came to the urban environment from a closed, feudal, paternalistic society, hierarchically structured, with little freedom of personal career choice. More nonwhites than whites made the migratory trip alone, the data suggesting that their solitary moves may be more plausibly attributed to social than to individual psychological factors. No comparative data are available regarding *fazenda* origins or solitary moves among nonpatient migrant Rio blacks as a whole.

HOUSING

The blacks had less adequate housing than the browns or whites. As indicated in Table 55, approximately a third of them lived in jerry-built shanties or *barracos* and had neither electricity nor running water in their homes. The majority of black patients lived in *favelas*, which while in urbanized areas were often in outlying suburbs. Proportionately more blacks than browns or whites also lived in rural neighborhoods in Rio State, necessitating long rides by train or bus for jobs in the more central parts of the city.

INFORMATION

With the disadvantages of illiteracy, little education, irregular and low-paying employment, and inadequate and remote housing added to those of color, the likelihood that blacks would be full participants in the information and cultural network of the community seems low. Table 56 bears out this supposition. Nevertheless, the majority of the black patients own transistor radios which, along with other media, make it possible for them to become familiar with the good things of life which they do not have. Approximately a quarter of the whites and browns attend movies at least monthly and these provide a regular though somewhat distorted window for them onto the United States and the world at large.

ORGANIZATIONAL PARTICIPATION

There are no major differences between color groups in regard to regular meeting with or participation in social welfare associations or agencies, trade unions, social or sport clubs, samba schools, attendance at soccer clubs or the beach. Seventeen per cent of the browns, as compared with 10 per cent of the whites and four per cent of blacks report attendance at dances on at least a monthly basis.

RELIGION

The finding that religious groups and the clergy constituted the single source of community contact more often used by blacks than those of differing color was not related to their immigrant status; more blacks than browns or whites were natives of the area. As shown on Table 57, more blacks than whites or browns admitted belonging to or attending Spiritist, Umbanda, or Macumba centers. These Afro-Spiritist groups are more characteristic of urban than rural settings. There are no differences between membership in established Christian churches according to color, and this is true for their apparently perfunctory attendance as well. Membership in religious groups of whatever nature apparently provides an important source of support and increased

self-esteem for these otherwise excluded individuals. (A fuller discussion of this issue is presented in the chapter dealing with religion.)

HOSPITALIZATION AND FAMILY DIAGNOSIS

As indicated in Table 58, most of the whites were seen at the
Casa Eiras, three-quarters of the blacks were seen at Casa Eiras
and none were patients at Botafogo. The group with the largest
percentage seen at Pronto Socorro were browns, suggesting a
population of browns perhaps slightly less consistently employed
than the blacks, in more urgent need of psychiatric attention, and
with less family support. The data on the acuteness of present illness, however, as shown in Table 59, indicate that the blacks constituted the most acute population. In keeping with this, only 28
per cent of the blacks in contrast to 42 per cent of the browns
and 55 per cent of the whites had had previous psychiatric contact, though not previous admissions. In other words, the whites
and browns had apparently demonstrated some capacity to live
outside of hospitals, with assistance despite continuing or intermittent symptoms. It may also be that the more poverty-stricken
and less educated blacks simply did not have the resources or
knowledge to obtain outpatient help. Since more live in poor, less
organized communities with greater tolerance for deviant behavior, the majority who are sick probably never come to psychiatric
attention. Thus, those admitted to the hospital may be considered
to have reached the point of decompensation so severe as to allow
for no alternative to removal from the community. Information
about symptom pictures, described below, suggests that the blacks
were, in fact, more floridly disturbed upon admission than the
others. Another reason for rapid admission may have been that
more had demonstrated physically assaultive behavior (see Table
60); this, in turn, may have reflected the predominantly male status of the blacks. While they more frequently admitted excessive
intake of alcohol (46 per cent as compared to 24 per cent of the
browns and 23 per cent of the whites), no patient in the sample
suffered from acute intoxication, delirium tremens, or chronic
alcoholic psychotic behavior. There was no reason to assume that

rapid hospitalization was owing to lack of family support or understanding because more of the blacks and whites (see Table 61)
than browns were accompanied to the hospital by family members.

About three-quarters of the white and black patients were
brought to the hospital by family members. Table 61 shows that
this was true for fewer browns. Added to the observations that
more browns were brought by family members because they
would not work, and that fewer of their family members knew the
details of their behavior, it seems that members of this group did,
in fact, receive less family support than either the whites or the
blacks. This presumption fits the less stable marital situation of
browns and is further supported by the fact that no black person
came to the hospital alone and in no instance was diagnosed by
his family as exhibiting unacceptable morally "bad" behavior. In
the sense that they were less a target of negative value judgments,
black patients appear to have received more family support than
whites.

Aside from inability to work and assaultiveness, the reasons for
hospitalization varied. Table 62 shows that whites were differentiated from the other two groups on the basis of depressive-
anxious or suicidal statements or acts. For all groups, the statements or acts leading to hospitalization were most frequently
made in the presence of family members.

In summary, hospitalization for all patients was generally
preceded by a build-up of tension in the families who accompanied them to the hospital, but the specific events precipitating
hospitalization varied with color. Acute externalized action in the
form of attacks against people and property activated the families
of blacks; failure to work more often precipitated the admission of
browns; and self-directed anxiety and depression, including suicidal ideas, more commonly preceded hospitalization in the whites.
An apparent low tolerance for inability to work, and possibly less
participation in the hospital admission process, suggest that
browns received less family support than blacks or whites. Blacks
were the least frequently labeled with negative value judgments
by their families.

Psychiatric and Behavioral Characteristics

DEPRESSION

As emphasized by the events leading to hospitalization, indications of depressed mood were relatively prominent among the whites, and often stimulated patients and family members to seek hospitalization. Table 63 however, reveals similar proportions of depressive symptoms in browns as well. Examination of the patients themselves showed that proportionately more browns and whites than blacks complained of sadness, weeping, suicide attempts, mood fluctuations and related feelings or thoughts. (The few statistically significant differences reflect the small number of blacks.) Depressive indicators appear to have been regarded less seriously by the families of browns than whites.

TENSION, ANXIETY, SENSITIVITY, AND FRUSTRATION

Browns, like whites, exhibited evidence of marked tension and anxiety more often and consistently than blacks. As indicated in Table 64, there were more frequent reports for browns than for whites, and usually for blacks, of impaired ability to work, concentrate, relax, or sleep. Thinking and memory problems, more prominent in browns and whites than blacks, are also shown on Table 64. These findings support the assumption that problems in recall, thought precision, decision-making, or freedom of thought also reflect the direct disruptive influence of anxiety or of attempts to deal with it. They are also congruent with the findings in Table 65 which show that environmental concern and angry or inferior feelings were most often reported by browns and least by blacks although no differences in this table are statistically significant. The same distribution is shown for impulsiveness in Table 66, while Table 67 demonstrates a similar distribution of attitudes toward others. Thus, browns were consistently more suspicious, and more often felt misjudged, stared at or talked about, and persecuted, as well as admired than whites, with blacks in intermediate position.

Browns more than whites or blacks, as presented in Table 68, also showed more tension, discomfort, and apparently conflictful dependency in relation to the interviewing psychiatrist. For his part, the psychiatrist described himself as neutral (in contrast to cheerful or sad), not empathetic, apprehensive, or annoyed more frequently in relation to browns. While differences in these respects are generally small and only a few are statistically significant, they are consistent. Members of this group, more than blacks or whites, demonstrated tension interfering with function, evidence of environmental frustration and conflict, suspiciousness, and feelings of harrassment and impulsiveness. More than the others, they elicited negative or uninvolved responses from the interviewers. And in the interview situation, fewer of them were rated as actively cooperative, or respectful.

Aside from these findings, differences in interviewer response according to color reveal institutionalized attitudes which may well influence the doctor-patient relationship. The psychiatrists reported greatest empathy and cheerfulness during interviews with blacks, presumably viewed in terms of a securely hierarchical, nonthreatening, dependent relationship. In sharp contrast, however, suggesting a depreciation of the blacks' complexity and intelligence and a feeling of greatest similarity with their own kind, the psychiatrists regarded the white patients as most interesting, friendly, and likeable.

THE BREAK WITH REALITY

Unlike the browns who were hypersensitive to reality considerations even though verging on the edge of irrational overresponsiveness, the blacks were marked by a higher proportion of behaviors suggesting a clearcut break with reality. This break, as a rule, appeared to reflect successful anxiety-reducing mechanisms, so that, except for insomnia, fewer blacks than browns or whites revealed evidence of anxiety, tension, or depression. Even though proportionately more blacks had committed physical assaults, fewer reported impulsive behavior or angry frustrated feelings, fewer felt badly treated or misjudged. Less anxiety and reality-based tension seemed to be associated with a greater tendency to deny reality and substitute fantasy. Thus, more reported what appeared to be auditory and visual hallucinations and more were disoriented in place and time. The most frequently reported sensory experiences, as noted in Table 69 were hearing voices and seeing people when others were unable to do so. For all the color groups, auditory experiences were the more common. The brown-skinned group were midway between the whites and blacks in the frequency with which they reported experiencing voices and people, seeing lights and color and unidentifiable entities, but at the same time, more browns than blacks reported experiencing unexplained noises which were not voices. This may reflect their tendency to be hypersensitive, suspicious, and to misinterpret. Religious, folkloric, or ghostly human and non-human entities were reported as part of their visual experience by more browns than blacks and by almost none of the whites. Following along this line, the intensity and importance of their apparent hallucinatory experiences are reflected in the pro-portionately higher numbers of blacks and browns who insisted on the reality of their experiences or who planned to act on the basis of them. Spatial and temporal disorientation followed the same pattern, as shown on Table 70. Very few patients, regardless of color group, were disoriented as to person.

SOMATIC PROBLEMS

Another group of complaints predominant among blacks, but not significantly so, concerned bodily sensations. As noted in Table 71, these complaints were not congruent with surface observa-tions of physical conditions. That is, in accordance with their superior economic status, fewer whites seemed poorly nourished or emaciated and more were neat and clean, but the examining psychiatrist thought the browns appeared weaker and unhealthier than the blacks, although the general nutritional status of the two groups seemed similar. The picture regarding psychophysiological complaints was mixed, as noted in Table 72, and no differences were statistically significant.

SEXUAL BEHAVIOR

Sexual activities were mentioned as a source of emotional difficulty least often by blacks and most often by browns, who, as noted earlier, reported consistent relationships with a mate less frequently than did whites or blacks. Thus, as described in Table

73, for browns, sex was more often a source of anxiety, shame, or guilt, and sexual impulses were more often regarded as too strong or too weak. At the same time, proportionally more browns (although a small absolute number) made grandiose claims about their sexual ability. For the whites, more of whom had had a consistent sexual partner, sexual performance was more often impaired by worries, changed by the present illness, or ineffective than it was for browns and blacks.

Deviant sexual behavior was more often reported by whites and browns than by blacks. There was no significant reporting of homosexuality as the leading or preferred pattern, although anal intercourse (with members of the opposite sex, sometimes in association with complaint of impotence in the male) and polymorphous variability were acknowledged without apparent reluctance.

Past Psychiatric History

A relatively small number of the many scheduled items of past history yielded suggestive information and, as shown in Table 74, none of the differences according to color were statistically significant. Previous events were more often regarded as sufficiently meaningful to be reported by whites and browns than by blacks. This apparent lack of available past history for blacks may be associated with their more prominent family instability and earlier independence in childhood.

As indicated in Table 75, more whites, though not significantly so, also reported a history of lapses or alterations in consciousness for all causes except head injury. In the last instance the blacks predominated. While the blacks, more of whom were male and exposed to more hazardous situations, were probably more often subjected to head injury, this cannot be substantiated. It seems equally probable that the whites, culturally more disposed to maintain conscious rational control, are made more anxious by lapses and are hence more prone to report them.

Discussion

The data support the conclusion that in terms of behavior and psychiatric symptoms the browns must be regarded as a psychologically separate group. In regard to some characteristics they may be classed with blacks and in regard to others with whites, but on the basis of many of their ways of thinking, feeling, and acting they appear to represent a distinct population. These characteristics are not corollaries of socioeconomic status as such, inasmuch as browns occupy an intermediate position between whites at the top and blacks at the bottom of the scale. Nor do they necessarily represent greater concrete economic frustration, for the browns' self-estimate of socioeconomic status as compared to their fathers and themselves a year earlier was similar to that of the whites. They seem, rather, to reflect the nature of their relationships with other people, their aspirations, and their place in the social context. Some of their behavioral and personality characteristics are expected concomitants of their less stable marital histories and less consistent relationships with parental figures, features which themselves require illumination. Others resemble people who are marginal in the sense of existing at the peripheries of two overlapping social systems. The concept of marginality with special reference to immigrant and socially visible minority groups has been examined by Goldberg (1941), Green (1947), Golovensky (1952), and Antonovsky (1956). Marginal individuals, as noted by Derbyshire and Brody (1964), may be upwardly mobile with one foot in their culture of origin and the other in the new culture, without a complete sense of belonging to either. For Rio de Janeiro browns, it is more legitimate to postulate a greater sense of being discriminated against as an aspect of their marginality, than it is for the blacks. The feeling of "lack of belongingness," coupled with marked sensitivity to rejection, a sense of isolation, and uncertainty about the motives of others with whom he must deal, are central features of the marginal man's psychology. These elements may also contribute to problems in sustaining a prolonged relationship with a mate, tolerating socially deviant behavior within the family, and recognizing the depth of depressive feelings in family members or friends.

Depressive symptoms, including suicidal ruminations and attempts, which occur with similar frequency in browns and whites are less easy to interpret. There is no reason to believe, in view of the apparently easy discharge of hostile tension, that depression in this group represents a turning of repressed hostile impulses against the self. While guilt is present in some individuals, the differences between color groups are not impressive and there was little evidence of any need for self-punishment. Two reasonable assumptions are that browns share with whites culturally determined needs for individual achievement and recognition which, if not satisfied, result in diminished self-esteem reflected in depressive symptoms, and that, associated with their upward and generally unsuccessful striving, there exists a degree of intrafamilial tension which interferes with sustained interpersonal closeness and warmth. Thus, loneliness and diminished self-esteem associated with unsuccessful status-striving, personal isolation, and lack of familial support are postulated as important for the development of depressive symptoms found to be more prominent in browns and whites than in blacks.

A special aspect of the problem of status-striving in a historically two-class society suffering from the sporadic inflation associated with uneven economic development, is its relative hopelessness. The population of this study is mainly poor. As psychiatric patients, they may be considered temporary dropouts from society and socioeconomic striving. They thus demonstrate in intense form the results of consistently disappointed hope. Striving for increased dignity and independence, they are repeatedly faced with their relative powerlessness. They are tempted to abandon the struggle, especially for a sense of inner dignity, and to accept passivity and dependence as a solution, but they are unable to do so comfortably. One way, then, of looking at the problem of lowered self-esteem and depression is to see it in terms of a chronic conflict between unattainable wishes to be independent, autonomous, and master of one's fate on one hand and unacceptable, dangerous wishes to lapse into absolute passivity with its connotations of worthlessness and (for men) lack of masculinity on the other. Depression, anxiety, sexual concern, and gastrointestinal symptoms are classic reflections of such a conflict.

A more positive and even militant black identity has not yet been regarded as important for Brazil's brown masses. Inevitably, the North American ferment has begun to stir at least journalistic interest in the possible social evolution of black or brown Brazilians as population groups of eventual political significance. This represents a serious deviation from the official policy, which looks to a continuing movement of racial assimilation—"whitening" —along the traditional road to a single, unified, "Brazilianized" population. The very few activities or meetings concerned with the question of a specifically black Brazilian identity, such as Abdias do Nascimento's *Teatro Experimental do Negro*, have been concerned almost exclusively with cultural matters. The expression "black power" has been tentatively used by some journalists, but its application has been difficult. This is partly because Brazilian blacks are too illiterate and economically submerged to form a base for such power, because of the symbolic interpenetration of the concepts of race and socioeconomic class and partly because of popular awareness of browns as a separate group. This is unlike the United States where many "Negro" leaders having lighter skins than many Brazilian mulattoes can be defined as Negro on the basis of origin alone.

Despite popular awareness of brown-skinned people as a group in some ways different from either blacks or whites, and despite the frequently quoted census figures showing that they constitute more than a quarter of the population, they have not been the subject of much specific social or psychological attention. Most authors, while using the differentiating labels, do not deal with them as a single group when discussing social phenomena of psychological interest. This follows the widely used literary phrase, *homem do côr*, or men of color, to categorize all those not regarded on bodily or social grounds as white. In the fall of 1968 a popular illustrated periodical, *O Cruzeiro*, underscored the potential significance of this group in an article entitled, "Mulatto: A White Negro." Here there was distilled a viewpoint, harsh in condensation, but direct and simple: ". . . in Brazil the Negro question has not been directly confronted, there has been a tactical accommodation on both sides in the hope that the skin pigmentation will disappear in time through the force of miscegenation. With the extinction of the Negro, his metamorphosis into mulattoes disguised as whites, the problem will cease to exist. The Negro will be acculturated, assimilated to the degree that he is whitened to the color of coffee with a little milk." The article predicts that when the mulattoes, "masked as whites and repudiating their color," finally overcome the problems of illiteracy and unemployment, the racist battles will not be between blacks and whites but between blacks and mulattoes. The article supplies additional background for an understanding of the browns' developing identity-crisis by referring to the stereotype the dominant whites have developed for this subgrouping, just as they have for the blacks. It is that ". . . of the *mulata* as a promotional object of erotic significance," a stereotype which makes it possible to forget all the virtues of this ". . . great human type by attributing to it purely and exclusively the elements of sexual attraction" (pp. 122–125).

The black patients (predominantly male) appeared less sensitive and suspicious in general, but a proportion equal to the browns felt persecuted by other individuals or groups. This feature was usually viewed by the examining psychiatrist as part of a psychotic syndrome. Perhaps the most striking difference between black patients and the other two groups was their higher frequency of behavior suggesting a clearcut break with reality, associated with lower levels of general anxiety and reality-based tension. They, more than the other two groups, expressed their psychological disturbances in plastic sensory terms and with reference to their outer rather than inner worlds. The loss of capacity to appreciate conventional reality involved in producing these symptoms was also reflected in the proportionally higher incidence among blacks of temporal or spatial disorientation. This finding is identical with that reported by Schleifer, Derbyshire, and Martin (1968) for poor blacks in comparison with whites referred from jail to public hospital in Baltimore because of psychotic disturbances. Possible elements contributing to this tendency include differences in literacy, education, available information, adherence to folk beliefs, available social support, power based on money or prestige, and channels of communication with sources of societal power. The apparently greater predisposition of Brazilian blacks to hallucinatory experiences, delusions of persecution, and disorientation may be plausibly linked to their relative isolation from the complex informational system of the modern world, rather than merely to the elements contributing to psychotic disturbances described just above. Such isolation reduces the likelihood of acquiring rational and achievement values, reflected in the importance given to time, to conscious planning, and to control of oneself and others. To this may be added greater willingness to abandon conscious control or to accept fantasy experience of various kinds as real and important.

The blacks seem to reflect, along with hallucinations and persecutory delusions, a tendency to "externalize" rather than "internalize" as a characteristic means of dealing with conflicts and anxiety. In this instance, the body, especially the head as the site of thinking processes, is a convenient place in which to localize the reason for discomfort or for things going wrong. When the body or an outside agency is established as the source of difficulty, a certain inner security can be maintained.

In view of the blacks real-life position at the bottom of the economic and prestige scale, their relative lack, compared to whites and browns, of anxiety and depression can only reflect the operation of adaptive and defensive mechanisms which protect them from being overwhelmed by anxiety, threatening retaliatory destructive impulses and other drives, and assist in establishing a stable, reciprocal relationship with their environment. Although their relationships with the dominant whites are superficially smoothed by well-institutionalized rules of social interaction, the overall human environment is essentially unfriendly. They are almost totally blocked in any effort to gain adequate housing, education, jobs, or dignity for themselves or their children. This ubiquitous social emasculation, similar to that postulated for black males in the United States, may be less painful and easier to deny and repress for the Brazilians. Their expectations are not yet so stimulated, and the tools for upward mobility are still largely unavailable. The discrepancy between real-life achievement and what can realistically be hoped for is therefore less. The ameliorating factors are few. Popular opinion and such works as *Black Orpheus* suggest that *carnaval* and participation in *escolhas de samba* assume compensatory significance. For our population of disturbed persons, often suffering relative social isolation, whose defensive and adaptive mechanisms are impaired and who must cope with psychiatric decompensation as well as poverty, these do not seem important. The relief provided by self-narcotization through alcohol, and the displacement of repressed anger generated by an oppressive social system toward family members and drinking companions are more significant outlets. These brief, violent eruptions toward their own kind appear as concomitants of passive conformity in relation to upper-class whites. These circumstances, plus the developmental experience more often encountered by blacks of absent or brutal fathers not providing adequate adult male models, make our findings of a comparative absence of sexual symptoms among black patients, as compared with browns and whites, surprising. Sex remains useful, in spite of the conflicts around masculine status, as a source of pleasure and human relatedness. Whether this reflects a greater functional development of one of the few sources of available satisfaction or a relative lack of guilt and conflict secondary to the failure to acquire certain middle-class standards while growing up is uncertain.

One other related possibility may also permit the black more sexual pleasure and protect him against the depressive feelings which were exhibited in almost equal measure by the whites and browns. This concerns his relative freedom from feelings of guilt, inadequacy, and fantasies or attempts at suicide. History and current circumstances conspire to keep the Brazilian black in Rio de Janeiro from significant self-determination. The "dependent child" aspects of the black's position in the social structure is fraught with speculation. Rather than himself becoming responsible for his own future and life course, his utter powerlessness forces his continued dependence upon luck, upon the unpredictable assistance of friends or strangers, and most importantly, upon the good will of the paternalistic whites, in whatever guise it appears. Basically he is not responsible for what happens to him or his family. Similarly, he is relatively less plagued by whatever superstructure of responsibilities burdens the sexual life of others. From this point of view, the symptom-producing conflicts between wishes to be independent on the one hand and dependent and subordinate on the other are not yet part of the psychosocial evolution of the Brazilian black man.

The salient characteristics of the white patients, just as with the white population of Guanabara as a whole, were socioeconomic. They were more privileged and more a part of the community than the blacks and browns in every respect. And yet, perhaps the leading comparative impression of the white patients was one of sadness and conflict which extended to their families. Thus, more of the white as well as the brown families expressed negative value judgments about their patient members. These findings support those of Hollingshead and Redlich (1958) in studies of psychiatric patients by social class. The possibility arises that the confluence of a number of cultural factors among whites increases their resistance to clear abandonment of reality testing even when inner states and observable behavior result in hospitalization. This may, however reflect less tolerance to disturbed behavior among the whites as well as easier access to psychiatric facilities, resulting in the admission of a less dramatically sick sample of the population.

One area in which whites exhibited more problems was that of sexual activity. Sexual functioning appeared to be more vulnerable to tension and anxiety than in the other groups, and the whites were more prone to describe it in terms of illness related to the psychiatric disturbance. The report of anal intercourse by more whites was associated with more frequent reports of impaired sexual functioning, particularly impotence. This suggests that anal intercourse was often a more effective sexual stimulator than vaginal intercourse, although there are some anecdotal suggestions that it may occasionally be used to avoid pregnancy.

The data reported from the Rio de Janeiro and Baltimore studies do not lend themselves to exact comparison. Nonetheless, it cannot be overemphasized that a major finding is the presence of symptoms of marginality in people of brown but not of black skin, a finding that has not been reported in the United States. This may be a consequence of the automatic social lumping together in the United States of people of all shades and color as "Negro" or "black." This total group as a whole exhibited indications of self-hatred and identity uncertainty in past years and now shows, with increasing frequency, the kind of tension and sensitivity which we have observed in Brazilian browns. Many observers see this as a result of the rapidly increasing upward social mobility of American blacks, in contrast to the still static economic depression and lack of social power of those in Brazil. In Brazil, the actual shade of mulattoes as a specific skin color appears to have sufficient psychosocial meaning to permit the differentiation of groups on the threshold of upward mobility with—at least among those becoming mental patients—a set of psychological sensitivities not yet apparent in the blacks.

CHAPTER 6

EDUCATION, LITERACY
AND PATIENT BEHAVIOR

THE BRAZILIAN elite are proud of their scholastic attainments, which they and the middle class that identifies with them seem to have achieved while perched on the shoulders of an uneducated, barely literate mass. Decades of efforts to establish general primary education notwithstanding, the proportion of literates has not outstripped continuing increases in population. To be illiterate is a major influence on individual development and behavior; to be illiterate means to be excluded from full participation in the cultural-informational network; to be illiterate in Brazil means political disenfranchisement, for only those who can read and write are permitted to vote. With rare exceptions, to have less than a primary education means exclusion from jobs in government or other bureaucracies which provide a toe hold on any career-ascension ladder. Literacy without formal education can produce serious frustrations in the form of increased expectations with no means of fulfillment; illiteracy produces its own kind of frustration through the stimulation of radio and television and the sights and sounds of the metropolis. Illiteracy and lack of primary school education in Rio de Janeiro are often part of a constellation of factors—rural origin, dark skin color, poverty—which contribute to the behavior observed in mental hospital patients.

A large United States literature suggests that children from "culturally deprived" or "disadvantaged" homes have impaired abilities to learn, to grasp concepts, and to pay attention to school work. That such studies have not been carried out in Brazil

173

reflects the social context of a country in development. The subtle impairments of children from literate though culturally bleak homes stand in sharp relief against the broadly inclusive school system and technical, automated society of the United States; the grosser deficiencies of children from illiterate, abysmally poor Brazilian families are not so clearly limned against the uneven educational background and the rural or hand service-dominated milieu in which most of them live.

As new industries develop, manpower needs draw rural migrants into the cities, and the factory becomes the newest arena in which inadequate performance and learning show themselves. While the country-man in the city provides a mixed source of amusement and despair for managers and foremen in the new plants, it remains to be seen whether the migrants' difficulties reflect fundamental problems dating from lack of childhood stimulation or whether they reflect transitory problems of adaptation (Brandão Lopes, 1967). Illiteracy and lack of education might be expected to influence the likelihood of Rio de Janeiro residents' becoming psychiatrically labeled. The impact of a culturally impoverished childhood, of exclusion and frustration in an already mobility-blocked social system, may force the acquisition of defensive and adaptive techniques or reinforce the passivity of those for whom there are no adaptive or defensive alternatives. This chapter will be concerned with the nature of the educational experience through which the study patients have been processed, its place in the social context of behavior (how it contributes to behavioral setting), and the social and behavioral characteristics of patients who have such experience and who are literate as compared with those who are uneducated and illiterate.

EDUCATION IN BRAZIL

THE PRIMARY YEARS

Formal education for the Brazilian begins officially at age seven. Nationwide data from the *Censo Escolar* (1968), however, show that taking all schools, rural and urban, into account, the maximum educational coverage does not occur until age 11, immediately after which attrition begins to leave its mark. (Forty-seven per cent of the seven-year-olds and 66 per cent of the eight-year-olds are enrolled in primary school. Increments are gradual up to 75 per cent at age 11, and then the proportions fall to 61 per cent at age 14.) Everyone is guaranteed four years of primary education. Many schools have added a fifth year, the *admissão,* to help students prepare for examinations which must be passed in order to enter secondary level. Under a law passed at the end of 1961, the primary school was extended to six years with the expectation that the first year of the secondary level, *ginásio,* would eventually be eliminated; so far, the fifth and sixth grades are available in only a few major cities. Educational opportunities vary widely according to region and to whether the child lives in an urban or rural area. Primary as well as advanced educational facilities and other business and cultural resources are most heavily concentrated in the "golden triangle" described in Chapter I. The four states, parts of which are included in the "triangle," Guanabara, Minas Gerais, Rio Grande do Sul, and São Paulo, account for between 50 and 60 per cent of the primary school population, a somewhat larger percentage of the secondary school enrollments, and about two-thirds of the university students. These numbers come almost exclusively from the big cities.

Two or three shifts of students daily are the rule in most primary schools. Shortages of schools and teachers are ubiquitous. Rio de Janeiro city, with one of the heaviest concentrations of educational facilities in the nation, is no exception.

Teachers often travel to several districts. They are harried and fatigued, pressed not only by awareness of educational needs but also, as are most other professionals, by the absolute necessity for several sources of income in order to meet the demands of continuing inflation. Because children are not bound to the primary school in the district in which they live, educated parents may engage in an anxious search for schools which are least crowded, have the smallest proportion of children from poor families, or the best teachers and facilities. It is never possible to find a fully satisfactory compromise as the following, somewhat extreme, example may show. The parents of a 10-year-old girl, living in the Catéte district not far from downtown Rio de Janeiro city, embarked on an extended, diligent exploration of possible primary schools for their daughter. Husband and wife have had some university experience, and the husband is a moderately successful businessman. Finally, at the urging of the child's maternal grandmother, they agreed on the public primary school on Rua Belford Roxo in Copacabana where the grandmother lives. This is considered an acceptable outcome even though the youngster must rise before daylight in order to make the early shift of classes and must change buses in the process of getting to school. The family is probably correct in considering itself fortunate to have completed registration early; despite the law guaranteeing universal primary education, such registration is often not easy to achieve. The school is pleasantly located on a cul-de-sac and its play yard is overshadowed by the steep cliffside of a *morro*. The students include children of lawyers, businessmen, and doctors as well as children who live in the hilltop shacks, which from below appear agglutinated to crevices or plateaus on the high rock. Some of the young *favelados* make the white female teachers anxious and present a problem in communication. Their parents seldom appear at meetings or appointments with the teachers who, in the face of their own frustration, conscientiously try to carry on. Unlike some slum children in the United States, students from the *morro* are not notably aggressive nor do they pose serious disciplinary problems. Indeed, they seem lost or unable to understand what is going on; they are pleasant, quiet, and a little embarrassed. Their usually uneducated parents are unable to help or to motivate them. Crowding and lack of privacy at home make it difficult to study or even to think but some of their problems simply lie in the lack of connection between the worlds of school and home. Their mothers and fathers (and they do not all have fathers at home) are working, and there is no one to look after them. Nonetheless, most manage to arrive reasonably well clothed and clean, and a certain proportion of *favela* parents are not only literate but ambitious for their children and place high value on available education.

While the traditional rigidity of the educational system has been subject to scrutiny especially since the early nineteensixties—the development of psychological services beginning in 1965 reflects this—the system is based on the classical European tradition of pedagogy and content-learning. This poses formidable obstacles for the first and second graders which, together with the lack of family help, result in a high rate of attrition. The first two or three years particularly, become clogged with repeaters; after a series of failures interest is lost and family pressures for the child's economic contribution mount rapidly. This situation is reflected in data summarized by Wagley (1963) from several sources. In 1960, 53 per cent of elementary school children throughout Brazil were attending the first grade, 21 per cent the second grade, 15 per cent the third grade, and only nine per cent the fourth and fifth grades combined. Anisio Teixeira estimated in 1957 that less than 10 per cent of Brazilian children complete the four primary school years. As Wagley stated, "It is quite clear that the elementary school system acts as a filter, making it impossible for the majority of the Brazilians to have the necessary qualifications for secondary education in any form" (p. 214).

In the city of Rio de Janeiro, where there are more facilities and greater pressures from families and authorities to attend school, the dropout proportion is somewhat lower than for the country as a whole. The nature of the problem, however, is similar, as demonstrated by the 1966 Guanabara primary school population figures: first grade, 30 per cent; second and third grades, 16 per cent; fourth grade, 15 per cent; fifth grade, 12 per cent; and sixth grade, six per cent. This situation may be compared with that of the Baltimore "inner city" which includes a predominantly Negro working-class population. Here the pattern is determined by strictly enforced laws requiring school attendance until age 16. In consequence, there are few dropouts during the primary years except for sick or retarded children who may be transferred elsewhere. Nonetheless, failures inevitably occur, especially among children whose families share the socioeconomic characteristics of Rio *favela* dwellers. Some such inner city children may be transferred to special schools. Others, however, who may be regarded as intellectually borderline, receive "social promotions" so that they do not fall too far behind their age groups. Capable of absorbing less and less, they leave the school whatever their grade level at age sixteen. The largest drop in Baltimore school registrants occurs between the ninth and tenth grades, and most of those who do not pass on to the tenth grade are 16 years old. Those who do make it are usually able to graduate, and there is great social pressure to do so; high school graduation in the

United States appears to have the social significance of primary
school completion in Brazil.

THE SECONDARY YEARS

The standard progression through secondary school includes
four years of *ginásio,* followed by three years of *colégio.* The *colégio*
level student may choose either a classical curriculum emphasizing ancient and modern languages and the humanities or, if he is
aiming for one of the scientific professions, one which offers a
more technical and mathematical preparation. Neither curriculum will act to constrain his university career should he progress
to that level. While every Brazilian state has at least one publicly
supported school in each of the secondary categories, about
two-thirds of the *ginásios* and more of the *colégios* are private. This
means that direct ability to pay, as well as the various social class
factors associated with financial status will determine who makes
the leap from the primary to the secondary level. After primary
school, lack of money for suitable clothing, books, equipment, and
transportation becomes significant. Most important, poor families
cannot afford the loss of income from a child who is in school and
not working.

In general, secondary, and primary school attendance across
the country is closely linked to degree of urbanization. Table 76
shows, however, that even in the almost completely urbanized
city-state of Guanabara, less than 30 per cent of youth of appropriate age are enrolled in secondary schools. This appears to
be due to a combination of financial and other class related factors; the percentage of manual workers' children so enrolled is no
higher in the capital cities of the rich southern states of São Paulo
and Rio Grande do Sul than in the poorer states of the North
and Northeast. Migration may also be a factor in this; the more
than doubling of São Paulo city's population between 1940 and
1960 followed to a considerable degree the arrival of unskilled
workers from small towns and rural areas in Bahia and the
Northeast. Their children had almost no chance for secondary
education, and most did not complete primary school. According
to Gouveia (1957), less than 20 per cent of the students in academic secondary courses in Sao Paulo came from working-class

homes. Some of these students attended normal schools—for elementary teachers' training—which are often free and offer good quality instruction. But the normal schools are attended mainly by middle-class girls, and the few available openings are sought by an overwhelming number of applicants. A larger proportion of working-class children was found in evening courses, primarily commercial and industrial, but here again their parents usually held skilled and supervisory jobs. The variability of admission examinations provides another element which militates against the education of the poor and the young who live in the cities. The tradition-oriented rigid examination requirements regularly result in a high proportion of failures throughout the country. In the capital city of São Paulo, for example, Gouveia reported a failure rate of 71 per cent for the public basic secondary courses as compared to a rate in the same year of 58 per cent in an "interior" city. This meant vacancies in the capital schools while the rejected applicants from poor families had nowhere to go. Private schools with inferior levels of teaching had admission examination failure rates of only 25 per cent. Financially capable students could attend these or even go inland in order to obtain the high school education necessary for university admission. Reviewing these data Gouveia (1957) makes a strong case for the proposition that " . . . educational facilities . . . perpetuate class related inequities . . . ." and that this poses a special problem when technological developments reinforce the relationship between salary levels and educational requirements (pp. 81–95).

Another insight into the social filtering process leading to secondary school enrollment is provided by a representative sample of *ginásio* and *colégio* students studied in Pôrto Alegre by Cunha and others as part of the present study. Their sample included 802 persons or two per cent of the secondary school population of that city, capital of one of the richest, most modern and highly developed Brazilian states. Almost none of these students were non-whites (two per cent were brown and one per cent black); almost none was employed even on a part-time basis; all had homes with electricity; only one per cent were without running water; and most lived in urban residential neighborhoods. They came from stable families. Of the 13 per cent of the families described as "broken," two-thirds were due to death and a third to *desquite* (the functional equivalent of divorce). The fathers were better educated than most Brazilian groups, with 30 per cent having had some university work. As an indication of the rapid rate of recent changes, however, 30 per cent of these predominantly middle-class fathers in a advanced region of the country had not progressed beyond the primary school level. These data support Gouveia's conclusion that the increasing availability of high school level education has not made an important impact on the children of working-class parents. The most apparent result seems to be increased educational experience for the children of the growing, but still relatively small, middle-class or bourgeois group. And even those with reasonable family and economic support appear to have difficulty in progressing through the system. While 24 per cent of the Pôrto Alegre students were in the first year of *ginásio*, only 12 per cent were present in the last year, and this was reduced to seven per cent by the last year of *colégio*. The high value placed on classical academic education is reflected in the fact that despite the considerable number of dropouts about 76 per cent of the group were taking courses necessary for university admission.

Alternatives to the academic secondary sequence, such as agricultural and industrial training, attract minimal numbers of students; for those oriented to educational achievement the goal remains traditional and manual work is still regarded as demeaning. Aside from normal school, the commercial course is a most popular alternative. Conducted by private organizations, these courses are usually of uneven quality. As Wagley (1963) points out, schools which prepare the student for much desired white-collar occupations and offer an escape from manual work are important agencies of social mobility.

The nature of movement through the school system up to the university level is illustrated by 1960 Guanabara census data (first published in 1968). The census lists a total of 1,600,200 persons over age nine according to educational achievement, beginning with completion of the primary level. Of this group of primary school graduates, 69 per cent had no further formal education. Percentages for other groups according to level completed are as follows: *Ginásial,* 17; *colégial,* 5; *normal ou pedagogice,* 1.7; *comercial,* 1.6. The remainder were divided between a variety of high school specialized training courses and university programs. The number of respondents who had not attended school at all was not given, but the 12 per cent of the Guanabara population over age nine described in this census as totally illiterate may be taken as a minimal approximation.

LITERACY AND THE EDUCATIONAL GAP BETWEEN SOCIAL CLASSES

The rapid increase of schools and teachers has not resulted in a marked increase in the proportion of literates. This is due in part to continuing migration from rural areas and in part to the birth rate which continues to be highest among the least educated. The approximate figure of 88 per cent literacy among Guanabara residents over age nine in 1960 has progressed little beyond that of 1950 when only 48 per cent of Brazilians of comparable age could read or write and over 84 per cent of the inhabitants of Rio de Janeiro city, then the Federal District, were literate. This high figure masks marked inequities within the Guanabara population as suggested by 1960 census data on a sample of *favela* dwellers, the 335,063 residents of 147 slum communities defined strictly on the basis of size and degree of urbanization. Covering less than half of the economically marginal people of Rio de Janeiro, in accordance with estimates of the Guanabara State Department of Social Services, they reveal marked gaps in education and literacy between *favelados* and other Cariocas. Only 55 per cent of the *favela* group over age nine could read and write 33 per cent less than the 88 per cent for the total Guanabara population. Data on schooling reveal similar relationships. Of a total of 274,781 persons five years of age or over, 44 per cent were listed as having had no instruction at all. Percentages according to years of schooling were as follows: between one and five years of school (some or all primary level) 54 per cent; between six and nine years (some or all *ginásio* level) two per cent; between 10 and 12 years (some or all *colégio* level) .3 per cent; between 13 and 17 years (some or all university or special course level) .03 per cent. In other words, almost none of the inhabitants had progressed beyond primary school. Approximately 16 per cent of those who did attend primary school, slightly more than eight per cent of the total *favela* group, had completed five years.

Within the primary school itself, comparative percentage figures of those attending each grade also indicate a high rate of attrition: first, 30 per cent; second and third, 23 per cent; fourth, 15 per cent; fifth, nine per cent. None of the *favelados* are listed as attending a sixth grade.

Four Rio de Janeiro State *municípios,* Duque de Caixias, Nova Iguacu, Nilopolis, and Sao Joao de Meriti make up the vast haphazardly urbanized industrial area called Baixada Fluminense, considered part of Greater Rio de Janeiro. In this concentration of 1.5 million people, mostly young and containing large numbers of migrants, at least half of the population between ages seven and 18 were not enrolled in school in 1967. Part of the problem, according to State of Rio statistics, lies in the absolute lack of facilities, with a deficit of 3,300 classrooms at the primary level alone. Another part of the problem, according to Dias (1968), writing in the *Jornal do Brasil,* lies in the poor health and poverty of children who could be students.

These differences within Greater Rio de Janeiro mirror those within the nation as a whole. The gap between the urban and rural, or as Poppino (1968) has put it, "the modern and traditional areas" has become progressively wider. Poppino and others have pointed out that these circumstances reflect on the one hand, the greater practical and prestige value attached to formal education in the more rapidly developing regions, and on the other, the difficulty in persuading qualified teachers to move into rural communities. Further, ". . . behind these difficulties lie such pervasive matters as . . . the relative poverty of the states and municipalities in the less developed regions of the country. As has always been the case, the rural student who wants more than the bare rudiments of a primary education must move to town (pp. 312–313)." If, however, the crescendo of population growth without concomitant development of services continues, "moving to town" may not much longer represent a solution.

SCHOOL MENTAL HEALTH FACILITIES

Given the filtering characteristics of the school system, the cultural gap which must be bridged by the poor child from a rural migrant or slum family, and the intense pressures under which

the middle-class aspirant must labor, one might expect a high incidence of psychological problems in the school population. Incidence data are not available, but a small beginning has been
made at providing mental health services and gathering information. The Department of School Health of the Secretariat of Education and Culture has established guidance centers (Centros Dis-
trital de Orientação Psicologica) in four of the 20 Rio de Janeiro
school districts. The one in Copacabana at the school on Rua
Belford Roxo, for example, was established in 1966. Its staff, all
part-time, includes three psychiatrists, two psychologists, a pediatrician, a social worker, an educational technician, and a secretary
and receptionist. Daily consultation hours are held in three
sparsely furnished rooms provided by the school. Referrals are
made by teachers, by the physicians (internists and pediatricians)
who cover all the school districts, or by families themselves. An
average of four months is required from the time application is
made until a child is seen. The presenting complaints, which most
often relate to learning difficulties, are frequently associated with
other emotional and behavioral problems. Evaluation, using interviews and psychological tests (including the Wechsler, Rorschach,
TAT and others), requires about a month followed by staff discussion of the case. Usually the Center's staff does not try to involve the teacher. If they had sufficient personnel they would like
to devote more time to orienting the teachers, perhaps through
some form of group therapy, but they feel that, as a rule, the
problem is with the family and they want the family to assume
responsibility. This usually means the mother, who always accompanies the child for interviews; fathers are almost never seen and
are regarded as virtually inaccessible.

The Center sees from 25 to 30 children per month, of whom
from one to six may be starting as new cases. Often they recommend psychotherapy, and if the family can afford it they are referred to a private practitioner. Otherwise the social worker may
see the child or his mother a few times. Group psychotherapy for
mothers was initiated in 1968. Perhaps the most impressive aspect
of the center group, representative of others, was the similarity of
its outlook to that of psychodynamically or "psychoanalytically
oriented" child guidance workers who deal with middle-class children in the United States. While the Centers were established at

the request of school doctors wanting help for psychotic, brain-damaged, or mentally retarded children, it is precisely these whom the staff will not accept. They continue to be referred to the large institutions where drugs and custodial care are the only alternatives. Staff members are sensitive to the impressive social determinants of many of the problems which come to them, but they are clearly happier and more comfortable when it is possible to make a psychodynamic formulation and think in terms of prolonged intensive psychotherapy.

THE UNIVERSITY YEARS

Universities in the modern sense were not developed in Brazil until after the first World War. They have still not assumed the highly organized form present in the United States and tend to consist more of federations of institutes and faculties, particularly those concerned with law, engineering, and medicine. The greatest period of expansion of university facilities began after 1950, and there is considerable pressure in local areas for their own institutions of higher education, largely because there is no tradition of acquiring university training away from home. The demand, which far exceeds the number of qualified teachers, appears more likely to produce schools comparable to United States junior colleges than those of traditional university character.

While few Brazilians reach the university level, these institutions help mold the structure of popular aspirations and partly determine the way in which people perceive and judge others as well as their own rank in the prestige system of the society. This is truer in terms of ideal patterns or the existence of emulative reference groups than in terms of possible concrete personal achievement. The number of places in Brazilian universities is small and entrance examinations (which are specific to individual institutions and do not have nationwide applicability) are rigid. When examination failures are subtracted from those whose talent, ambition, family connections, and class and financial status have brought them to the doorway, those who matriculate form a tiny group indeed. Nonetheless, the professional class as well as the old land-holding and the newer business-owning elite who have been university students exert an influence on national life disproportionate to their numbers, and through them, the university experience exerts its influence. In the mid-60's, rising to a peak in the summer of 1968, university students were increasingly visible protesters against the rigidities of a system which limits entrance to a select few and perpetuates archaic aspects of the curriculum and the teaching process. Invasion of a number of universities by military police, broadly reported in the press, has brought the former more than ever to the attention of the man on the street.

Census figures for 1960 showed approximately .001 per cent (393) of all Guanabara residents between the ages of 30 and 34 with some university education. This was the age range which revealed the highest proportion of university attendance; Guanabara and Sao Paulo, together, include almost 42 per cent of all university level students in all of Brazil. The socioeconomic characteristics of first year university students have been described by Monteiro de Castro (1966) on the basis of 18,230 returns to a detailed questionnaire. Her 1965 sample covered college level institutions in Fortaleza, Recife, Salvador, Belo Horizonte, Niteroi, Rio de Janeiro, São Paulo, Curitiba, Pôrto Alegre, and Brasilia, cities which together include 90 per cent of all Brazilian university students. The typical student was male (65 per cent of the total), single, aged 18 to 22, and born in an urban area in the state where he was attending university. Less than half had entered university immediately after secondary school graduation and two-thirds had attended courses preparing them for entrance examinations. More than half, 52 per cent, were born in the city in which the school was located, and another 17 per cent had lived there for 10 years or more. Their families were largely intact except for the loss of 13 per cent of fathers through death, and more than half the students lived at home. (Another recent survey by SPLAN [Jornal do Brasil (August 18, 1968)]—Sociedade de Pesquisas e Planejamento—indicated that 60 per cent of university students live with their immediate families or relatives and another 10 per cent with their wives.)

The parents of these students were better educated than the majority of Brazilians: 23 per cent were university graduates. Even in this group of fathers, however, 30 per cent had not gone beyond primary level, and the figure is considerably higher in certain areas, particularly in the Northern and Eastern states. While this suggests a degree of upward intergenerational mobility in spite of the obstacles posed by low financial and social status, the relatively high proportions of fathers with little education is probably due to the overall lack of school facilities.

A major student complaint, described in the previous noted *Jornal do Brasil* survey and reflecting the weight of tradition interfering with university reform, concerned the "advanced age" of many professors "who still did not know of the atomic bomb or that Victor Hugo and Alencar had died many light-years ago." The students spoke particularly of their wish for livelier instructors disposed to take new approaches to the Brazilian "social and political reality" (p. 24).

THE SAMPLE

The patients were divided into major categories on the basis of literacy and education. Fifty-seven per cent, designated in the tables as Group I had not completed the primary grades. One-quarter of this Group had never attended school. The 43 per cent of the entire sample designated in the tables as Group II had progressed beyond this level. This is considerably less than the 62 per cent of the total Guanabara population, which according to the 1960 census graduated from primary school. Their distribution is listed in Table 77. The patient group, however, contains proportionally fewer persons with no formal education at all than the *favela* population of which 44 per cent, as noted above, never attended school.

Three literacy categories are used in the accompanying tables. Group I, including 15 per cent of the patients, is illiterate. Approximately half of these could sign their name or make change; the other half could do neither. Group II includes the 14 per cent of the patients who could read and write with difficulty or at a simple level—the partly literate. Group III, the large majority at 71 per cent, could read and write with relative ease. This figure, between the 55 per cent level for the slum dwellers and the 88 per cent literacy figure in 1960 for all of Guanabara, indicates an overrepresentation of nonliterates as well as the uneducated in the patient sample. Whether or not this is true for the Rio public and

INPS mental hospital population at large is not known, but it seems probable.

The relationship between education and literacy is shown in Table 78. Forty-one per cent of the literates had not graduated from the primary level. This confirms the commonsense expectation that intelligent people with some drive and opportunity will learn to read and write regardless of lack of early education. The following two detailed examples give an idea of the social and psychiatric constellations regularly encountered in the illiterate, uneducated patient population. One case is white, male, and was seen in Casa Eiras. The other is brown, female, and was seen in the Pronto Socorro.

A 34-year-old white, married, totally unschooled, illiterate, unskilled factory worker came to Casa Eiras accompanied by his brown 37-year-old wife, of three years with whom he had lived for another two years before having a civil ceremony. Aside from the patient, she, a partly literate second grade graduate, and a skilled seamstress, was the principal informant. The patient had been born and reared in a small village in rural Paraiba in the Northeast. He had worked assisting his father, an illiterate, unschooled, paid agricultural laborer, until at age 18 he migrated alone to Rio in a truck (a *pau-de-arara*) to find work and, possibly, adventure. His mother, 70, illiterate, and unschooled, is now living in Rio with one of the patient's nine brothers. She spends the major part of her time as a Macumba devotee. Another brother has been a patient in Casa Eiras because of seclusiveness, threatening behavior, and an episode in which he broke all the furniture in his house. The patient, his wife and her mother, occupy a four room *barraco* with a kitchen and bath area, but no water or electricity, in the industrial zone of Manguinhos in Rio city. He owns a radio, which, apart from word-of-mouth, is his sole source of outside information. He has no religious affiliation and attends no services of any kind, although his wife identified herself as an adept of an Afro-Brazilian cult center which she attends on holidays and special occasions. He attends no amusements now but he used to be part of a samba school when he was young, and before becoming ill he regularly attended the movies. While he likes to gamble, he rarely does so. Admission was precipitated by his physically attacking his wife during a "nervous crisis." She regards him as mentally ill and believes hospitalization to be necessary.

Symptoms had been developing for approximately six months. At times the patient was quiet and seclusive, a marked change from his usual behavior. On other occasions he said that he saw fire, animals, and neighbors "making macumba" in order to kill him. He complained of pain in the head, and occasionally said he had "wadding" in his head. He was irritable with his wife and said that she was "against" him. He was insomniac, ate little, wept easily, and "wanted to fight with the whole world." She attributed his mental illness to his becoming "very upset" after having been laid off from work approximately 11 months earlier and to an explosion in their neighborhood three years ago which had destroyed their former shanty; she also said he had been "nervous" as long as she had known him. The discharge from work was apparently due to "nervousness." The patient has since searched unsuccessfully for other jobs and failed some qualifying tests. He has been preoccupied with his financial obligations.

He reported a severe blow on the head in early childhood, associated with much blood loss, followed by three hours of unconsciousness. The routine physical examination given to all study subjects revealed no neurological findings except for a depressed scar suggesting a badly healed skull fracture. The patient said he had "always carried some pressure" in his head. He has been unable to work in school and had tried for a time to study with a "private teacher," but "I could never remember anything I learned." During the interview the patient was tense, uneasy, and only moderately cooperative. He appeared to have difficulty remembering both recent and remote events. While his memory was never good, he felt that it had become less reliable in recent months and that his ability to think was similarly less intact. He was temporally disoriented as to day, week, and year. He complained of palpitations, tremors, vertigo, and feeling badly throughout his body as well as of head pain. He felt that people were criticising and belittling him, was preoccupied with the loss of his home three years earlier (at which time, he said, his most severe head pain began), and had thoughts of throwing himself under the wheels of a train. From time to time he heard voices, mostly of unknown persecutors, although at times he identified these with practitioners of macumba. Sometimes the voices screamed: "Take care." Or, "We have seen you!" For five months he had been unable to maintain erection sufficient for intercourse, and was concerned about his diminished interest in sex.

A 28-year-old brown, married (civil ceremony), unschooled, illiterate housewife, who had formerly worked as a maid, was brought to the Pronto Socorro one month after the birth of her last child by her 37-year-old white husband of eight years. He is a stonemason's helper and *biscateiro* who continues to raise bananas on a small piece of land in Conceiçao de Jacarai in Rio State, from where they had come. The husband, illiterate and unschooled, was the principal informant aside from the patient. The patient had begun to work as a paid field hand at age 12. She was regarded by family members as a very "respectful and obedient" child, but had been removed from the first grade because "she was not able to learn." Of her 13 siblings, nine survive. Her father, an illiterate and unschooled fisherman, died from "startle" when she was 21. "He was fishing when he saw a very big fish persecuting him and trying to turn the boat over. He was not healthy anymore and his heart became all shook up." Her mother lives, at age 50, with a mate by whom she has had one child. Also illiterate and unschooled, she does daily agricultural labor on a small rented farm. She has been in touch with the patient and her husband since the onset of the present illness and revealed the hitherto unknown fact that she had been psychiatrically disturbed for a short time in her youth: "She doesn't know what happened to her . . . it healed by itself." Both parents, as was the patient, were indifferent Catholics and none acknowledged attendance at other religious centers. None of the patient's siblings had completed the first grade of school and none were more than partly literate. Although the oldest of the patient's four children was seven, no plans had been formulated for him to attend school. The patient, her husband, and their then two children had migrated into Rio city by train five years earlier (placing them in the recently migrant category for purposes of data analysis) along with two friends and a brother-in-law. The move was motivated by the husband's conclusion that he could not support the family by his small banana-raising enterprise. They live in a house with electricity and piped water in suburban Campo Grande. Husband, wife, and children sleep in the living room, while one of the patient's sisters and a sister-in-law share the small bedroom.

The patient's major source of outside information had been the radio, but for the 10 days preceding admission she did not listen and forbade the rest of the family to do so. She had always been on good terms with her neighbors, especially those who had moved into the city from the same rural area, but 10 days earlier had become suspicious and hostile, feeling that they were laughing at her and talking about her. She had never acquired the same feeling of status in Rio city as in her native village where she had been on friendly terms with the mayor and his family. There, the local policeman had also been her *compadre*. Her chief outside amusements since moving had been attending movies two or three times yearly. Before marriage she used to dance at family parties and religious celebrations, and before migration used to go to the beach at least once weekly. She had always gotten along well with her husband until the present illness, when she threatened to strike him. Believing her to be suffering from a mental illness, he had taken her, a day earlier, to visit her brother-in-law who lived nearby and had come to the hospital from there. He said that she had seen men and women on the wall "winking" at her and persecuting her and that she had attacked him because he would not defend her against them. She talked and laughed by herself, destroyed objects in the home and uttered obscene words. All this behavior took place before neighbors and relatives alike. All believed her to be ill, but had no theories about the cause of the condition, although they related it to pregnancy. During the seventh month of her recent pregnancy (three months before admission) she was transiently more aggressive than before and accused her husband of infidelity. Shortly after this a fall on a staircase resulted in a deep head wound. After delivery, the formerly transient attitudes, especially of aggressive jealousy, seemed to become crystallized. When angry, she "frothes with a lump in her throat and her skin becomes very red . . . she gets back on the children." Neither her husband nor the other relatives and neighbors, however, had regarded her as sick until the onset of acute socially disruptive symptoms 10 days earlier.

In the interview the patient seemed preoccupied, distractible and hypervigilant to outside stimuli. She often paid little direct attention to the psychiatrist, and according to him, spoke "in a loose and heedless way." She was thin and dirty, with clothing in disarray, and she appeared weak and tired. Moods of seriousness, worried tension, and apparent cheerfulness occurred in rapid succession. At the same time, she communicated in an intelligible and often self-protective manner. She described herself as being in her "post-birth" period, and said her husband was the major source of trouble because he was "very jealous" of her. She offered no specific complaints aside from low back pain. General suspiciousness, apprehension about the motives of others, and vague complaints of persecution recurred throughout the interview, but were not crystallized, nor did they fit together in a system. She believed that her husband, her newborn daughter, and most people around her could read her inner thoughts and feelings. At one point she noted that she would not eat a fish which her husband had brought home for dinner, but did not specify the reason. In response to questions about sex she noted that she would not permit sexual relations until 40 days had elapsed following delivery (now approximately 30 days past). She said that she was restless due to many worries, but would not divulge their specific nature. Much of what she said was not logical, and much time was spent ruminating about her children who annoy her and her brother-in-law, who she insists is known to the doctors. She was disoriented in place, believing herself to be in her home neighborhood of Campo Grande rather than in Engenho de Dentro, but knew that she was in a hospital ("where people get needles and blood tests"). She said that her daughter was born on October 31st and that the date of the interview was October 18th. Toward the end of the two-and-a-half-hour interview it was possible to construct her own subjective view of things. She stated that she was not ill and had been forced to come to the hospital by her husband, who, along with the newborn baby, is jealous of her. This jealousy is expressed through "twinklings" when other people talk to her. This sometimes happens on the streets because "people love babies." She said that after the baby was born her husband insisted they go into the center city to buy furniture. Instead, they went to her sister's home in Campo Grande, where she helped her sister so much she became indispensible to her.

Her sister's children are in great danger of something happening
to them because they are so excitable.

SOCIAL CHARACTERISTICS

SOCIOECONOMIC INDICATORS

Table 79 shows that the least educated (less than primary) are
almost evenly divided between the skilled and unskilled manual
occupational categories. The more educated are divided between
the skilled manual and nonmanual occupations. Literacy as well
as education is directly related to occupational status. Twenty-
four per cent of the literates in contrast to none of the illiterates or partly literates are in the top three occupational classes.
Of the remainder, most are skilled manual workers. The partly
literate who can read and write "at a simple level" are distributed
in a manner identical with the totally illiterate. Less than half the
number of literates, however, are unskilled with the difference
made up by a slightly higher proportion in Class V as well as
Classes I through III. While many skilled manual workers, including drivers, policemen and others in responsible positions, are relatively uneducated, they include those whose motivation and
ability have resulted in their becoming literate.

Another index of socioeconomic status is housing. Table 80
shows that although the total numbers are small the less educated
have fewer essential services, less space and privacy than the more
educated, and are more apt to live in a shack. The distribution is
similar for literacy, with clear progressive differences from the illiterates to the literates with respect to the nature and amount of
housing and the presence of services. The differences are least
marked with regard to privacy. This is related to the high cost of
adequate housing in Rio de Janeiro. The maintenance of an
apartment or a small house with all essential services requires a
sufficiently high and regular income so that even the partly literate can not often affford it. Privacy, even in the sleeping room,
was a luxury reserved for just over half of the literate group.

As indicated in Table 81, a relatively small number of the patients lived in *favela* communities. This was about half the number of those with neither electricity nor running water whose sub-

standard housing was not located in an area defined as a *favela*. Significantly more of the uneducated and illiterate, however, were *favela* dwellers. At the opposite end of the scale, proportionately more of the educated and literate, including the partly literate, occupied the urban residential areas. There was a considerably overlap between groups, however, which was even more marked in the relatively stable suburban working class neighborhoods. Somewhat more of the uneducated, and nonliterate lived at a distance from the city center either in the State of Rio or in small Guanabara towns regarded as part of greater Rio de Janeiro. These living area characteristics of the psychiatric patient population confirm what is generally known about the Rio de Janeiro population at large: (1) the poor and uneducated live mainly at a distance from town, commuting to work with considerable delay and discomfort, unless they choose to live in a *favela;* (2) no neighborhood is homogeneous, and almost any given block may contain people of widely varying status according to almost any criterion.

Table 82 indicates how the patients themselves regarded their socioeconomic stability. More of the literates and the better educated (but these last not significantly so) felt their status to have improved during the preceding year, and more of the nonliterate and the less educated felt that it had declined. While about 60 per cent of the patients reported no change in either direction, the data confirm the impression that the potential for economic betterment is established relatively early in life both by formal education and the ability to read and write. The better educated, unlike the United States Negro patients described by Parker and Kleiner (1966), did not report more aspiration-achievement discrepancy.

MIGRATORY STATUS

Data on this point are summarized in Table 83. Migrant status as such does not vary with education or literacy. The uneducated and illiterate patients include proportionately more, however, who arrived in Rio de Janeiro after maturity; that is, were not reared in the area. Significantly more of the illiterate and partly literate also had migrated within the preceding five years; their

characteristics in relation to the literate may be expected to resemble those of the recently migrant in relation to the settled patients described in a preceding chapter. For the less as compared
to the more educated, however, although proportionately more
had been residentially mobile within the area, the difference in
recency of migration was significant only with the division point
at the ten-year level; that is, the uneducated patients as a group
had been in Rio longer than the illiterate. Social-behavioral
differences according to education are not the same as those according to recently migrant-settled status. Reading skills were
evidently acquired in time by those without formal education as
part of adaptation in the urban environment. It is possible that a
matched sample of uneducated nonpatients, presumably more
successful copers than those who became patients, would show
even less illiteracy.

The large majority of less educated and nonliterate migrants in
comparison with the more advantaged came from rural settings.
These findings for all migrants representing 55 per cent of the
patient group, support the impression that an important segment
of the uneducated and illiterate Rio de Janeiro population has
been reared in rural areas with inadequate school facilities; they
probably retain other features of country-reared people as well.
More of the uneducated left their former homes because of lack of
jobs and, along with the nonliterate, had changed the nature of
their work after the move (although in every instance it remained
in the unskilled manual category). The nonliterate, as the recently
migrant (within five years) with whom they overlap, came to Rio
more often than the noneducated for personal-emotional (rather
than occupational) reasons. The frequency of these reasons, however, unlike the case for the recently migrant versus the settled,
did not vary with literacy status to a statistically significant degree. More, too, had made the journey alone. It seems probable
that earning little, they could not afford to bring their families to
Rio until a new job had been obtained.

DEMOGRAPHIC CHARACTERISTICS

As shown in Table 84 significantly larger proportions of the
literate and the educated were white. Among the uneducated and

the nonliterate proportionately more were nonwhite, but there were no significant differences between browns and blacks whose behavior, as noted in Chapter IV, was in a number of instances markedly disparate.

Larger families of origin and more children of their own characterized the uneducated. This last was partly due to the fact that more of them (75 per cent of the uneducated versus 60 per cent of the educated) had consistent mates. This in turn may be owing in part to the tendency of the educated to be younger—more under 25 years old—than the uneducated, explicable on the basis of increases in schools and teachers in Rio during recent years. Otherwise the results fit the familiar equation between large family size and lack of education. In contrast to the relation with educational status, childhood family size did not vary according to the patients' literacy. This may be because literacy more than education is determined by personal rather than familial or community values and the availability of schools. While marital status did not vary with literacy, child-producing literates had fewer offspring than nonliterates.

Table 85 reveals no significant differences in religious participation according to education or literacy. Thirty per cent of the illiterates said that they at least occasionally attend Afro-Brazilian cult or Spiritist sessions.

CHILDHOOD INFLUENCES

More of the illiterate than the literate, as shown in Table 86, appeared to come from less stable childhood situations. Fewer reported sibs by both parents or were reared by both parents, and more reported the father had died before the patient was 12. The variability of data in this respect, however, made differences not statistically significant. Figures for the educated and uneducated in respect to childhood family stability and death of the father before the patient was 12 years old were virtually identical. This again suggests that prevailing community values and the availability of facilities were more important in determining educational achievement than the individual psychological factors of the kind which might stem from family disorder during developmental years. Within the most favored groups, however, the chief disciplinarian was the mother, who presumably had more time and energy for childrearing than the mothers of the less educated and nonliterate.

The data in Table 87 indicate that parental literacy may be more important than family stability as such in determining the education and literacy of children. Proportionately more of the fathers and mothers of the better educated and the more literate could themselves read and write. This was true although formal education within the parental generation was too limited to construct comparative groups. This finding supports the suggestion in Table 86, although the data were not statistically significant, that literacy—in contrast to education—in this patient-population is related to family stability and to the kinds of family values and interests reflected in parental literacy in the absence of educational opportunities. In a developing country, without a firm tradition of compulsory public education, cultural transmission must depend more upon families than other social institutions.

As indicated in Table 88, more of the fathers of educated and literate than uneducated and nonliterate patients worked in the top five occupational categories. No fathers of illiterates, in contrast to fathers of the uneducated, were represented in the top three categories, and there is a greater range of differences according to patient-literacy than patient-education in regard to paternal representation in occupational-Class V. A clear majority of fathers of the less educated and, to an even more marked degree, the illiterate groups were at the lowest occupational level.

There were no marked differences in parental religious affiliation according to education or literacy.

INFORMATION AND SOCIAL PARTICIPATION

Access to major sources of general information is listed in Table 89. Radio ownership, mainly of transistors, was almost universal. The majority of the less educated and the illiterate described the radio as their only source of general information. Ownership of other information sources or attendance at them was uniformly more frequent within the more educated and literate groups, except for the cinema. Those with more schooling were proportionately more frequent movie-goers, but this was not true for the literates, again suggesting the formal characteristics of the educational dimension as compared with the personal achievement characteristics of the literacy dimension. At the same time, over twice the proportion of more educated and literate than of the others were sometime movie-goers. While sheer lack of money may have contributed to the large proportions of the uneducated and illiterate who never attended movies, Table 90 shows that this did not keep them from attending soccer games.

These data confirm the common-sense expectation that people with little schooling who cannot read are only peripheral participants in major aspects of the surrounding culture and suffer relative informational deprivation. The degree to which personal conversation and other auditory input as by radio, supplemented by combined audiovisual input as through television, can compensate for what is lost by being unable to read is uncertain. Other factors besides the economic (lack of curiosity or deficient ability to assimilate information) may result in decreased exposure of the noneducated, nonreading public of Rio to general informational media.

It was expected that the nonliterate and less educated, especially since they included more recent migrants, would have less support than the others from friends or relatives. However, as shown in Table 90, the differences between groups were not significant in contrast to the recently migrant–settled differences shown in Chapter IV. This indicates again that while the recently migrant and nonliterate groups have much in common, they nonetheless reflect different behavior-determining factors within the patient population. Contact with institutional support sources showed the same pattern as for other groups divided on bases related to socioeconomic status. The literate and the more educated, presumably with least need, reported more contact with welfare workers and more use (although at an extremely low level) of organized welfare services. Use of services which are scarce and often hard to locate seems determined mainly by the applicants' possession of knowledge and skills. Those outside of the informational-cultural stream, with the most intense need for assistance, are least likely to find it. The two educational subdivisions do not differ from each other with respect to participation in dances or the major Brazilian spectator sport of soccer. Smaller proportions of the literates, however, report frequent attendance at soccer games or dances, a clear indication that economic factors alone do not determine attendance at activities requiring payment.

HOSPITALIZATION AND FAMILY DIAGNOSIS

As illustrated in Table 91, more of the literate and the better educated had had previous contact with psychiatrists. Conversely, the less educated and the illiterate had fewer such contacts, reporting illnesses of shorter duration and presumably greater acuteness. While more (though not significantly so) of the native than the migrant (noted in Chapter IV) had had previous psychiatric (outpatient) contact, there were no differences in this respect, or in duration between the recently migrant and the settled. As noted in Chapter V, the illnesses of the blacks before hospitalization were more often of relatively shorter duration than the illnesses of the whites; this was not so for the browns.

Half the illiterates were encountered at the Pronto Socorro, as were 38 per cent of the part-literates and nine per cent of the literates. Similarly, 36 per cent of the less educated, in contrast to eight per cent of the more educated, were seen at the Pronto Socorro. These findings, reflecting job constancy and community integration, are similar to those for the recently migrant and nonwhites, and within this last group more so for the browns than the blacks. There was no reason to believe that rapid hospitalization represented lack of available family support, since approximately equal proportions of all groups were accompanied to the hospital by family members. But, as in the case of recent migrants, some inability to sustain an economically unproductive person is suggested by the higher proportions of the illiterate and uneducated who were brought to the hospital because of failure to work. This is similar to the findings regarding browns, more of whose hospitalization was precipitated by failure to work than was true for whites and blacks.

There was a clear predominance among the less educated and nonliterate of paranoid statements, physical assaults (as in the case of the predominantly male blacks, but not the whites or browns) and threats, as reasons for hospitalization. It seems likely that these events as precipitants of hospitalization reflected the patient's behavior as much as they did the relatives' sensitivity, inasmuch as higher proportions of illiterates than literates (though not of the less educated) were also admitted because of anxious and depressive symptoms. Contrary to expectation, other forms of bizarre or clearly psychotic behavior were also more often listed as precipitating hospitalization among the more educated and literate. In these respects the data for education and literacy differ from those for migration. The only significant difference between groups, other than failure to work, was in respect to anxious, depressive symptoms as reasons for admission; proportionately more of the settled than the recently migrant cited such reasons.

The diagnostic impressions of families are summarized in Table 92. Significantly higher proportions of the less educated and nonliterate families regarded the patients as suffering from mental illness. Conversely, a few more of the better educated and literate regarded the patient's disturbance as being due to life stress, or they classified it as strange or peculiar. This preponderance of mental illness labels among the presumably less sophisticated is surprising, and does not fit the limited United States data indicating that poorer and less informed people are more apt to look at seriously disturbed behavior as adaptive or bad rather than sick.

PSYCHIATRIC AND BEHAVIORAL CHARACTERISTICS

TENSION, ANXIETY, SENSITIVITY AND FRUSTRATION

During the interviews, as indicated in Table 93, the better educated and literate patients were more frequently cooperative, friendly, and relaxed, and less often fearful, avoidant, and distractible. More of them actively sought advice and attention and were regarded as dependent in attitude without anxiety. The less schooled and nonliterate seemed ambivalent and conflictful; they more often stated a wish not to be helped and, at the same time, like the recent migrants, more often expressed strong unsatisfied wishes to be cared for. The majority of patients, however, revealed neither a strong tendency to be independent or dependent. The literates appeared more behaviorally stable than the nonliterates. That is, they more often showed no behavioral change between the beginning and end of the interview. Most patients did show some such change, either in the direction of decreased anxiety and improved reality contact or increased hostility and uncooperativeness.

Table 93 also shows the reaction of the psychiatrists to the patients. Without exception, more of the better educated and literate patients elicited positive, empathic, cheerful responses, while more of the less educated and illiterate elicited (although the frequencies were low) distant and hostile feelings. The less positive interaction of psychiatrists with patients who differ markedly from them in education and language usage may well determine the quality of behavioral data of all kinds. The more frequently noted interview anxiety of the nonliterate, for example, may have been accentuated by the nature of the psychiatrist's response.

Most anxiety symptoms were not differentially distributed according to literacy or education. Table 94 does show, however, that, more of the better educated and literate complained of constant diffuse anxiety or fear of loss of control over specific actions; more of the illiterate and less educated individuals complained of fear of disease in some organ (as noted for low SES patients in a number of other studies), and more expressed worry of some kind about relatives. The degree to which these concerns were related to their real-life problems is unclear. (There were no marked differences between groups regarding worries about jobs, money, or housing.) Interference with function due to anxiety, while reported in some respect by a half to three-quarters of the patients, was not distributed consistently according to education and literacy. As shown in Table 94, illiterates significantly more often complained of difficulty in clear thinking. This last was also present more often among the less educated.

Hostile tension, impulsivity and feelings of frustration, inferiority and interpersonal discomfort, as indicated in Table 95, were reported by proportionately more of the partly literate. It seems plausible to assume that this group, not fully capable of reading and writing but more ambitious and advanced than the totally illiterate, might suffer from some of the difficulties of upwardly mobile, marginal persons. Similar findings, as noted in Chapter IV, were found for the browns in contrast to white or black patients, but, as noted in Chapter V, were not found with the population divided according to migratory status. The illiterates most frequently denied or did not mention the existence of angry feelings. This does not mean insensitivity to frustration, although the total numbers are low; more than the fully literate, both they and the part-literates indicated awareness of the discrepancy between what they would like to achieve and what they had actually accomplished. The apparent lack of hostility among the illiterate is most easily explained as owing to the lowest-class person's habit of passive subservience or evasion with members of the privileged classes.

DEPRESSION

As indicated in Table 96, several depressive features were more prominent, although not usually to a statistically significant degree or markedly so, among the illiterates. (There were no differences according to education.) These were mainly slow, sad, or dull interview behavior, as well as feelings that something bad was going to happen to them or that they would not be cared for both realistic possibilities. Similarly, their feelings of body weakness or inferiority could be reality-based. Again, these findings did not characterize the recently migrant as a group. Feelings of guilt, related generally to failure to achieve, were most prominent among the partly literate. These findings may be associated with those listed in Table 95 suggesting greater anger and frustration within this group, intermediate between the nonparticipants and the full participants in the written information system.

THE BREAK WITH REALITY

Table 97 lists a variety of suspicious or paranoid statements, all of which were made more often by the nonliterate than the literate patients, but were not related to educational level. Differences within the nonliterate group, i.e., between the illiterate and the partly literate, as indicated in the table, are variable and not consistent in direction. The lack of differences in association with educational level reinforces the suggestion that formal education alone is of less weight than the range of possible factors contributing to failure to learn to read or write. These factors might include, in addition to educational opportunity, motivation, psychological or socially based learning inhibitions, absence of family support, or innate or acquired impairments in sensory, perceptual, or other functions necessary to learning.

Hallucinatory, in contrast to paranoid phenomena, as noted in Table 98, were reported by larger proportions of both the less educated and the illiterate, with more of both groups insisting on the reality of their experiences or planning action on the basis of them. The proportions of partly literate were usually midway between the literate and illiterate or closer to the latter. Misinterpretations and illusory phenomena were significantly more often reported by the illiterate patients. It seems likely that deficient early programming combined with deficient current informational input may increase proneness under stress to substitute a self-produced sensory environment for external reality. This vulnerability, originally reinforced by religious-magical beliefs in rural areas, would reach maximum proportions under the impact of geographical relocation to a strange environment. These data are congruent with those in Table 99, showing that spatial and temporal disorientation are more common for both the less educated and the nonliterate. The possibility that the more prominent and ego-syntonic hallucinatory phenomena, combined with illusions and disorientation, among the illiterate may be due to a greater prevalence of alcoholism in this group was discussed in earlier chapters. While chronic heavy drinking is considered to be more usual among the poor and illiterate population at large, and may well have contributed to the development of hallucinations in this patient sample, few admitted to problem drinking and none were admitted suffering from acute or incipient delirium tremens. Alcoholism was not reported as a problem more frequently by any of the subgroups in this study.

SOMATIC PROBLEMS

As noted earlier, the less educated and nonliterate expressed more anxiety about organ disease and more often regarded their bodies as weak and inferior. Table 100 shows that significantly more of the less educated complained of physical pain and discomfort. This was also true, though not significantly so, for the illiterate who more often complained that their physical movements were slowed and of feelings of fatigue and weakness. These symptoms may also be regarded as depressive indicators. In general, somatic complaints seem more characteristic of the nonliterate and may be rationally related to inferior medical care, poor nutrition, and the greater physical hardships which they endure. The feeling of something strange in the body reported by few people, significantly more often in the nonliterate group, was usually presented with a quality of reluctantly admitted belief, suggesting that it may have been delusional. Psychophysiological complaints occurred with the reverse distribution, although the differences were not statistically significant and the total number of patients involved was relatively low. There were proportionately fewer such complaints among the illiterate and more among the partly literate and literate. Faintness or dizziness, and sweating and hot flashes were most frequently reported by the partly literates.

SEXUAL BEHAVIOR

Differences according to education or literacy were not remarkable in most respects. As indicated in Table 101, however, sexual symptoms were significantly more frequently reported as part of the present illness by the literate patients (in contrast to the finding of more sexual problems related to the present illness among the recently migrant). Intense, uncontrollable, or fluctuating sexual impulses were least frequently reported as problems by the illiterate. These findings are similar to differences between white and black patients. They do not, however, overlap with those for color in general, since, as indicated in Chapter V, sexual difficulties were most prominently reported by the browns, whose literacy level more closely approached that of blacks than whites. In other words, the presence of sexual difficulties with regard to literacy appears to occur independently from its presence with regard to color or migrant status.

Past Psychiatric History

Few of the past-history items yielded differences, and, of these, more could be identified according to literacy than education. In several instances the highest proportions of earlier traumata or difficulties, as indicated in Table 102, were noted within the partly literate group. This raises a question of the possible etiology of partial literacy. Does, for example, the marginal significance of partial literacy, as suggested earlier, contribute to anger, sensitivity, and impulsivity, or might the failure to achieve full literacy as well as the occurrence of other problems among the nonliterate be more the result of childhood head injury or illness? Childhood and adolescent rages and sleep disturbances were equally frequent within the partly literate and completely literate group, and the latter were almost never reported by the illiterate. Or, again, can the figures be an artifact of reporting, i.e., might the reportedly higher incidence of earlier trauma in the partly literate be a function of their greater degree of tension and disturbance at the time of reporting?

Discussion

In this sample, illiteracy more than lack of education appears to be associated with the broadest and most incapacitating spectrum of symptomatic or maladaptive behavior. There are few published observations, however, as a background from which to view these data, and it is usually impossible to separate lack of literacy per se from the matrix of associated factors in which it is imbedded. Carothers (1959), for example, has noted infrequent delusional systematization in nonliterate African schizophrenics whose usual psychotic pictures included mental confusion, often with excitement or panic, and externally directed violence. He tied this response pattern to tribal social organization as well as nonliteracy: ". . . a man comes to regard himself as a rather insignificant part of a much larger organism—the family and clan—and not as an independent self-reliant unit . . . a meaningful integration of a man's experience on individual personal lines is not achieved" (p. 308). High activity and freely expressed, outwardly directed hostility have also been noted as characteristic of the psychotic behavior of nonliterate peoples by Opler (1956). These he considers in part a consequence of the "lack of systematized fantasy or delusions acting as ego-defenses" (pp 45–46). Confused excitement (often combined with homicidal behavior and little depression) was regarded, too, by Benedict and Jacks (1954), as frequent among nonliterates. They concluded that the hostility of nonliterate psychotics tends to be directed outward in contrast to the situation in literate Western cultures, where mechanisms of conscience (superego) and the incorporation of supernatural authority figures are more highly developed (p. 387). Wittkower and Fried (1959) summarized the comments of various observers of schizophrenics in preliterate cultures in terms of ". . . paucity of content, the shallowness of affect, the lack of psychogenic precipitating factors, and . . . gross dilapidation of habits . . ." (p. 494). These features are regarded by Yap (1951) as related to the likelihood that the " . . . richness of psychiatric symptomatology is dependent on the intellectual and cultural resources of the patient" (p. 326). They are, therefore, according to Yap, less associated with specific aspects of the primitive state than with differences "between the educated and the uneducated in any culture."

The more systematic findings of Leighton (1963) and Field (1960) offer a contrast to these observations. Leighton et al. on the basis of community studies among the Yoruba of Nigeria, were less impressed by the presence of excitement and activity in nonliterate Africans than the above authors, who limited their studies to mental hospital patients; they were impressed rather, by the overall resemblance of psychiatrically labeled behavior in the community at large to that encountered in literate western societies. They did, however, note a correlation between the progress of education and modernization, and the higher proportion of educated people in more integrated village societies which seemed to yield proportionately fewer psychiatrically disturbed people than less integrated villages. Field (1960), in Ghana, noted the possibility that within the predominantly nonliterate population it was the literates who were more vulnerable to psychiatric disorder. They did, indeed, have heavier demands made upon them and were often disappointed that "the rewards of literacy are so meager compared with the worries" so that they sometimes envied their "relatively carefree illiterate brethren," (p. 53), but their conflicts were manifest and not associated with mental illness. Although the literate schizophrenics observed at Ashanti shrines and in their home villages were not more numerous than the illiterate, they were "more conspicuous." The difference is illustrated in the case of two schizophrenic brothers. One, an illiterate farmer, "is withdrawing gradually and unobtrusively into mental disintegration." The other, a literate teacher, "is fighting off, with courage, insight and suffering, repeated acute attacks, apparently precipitated by the stresses of his literate circumstances" (p. 453). In these respects, Field's observations confirm the shallowness and lack of content and systematization of psychotic ideas, although not the outwardly directed violence reported by the various authors above.

The very few acutely excited or violently hostile patients appearing at the Pronto Socorro during the period of data gathering were excluded from the present sample because they were dealt with by immediate heavy sedation and electroshock treatment. No such patients were admitted to the Casa Eiras at the time, and among those already in the hospital, clearly hostile, forceful, outwardly directed behavior was a rarity. (The assaultive behavior more often reported by families of the uneducated and non-literate as precipitating the decision to come to the hospital was never present by the time the hospital was reached.) In this Brazilian patient population it seems unlikely that continuing uncontrolled violence, a behavioral form eliciting strong cultural disapproval, would prove upon investigation to differentiate the literate from the nonliterate. Other differences were noted, however, between these groups in the sample. In contrast to the observations of Benedict and Jacks, above, the illiterate (although not the uneducated, 50 per cent of whom were literate) more frequently complained of depressive symptoms, insomnia, feelings of weakness, restlessness due to worries, and premonitions that something bad was going to happen. There was no evidence in this group of less guilt, self-criticism, uncomfortable awareness of personal inadequacy, or other indications of inadequately internalized social standards or poorly developed conscience mechanisms. This is true, although to some extent these patients resemble those described by Carothers, above, in regarding themselves as relatively powerless units of the society and family. The opposing trend is present also, however, in the form of the Latin emphasis on the importance of personal dignity and manly virility.

The illiterate (but not the uneducated) also more often exhibited paranoid behavior. As reported by observers of preliterate cultures, the delusional content was often fragmented or not extensively organized, but this characterized most of the patient sample, and clear differences in this respect were not found according to education, literacy, or other related social class indicators such as occupation. (This phenomenon has also been noted in a psychotherapeutic study of a small number of young adult Negro males, all literate though not educated beyond high school, reared in a United States inner city slum [Brody, 1961]). Significantly more of both the illiterate and the uneducated also complained of difficulties in clear thinking and exhibited spatial and temporal disorientation, a characteristic of the recently migrant and the blacks as well. In this instance, as for the "primitive" tribesmen described above, greater vulnerability to disruption of thought processes seems characteristic of those less accustomed to using these processes in the service of adaptation, those with less complex and extensive information at their disposal, and with less continuing involvement in the symbolic-meaningful experience of the dominant society. The illiterate and less educated also exhibited more hypochondriacal concern about organ functions, anxious concern about their relatives (who were more important to them because they had fewer friends than the others), and hallucinatory phenomena (which they insisted were real and required action). This last, along with the observations of Field, above, suggests less "struggle" against the psychotic process; the hallucinatory phenomena are pervasive and ego-syntonic, creating little or no anxiety or sense of being alien in the least educated and literate.

The quality of interview interaction was congruent with the attitudes and symptom pictures brought by the patients. The uneducated and nonliterate were more often fearful, avoidant, distractible, and clearly conflictful about their wish to be helped. Their traditional wish for, or expectations of, concrete assistance from representatives of the more powerful upper class were mingled with hostility and fear of closeness. For their part, the psychiatrists reported they felt less empathic, cheerful, and comfortable with uneducated and nonliterate patients and more distant and hostile than with those who were better educated and literate. This clearly suggests a mutually reinforcing pattern of negative interaction.

The observations reported here may perhaps be understood less as the behavior of primitive people than as that of people on the margins of modern society. They are familiar to students of the poor and those excluded from full participation in the value and symbol systems of the dominant society of whatever country in which they live (Brody, 1966). In this sense, the illiterates—the most culturally excluded and distant from all sources of societal power—emerge as the most significant minority group in metropolitan Rio de Janeiro. Within this patient sample in a metropolis with large populations of recently migrant, uneducated, and nonwhite persons, lack of literacy appears as a major element separating one segment of the deprived population from the rest. Illiteracy decisively limits communication, the inflow of information, and reciprocal relationships with more dominant members of the society. Illiterates as a group do not have the institutionalized ways of reciprocally relating with dominant persons, characteristic of the blacks. These last constitute a socially visible population segment with a historically defined set of interpersonal rules determining a complementary way of relating to whites.

The illiterate also has the least available information allowing him some independence from environmental stresses. It has been suggested earlier (Brody, 1968) that behavioral vulnerability to shifting environmental circumstances is greatest in the absence of currently useful information as well as in the absence of a stable system of longitudinally acquired reference points which permit the categorization and evaluation of new information. Singer (1962), for example, has shown that an adequate explanation (information) about physiological changes in response to injected adrenalin protects the subjects' affective response from influence by directive external cues. In the absence of such information, mood is more dependent upon environmental factors. At the longitudinal level, behavioral disorganization may be related to defective symbol and concept learning (Brody, 1969d). Such disorganization, that is, psychotic behavior, may be described as dedifferentiation or the abandonment of complex in favor of more simple ways of perceiving, making discriminations, and processing information. The outcome, as observed in the present patient group, can be animism, a tendency to magical thinking, or a tendency to react to people not as individuals but in terms of gross categorizations, such as being a member of a class of strange or dangerous persons. In fact, this is one definition of paranoid behavior. Dedifferentiation also involves a diminution of the capacity to distinguish between self and nonself, between the world of independent objects and attitudes and expectations concerning such objects, again a characteristic of paranoid behavior. The greater frequency of disrupted thinking processes and of disorientation among the illiterate was evidence of disorganization with less clearly defensive value. It has been postulated (Brody, 1968, 1969d) that vulnerability to cognitive dedifferentiation is related to defective or distorted participation in what Kroeber and Parsons (1958) call the "symbolic—meaningful systems," i.e., the culture, of one's society. This might occur as a concomitant of low socioeconomic status, cultural exclusion, rapid social change, migration, or as described by Leighton and colleagues (1968), membership in a disintegrated society with ineffective communications, few associations, broken families, and inadequate leaders. The "cultural symbols" —concepts, images, events, language, and objects—described by Jaeger and Selznick (1965) as "carriers of connotative meaning," provide criteria, as they are learned by the maturing members of a society, against which behavior may be measured according to a hierarchy of preferences. They provide reference points around which social identities are organized and influence the ways in which members of a society categorize and conceptualize their experience of themselves and others. They permit a classification and ordering of experience, and as Parsons (1952) put it, in his discussion of moral standards, stabilize "cognitive definitions of what persons are in a socially significant sense" (pp. 22–23).

Conditions of rapid sociocultural change require changes in role patterns, new categories for organizing experience which must be made continuous with past personal histories, and new personal and social referents. These may be expected to maximize the behavioral reflections of defective symbol and concept learn-

ing and dependence upon or vulnerability to environmental factors. The adaptive requirements of life in a developing society
were combined with the circumstances of recent rural-urban migration for 28 per cent of the present patient population. This
would be expected to result in particular vulnerability to behavioral disorganization for those whose innate problems, plus a developmental period characterized by defective participation in the
symbolic-meaningful experience of the society, resulted in their
illiteracy as adults. As noted above, the recently migrant
patients—those hospitalized within five years after moving to the
metropolis—were 29 per cent illiterate and 52 per cent literate in
contrast to nine per cent illiteracy and 74 per cent literacy for the
settled and an 88 per cent level for the unhospitalized Guanabara
population at large. (There were no significant differences regarding part literacy). People who are socially and economically powerless, not fully informed, and at the mercy of others, tend to be
vigilant, suspicious, anxious, and depressed. Along with preliterate groups or those prone to magical thinking, those who have
grown up with a regularly reinforced perception of themselves
and their parents as having little power or self-determination in
the face of overwhelming supernatural or human forces tend to
externalize, to place the blame for their discomfort on outside
sources. Such sources, already existing in the culture, are convenient targets for the projection of unacceptable inner feelings and
wishes. The body, too, is a legitimate source of anxious concern
for poor people who depend on their physical strength for survival. Body concern also provides many with their customary way
of integrating a variety of otherwise inexplicable subjective phenomena. Highly visible and dramatic psychiatric symptoms, often
involving body dysfunction, can also have important communicative functions for deprived persons with otherwise blocked access
to sources of help and societal power. For them, the social role of
patient may also have particular conflict-resolving value and offer
considerable secondary gain. Feelings of depression, although they
may include elements of guilt, seem less related in this group to
strongly ingrained concepts of personal responsibility or to inwardly
turned hostility than to loss, deprivation, hopelessness, and despair of achievement in the face of insurmountable odds.

The behavior of the partly literate poses some special problems.

They emerged to some degree as a separate group in terms of the quality of their symptoms. Feelings more frequently reported by this group than by either the literates or the illiterates included: hostile tension, impulsivity, frustration, inferiority, interpersonal discomfort, feelings of guilt—especially about failure to achieve, and actual bodily pain or discomfort without obvious cause (rather than hypochondriacal or somatic anxiety). Like the illiterate, they more frequently than the literate exhibited paranoid behavior. It is plausible to assume that this group, more ambitious and able than the illiterates but not fully fluent in reading and writing, might be particularly vulnerable to self-doubts and criticism and to the criticisms of others. In this respect they would resemble other marginal groups. They might also be more likely to develop retaliatory protective hostility. Their expressions of irritability and anger are in sharp contrast to the almost complete absence of such hostility among the completely illiterate, who seem to behave in the traditionally subservient manner with more advantaged and powerful persons. Some doubt is cast on this idea, however, because of the more frequent reporting of head injury or serious illness in the childhoods of those who became partly literate. It is possible that such early trauma might contribute both to their inability to become fully literate and their hostile sensitivity.

The higher incidence of psychophysiological symptoms and of obsessive concern with behavior control reported by the educated and literate have been noted in upper-class as compared to lower-class groups in general. A variety of speculative explanations for these phenomena have been offered, ranging from the child-rearing experience of the upper- and middle- in comparison with the lower class, to lack of freedom to fully express feelings at a verbal sharing level, to comparative sophistication in choosing symptoms to achieve certain unconscious psychological aims. The literate and better educated, more of whom exhibit these symptoms, also work in more socially demanding environments, which, like the family environments of their childhood, require greater degrees of behavioral control than the developmental or current milieus of the less educated.

In Brazil as well as in the United States, symptom pictures and psychiatric constellations are linked to a person's capacity to understand and manipulate symbols, his level of general knowledge, the requirements upon him for social control and conformity, and the range of social and individual concomitants of literacy and education beginning with genetic endowment and childhood experience. In this patient population, recent migratory status, especially from rural areas, is a frequent concomitant of lack of education and particularly of illiteracy. These elements, contributing to unfamiliarity with the social context and lack of skills necessary to cope with it, might be expected to maximize the effects of lack of literacy per se. Differences between educational and literacy subgroups according to whiteness are also statistically significant. Psychiatric differences according to education and literacy (excluding part-literacy) appear to reflect the consequences of color-based cultural exclusion, and the unfamiliarity, coping stress, and rural backgrounds associated with recent migration, as well as the problems of absent skills and information, as such. Lack of literacy, seen as a concomitant of defective participation in the symbolic-meaningful experience of the society, however, is regarded as the crucial item characterizing the most psychiatrically vulnerable segment of this generally deprived patient population.

CHAPTER 7

OCCUPATION, INDUSTRIALIZATION
AND PATIENT BEHAVIOR

WORK AS PART OF THE BEHAVIORAL SETTING

OCCUPATION is the most widely accepted index of socioeconomic status in 'Brazil. Because education is so unevenly available and inherited wealth a rarity, in this chapter occupational category will be regarded in part as a general SES indicator. In terms of the Rio de Janeiro behavioral setting, particular interest will be focused on the differentiation between unskilled and skilled manual labor, and between manual and nonmanual occupations as corollaries of health and illness, life-style, personal satisfaction, and self-esteem. Attention will also be paid to the process of evolution into new occupational and therefore social roles which characterizes large masses of Brazilians, especially those migrant from rural into urban areas.

It is difficult to achieve an accurate picture of occupational distribution in Brazil. Many people hold more than one job, and underemployment is common. Some, especially the self-employed and those in rural areas, are only partly represented in the census figures. Nationwide data usually combine everyone aged 10 and over, thus tending to obscure certain patterns because children and women may not work fulltime or in capacities identical to those of men listed in the same occupation. Many firms discriminate against adolescents under the age of 18 because at this age Brazilians are not only subject to military conscription and under the law must be re-employed upon discharge, but they must also be paid the minimum wage—at least theoretically. Many boys of 14 and 16 are hired at fractions of the minimum wage and discharged before the passage of a full year so that the employer can

213

avoid paying the required year-end bonus amounting to one month's wages.

NATIONAL AND RIO DE JANEIRO DISTRIBUTIONS

Outside of the few metropolitan centers, mainly São Paulo and Rio de Janeiro, the largest number of Brazilians continue to be engaged in rural occupations. The best available national data (the 1950 census) show almost 60 per cent of the active labor force as agriculturists of one kind or another, in contrast to less than 10 per cent engaged in industrial work. As Furtado (1963) pointed out, the average per capita income for the nation in 1960 was estimated at no more than $300, with a range extending from approximately $1,000 in São Paulo city to under $100 in rural parts of the Northeast. The State of Guanabara registered about 300 per cent of the national average income between 1950 and 1960.

The low per capita income is due in part to the fact that about 1.5 per cent of the large plantations control over 50 per cent of the land. In 1968, according to the Instituto Brasileiro de Reforma Agraria (*Jornal do Brasil,* 9/1/68), *latifúndias* of 2,500 to 250,000 acres each, in the hands of 13 per cent of the rural proprietors, occupied 81 per cent of the total national territory. Approximately 85 per cent of the workers on these plantations were designated tenant farm laborers, mainly sharecroppers. *Minifúndias* of between 25 and 250 acres, owned by 87 per cent of the proprietors, occupied the rest of the farming land. Smith (1963), following recomputation of 1950 census data, found that fully 94 per cent of those engaged in agricultural activities were classified as "laborers and hoe workers." The economic status and the nature of the occupational struggle experienced by workers on the land—the major reservoir of those who, migrating, have come to constitute almost one-half of greater Rio de Janeiro's inhabitants—are suggested by several studies summarized by Ellenbogen (1964), and are reflected in the personal histories of patients in the present study. Harris' (1956) study of villages in the Eastern Highlands of Bahia in the early nineteen-fifties gives a picture of how small farms and sharecropper's plots operate. In none was the plow used; the advantages of using fertilizer were known but rarely practiced because of the scarcity of animals; seed selection and crop rotation were largely unknown. Harris placed considerable emphasis on human factors in this situation, including the pattern of individual action rather than group cooperation, timidity over the prospect of an indisposable surplus, and the "extreme dissection" and scattering of arable land due to the inheritance system (p. 88).

Rural workers moving to Greater Rio de Janeiro have almost uniformly experienced a change in the nature although not in the overall category of their jobs. Thus, Instituto Brasileiro de Estatistica da Fundação data based on the first three months of 1968 indicate that for Guanabara and Rio State combined only nine per cent of those who were actively employed worked in agriculture. In 1966, 44 per cent of all Guanabara employees were classified in the Anuario Estatistico as working in "industry" including construction. In the same year, government employees, including military, health, welfare, education, legislative, justice, and administrative personnel made up slightly more than 20 per cent of the economically active population of the state. The rise in the proportion of factory and other industrial workers in Greater Rio de Janeiro during the past decade is part of the national picture of progressive industrialization described by Briggs (1963) and Furtado (1963).

EMPLOYMENT AND LIVING COSTS

In 1966, only 33 per cent of the national population were economically active, and just over 70 per cent of the economically active were being compensated with nothing more than the minimum wage. In Guanabara in 1964, 88 per cent of all working women and 80 per cent of all working men earned less than double the minimum wage (*Desenvolvimento e Conjuntura*, 1966). These earning levels become more telling when they are understood to be the sole source of income for others in addition to the wage earner and when they are examined in relation to the escalating cost of living. Living costs went up 45 per cent in Guanabara in 1965 and 41 per cent in 1966. Rent increased 111 per cent in 1965 and 73 per cent in 1966. During the same period, the cost of food increased 40 per cent and 32 per cent, the cost of clothing increased 29 per cent and 34 per cent. The only solution for the Carioca earning a minimum wage appears to be to work progressively longer hours in the hope of stabilizing the proportion of his income going for essentials. In the beginning of 1967 he had to work five hours longer in order to buy the same amount of merchandise purchased at the beginning of 1966. Since he could not work more than he already did, this meant a reduction of buying power with its related negative effect on production. A standard for comparison is provided by the highest paid classified federal employee (*funcionário federal*), who in 1967 had to work for 17 days in order to pay the rent of a one-bedroom apartment in Copacabana. The rent for a three-bedroom apartment exceeded his total monthly income (*Desenvolvimento e Conjuntura*, 1967).

A final item, rarely considered but important for a worker who must commute long distances from his suburban home to a job in the city center, is the cost of travel. An example of a *funcionário público* in 1968 is a 33-year-old white man employed by the Federal University, who had migrated into Rio from Alagoas 13 years before. Married, with two children, he earned 180 New Cruzeiros monthly, about 30 per cent over the minimum wage. Of this he devoted approximately 40 New Cruzeiros, 22 per cent of his monthly wage to commuting (with an occasional snack), a trip of more than an hour between his job and his home in Duque de Caixas.

ECONOMIC GROWTH AND RURAL CHANGE IN RIO DE JANEIRO

The nature of individual behavior associated with occupational status is illuminated by a scrutiny of recent changes in the rural areas of Rio State peripheral to the urban center. Comparative data from 1953 to 1962 were collected by Haller (1967) in four *municípios* (roughly equivalent to a United States county) varying in distance from between 60 and 120 kilometers from the city center. This period was marked by increases of 15 per cent in the number of non-farm workers and six per cent in farm wage laborers; small farm operators decreased by three per cent and sharecroppers by 18 per cent. The important occupational shift, representing what continues as an accelerating process in the country as a whole, is the transformation of sharecroppers into proletarians, i.e., people who work for others in return for money. This is of particular interest since it involves giving up whatever security and nonmonetary benefits the sharecropper may receive from his *patrão*, the landlord. At the same time, the feudal-like relationship with the landowner may often offer little in the way of real support and, as noted in the chapter on migration, may even be perceived as a form of slavery or serfdom. Proletarianization can also mean a shift from self-employment as an artisan or small farm holder to salaried employment. Whatever the change, it seems likely that wage workers will develop increasing self-awareness as members of a class held together by a need to relate purposefully to employers to whom they are no longer tied by submissive personalistic bonds; the fixed link to a paternalistic *patrão* will be replaced by impersonal, rational, and negotiable relationships.

The move of individual workers to different occupational statuses and the multiplying transactions between center and periphery are reflected in an increasing participation of the population in the surrounding culture. If, indeed, social powerlessness, distance from sources of power, and lack of information increase the likelihood of disturbed behavior, increased social participation might be assumed to promote optimal function. Haller's data show that such increased participation did occur, although at a modest level. Increases of between six and 17 per cent were found in a number of indicators such as formal education, literacy, having children born in a hospital, and sending them to school. The index that increased most sharply was radio listening at levels of from 17 to 46 per cent for the four occupational categories (farm operators, non-farm workers, sharecroppers and farm wage laborers). The index which showed no change was consulting trained medical personnel in case of illness, which was already being done at a high level in 1952.

OCCUPATIONAL POSITION AND SOCIAL MOBILITY

Hutchinson and co-workers (1960) have been interested in structural mobility and in mobility involving ascent of the existing socioeconomic ladder. The former is a consequence of industrial development creating new positions for skilled or semiskilled workers. The latter requires a certain flexibility in the social structure and, therefore, has not been marked. Those who have exhibited the ambition and drive necessary for such upward mobility have been largely of foreign birth or the children of European immigrants.

In order to carry out a study of intergenerational mobility in São Paulo, Hutchinson (1960) devised the six-level scale of occupations used in the present study. The bottom or sixth level includes the lowest prestige, unskilled manual occupations. The bulk of Class VI are unskilled construction, street repair, and agricultural laborers—mainly those described as "using the hoe"—as well as unskilled factory workers. Certain other categories, such as garbage collector and stevedore, are included. The inclusion of waiters in this category, especially in highly urban centers such as São Paulo and Rio de Janeiro, adds a diluent since they are mainly literate and in some respects skilled. Nonetheless, because they serve others by carrying and fetching, they are in a low-prestige category. It seems unlikely in view of their small numbers that their inclusion significantly influences data about Class VI workers in the present study.

Class V, the artisans or skilled manual workers, constitute the most potentially mobile and influential group. These include carpenters, mechanics and other craftsmen, skilled workers such as chefs, transportation workers such as taxi drivers, train and bus conductors, truck drivers, policemen, and skilled agricultural workers, as well as an increasing number of machine operators or production line *operários* in factories. Some uncertainty surrounds the classification of this last group, however, since unskilled assembly-line workers may often describe themselves as *operários*. Taken together, Classes V and VI cover the bulk of all economically active persons in the country and in the present patient population.

Class IV includes the still small number of factory supervisors, construction foremen, and skilled technicians, in addition to small farm owners. Again, the addition of the farm owners may result in the inclusion of essentially unskilled people who have inherited a small piece of land. These amount to a small number in the overall occupational census, however, and are virtually unrepresented in the patient population under study. The "skilled technician" group is confined to Class IV, along with construction foremen and factory supervisors, thus reflecting the continuing lack of a significant group of highly trained technicians to write computer programs, operate sophisticated regulation systems, and perform other tasks requiring education and judgement but not involving the direct supervision of others. The prestigious technical person in the United States is almost always a university graduate, and this would, in terms of general skill, knowledge, and economic capacity automatically place him at the Class I or II Brazilian level.

Hutchinson's three top groupings resemble many attempts at occupational classification in the United States. Class I includes members of the liberal professions, major creative artists, executives, and owners of large businesses and landholdings. Class II includes proprietors or managers of medium sized businesses, factory managers, and school administrators below the university level. Class III encompasses small business administrators and proprietors, minor government administrative personnel, clerical workers, salespeople, the clergy (nonexecutive) and primary school teachers.

Hutchinson (1963) demonstrated that in São Paulo (and he believes the situation to be similar in Rio de Janeiro), there is a general tendency for the "average status" of the filial generation to be higher than that of the paternal generation, the result, in at least two-thirds of the cases, of "structural" factors, mainly new opportunities in the Class V skilled and semiskilled categories. An important part of this upward mobility, however, is based on the achievements of the foreign born: whereas the occupational status of 40 per cent of this of male adults exceeded that of their fathers, 69 per cent of these had fathers of foreign birth. Kahl's (1966) data, too, indicate that the fathers of upward mobile managers and skilled workers in the early 1960's were likely to have been born outside Brazil. Seventeen per cent of Hutchinson's cases were in occupations of lower status than their fathers. Proportionately more of those who themselves were born in Brazil were downwardly mobile than were those who had immigrated into the country. His final calculations, separating out factors due to age and initial status, led him to a figure of 15 per cent each for upward and downward "exchange mobility," (i.e., due to replacement of others within the existing occupational structure). These figures were smaller than those for the United States, Great

Britain, France, and Italy in 1949, the period closest to that in which his data were gathered. His final conclusion was that industrial growth in Brazil, up to the time of his research, had not resulted in a breakdown of class barriers or increased fluidity in the social structure.

Some of the problems involved in attempts to climb the socio-economic ladder beyond the factory operative level are noted in Pereira's (1965) interviews with workers who found their ambitions blocked by real-life obstacles. The importance of education was repeatedly stressed. As one man said, " . . . the *operário* might be able to change his class through study or through money. But he has to have education. This depends on how much courage he has to start out working for himself." Another, " . . . the only way to change class is by studying a good course. This changes a person's relationships completely. The *operário* passes on to become something different. I have a cousin who from being a painter moved to study and became an accountant." But this hopeful note was not often sounded: "One can never reach a higher class. In order to be of middle class a person must study in order to have a different kind of employment allowing a better life." Or, "Unhappily the *operário* is never able to belong to a higher class because the pattern of his life is very low and his salary is low. In order to raise his class he must have more money in his hand and more learning" (p. 152). Kahl (1966) also reported a strikingly high evaluation placed on education by workers at all levels. Both skilled factory operatives and *favelados* rated the right to a free education of first importance alongside the right to equal treatment before the law. Only managers who had had the best education available in the country rated free education in second place, but they too placed it above such other rights as having an effective voice in politics, a minimum wage, and access to state social services.

THE SMALL ENTREPRENEUR IN RIO DE JANEIRO

The highly individual orientations of rural and small-town Brazilians noted by Harris (1956), Wagley (1963), and others, and their reluctance, indeed, their inability to function well as part of a collectivity appear at first glance to have been transplanted to the metropolis. The relative number of specialized craftsmen and individual purveyors of goods and services in the urban setting is not so great as it is in the interior villages where manufactured goods have not completely supplanted home industry, but it is nonetheless impressive to observers from countries where daily goods are predominantly supplied by centralized production and delivery systems, and where a fairly well educated labor force finds steady employment and career opportunities in industry. Because the wish to be "on one's own" or independent of a boss was regularly encountered in conversations with the Class V and VI patients in the present study, some aspects of the small entrepreneurial picture will be described here in detail.

The uneducated man who wishes to avoid hard manual labor or who·cannot keep a job may *fazer biscate*. This term refers loosely to pick-up work, usually on a daily basis. The *biscateiro* may be seen on the beaches where, with stock obtained from a central source, he trudges barefoot, dressed in shorts or green overalls bearing the name of his product, back and forth along great stretches of sand peddling popsicles, ice cream bars, lemonade, or cold *mate*. This last is the bitter tea of the Argentine pampas and the *gaucho* country of southern Brazil in the State of Rio Grande do Sul. He may balance atop his head a cartwheel basket or box containing pineapples which, upon request, he will slice with a *machete*. On the beaches, along their adjoining streets, or on corners in the Centro district, he may peddle balloons, small toys, kites, or almost any conceivable item which he may buy in the morning and try to dispose of by nightfall. Women, usually black, sell confections of sugar and coconut or other foods usually identifiable as Bahian. Children, one step removed from begging, make their rounds, especially through restaurants and busy theater areas at night, selling candies or chewing gum. The population of mobile or transitory peddlers is uncounted. They are economically marginal but they have the satisfaction of not being under orders, of not wielding hoes or pickaxes, of being, in fact, "in business," however minute and ineffective, for themselves. The same is true for the individual venders of services. Shoes are shined by a ragged army of seven- to 14-year-old boys from the *favelas*. Others watch cars while their owners are away. The older service venders are encountered less frequently but the cry of the

THE LOST ONES

knife-sharpener is still heard in the city. On a late afternoon, a gray-haired man with his pedal-driven grindstone supported by a frame mounted on two bicycle wheels, uttered his characteristic long-drawn-out cry and waited for the local housewives to appear. The women of Ipanema in their comfortable apartments surrounding the Praça General Osorio do not regard this hand-operated service offered by an independent, itinerant artisan as a twentieth century anomaly. They are accustomed to dealing with individual entrepreneurs who "take orders from no one but themselves."

Some housewives in this well-to-do section of Ipanema buy part of their food in the supermarket, but this is a recent development. Most continue to go where they believe they will find "the best" in meat, fish, vegetables, or baked goods. In the streets immediately surrounding the Praça, the supermarket competes with a large series of overlapping, duplicating, competing retail outlets differing mainly in terms of the human qualities of their managers and the subtle variations in their products. The *feira,* the mobile street fair or market, is held in most city neighborhoods on an approximately weekly basis. Here, in an expansive array of temporary stalls, the housewife can buy fish, meats, and almost anything else from fresh flowers through bananas to dried black beans or herbs. Many, feeling that they somehow obtain better buys for their money in this unregulated (but actually no cheaper) melange of colors, people, and odors, prefer to wait for the *feira* rather than patronize established groceries.

The repetition of services and the competition by individual small operators for neighborhood business is not confined to food outlets. Within the restricted range of four intersecting streets surrounding the Praça Osorio, and extending for a block in each direction in a heavily residential area, for example, there are two locksmiths who announce keys reproduced in minutes, two shoe-repair stalls, several small household-repair businesses for plumbing, electrical fixtures, and furniture, two stores selling school and art supplies, four newspaper and magazine stands, a hardware and sundry store, and a dozen shops for clothing, furniture, textiles, dishes, records, appliances and more. Some have several employees, but most are operated by the owner assisted only by members of his family.

Within the stores themselves, as with other "business" contacts, every transaction with a customer involves some personal interchange. There is no evidence of hurry or disdain for small purchases, and the opportunity for conversation between customer and sales person is maximized by the number of steps required to complete a purchase. In addition to individual establishments in conventional urbanized areas, all depending to some degree upon the development of a personal relationship between owner and client, are the small stores and bars found within the city's *favelas*. Since their operators buy their supplies at retail prices from other stores, they pass on a markup to their customers, who pay without protest for the privilege of dealing with familiar persons who may extend credit.

DOORKEEPERS, MAIDS AND WATCHMEN

The entrance to each apartment building is manned by, a *porteiro* or two—porters or doormen who scrutinize all who enter or depart and spend much of their day sitting on a chair by the entryway, listening to transistor radios or chatting with friends. Their other tasks, small maintenance jobs or activities necessary to the upkeep of the building, generally occupy little time. The city is dotted with slow-moving construction jobs and reinforced concrete skeletons of buildings temporarily abandoned for lack of money. Each of these also has its contingent of *porteiros* who function as watchmen and remain on duty after working hours and on Sundays, standing or squatting at the entrances to the fences which surround the excavations or scaffoldings. The *favelados* keep a constant lookout for materials which can easily be carried off and sold or used to improve their own dwellings, and the *porteiros* must try to prevent odd bits of lumber or other construction material from disappearing from the site. When work is not in progress, watchmen may be seen sitting patiently on the street near the mobile equipment which can be stripped of rubber or removable parts.

The ubiquitous household employee is the *empregada doméstica* (household employee, or maid, usually known simply as the *empregada*). These women, most often brown or black, are available to their employers most hours of the day and most days of the week.

The usual middle-class Rio apartment contains a maid's quarters, a sparsely furnished room scarcely large enough to turn about in and opening onto the rear balcony, where washing is done and hung and where the service entrance to the apartment is located. For the equivalent of 20 United States dollars weekly, and often less (since the minimum wage laws are not yet fully observed), the maid accomplishes major tasks with little equipment and much physical effort. She may go home at night, or sometimes just one day weekly, to visit with her family in one of the *favelas.* Or she may be single, a migrant who looks to her master or mistress, her *patrão,* for whatever emotional as well as economic security she can. In a large number of instances, the mistress does develop a real feeling of responsibility, and if the *empregada* becomes ill will care for her and even hire another to look after the house. This is not universal, however, and the relationship appears to be vulnerable to disruption in case of mental illness. The physician in charge of the female unit at the Pinel Hospital said that few of the domestics who were patients there would return to their employers because they were ashamed and embarrassed to do so.

The role and status of the *empregada,* who according to various estimates makes up approximately one-third of female workers in Guanabara, is changing, however slowly. In the nineteen-fifties almost all lived in their employers' apartments and were practically without rights. Since the largest proportion were illiterate and unprotected by minimum wage laws, they were "extremely exploited" even in the eyes of a dispassionate Brazilian observer accustomed to paying low wages for long hours. Three factors seem responsible for the change. First, with the increasing number of people able to afford help, the demand began to exceed the supply, and by the late 1960's it became harder to find a reliable, effective person. With increased demand the *empregadas* have become aware of their own leverage. Coupled with the second factor, their increased educational level, they are now more prone to "discuss the price" rather than to passively accept whatever is offered. A third factor is the increasing availability of factory and other work offering on-the-job training for people capable of becoming at least semiskilled workers. Some of the women have taken such employment in preference to housework, but others, have become housewives. Because their husbands are regularly salaried in a manner rarely encountered 10 years earlier, they have a more stable domestic existence than before and can afford to work only part-time while devoting more attention to their own homes. Many of these women, with little education themselves, have the goal of completed primary education for their own children and feel themselves to be increasingly participant members of the society.

THE FUNCTIONARY

The city's office buildings, government establishments, and educational institutions all maintain what appear to the North American eye to be veritable squads of men who act as *funcionários* of one kind or another. Those at the lowest level hover in the background waiting to be given a message to deliver, a visitor to guide, some information which may be laboriously copied or transmitted elsewhere by word of mouth. In contrast to the *porteiros* who dress informally, these men conform to the white collar mold. Their suits may be shabby and their shirts frayed, but they wear neckties and keep a shine on their shoes. Some cover their clothing with blue smocks during the day. Clothing, as well as deferential speech patterns, announces one's status to others. The jacket and necktie, even in the hot muggy days between October and May, are part of the jealously nurtured image of the non-manual worker; his white shirt and shined shoes often seem more important to him than the correction of his functional illiteracy. (The status significance of clothing is seen in the general attitude toward men wearing short pants. Shorts are seen on a few more upper-class males in the beachside districts of Copacabana, Ipanema, and Leblon than heretofore but they are still rare and, along with rubber sandals, are associated in the minds of Cariocas with street-repair gangs and construction laborers. These latter, often dark and barefooted, with stocking caps or forehead bands to keep the streaming sweat from their eyes, are the urban equivalent of the man with the hoe who inspires such contempt from small-town dwellers.)

At a slightly higher level a *funcionário* may be stationed behind a typewriter or at a telephone. Some may be secretaries of high capability but the same general term can describe a clerk with quite limited decision-making responsibilities, such as searching for records and on the basis of what is discovered referring an applicant on to another office. The series of offices through which people must so often go in the course of conforming to the regulations of an overgrown government bureauracy—to get proofs of birth or military service, to obtain working papers, to apply for various social security benefits—can transform applicants into supplicants, and the clerks, themselves, occasionally show the strain of wasteful repetition. The dignified middle-aged man in dark suit and rimless spectacles who sat behind a barred window all day processing passport-renewal applications, showed no emotion at first encounter. A sympathetic comment, however, about his difficulties in lining up the complicated series of multicolored tax stamps (previously purchased at another window) which had to be tediously moistened and pasted into the passport, released an indignant flood of words culminating in an explosive, "*arcaico!*"

The boredom and frustration endured by people capable of more complex and varied tasks in order to have an assured though small income and avoid the ignominy of manual labor, leads to behavior which is described in deprecatory terms. The almost careful avoidance of doing more than is expected of one reflects the lack of a sense of purpose to the work and the fact that upward mobility in the system, if it ever occurs, will more probably be the result of personal connections and *pistolão* (pull or pressure exerted by relatives who know the boss) than of commendable performance. Citizens who must deal with the offices of large systems, particularly in the government bureaucracies, pick their times so as to be sure the *funcionários* they must consult are "not out having a *cafezinho!*"

The Evolution of New Occupational-Social Roles

INDUSTRIALIZATION AND RURAL-URBAN RESOCIALIZATION

Rio de Janeiro's individual entrepreneurs represent the continuing force of the past. *Funcionários* and *porteiros,* although often part of impersonally organized systems and despite many persisting relationships with a *patrão,* also represent the underemployment and human surpluses of a society in development. But the Brazilian in general, and the big-city dweller in particular, is becoming more conscious of himself both as an individual with rights regardless of the patron's wishes, and as part of an occupational group with shared problems and values. ·He is beginning to understand his capabilities, but he is not always ready to engage in joint action in order to achieve shared goals. This dawning understanding reflects the major occupational change of the 1950's and 60's: the gradual development of a new class of industrial workers or factory operatives, *operários*. Between 1920 and .1960 the number of such workers engaged directly in production (excluding unremunerated family members and those in maintenance, transport, and other services) increased by 579 per cent in comparison with a total population increase of 232 per cent.

The *operário* (as will be discussed later) has not yet demonstrated a clear sense of solidarity useful as a basis for social action. As the case histories reported by Pereira (1965) show, in defining himself in terms of his participation in the productive process and in relation to the figure of the *patrão* (the plant owner), he at least hints at a developing sense of recognition of others of his own kind: ". . . whoever lives on wages is an *operário* . . . the foreman is an *operário* because he does almost the same thing as everyone else and also takes orders and receives wages . . . the chief is an *operário* because he is not the owner, not the employer . . ." (p. 143). This definition includes some of those who work in the country, namely, the man who may be called the *trabalhador rural autônomo,* preserving a degree of freedom and independence from the *patrão* because he is paid in cash. With time, the farmer becomes a *faxineiro* (a worker, like a soldier on fatigue duty) in mechanized and routinized agriculture, the stonemason's assistant becomes a truck driver. These and others undergo a gradual resocialization determined by the psychosocial requirements of the industrializing milieu. This development is true to a much greater degree in the city. In 1960, approximately 85 per cent of all employees listed as *operários* lived in urban areas (excluding the almost totally urban construction and public utility workers). Some of these had been small urban proprietors. Following the persisting value orientation, a number who had previously been in factories tried working for themselves after they had accumulated some money. As a furniture factory employee said ". . . people who work for themselves have a better life and more liberty." Typical histories show attempts to manage little shops, drive trucks, or operate bars which failed; expenses were too high, or the earnings were simply not sufficient to support a family. At that point the regular wages and social security benefits of factory work become more attractive.

So far, the main source of beginning workers (not foremen or supervisors, who are more often city bred) has been the country. The resocialization of such persons into what Pereira calls the *personalidade-status trabalbador assalariado* (salaried worker's personality) has been in part the result of the urbanization of rural personalities. For country people, the valued ways of earning a living are those which offer the greatest promise for reducing discrepancies between reality and aspirations stemming from an urban life-style: aspirations which are acquired mainly via the transistor radio, relatives, and friends who return from working in urban centers, and the people in nearby market towns. The residents of these communities, who perceive themselves as profoundly different from the inhabitants of surrounding farms and villages, are oriented to the coast, the federal and state capitals, and Europe.

Rural workers are attracted to paid factory labor, as noted in Chapter IV, in part because of the city's facilities. Industrial work also represents a situation in which, as Pereira's subjects noted, a man may do "clean work," know the "value of his rights," be "more respected by others," be "better treated by the *patrão*," lead "a more dignified life," "live more comfortably even though he doesn't earn much," and, above all, "work without needing to use a machete" (p. 149). The gradual climb up the occupational ladder involving rural-urban migration is illustrated in some of Pereira's interviews. The work histories are representative of those in the present study. A 27-year-old man, for example, with two years of primary school, had helped his father on a small farm in Pernambuco until he was 19. Then he came to São Paulo where for a year he worked as a stonemason's helper. At that point he made the transition to working with mechanical things and spent three years as a locksmith's assistant. At the time of his interview he had spent three years as a mechanic's aide in a small machine-tool plant. He stated his case quite simply: ". . . the first months were quite difficult but after one or two years I overcame the problem. When I first came I didn't even know what a drill was. Now I know." Other comments by a variety of workers indicate the nature of the transition which must be made: ". . . work on the *roca* (the land) is brutal, you don't need to know anything. In industry everything is electrical, and it is very hard for men to learn . . . here the tasks are different, they have to change their entire way of thinking . . . the *pessoa da roca* (man of the soil) knows nothing of machines. He doesn't know how to read or write. He doesn't know a meter either. He is not able to become anything . . . people from the soil have a different *jeito* than the townsmen." (pp 169–171). As noted earlier, the word, *jeito*, in its narrowest sense may be taken to mean "skill." It is usually used, however, to indicate a way of circumventing authority and of "finding a solution" to sticky problems which require flexibility, shrewdness, and some talent for interpersonal dealings and manipulation. In general, the city bred *operário* sees his country-bred benchmate as shy, stupid, untrained, ready to accept any kind of job, feeling inferior, and totally without *jeito*.

Brandão Lopes (1961) paid particular attention to rural migrants' styles of participation on the production lines in a São Paulo factory. These people often came from quasisubsistence economies based on traditional forms of behavior. Nonetheless, all considered a 10-hour factory day easier than agricultural work, even though it meant working apart from family members and required that their freedom to stop working at will was restricted. They consistently expressed, in various forms, disparaging feelings about physical labor— *trabalho mais bracal,* unskilled heavy manual work—but at the same time, the value of working for one's self— *trabalhar por conta propria,* or "on my own," *por minha conta*—contributed to high personnel turnover and low working efficiency. Thus many used their free time to buy and sell on the side, motivated primarily by the hope of accumulating enough money to abandon the factory, usually for independent commercial activity. The latent desire for independence continues to influence the behavior even of those who remain in a job for several years, and, as Brandão Lopes (1961) noted, ". . . any cause of dissatisfaction may bring this to the surface and so affect his conduct" (p. 242). At this point the wish to receive dismissal compensation as a start for an independent business may motivate a deliberate lowering of output in order to be discharged. For its part, management, with the idea that all employees become inefficient after some years, begins to discriminate against semiskilled and unskilled workers (who are easily replaced) even before lowered productivity becomes apparent.

Another contributor to the rural migrant's difficulties in adapting to the new environment and his persisting wish for independence may be the nature of his former relationship with the *patrão*, the owner of the land on which he was forced to gain a living. While the relationship fostered a degree of passivity and probably gratified certain dependent needs, it was inevitably conflictful. It led to debt-dependence, and, as Pearse (1961) has stated, the countryman "was obliged to accept a situation in which he was an inferior partner to a contract . . . all the weight of advantage was on the side of the *patrão*" (p. 201). In town, while distressed at the lack of a personal relationship with the boss, the rural migrant finds that the government has become his protector, guaranteeing him a minimum wage and a variety of social welfare benefits. Yet his assurance depends upon continued employment by the anonymous factory, a state described by Pearse as ". . . the powerless independence of the urban worker who is linked to the power-center solely by the cash wage nexus . . ." (p. 202).

Additional light is shed on the relationship between industrialization and individual behavior by Kahl's (1966) comparison of the attitudes of top-level executives attending a management course, highly skilled workers in a single São Paulo plant, and Rio de Janeiro *favelados*. While the workers approved it, *favelados* and managers joined in deploring the loss of personal contact between employers and workers accompanying industrialization. The skilled operatives emerged, in general, as more unconditionally committed than the managers to the work and organizational values of the modern industrial enterprise. Competition was least sought by the unskilled *favelados*, most of whom were not committed to their present jobs. Like the operatives, but unlike the managers, they wanted eventually to go into some type of independent work.

THE DEVELOPMENT OF OCCUPATIONAL COLLECTIVITIES

Among the background elements contributing to the migrant's adjustment problems in the work situation is the absence of experience in collective action beyond kinship and immediate neighborhood relationships. Relating on the basis of similarity of position in the industrial structure is totally new, although as indicated above, the *operário* soon learns how to define himself in relation to others. The union itself is perceived as something made not by him, but for him by others. Joint action according to Brandão Lopes (1964) is still more often based on personal friendship or kinship relations rather than formal membership in the group of workers. Reluctance to become involved in movements to elevate wages or working standards, ". . . because I have nothing to do with this," was especially marked among those coming from Bahia and farther to the Northeast, vitiating attempts by the city-reared to initiate joint action. A clear animosity between these groups was apparent. At the same time, however, there did exist a vague solidarity on the basis of shared latent and vague conflict with *"os patrões"* (the owners or the bosses). In case of discord between an *operário* and high-level management, for example, his companions, workers of equivalent rank, watched the conflict with interest, expressed satisfaction if the *operário* won his point, and avoided anything which would impair his case. In 1957, when Brandão Lopes was gathering his data, there were no production norms developed by the workers as a group. The main influences were individual interests and traditional values and patterns internalized while growing up in the rural communities. Traditionally then, there is a lower limit of effort, ambiguously defined in terms of *cumprir a obrigacão* (to do one's duty) in the sense of not becoming too careless or flagging, and an upper limit, *a gente não deve se matar* (one should not kill oneself working). If the worker did become careless or deliberately reduced his production there were always employees in less well-paid jobs wanting to work on the line; even on the most difficult machines, training required no more than a month. Substitution, therefore, was easy—at least when consent was not legally required because of the definition of a particular job—and most workers' persisting individual orientation prevented a group reaction against it.

The transformation in the late 1950's of *operário-patrão* relationships in two small-town factories in the interior of Minas Gerais is described in another volume by Brandão Lopes (1967). His findings are relevant to the present study, for they indicate the cultural evolutionary process through which the large majority of patients are going in regard to the human environment of work. In the factory described by Brandão Lopes, employees were traditionally selected and promoted on the basis of a network of personal loyalties; they themselves expected concessions regarding the hiring of relatives, time off on special occasions, and so on; conflicts were reduced and resolved on the basis of direct and personal arrangements between workers and supervisors, and some workers would bypass foremen and go directly to the owners. These latter occupied important political positions in the community which made their power over the workers almost absolute. Then, external events interfered with the pattern of paternalistic domination and submission. There occurred a crisis in the textile industry involving prices of raw materials as well as finished goods, competition increased, the price of labor went up, and new labor legislation was enacted. The owners met the crisis by lengthening the working day, requiring higher production levels, increasing the rent on company-owned houses, and using more minors and women. They did not recognize the new legislative standards. This generated a slowly developing feeling of rejection and resentment among the workers, who finally, and with a great deal of inner as well as interpersonal conflict accompanying the rupture of traditional emotion-laden relationships, formed a union. With the formation of the union and the worker's awareness of his own potential power, the decomposition of former patterns accelerated. As Brandão Lopes noted elsewhere (1966): "Even using the union's president for voicing one's grievances is a disloyal and rebellious act in the eyes of the traditional employer. The ties of obligation and loyalty have been broken. A cumulative circular process of change is established, and behavior and relationships get farther and farther away from the patrimonial patterns. The process is irreversible; the slow dissolution of patrimonial ties results" (p. 72).

Collective action expressed in the form of strikes has been increasing. It has even extended to such traditionally static individuals as bank clerks. Their union, the Sindicato dos Bancarios of Rio State (primarily in Niteroi), for example, threatened in August, 1968 to paralyze all banking operations in that area if demands for wage increases and a 10 per cent emergency bonus were not met. In the same month, the fiercely independent taxi drivers *(motoristas de taxi)* of Rio de Janeiro city staged a two-day strike preceded by noisy hornblowing processions through the streets and an unsuccessful attempt to block all traffic on one of the main thoroughfares. In this instance, however, the strike was not precipitated by financial considerations but by the inefficiency of the police regarding a series of murders of drivers in the hours surrounding midnight.

Collective action is gradually expanding to rural areas. An example of agricultural workers banding together for self-protection in this respect is the Association of Northeasterners of Ituituiaba (described in the chapter on migration).

In the summer of 1968, the press reported (still on the back pages) the incarceration in a private prison and physical punishment inflicted on workers in a ceramics factory in Chiador in the Zona da Mata of interior Minas Gerais. This treatment followed breakage of finished ceramic pieces, reporting late for work, not buying food or other supplies at the company store, and other activities which displeased the managers. The harsh situation finally resulted in the arrival of a busload of workers at the headquarters of the civil construction and industrial union in Juiz de Fora some distance away, and the eventual referral of the matter to a district court. Several features make this case instructive, beginning with the fact that it can still exist in modern Brazil. None of the author's professional colleagues doubted the veracity of the story (which was finally checked by officials from the Secretariat of Security). They all agreed, that similar, although less extreme, situations probably existed which did not receive such publicity. The exploitation of manpower, with little regard for individual rights, appears to be facilitated by the workers' passivity especially in relation to a powerful *patrão*. In the Chiador case a bizarre note was added because the managers were 17-year-old twins, sons of the owner and nephews of a well-known ambassador. According to newspaper accounts, their behavior was influenced by exposure to too many *"revistas de cow-boy."* Even temporary submission to such treatment at the hands of capricious adolescents, whether of a powerful high-status family or not, would be unthinkable in most industrialized modern countries and probably in urban Brazil. It was possible in part because of the isolation of the factory located on a large *fazenda.* The 104 factory operatives had been recruited from the ranks of the "hoe workers," and most still lived on the land where they had once been sharecroppers. The main point, however, is the eventual development of an orderly collective appeal to higher authority by workers, who only a few years earlier might have been inclined to preserve their relationships with the owner and suffer in individual silence.

In general, the large masses of rural workers have been relatively unmoved by calls for agrarian reform. This is partly because increases in wages and buying power have had a powerful impact on people who were formerly in the functional status of serfs. Caido Prado Jr. (1964) regarded the new buying power of the utterly deprived sugar workers of the Northeast as resulting in an "emptying" of the "revolutionary character" of their demands. In January and February of 1964, these workers, among the most miserable and exploited in the nation, by virtue of their own organization, achieved an almost tenfold increase in wages. Rural laborers who had hardly known of their existence began acquiring beds, sheets, trousers, transistor radios, and even items for self-adornment or for improving personal appearance—*artigos de toucador,* (literally, articles for the dressing table), all of which have significant implications for the growth of self-respect, a sense of viable identity and social power, and increased ability to communicate. The tendency to act collectively in time of crisis, a tendency which contrasts with traditional value systems, is also reinforced. A chain of circumstances, each of which contributes to the increasing self-determination of workers as individuals and in groups seems to follow any modification in the original premise. As Furtado (1963) pointed out, putting sugar workers on a wage basis meant a change in their spatial distribution. They were no longer scattered over the land on small shares of the owner's property on which they had planted subsistence crops. Instead, they were gathered into hamlets along the roads, thus facilitating communication among them, with the resultant more rapid spread of ideas and the emergence of leadership where none had previously existed.

Occupational Outgroups and Rehabilitation— the Unhospitalized Mentally Ill

THE LOWEST RUNG. SERVICO DE RECUPERAÇÃO DE MENDIGOS

Begging is an important means of survival for many in a society with the largest absolute numbers of illiterates and migrants or wanderers of any nation in the hemisphere. Beggars or *mendigos* constitute a major pool of the unidentified mentally ill and, as suggested below, their separation from responsible relatives contributes to their underrepresentation in the mental hospital population. The mulatto child from a nearby *favela*, the gaunt-faced, tan-skinned young woman holding a dirty infant, the stubble-bearded, shabby man of middle age or older—these, as they extend their hands with palms turned upward, are familiar figures on the streets of Rio de Janeiro. Beggars may be roughly classified into three groups: the professional, the occasional, and the sick. The professionals include some who have developed a routine, or a "story," who usually have a favorite post in an area with many passersby, and who follow regular hours like other self-employed persons. The occasional beggars are those who are intermittently or seasonally employed, who have migrated and been unable to find a steady source of income, or who have experienced a business failure or been discharged from a job. Some of these last have already been through a rehabilitation center and are unable to find work. The occasional begger becomes enmeshed in a process from which it is increasingly difficult to extricate himself. Without money he doesn't have a place to go to wash or shave. He needs a haircut. As he becomes dirtier and more unkempt it is harder to find a job. Discouraged, he may begin to drink, or more frequently resume the drinking which was often a cause of his unemployment.

The sick category is mixed and overlaps with the others. Some in this group are acutely ill, while others may be chronically mal-functioning, e.g., they have anemia secondary to malnutrition or parasitosis, or bronchiectasis, or some other physical disorder re-sulting in weakness, fatigue, and lack of ambition. In this catego-ry, too, are the chronic schizophrenics, mild mental retardates, and people with borderline cerebral deficit following injuries, strokes, or degenerative changes. Some of these have developed stable routines and locations; others are wanderers. To an extent they are semiprofessional beggars.

In the middle 1960's, national attention was drawn to beggars as a group after the Rio de Janeiro police killed several by throw-ing them from a bridge. Stories circulated about secret murders and other police methods for dealing with the *lixo humano,* human garbage, or as more technically oriented persons called them, members of the *classa marginalizada.* These were the people who, when they did work, would *fazer biscate* and who when they were sick or otherwise unemployed would beg. The public outcry fol-lowing the police murders stimulated the opening of the service for the Recuperation of Beggars, a unit of the Guanabara Secretariat of Social Services. This department opened it doors in 1966, along with a dormitory shelter accommodating several hundred people, the Abrigo Cristo Redentor (Shelter of Christ the Redeemer) which takes care of some of those who at other times find tempo-rary shelter in the Albuergue Joao XXIII.

The Service has three sections. One is concerned with picking up potential inmates. Its two cars are in full-time use, cruising areas of town most frequented by beggars or going out in re-sponse to calls. The police are now expressly prohibited from col-lecting or otherwise participating in the process. A second section provides social service care. This may be making contacts with family members, referring the beggars to other agencies, helping them return to their home communities, and making arrange-ments for employment. About 80 per cent are sent on to other public or private agencies. The third section is for medical, in-cluding psychiatric, service and employs a psychiatrist for four hours each day. Approximately 40 per cent of all the beggars coming to the Center as of mid-1968 have required hospital eval-uation of medical or psychiatric conditions, and 10 per cent have been actually hospitalized or admitted to public institutions.

In addition to these three sections, a rehabilitation center located along with the Abrigo in the suburban district of Bom Successo, was started in 1967 in Campo Grande in Rio State. This is an old *fazenda* on which shops for vocational training and facilities for acquiring agricultural skills are available. After a pilot period, it acquired its first group of long-term rehabilitees in May, 1968, and by August was operating with 230 clients in residence. Unpublished statistics for 1967, its first full year of operation, show that there were 3,151 admissions to the Beggar's Service, of whom 23 per cent were repeaters. Three per cent of those admitted left without permission because, according to staff members, they were afraid of being killed by the police.

The clients were predominantly male (65 per cent), but included 253 children—usually accompanying their mothers. Color statistics were not kept, but approximately two-thirds of those seen by the author at the Service in August, 1968 were shades of brown, with the remainder divided between white and black. They were older than the population at large. Twenty-four per cent were over 50, with another 24 per cent between ages 41 and 50. This suggests that for many begging is a means of coping with the social deterioration and inadequacy which accompany loss of youthful vigor and optimism. Only 23 per cent of the beggars were less than 30 years of age and none, in comparison with the 50 per cent of all Brazilians, were less than 18 years of age.

Ninety-seven per cent were migrants, with the greatest number —64 per cent—coming from the East, chiefly Minas Gerais and Rio State.

According to the psychiatrist at the Abrigo Cristo Redentor, in the six months' sample following July 1, 1967 he saw approximately a third of the admissions for consultation. Of these, 43 per cent were diagnosed as alcoholic, and he felt that another 15 or 20 per cent could be regarded as having drinking problems. Twenty per cent of admissions referred to the doctor were schizophrenic. These alcoholic or schizophrenic persons, mainly male, included about 10 per cent of the entire population, and most were of middle-class origin. A typical story was that they had lost their jobs, and shocked and dismayed their families by their behavior. Most had been taken to folk healers early in their psychotic career and had become worse. Many had been hospitalized at least briefly in private sanitoria. When money was no longer available for this support they were not, as might have been the case in the United States, sent on to public facilities. Instead, most were allowed to wander away from home without restraint, and their families made no effort to maintain contact with them. The social worker said that most families are not interested in resuming contact, although they may be willing to do so if the client is in the process of apparently successful rehabilitation, and especially if they become convinced that he is serious in his wish to give up alcohol. The remainder of the psychiatric consultations were divided between mental retardation (nine per cent), cerebral arteriosclerosis (nine per cent), and those for whom no diagnosis could be made or who were sent to the Pronto Socorro for further observation (11 per cent). There were a few cases each of senile dementia, general paresis, and epilepsy.

The outlook for those who pass through the Beggar's Service is uncertain. They remain at the Abrigo as long as necessary for the collection of social data and the medical or psychiatric evaluation. Those who have acquired skills at Campo Grande have had no difficulty acquiring jobs, either as paid agricultural laborers, or in the city as carpenters or construction workers. The doctor, however, was not optimistic about their not relapsing into alcoholism, and he was especially impressed by the qualities of passivity and dependency which reduced the likelihood of their attaining self-sufficiency.

VOCATIONAL REHABILITATION AT EMAUS*

The Communidade de Emaus do Brasil is a center for the rehabilitation of homeless men. It is patterned after one in Paris, and there are similar centers in Argentina and Chile. Operated by the Banco da Providencia, described in the chapter on mental health services, it was founded in March, 1963 by Dom Helder Camara. The center will be described here in some detail since it represents another concentration of people who, given family support and

---

* Emmaus House in New York City is the name taken by a group of young intellectual radical Catholics, led by members of the priesthood, which maintains a special interest in civil rights, protest, and antiwar movements. Emmaus (or Emaus depending on language) is known as the place where Christ was recognized by his disciples only after they had broken bread with him.

the proper combination of chance, might also have become mental hospital patients. The milieu-therapy aspects of the center also reflect the cultural pattern of relating to an authoritative, hopefully benevolent patron.

"Emaus," as it is popularly known, is located on the road to Petropolis about 45 minutes from the Centro. It is surrounded by a high whitewashed stucco wall with an entry road barred by a railroad gate. The gate house is manned by two residents who must call the main office for permission before allowing visitors to enter. The community, including dormitories, mess-hall, shops, offices, and a large meeting hall, stands on about five acres of ground bordering a refuse cluttered marsh which merges into the placid scummy waters of a river extending south of Rio de Janeiro city. Part of the site is filled land, and Emaus has permission to reclaim as much as it can.

During 1967, 697 men had been in residence at Emaus for varying periods. The reduction from a high of 927 seen during 1966 occurred because so many were reluctant to leave; they had no homes to which to return and they had formed positive attachments to the community. At any one time there are about 300 residents, of whom approximately half are returnees. Their average age is in the late twenties and there are usually about 30 adolescents with a median age of 16. In mid-1968, about two-thirds of the group were unmarried, and the same proportions were illiterate and black or brown. Two-thirds were migrant, with half of these coming from Minas Gerais or Rio State and half from Bahia and the Northeast. Most arrived through the headquarters of the Banco da Providencia or the Albuergue Joao XXIII (described in the chapter on migration).

The community operates on a strict daily schedule. The rising hour is six A.M. with coffee, milk, bread and butter served at 6:15 A.M. Work begins at 6:50 A.M. and, with a brief interruption for lunch, continues until four in the afternoon. Dinner is at five P.M., lights out and silence at 11 P.M. Punctuality at meals is rigorously enforced, and anyone five minutes late does not receive a tray. Discussion of religion and politics is forbidden, nor are political or religious newspapers or magazines permitted on the grounds. This is regarded as consistent with the community's function as "a center for reeducation—professional, moral, and civic." The work with which the days are filled serves as vocational rehabilitation and as a means of sustaining the community. The bakery, kitchen, laundry, and several other sections take care of the needs of the residents. In addition, products are sold through the annual *Feira* of the Banco da Providencia, and occasionally elsewhere. These are produced in shops for carpentry, upholstery and mattress making, tailoring, shoemaking, and cabinet making. Men assigned to the bricklaying, electricity, machine repair, and transport sections are actively at work expanding the community; Emaus residents have built all the structures on the site. At the time of the author's visit, a group of men were adding an extension to one row of shops. They were raising, tile by tile, without benefit of a plumb line, what was to be the front wall of a medical consulting office. They worked slowly but steadily, using crude hand tools of the kind seen on many Brazilian construction jobs. In addition to the working sessions, all illiterates are required to attend classes in reading or writing. Plans are underway to initiate a "cultural program." This will be implemented by the creation of a library in just completed space, and by a series of lectures and discussions in the recently completed meeting and recreation hall.

Members of the community receive housing, meals, clothing (made on the grounds), medical and dental care, and a weekly allowance equivalent to about $2.00 in U.S. currency. Gambling is forbidden. For the first eight days no privileges are granted. Afterward they may be absent from Saturday noon until six A.M. Monday, but not during the week except with specific permission. If they are not back by the required hour they are automatically discharged. Admission and departure from the program are voluntary, but if a man leaves without discussion with the director he loses the privilege of being readmitted.

There is no fixed duration of stay. After three months (but it may be six or 12), if a man seems to have acquired "good work habits" and the necessary skill he is referred to the Banco da Providencia for job placement which is never a problem. The need for people with the basic elements of literacy and a few manual skills is constant. These men are not trained for work in a fully industrialized or technical society, but Brazil has not yet reached the position of the United States where the "hard core" unemployed, mainly literate with manual skills, are unprepared to fill openings requiring complex decision-making or high-level technical tasks. Graduates of Emaus are needed in small plumbing, baking, lock-repair and similar establishments as well as in the small factories in the peripheral zones of Rio de Janeiro. This is still a society in which, for example, it is difficult to buy inexpensive standard sized mattresses of good quality—a housewife will go to an upholsterer to have one made and the upholsterer's assistant might be a former resident of Emaus.

One life story of a better educated Emaus resident was that of a staff member, an *adjunto*, who had arrived in search of help a few months after the community opened. Now in his fifth year, with the community, he did not, despite a gray complexion and bloodshot eyes, appear to be more than 40. He had arrived in Rio from Bahia at age 16, lived with an older brother, completed secondary school, and become a salesman. Repeated drunkeness, however, resulted in his losing one job after another until he was finally reduced to the life of a semivagrant. Coming to the Banco da Providencia to try to arrange a loan, he had been referred instead to Emaus. Although he had often thought of leaving, he was satisfied with his life as a responsible *adjunto* and anxious about living alone and becoming self-sufficient. Now, however, a new career possibility had opened up. In December, he and several others who had been there for similar lengths of time, all members of the directive group as section chiefs or entrusted with tasks of a semipermanent nature, were going to form a cadre of men for a new Emaus community, either in Belo Horizonte or São Paulo.

The atmosphere of the community stemmed from its director, a stocky French engineer in his mid-forties with light sparkling eyes and rapid, spirited speech. He had been working in Brazil for three years and was ready to return home when he had been recruited for the job. He had consented to stay for a year in order to get the community started, but quickly became so involved that he decided to remain. He described the program with tremendous enthusiasm, using such expressions as, "the men really work," and "there is real discipline though it is voluntary." He described his administrative system as "pyramidal," with decisions going down from him through section chiefs concerned with discipline, work coordination, and general service, and on to the specific shop-oriented groups. As he put it, "The men here have suffered so much ... they are submissive ... not accustomed to making their own decisions." It was clear from his manner and the way in which the residents responded to him that he was in the position of a stern, benevolent, loved and even charismatic father, inviting no participation from anyone else in the process of making decisions and in some respects holding the whole system together through the force of his own personality. He made a point of keeping in touch with as many Emaus "graduates" as possible, once a month touring nearby factories and shops, the "faithful clients" who employed them. He reported with great gratification that Emaus alumni sometimes returned to visit, even when on army leave. There seemed little doubt that he satisfied the workers' and residents' need for a strong paternalistic *patrão*. His attitudes were rational, supportive, and uncompromising. Thus, while acknowledging the great prevalence of problem drinkers among the men, he said he did not regard heavy drinking as "alcoholism—a disease," but, like most deviant behavior, a reaction to life stress, deprivation, and frustration. In a supportive, disciplined milieu with suitable rewards for good behavior, he felt there should be no problems. As confirming evidence he noted that of 300 men who departed for the weekend only eight returned intoxicated.

The director expressed great pride in the equipment and buildings created by the residents and in their developing capacities. Later this pride was echoed by the *adjunto* as he escorted the visitors around the various sections, and by the subchiefs, all of whom insisted on demonstrating the products created by the men working with them. At noon the men ate in the large mess hall at crude tables, each seating four to six people. They served themselves cafeteria style on trays which, on the day of the visit, contained copious servings of spaghetti with tomato sauce and a stew made with tomatoes and tripe. Afterward, in the brief rest interval, they talked quietly with each other or sat alone. They wore shapeless blue drill shirts and trousers, and rubber sandals—all of their own manufacture—or old clothes of their own, sometimes shorts. A few were in a small garden which they had made themselves. In the dormitory for *menores* (minors) youngsters leaned against their doubledecker bunks. These, with ancient, baggy straw mattresses, were scattered at random over the room. Nonetheless, the boys, like other members of the community, seemed to have feelings of personal achievement, and especially of belonging, feelings which must have been rare in their lives just prior to admission.

THE PATIENT SAMPLE

The largest number of patients in the study population, 43 per cent were in the Class V category, skilled manual workers. These included some factory operatives, mechanics, repairmen, chefs, carpenters, certain construction workers, e.g., stonemasons, and others who worked in shops and small businesses and whose primary concerns were with objects. Also included were those such as policemen, railroad conductors, truck and taxi drivers, who, while operating machines, dealt significantly with other people. The predominance of Class V workers in the patient sample is due to the fact that so many came from the INPS service of Casa Eiras. Upper-class patients are more apt to be found in private and Class VI patients in public mental hospitals. Twenty-nine per cent of the patients were in Class VI, the unskilled manual category. This included irregularly employed *biscateiros*, laborers mainly in construction and road repair, factory workers, *porteiros*, and others. Three per cent of the sample, including the occasional full-time student, were considered unclassifiable. In order to provide a group sufficiently large for analysis, the 25 per cent covering Hutchinson's Class I through IV were combined. These were concentrated mainly in Class IV (8 per cent) and III (13 per cent) of the entire sample. These two categories included factory and construction supervisors, skilled technicians, secretaries and clerks, government *funcionários*, primary school teachers, and small proprietors and managers, i.e., individual commercial entrepreneurs. Class I and class II, with two per cent each of the total sample, contained professional men (including writers and artists and executive clergy), business executives, higher level educators and primary school executives, and factory managers. The top three classes appear to share similar attitudes and values. Class IV, with the factory supervisors, may occupy an intermediate position in this respect between the artisans and the white-collar workers.

Only 15 per cent of the entire group admitted to holding a regular second job, including seven per cent in Class VI and three per cent in Class V categories. These were typically "independent" activities outside of organizational contexts. All of those in Class VI, however, and the majority in Class V acknowledged irregular or occasional paid work as private contractors outside of their usual occupations. (*Biscateiros* by definition have many independent small jobs.)

Female patients with no primary occupation other than housewife were categorized in accordance with the employment status of their husbands or, for the one per cent unemployed and unmarried, of their fathers. Of the 35 per cent of the total sample which was female, 53 per cent classified themselves primarily as housewives and were tabulated according to their husbands' occupational status (even though some did part-time work outside the home). Forty-three per cent reported that they engaged in outside employment and functioned secondarily as housewives or, if unmarried, as homemakers; these were classified according to their own occupational status. Three per cent were listed as unclassifiable or undetermined. With these considerations in mind, 97 per cent of all the female patients were classified as follows: Class I-IV, 26 per cent; Class V, 47 per cent; and Class VI, 24 per cent. This distribution is virtually identical with that of the men. The employed wives of Class VI (nonpatient) husbands were, themselves, almost exclusively in positions of that category, mainly as domestic *empregadas*, or unskilled factory workers. While this was true for many of the patients who had Class V husbands, a few more of these were employed in clerical or skilled manual positions rather than as maids or houseworkers. This is a group more interested in education and prestige and apparently poised for upward mobility.

Three per cent of the total patient population who prior to migration had worked only as housewives began outside employment after coming to Rio de Janeiro. Another 11 per cent (male and female) of the total classified themselves as permanently unemployed prior to migration. A number of these had succeeded in finding work in the city; thus, only 3 per cent of all of the patients stated that they were permanently unemployed at the time of the study. An additional 3 per cent described themselves as retired or permanently incapacitated. Forty-two per cent said that they were temporarily unable to work because of their present illness. In general, the patients appear to have been relatively constant in their occupational activities, aside from shifts associated with migration. Less than one per cent reported any change in basic occupational category after young adulthood, although many had changed jobs within occupational classes. Only six per cent said that they had changed permanent jobs as part of an active search for socioeconomic betterment. Another 13 per cent had had several jobs, but always "doing the same thing" in different contexts. Approximately two-thirds had always answered directly to a *patrão*. In spite of wishes to be "independent," only five per cent said that they had never been employees and would never consider working for someone else. In contrast, 17 per cent reported that their fathers had always been self-employed and had never wanted to be an employee. Of the fathers, half had always answered directly to a *patrão*.

Each patient had his own occupational story, different in detail but similar in pattern to many others. An example of an employed unmarried woman is a white fourth grade graduate of 24 who lives with her parents, four brothers and three sisters in Madureira in the home where she was born. At age 18, motivated by a wish for independence and against her parent's wishes, she went to work for the telephone company. At first she was a *funcionário*, a low-level clerk, but she soon became a switchboard operator. She is proud of her work and her financial capacity, accepting as a matter of course her continued residence at home.

Another unmarried woman, a white 23-year-old, lives with her mother and two brothers in Aboliçao in the urban zone of Meier, the area of her birth. She completed primary school and has been working since she was 16, full-time since age 18. She has been a part-time *empregada* and a waitress, but didn't like being at the beck and call of a mistress or of customers. For three years she has been an unskilled *operária* in a lamp factory, stating that she prefers the impersonality of the supervisory system. She says that she earns more than her late father, although he was a mechanic.

An example of the way in which newly available factory positions for women increase the likelihood of friendship and social activities outside the extended family is seen in the following. A recently married woman, a brown 21-year-old from Paraiba, came with her parents and siblings to Rio de Janeiro when she was 10 years old, having terminated her schooling with the second grade. By the time she was 14 she was almost completely self-supporting as an *empregada*. By 18 she was bored, felt restricted, and heard from her friends that factory work paid more and was less constraining. She obtained an unskilled job as an *operária* making ceramic tiles. The work and the relatively low pay are unimportant to her because she has made good friends among her co-workers and has a husband who also brings home money from his job as a construction worker. They and their three-month-old baby live in a *vila* in the industrial zone of Meier.

An example of an unemployed woman is a brown 22-year-old third grade graduate, who, coming from Espirito Santo during childhood, lives with her parents and four brothers in a *vila* in Nilopolis in Rio State. She assumes much of the responsibility for cooking and cleaning house for the family. Her father, in his early fifties, was a paid farm laborer before migrating. Now he is a skilled manual worker for the railroad.

An example of a downwardly mobile person is a white 30-year-old bachelor, a graduate of the second *ginásio* year, who left school because of family financial difficulties. Born in Meier, he now lives with his parents in Botafogo. He works as a *porteiro*, and is upset because he is worse off economically than his friends whom he knew in school. His father, a transplanted Pernambucano, is a career army officer (Class III) now in reserve status.

A person upwardly mobile within his father's class is a white 35-year-old bachelor, a fourth grade graduate born in Mangue, who now lives in Tijúca with his married sister and her family. A typesetter, he is satisfied with his work and proud of being considered a "high grade professional." His father was a Class V *funcionário*.

An illustration of the drive for independence is seen in a white 33-year-old married man, born in the residential Vila Isabel section of Tijúca, who still lives there with his wife and six children. A graduate of primary school, he is a fireman skilled at handling the high-pressure water apparatus. He also raises pigeons, describing this as working for himself, *"por conta propria."* Nonetheless, he is dissatisfied, feeling that he has been slipping economically and is worse off than his father was at his age. His father, now in his early sixties, is retired from a job as night watchman at a mental hospital.

Another example of someone with a second regular job is a white married 35-year-old bookkeeper, a *colégio* graduate with three children. He also works regular hours as a clothing salesman but he is worse off economically than last year. This is partly because, having moved out of his father-in-law's house, he must now pay rent.

Frustrated strivings for upward mobility are illustrated by a white 40-year-old primary school graduate who had worked for his father on a small farm in Paraiba since early adolescence. Later he moved into a small town and was apprenticed to a stonemason. At the age of 30 he migrated south to São Paulo, but after several months decided that he could not make a living and came back north to Rio de Janeiro. Although he is supporting himself, a wife and two step-daughters, he is not satisfied with his occupation and is thinking about "studying" to improve his status. He is pessimistic about this, however, believing that he is too old to try something new and that, anyway, the acquisition of more education will not guarantee a better job.

Approximately 30 per cent of the male patients spoke spontaneously of previous hopes for upward occupational mobility; almost all had been uniformly unproductive of sustained results. A streetcar conductor had, upon migration from another city, obtained the same job in Rio. He was bored with the work, but didn't think he could get a better job. A shoemaker, attracted by the public acclaim, had daydreamed for several years of becoming a fireman. A railroad-crossing guard beleaguered by the expenses of an enlarging family had made several job shifts, all within Class VI, during the five years preceding hospitalization, in an unsuccessful attempt to improve his financial status.

Social Characteristics

The following analyses are for three basic groupings of patients according to occupation. They will be designated in terms of Hutchinson's classifications: I-IV, V and VI. Fifty-two per cent of those in Class I-IV are in Hutchinson's Class III. These are low-

level administrative, commercial and clerical personnel, small proprietors, primary school teachers, and non-executive clergy, i.e.,
according to United States' terminology, the white-collar class.
Thirty per cent are Class IV, the skilled blue-collar and supervisory
class. Eight per cent and 10 per cent are in Classes II and I respectively.

SOCIOECONOMIC INDICATORS

Data on literacy and education are shown in Table 103. The
distributions are as expected, with a direct relationship between
increasing occupational status, literacy, and education. The overlap is not complete, however. Only 28 per cent of those in Class
VI, for example, are totally illiterate, and a surprising 6 per cent
of those in Class I-IV are not literate. Similarly, although less
surprising in view of the inadequate educational facilities, almost
a quarter of those in Class I-IV had not completed primary
school. Class V, as in respect to most other indicators, occupies an
intermediate position.

Housing, as shown in Table 104, was also directly proportional
in terms of quality and space to occupational level. Between a
quarter and a third of the Class VI workers lived in shanties or
had no essential services. The Class V workers were closer to those
in Class I-IV in terms of housing.

Table 105 reveals several trends with respect to area of residence. More than half of those in Class I-IV lived in urban or residential areas, in contrast to Class VI of whom more than half
lived in suburban or industrial districts. It had been expected that
more of the stable Class V workers would inhabit the suburbs,
but while their concentration approaches that of Class VI, the
balance is swung by the 40 per cent of them who live in urban
and residential districts. Relatively few in Class VI lived in neighborhoods known as *favelas*, even though, as noted above, from a
quarter to a half inhabited *favela*-type housing. Approximately a
third, the highest proportion of any occupational group, lived in
peripheral small towns or semirural areas within Greater Rio de
Janeiro, many of which are in Rio State. In this respect Class VI
workers overlap with those who are recently migrant and nonwhite. Those in the least skilled and remunerative jobs occupy

the least expensive dwellings at the greatest distance from the city center, save for the marginals, regularly employed workers who have made homes in stable centrally located *favelas* (some of which have been established for as long as 35 years), and transitory occupants of lodgings in the obsolescent central districts. While the peripheral dwellers must spend long hours getting to their jobs, they sometimes have the advantages of being able to maintain small gardens and a chicken or a pig to supplement their meager rations. Some *favelados* also keep an animal or two for food.

SOCIOECONOMIC MOBILITY

Despite frequently voiced wishes to be better off, the sample as a whole was not characterized by consciously expressed occupational discontent, nor had the patients' lives in the year before hospitalization been marked by major economic reverses. Thirty-six per cent of the total patient group described themselves as content with their occupational accomplishments and only 19 per cent as discontent. The remainder declared themselves neutral or were unable to give a definitive response. Of the total group, 37 per cent each felt their economic status to have improved or declined in the year preceding hospitalization while the remainder believed it to have remained stable. Forty-four per cent of the sample regarded their economic status as better than their fathers' and only 20 per cent as worse, with the remainder unchanged or unknown. The constant presence of unremitting work in their lives is suggested by the finding that 18 per cent of all the patients and at least 25 per cent of their fathers (for whom the data was undetermined in 47 per cent of the cases) had begun to work for money prior to age 14.

The patients' estimates of their socioeconomic status according to occupational category, as it progressed during the preceding year and as it compared with that of their fathers is shown in Table 106. Similar proportions in all groups felt their status to be lower than their fathers'. These subjective ratings are virtually identical with data on paternal occupation in Table 110 showing that 23 per cent of Class VI and 19 per cent of Class V workers had indeed experienced downward intergenerational mobility:

their fathers had been in Class V or Class I-IV. The similar proportion, shown on Table 106, of 18 per cent in Class I-IV also reporting socioeconomic inferiority to fathers must be assumed to have remained in the same occupational category while earning less money or to have dropped from the professional-executive to the white-collar or supervisory level. In general, these downward mobility figures for the patient sample resemble those reported by Hutchinson for the population at large. Eleven per cent of the entire patient sample (excluding those within Class I-IV) were downwardly mobile.

More than half of Class I-IV, and about a third each of the skilled and unskilled manual workers rated themselves as having achieved higher socioeconomic status than father. Table 110 shows that approximately a third of those in Class I-IV had, in fact, experienced upward intergenerational mobility, in equal proportions from Class V and VI. Only a little over half of them had had the advantages of their present level during childhood. Approximately a third of Class V, a proportion similar to the subjective reports of improvements (Table 106), and almost twice the proportion who had descended from fathers in Class I-IV, also showed upward intergenerational mobility from Class VI (Table 110). The number of those in the total patient sample in higher occupational categories than their fathers (excluding changes within Class I-IV) was 23 per cent.

While downward intergenerational mobility may be plausibly considered a consequence of psychiatric illness, such illness, as noted above, did not prevent upward mobility into Class I-IV and V by 23 per cent of the patients. The degree to which this may be considered structural mobility, i.e., a consequence of the increasing number of skilled and white-collar jobs to be filled, is unknown, but the data presented earlier suggest it as a major factor. As shown in Table 106, significantly fewer in Class VI felt that they themselves had improved, while fewer of Class I-IV rated themselves as having declined during the past year. Class V self-ratings in this respect indicate more feelings of improvement than in Class VI and more of decline than Class I-IV. The remote possibility of upward mobility via study and greater effort was touched upon during interviews by approximately a quarter of the men and none of the women. In almost every instance, rumination on this subject was discouraged, tentative, and inconclusive.

MIGRATORY STATUS

As indicated on Table 107, Class VI workers were more often than those in the other classes relatively recent arrivals into the area and came after maturity. That is, they were not socialized or educated in the Rio environment. More than a third of those in Class VI had migrated into Greater Rio de Janeiro within the preceding five years. Four-fifths of Class VI migrants and smaller proportions in the other groups had come from rural areas. Class V migrants were closer to members of Class I-IV in this respect than to Class VI.

While it is true that significantly greater percentages in the two lower categories migrated because of lack of jobs, the differences between VI and V are not large. Of the total Class VI group, more than a third had changed specific jobs after migrating, but almost all remained in the same occupational class. The shift from agricultural labor, "with the hoe," was mainly to carrying and hauling or construction activities (bricklayer's helper) in the city. Of the Class V group, 17 per cent were upwardly mobile from Class VI and two per cent downwardly mobile from Class IV in consequence of migration. All of the six per cent of Class I-IV who had changed occupations after moving had ascended from their premigratory statuses. There were no shifts among those previously employed in the top three categories. In other words, those people with skills and the highest level occupational records before migration were employed in similar capacities after coming to the new environment.

In summary, downward mobility associated with migration was negligible. In contrast, 16 per cent of all migrants had achieved upward occupational mobility in association with their move to Rio. The eight per cent of all of the patients whose upward mobility was associated with migration, constitutes approximately a third of all of the occupationally ascendant in the sample.

DEMOGRAPHIC CHARACTERISTICS

The familiar direct relationship between skin color and socioeconomic level is demonstrated in Table 108: the proportion of nonwhites increases with descending occupational status. There are no statistically significant differences according to age or sex.

Proportionally more of the Class V workers were married, perhaps reflecting a more stable and conventional social situation for
these upwardly mobile persons than for either of the other two
categories. The Class VI workers, more of whom came from poor
rural families, report larger families of origin than the others.
Similarly, more of them than the Class I-IV patients, of whom
equal numbers were married, report having produced four or
more children.

Data on religion, reported in Table 109, show that more of the
Class V and VI workers (in similar proportions) than those in
Class I-IV have embraced Protestantism, Spiritism or an Afro-
Brazilian cult in place of Catholicism.

Table 110 shows that to a significant degree the proportion of
illiterate fathers increases with descending occupational status,
while the proportion of literate fathers increases with ascending
status. Proportionately more patients of skilled or nonmanual status had literate fathers.

INFORMATION AND SOCIAL PARTICIPATION

Table 111 shows that ownership and use of informational media increase with ascent up the occupational scale as with levels of
education, literacy, and skin lightness. The use of newspapers,
magazines, and books is similar in the two lowest occupational
classes, which fits other data indicating a major break in educational achievement accompanying the step from manual to nonmanual jobs. The fact that fewer Class V than Class VI patients
are regular movie-goers may indicate that they have other sources
of amusement or other responsibilities.

Table 112 also adds support to the picture of Class V workers
among the patients as having beeen more thoroughly integrated
into their communities than the others. As noted earlier, those
who need it most, in this instance Class VI workers, appear to
have least contact with the clergy and with welfare agencies.
Despite the overlap between recent migratory and Class VI status, the Class VI workers, unlike the recent migrants as a group,
did not report most frequent attendance at dances but the soccer
data confirm the supposition that relatively more of the manual
working classes than the nonmanual are regular fans.

HOSPITALIZATION AND FAMILY DIAGNOSIS

The bulk of Class V patients, 86 per cent, were seen at Casa Eiras, reflecting the fact that most were employed with social security coverage for illness through a contract between the INPS Institute to which they belonged and that hospital. The relatively small proportion of Class VI workers seen in Casa Eiras occurred because 36 per cent were admitted at the Pronto Socorro. Only 10 percent of Class I-IV patients were seen in the Pronto Socorro; they made up the highest proportion of any occupational group, 16 per cent, seen in the private Sanatorio Botafogo.

Table 113 shows that the only circumstance precipitating hospital admission in comparable fashion for all deprived groups is paranoid, externally directed behavior. This was a leading reason for admission among the illiterates, the uneducated, and the recently migrant as well as the Class VI workers. There was, however, no consistent indication that physically expressed or "acting-out" behavior was a more important event leading to admission in the Class VI than the other occupational groups. In fact, physical assaults were equally divided among the groups, with more of the Class I-IV than the manual workers admitted because of bizarre acts. Additional evidence suggesting Class V as a psychologically "middle-class" group tending to internalize problems and with families sensitive to evidence of depression, is seen in the fact that proportionately more, though not significantly so, of these workers than those in I-IV or VI were admitted following anxious, depressed, or suicidal behavior. Interviews, however, as noted below, revealed more actual suicidal thoughts and threats among Class I-IV.

Table 114 shows that more of the families of Class V patients labeled their behavior in terms of illness, mental or physical. Class I-IV families thought most, in terms of reaction to life stress rather than illness and Class VI did so least.

PSYCHIATRIC AND BEHAVIORAL CHARACTERISTICS

TENSION, ANXIETY, SENSITIVITY, AND FRUSTRATION

In the interview itself, differences in the patients' tension and anxiety as well as social class were reflected in the psychiatrists'

subjective responses. Table 115 shows that the interviewers invari-
ably felt more involved, cheerful, and interested with those in
Class I-IV, liked them and felt liked by them. In most instances
there were few differences between their responses to Class V and
Class VI, in spite of evidence suggesting the former as a more socially conventional group. In other words, there was a clear break
in terms of the interviewer's feelings and attitudes between the
manual and the nonmanual workers rather than between the
skilled and unskilled manual. The single finding of statistical
significance was that proportionately fewer of Class V were regarded as hypervigilant or distractible. These results are impressive because they do not fit the interviewers' biases. As suggested
by their subjective responses, the data do not follow a clear continuum from least to most deprived. They appear, rather, to reflect
some specific characteristics of the skilled manual worker group in
contrast to the others. These may plausibly be inferred as increased security and a sense of positive identity.

Anxiety symptoms are listed in Table 116. Environmentally
(job) related worries increase significantly—consistent with reality
considerations—as occupational level decreases. Diffuse anxiety,
and fear of loss of control over specific acts, this last to a
significant degree, were most frequent in Class I-IV. These
findings generally fit previously reported tendencies for more educated upper-class people to exhibit obsessive tendencies while the
less educated focus more on body function. In general, the functioning of Class VI workers was more disrupted by anxiety than
that of the other two groups. As indicated above, however, there
is no consistent progression up the occupational scale and Class V
appears more stable in some respects than Class I-IV.

Other indications that Class V is less vulnerable than either
Class I-IV or VI are found in Table 117. Significantly fewer exhibited interview hostility or felt that others regarded them as
mentally or morally inferior. Fewer, although to a lesser degree,
reported significant achievement/aspiration discrepancies, felt
uncomfortable or isolated with others, or engaged in impulsive
acts. There were no marked differences between groups in regard
to the expression of anger.

DEPRESSION

Table 118 shows that between a quarter and a third of Class I-IV expressed suicidal fantasies, wishes, or threats—considerably more than members of the other two groups. There were no marked differences, however, between groups in the frequency of reported suicidal attempts. Similarly, more of the Class I-IV were self-accusatory and felt inadequate or guilty than members of the other two groups, which did not differ markedly in this respect.

Class V rather than Class I-IV patients were more open in expressing feelings of sadness and depression to the interviewer, though not significantly so. This is congruent with their more frequent reporting of high-intensity feelings as a problem. Conversely, fewer were rigid, flat, or apathetic during the interview, and fewer reported absent or dulled feelings. Despite these differences in expression, however, comparable numbers of Class V and Class I-IV patients said they often felt sad and like weeping. In the face of the high proportions of illiterate and recently migrant in Class VI, this occupational group, in comparison with the others, failed to show a proportionately greater frequency of depressive symptoms. The only depressive indicator more frequently reported by Class VI patients concerned body weakness and inferiority. These findings suggest that depressive feelings should not be regarded in a unitary way, but that their components may vary differently in respect to social class linked factors. Thus, physical symptoms would be more important to manual workers dependent upon their bodies for livelihood, while guilt and inadequacy would be more relevant for upper-class persons driven by internalized aspirations which they cannot meet. An alternative conceptualization would not refer to "components" of a depressive constellation, but rather to the means of expression of depressive problems via action, thought, feeling, or sensation. This would be concerned with channels of emotional, physical or cognitive communication, or tension discharge sanctioned or inhibited in particular social strata.

THE BREAK WITH REALITY

Differences between groups in the expression of general paranoid feelings were small. Table 119 reveals statistically significant differences in feelings of being stared at or talked about, and that others are not trustworthy. For every indicator, the most frequent reports of paranoid feelings come from Class VI but there is no general progression from highest to lowest occupational status. Fewer or similar numbers of Class V than of Class I-IV make paranoid statements. Again, the evidence suggests that occupational status is related to behavior in a manner somewhat different from educational or literacy status. Class VI exhibits the suspiciousness and outward orientation of the culturally disconnected, as seen in the groups divided on the basis of literacy and mobility. Class V members, many of whom are also poorly educated and nonliterate, seem, however, considerably more secure and exhibit a greater sense of personal worth. In other words, achieved occupational status appears to outweigh illiteracy and lack of education in reducing vulnerability to paranoid behavior in this patient population.

Class VI patients as listed in Table 120 report markedly more hallucinatory phenomena than members of the two other groups. This finding resembles that found among illiterates, recent migrants, and blacks. Slightly more than half the Class VI patients, approximately twice the proportion of those reporting from the other group, heard voices; and more than a third, or over three times the proportion of the others, hallucinated human figures. Approximately three times the proportion of the other occupational classes insisted on the reality of their experiences, and five times as many planned specific action based on them. Such insistence and planning sometimes accompanied an acute episode, but more often was part of a chronic psychotic picture or a retrospective comment about an acute episode which had precipitated admission. Proportionately more also reported less well-crystallized visual (but not auditory) experiences, i.e., of lights or amorphous figures; and more tended to misinterpret stimuli during the interview. Some of these differences may be associated with the higher incidence of religious, folkloric, or ghost-connected phenomena in this group. The reported frequency of hallucinatory experience for Class V and Class I-IV patients was virtually identical.

Problems in orientation which may be related to the frequency of hallucinatory experience, especially in the presence of brain damage or toxic states, are listed in Table 121. These occurred most often at the lower occupational levels—among illiterates, recent migrants, and blacks—and decreased progressively as the scale was ascended. Temporal disorientation of at least a transitory nature was reported or observed in 42 per cent of the Class VI patients. This figure is almost twice the frequency for those in Class V, and more than three times that of Class I-IV.

SOMATIC PROBLEMS

As noted earlier, Class VI patients expressed more organ anxiety than members of the other two groups. The general tendency of unskilled manual workers who have become psychiatric patients to complain about their bodies more than those at higher occupational levels is shown in Table 122. Without exception, Class VI patients reported more symptoms of a somatic, hypochondriacal, or psychophysiological nature than Class V patients. This was true to a statistically significant degree for any physical pain or discomfort, headache, fatigue, and dizziness. There is a progression with descending occupational status of concern about the head, but in most other respects the two manual categories tend to resemble each other in the proportional frequency of typical complaints. As in the case of depression and some aspects of interview behavior, these findings are not identical with those of the population divided according to literacy, mobility, or color. They suggest that being illiterate, nonwhite, or recently mobile may be important determinants of the behavior of unskilled manual laborers, but that the fact of depending upon such labor for survival is the key element which results in the higher reporting for this group of all kinds of body related symptoms.

SEXUAL BEHAVIOR

Approximately 30 per cent of each group stated that their current sexual pattern was associated with their present illness, and about 40 per cent reported that worries interfered with sexual functioning. Table 123 indicated a statistically significant difference with respect to long-term monogamous relationships. Reported most often by Class V patients, these support the impression that this group is perhaps the most socially stable of the three. The significantly higher proportion of sexual concern among the literate and educated with its converse, is not reflected in these data. This probably is in part due to the higher proportion of browns (with sexual problems) within Class VI.

Past Psychiatric History

As indicated in Table 124, Class I-IV reported significantly more childhood sleep disturbances, perhaps because these were more noticable in their family settings. More of Class VI, the unskilled manual workers, reported histories of head injuries with loss of consciousness, which could be due either to lack of preventive care or to the greater hazards to which they were exposed. Conversely, it is possible that for some, the early trauma produced the conditions resulting in their remaining at the lowest occupational level. The degree to which such injuries or cerebral malfunction predisposed them to loss of reality contact in the event of high anxiety, mental illness, or intoxication is uncertain. It may be recalled, however, that such findings did not characterize the illiterate but rather the partly literate. As noted earlier, cursory physical and neurological examinations performed on all study subjects yielded no consistent findings according to any social category.

Discussion

In general, education, literacy, lightness of skin, ownership and use of informational media, residential stability, and the nature and location of housing in the patient sample vary directly in quality and degree with ascending occupational status. But while Class I-IV are almost exclusively white, suggesting that dark skin is an obstacle to occupational advancement, all three occupational categories include patients at all levels of literacy and education. The same is true for housing and area of residence.

The skilled Class V workers tend more often than members of other groups to be married. They are less frequent movie-goers, closer to their neighbors, and have more useful and friendly contact with clergy and welfare workers. These findings suggest that

Class V persons, as represented in the patient sample, may be considered a type of pre-bourgeois, better integrated into their community, and perhaps with more stability and security than the shopkeeping or white-collar class in an inflationary economy and a society in which skilled labor retains high importance and desirability. Consistent with this is the finding that Class V families more often attributed patient behavior to illness than to value-related judgements. Occupational stability at this level is not, however, associated with stable membership in the Catholic church. Consistent, formal, practicing Catholicism still appears associated with membership in the highest occupational statuses closer to traditional sources of power.

The interviewers' confort, interest, and empathy, as expected, were greatest with Class I-IV, who were most similar to them, and whom they rated as most "cooperative." Class V patients, nonetheless, were more secure, less anxious, less hostile, and less rigid, flat, or apathetic during interviews than those in either of the other two categories. Similarly, fewer complained of feelings of inferiority, social discomfort, or isolation.

The behavioral findings also fit the impression, based on social charactcristics, that occupational Class V constitutes a relatively stable, affectively involved, but not burdened, personally concerned, conforming, achieving segment of the developing social structure, perhaps comparable in terms of values and approved behavior to a mixture, although not yet crystallized, of Hollingshead's United States social class III and IV (Hollingshead and Redlich, 1958). Anxiety and depression do not disrupt their usual behavioral patterns so easily as in the unskilled group, there is less tendency to externalize and project, and less tendency to either withdraw or attack. At the same time, while showing their depression, they are less self-destructive, impaired by guilt, or withdrawn than the nonmanual groups.

In a few respects the symptomatic behavior of Class V patients resembled that of Class VI or could be placed on a continuum between VI and I-IV. Thus, environmentally related worries, e.g., about jobs, increased with descending occupational status. The same was true, although less markedly so, for anxiety attacks, organ anxiety, and insomnia.

In a number of respects findings in this chapter resemble those in the United States in which occupation is a key element. Kornhauser (1962) demonstrated that the higher the occupational level among factory workers classified by skill levels and variety of work operations, the higher were scores indicating "good mental health." His findings also suggested that occupational mental health differences persist apart from the influence of education. In his study, proportions of workers having good mental health, consistently decrease from higher to lower level occupations within each of three educational categories (grade school, some high school, and high school graduation). For youthful workers, the magnitude of differences in mental health according to occupation was very nearly the same, regardless of education. Among middle-aged workers, mental health was best among those high in both education and occupation, and poorest for those low in both education and occupation. Differing with the suggestions of other investigators, Kornhauser concludes that the occupation-mental health relationship is independent of the pre-job background or personality of the men who enter and remain on the several levels of work. This conclusion is based partly on the findings about education and partly on the results of an extensive investigation into childhood conditions, behavior, attitudes, and aspirations. In short, his study suggests that mental health is dependent upon factors associated with the job. Some of these may be: lower pay, economic insecurity, lack of self-determination, unpleasant working conditions, relations with supervisors, monotony and repetitiveness of work, status considerations, and mobility blocked by social factors. The world of the Rio de Janeiro Class VI worker includes all the negative elements found in that of the repetitive semiskilled worker in the United States (the lowest in Kornhauser's study), plus the physical weight of fatigue, inadequate protection from injury or special hazards, and for many, the psychological problems of illiteracy and rural background.

McMahon's experience (in Riessman et al., 1964) with unskilled United States factory laborers coming for consultation about their sons provides a population similar to the regularly employed Class VI Brazilians. Most of them verbalized complaints about themselves of a physical or work nature. To feel tired or "weak" after a hard day's work was not incompatible with their masculine self-image. Later, however, in contrast to the Brazilians who generally deprecated physical labor and spoke constantly of their wish to be "on their own," the counselor found it easy to elicit "the pride that these men felt in their manual work, provided they were given cues about the author's interest in the exact nature of their daily task." What the father "did" was " . . . one slice of his 'adequate' profile." At the same time, they deprecated their value as occupational models: "Can I ask my son to be like me—a factory worker?" (p. 298).

Srole et al. (1962), in the Midtown Manhattan Study, provide perhaps the most complete data of comparative interest. Their home survey sample of non patient respondents aged 20 to 29 revealed that differences in the "sick-well ratio" (mental health) were significantly tied to differences in the SES of their parents. Except for generalized tension-anxiety, all symptom dimensions revealed a significant inverse correlation with SES origin. Downward on the parental SES scale, for example, there were increased tendencies to somatization and psychophysiological symptoms, depression, hostile suspiciousness, self-isolating tendencies, and rigidity and immaturity (suggesting difficulties in impulse control). It seems plausible to infer that these differences "were predominantly implanted during the preadult stage of dependency upon parents and were brought into early adulthood rather than initially generated there" (p. 216). At all age levels the sick-well values are progressively larger as SES origin descends. Thus, " . . . progression through adulthood carries in its wake further precipitating or aggravating pathogenic effects for the vulnerable people from all SES-origin groups" (p. 220), and the greater vulnerability of those of low SES origins is maintained. On the basis of a literature review and their own experience, Srole and his colleagues postulate that upward mobility requires appropriate aspirations and efficient personal mobilization, for both of which sound mental health is important; they suggest further that accomplished upward mobility and its rewards increase mental health, while downward mobility and its associated deprivations and rewards have the opposite result. Their data confirmed these postulates, with marked increases in the sick-well ratio down the scale from upward to stable to downward occupational mobility in relation to fathers. Healthier sons replicated the positions of fathers in the top occupational positions, while the less healthy sons more often moved down to be replaced by healthier men ascending from fathers at lower levels. These investigators suggest that in general "those in the ascending traffic stream are subsequently less likely to show exogeneous deterioration in mental health than those in the descending stream" (p. 228), an idea confirmed by their finding that personal SES is even more sharply related to adult mental health than is parental SES.

Compatible findings with psychiatrically labeled persons have been reported by Turner and Wagenfeld (1967) in Monroe County, New York. They showed that substantially smaller numbers of schizophrenics are upwardly mobile in respect to occupation and a greater number are downwardly mobile relative to their fathers than in the general population, and that downwardly mobile schizophrenics show a more severe drop than downwardly mobile nonschizophrenics. At the same time, while a small percentage of the schizophrenic sample showed downward movement within their own work histories, the large majority, 83 per cent, were surprisingly stable in terms of the character of jobs held. In other words, they found a downward social drift for the sick individual—presumably following the onset or intensification of symptoms—to be a relatively minor contribution to the heavy representation of schizophrenic patients in the lowest SES. They conclude that the major factor in this overrepresentation is social selection, i.e., the failure of persons destined to become psychotic to gain the expected occupational level in spite of educational and other advantages.

Langner and Michael (1963), in the second volume of the Midtown Manhattan Study, delineated a relationship between SES, mobility, and specific patterns of psychiatrically labeled behavior. Low SES persons in their study showed proportionately more delusions, withdrawal, dissociation, rigidity, suspiciousness, and dependency. They did not plan ahead (a characteristic associated with fatalism) and were more prone to depression, feelings of futility, lack of belongingness, friendlessness, and lack of trust. At the same time, they were more authoritarian in their attitudes, stressing obedience, power, and hierarchical relations. The high SES persons showed more anxious, worrisome states, hypochondriasis, self-dissatisfaction, and various signs of tension. Downward intergenerational mobility was associated with character disorders or disturbances in personality traits, and such persons were more apt to be alcoholic than the static lows. The upwardly mobile in comparison to the static highs, were more likely to be obsessive-compulsive or schizoid, but less suspicious, rigid, or depressive than those in their stratum of origin. These findings for nonpatients in the community resemble those of Hollingshead and Redlich (1958) for identified patients in a treatment or custodial relationship. Among the character traits associated with downward mobility noted by both investigative groups are depression, rigidity, and suspiciousness. On the basis of their own findings and those of others, these authors suggest that low SES persons in their sample are characterized by (1) a weak superego, (2) a weak ego with lack of control or frustration tolerance, (3) a negative distrustful, suspicious character with poor interpersonal relations, (4) strong feelings of inferiority, low self-esteem, fear of ridicule, and, (5) a tendency to act out problems with violent expression of hostility and extra punitive tendencies. They associate these characteristics with failures of child rearing, including training for redirection (or, following Hollingshead and Redlich, sublimation), training for a sense of identity (including constant reminders of one's replaceability and lack of uniqueness), and training for communication.

Another dimension to the behavioral analysis of people in the lower income strata was added by Miller (1963 in Riessman et al., 1964). His basic categories include those who are poor but both economically and familially stable; the strained, with an unstable family pattern including life-cycle problems, i.e., "wild" younger workers or alcoholic older ones who disturb family functioning; the copers, who, while having serious economic difficulties, manage to keep themselves and their families intact; and the unstable. This last is "a category of unskilled, irregular workers, broken and large families, and a residual bin of the aged, physically handicapped and mentally disturbed" (p. 146). Their life "is crisis-life, constantly trying to make do with string where rope is needed." These factors lead to a chronic pattern: "Low-paid and irregularly employed individuals do not develop an image of the world as predictable and as something with which they are able to cope. Controlling or directing events appears . . . an unattainable achievement. When they suffer long-term unemployment, they are less likely than other unemployed who have had the experience of fairly regular employment to maintain a personal stability" (p. 147).

The psychiatrically significant behavior of the three occupational Brazilian groups resembles many although it is not identical with United States findings. In particular, behavior does not necessarily vary directly with descending SES. Some differences also appear related to the harsher environment and lower degrees of competence of the bottom-rung Brazilians, i.e., in terms of illiteracy, almost absolute lack of education, and relative failure of collective organization leading to marked powerlessness and hopelessness. Thus, for example, the lowest occupational class of Brazilians most often presented hypochondriacal or body-related complaints. Specific psychiatrically labeled behavior according to occupation overlaps to some degree with that of the patient population divided according to indices of socioeconomic status and cultural integration described in previous chapters. It may be seen, however, in a particular association with occupational category as related (1) to having achieved a relatively new and satisfying status with the promise of further improvement and of an increasingly strong and stable sense of identity (Class V), (2) to having been unable to advance or having dropped backward on the occupational ladder, due either to extrinsic environmental factors or to intrinsic, intrapsychic, or personal factors and struggling for economic survival from crisis to crisis (Class VI), and, (3) having acquired status mainly by virtue of parental help and more favorable early conditions and now being threatened by changes in social structure, values, and interaction patterns incident to industrialization (Class I-IV).

Members of all categories in this study are temporary psychiatric drop-outs from the occupational struggle. All are subject to severe and continuing economic stress. The quality of stress, however, differs between groups. For Class VI it is the effort to maintain marginal status, to earn or scavenge enough to obtain an inadequate diet, inadequate shelter, and to survive. For Class I-IV it is the battle to stave-off the threat of a declining standard of living in the face of inflation, and to deal with the constant frustrations experienced by educated people with middle-class aspirations who lack the money to achieve them. Perhaps the stress is least for Class V, the members of which may be assumed to have achieved and acquired more than in the past, to be more adequately integrated into the society than Class VI, and to conceive of themselves as moving in an upward direction rather than just trying to survive or fighting against imminent downward mobility.

CHAPTER 8

HOUSING, URBANIZATION,
AND PATIENT BEHAVIOR

THE GRADUAL development of self-awareness among the slum dwellers and their first tentative moves in the direction of power is a significant evolution within the Rio de Janeiro setting. The morphology of the city and its various subareas were described in detail in Chapter I. Like all the great cities of Latin America, Rio de Janeiro is inundated by a population whose growth has outstripped the pace of industrialization. The city cannot offer its newcomers the job which they require in order to rent, purchase, or build adequate dwellings for themselves and their families. Thus, less expensive and undesirable sites in central urban and some predominantly industrial zones, as well as rural parts of adjoining Rio State (included in Greater Rio), have become the home area for many of those at the lowest socioeconomic levels, including recent immigrants from the country. Moreover, the local government is incapable (in part because of an insufficient tax-producing population) of furnishing the supporting services needed to "urbanize" its growing edges and pockets. The conversion of an agglomeration of shanties, erected without regard for order or accessibility, and without electricity, sewers, or running water, into living space which might encourage the healthy development of families and communities seems an enormous task. When the shantytowns, which themselves house from 20 to 25 per cent of those who constitute the metropolis, are added to the substandard dwellings in more established neighborhoods, the outlook for immediate relief seems dim indeed.

THE FAVELAS

The growth of slums or *favelas* is perhaps the most characteristic aspect of Rio de Janeiro's disorderly urbanization. Only a small proportion of the study population comes from defined *favelas*, but those coming from substandard housing live in neighborhoods which share many *favela* characteristics. The *favelas* as physical and social realities are salient features of Rio de Janeiro as a context of behavior. Squatter's shanties, rural in appearance and clinging to hillsides or clotted in lowlands, fill the interstices between the sea, the uninhabitable mountainous rocks, the gleaming skyscrapers, and the residential quarters. Pearse (1961) credits a writer for the weekly *Manchete* with the history of the name given these slums by veterans of the late nineteenth-century War of Canudos. While pressing their claims for pensions, they chose to live on Providence Hill overlooking the War Ministry. They called it Favela Hill, from which the final assault was made on Canudos; this last so called because of the bitter, stinging *favela* plant growing on it. In the same era, immediately after Emancipation in 1888, according to Costa Pinto (1952), many recently freed slaves also settled in the Rio hills.

The National Census Service has adopted relatively strict criteria for the definition of a *favela*. It is an "urban agglomeration" possessing in whole or in part the following characteristics: more than 50 dwellings, predominantly rustic, made of sheets of tin, zinc, boards, tar paper, or scrap material; constructed without licensure or supervision on land controlled by third parties or of unknown ownership; mainly without a sanitary network, lights, telephones, or running water; in an area not officially urbanized in the sense of being numbered, surveyed, or plotted. By the time of the 1960 census there were 147 settlements of this nature, all with specific names. These contained 335,063 persons. This massive figure represented approximately 10 per cent of all city residents and an almost 100 per cent increase over the past 10 years, but even so, it is not generally regarded as an accurate representation of current substandard and "un-urbanized" housing in the area. A survey conducted by the Instituto de Pesquisas e Estudos do Mercado in 1957 reported that 650,000 of the population (then two million) lived in *favelas* (Pearse, 1961). A 1961 police report published in Correio da Manha (Bonilla, 1961) put the number of Rio *favelas* at 194 and estimated their population at close to one million. In December 1967, the Fundação Leao XIII, the major Guanabara state-supported operational agency of the Secretariat of Social Services, identified 230 *favela* neighborhoods including an estimated 162,741 dwellings and 757,696 people. In 1968, representatives of the Secretariat of Social Services, not concerned with the narrow criteria of the census, informally estimated the number of *favelas* in Greater Rio de Janeiro (including some parts of Rio State) at approximately 350. These identifiable settlements, together with smaller clusters of similar dwellings wherever unclaimed space permitted, were thought to contain from 900,000 to a million people, or between a quarter and a fifth of the metropolitan population.

Favelas originally grew as a result of natural population increases, but migration was to become a more important contributor to their growth. In 1930, two major factors led to increased migration into the city, especially from nearby states : A sudden fall in agricultural prices made it increasingly difficult to survive in rural areas; at the same time, the government supported the growth of new industry. Moreover, many families were expelled from slums leveled in the old central sections of the city. As tenements and collective dwellings, often in formerly luxurious mansions, were torn down and replaced by business buildings, some lower paid workers moved to the suburbs, but many resettled on the hills. According to the United Nations report on the World Social Situation (1957) this movement first assumed large dimensions in the 1930's. Increasing land values which made most suitable building areas unattainable, the central location of available jobs, and the drastic inadequacy of bus and rail transport continued to stimulate the search for space within the city itself. The *favela*, then, became for the displaced city worker, and for the immigrant, as Pearse (1961) put it, "a means of establishing himself and his family as an unbroken unit in the shortest possible time, and with the least possible outlay, in his own house, in conditions similar and sometimes superior to his country home" (p. 195).

The shanties found in *favelas* and in vacant spaces throughout the metropolis have been classified in terms of the main materials from which they are constructed: *Casa de alvenaria* (of masonry or brickwork); *casa misto* (made of a hodgepodge of materials); *casa de pau-a-pique* (a mixture of sticks, stones and dried mud, sometimes strengthened with plant fibers, with some qualities of adobe—a type of home often seen in rural areas). In general they represent, as Pearse noted, " . . . the intrusion, into the interstices of an urban system of life, or rural standards of housing . . ." (Ibid).

Some characteristics of *favela* housing may be abstracted from the 1960 Guanabara Census data which include information on 69,690 private dwellings in *favelas*, defined according to the criteria noted above. The median occupancy level (present in 19 per cent of the dwellings) was four people, but the range was wide and 13˙per cent were occupied by eight or more individuals. Three rooms were the average and about half the space in each shanty was used for sleeping. Approximately 23 per cent of the dwellings were attached to the general water supply, but only 14 per cent of the total had a faucet inside the home. Another 10 per cent depended on their own well or spring. Inhabitants without these facilities carry their water, often up long flights of stairs, from communal pumps. The pumps are social centers and the women who carry the water, in old olive oil or other gallon tins balanced atop their heads, expect to spend some time gossiping and resting while awaiting their turns. The pump areas are also used for washing clothes which are then carried back up to the shanties where they are hung out to dry. Fifty-five per cent of the dwellings were described as having sanitary installations. These ranged from toilets attached to septic tanks, to simple drains into sewers, and plain dug trenches. The remaining 45 per cent of the homes did not have even this last rudimentary facility. Excretion is regularly performed elsewhere, judging from the visible remains under bridges, in erosion gullies or gutters, or wherever minimum privacy can be achieved. Almost 94 per cent had some kind of cooking stove, mostly burning oil or kerosene. Seventy-eight per cent had at least one electric light, but the number attached to the general electrical system was not recorded. Radios were owned by 60 per cent of the *favelados*, refrigerators by seven per cent, and television sets by one per cent.

The long-established central sections of Rio still contain over-crowded multifamily units and lodgings for unattached men. Some of the terms designating these are : *cortiço* (literally, "bee-hive," a unit of which is described as "a rented room of the lowest class in a private home"); *cabeça de porco* ("pig's head" or a flop-house bed); and *vaga no quarto* (a room which must be vacated for other sleepers during the day). Among the crowded and more popular types of units found most often in peripheral parts of the city are the *vilas* in which rows of one-to three-room dwellings open onto a common courtyard or corridor. These are ostensibly occupied by single families, but upon closer inspection often prove to contain at least two, usually united by ties of blood or marriage.

Nineteen-sixty census data for the non-*favela* neighborhoods of Guanabara offer some standard for comparison with *favela* hous-ing. Of 708,218 private dwellings, 75 per cent, or more than three times the proportion in *favelas*, had piped water (almost all with at least one inside faucet). This compares with a PAHO (1961) estimate of approximately 50 per cent of the total Brazilian ur-ban population with water service in their homes. Ninety-three per cent, 15 per cent more than in the *favelas*, had at least one electric light, and 89 per cent, or 34 per cent more than in the *favelas*, had some type of sanitary installation. Non-*favela* housing differed markedly according to location. While water, electricity, and sanitary facilities were present in over 90 per cent of the ur-ban non-*favela* homes, this was true for only seven per cent of those in the suburbs (approximately eight per cent of the total houses surveyed). They were present in only one per cent of those in rural Guanabara (approximately two per cent of the total houses surveyed). In other words, in the 1960's substandard hous-ing was general in suburban Rio and the rule in rural parts of Greater Rio de Janeiro. None of the patients in the present sam-ple who reside in rural areas, mainly of adjacent Rio State, have homes with electricity and piped water. This supports the general observation that the quality of *favela* housing resembles that to which countrymen have previously been accustomed before mi-gration and, in fact, often represents an improvement. Even the communal pump and the long walk with household water can at first be better than dependence upon an irregular and polluted river or well. With time, however, the countryman turned city slum dweller becomes sensitive to the discrepancy between what he has and what he might have, to what he has seen in his daily contacts.

Five per cent of the non-*favela* homes described in the census depended on their own wells or springs, leaving 20 per cent using other sources or not responding. Most had a stove, generally operated by gas. Radios were owned by 85 per cent, almost half had refrigerators, and approximately 27 per cent reported television ownership. Occupation density was similar in non-*favela* and *favela* homes although, on the average, the former were one room larger. The median occupancy of these homes were four persons, the number living in 17 per cent of them. Approximately 10 per cent were occupied by eight or more persons. The average number of rooms per dwelling was four, with an average of two used for sleeping.

These figures make it clear that much housing outside of the *favelas* is also substandard in the sense that it does not provide the basic facilities, and overcrowding appears to be the rule. As indicated earlier, high rents make it almost impossible even for the regularly employed clerical worker or *funcionário* to obtain adequate space for his family.

SOCIAL CHARACTERISTICS OF SLUM DWELLERS

The quality of housing is only one aspect of *favela* life. As indicated in earlier chapters, Guanabara *favelados* have less education, less skilled employment, are less literate, and are more often migrants and recent migrants than other Cariocas. There are other studies (e.g., Aspectos Humanos da *Favela* Carioca [1960]) which suggest in Bonilla's (1961) words, that "as a group the *favela* population is on the wrong side of every standard index of social disorganization whether it be illiteracy, malnutrition, disease, job instability, irregular sexual unions, alcoholism, criminal violence, or almost any other on the familiar list" (p. 5). Statistics over several years from the Brazilian Public Health Service indicate especially high rates of tuberculosis, venereal disease, and deaths from respiratory and other infections in these areas. Again, however, as in the case of housing, much of what is reported for the *favelas* also characterizes vast poverty-stricken rural areas of the nation. A wide audience has become aware of the hardship, social disorganization, and brutality of *favela* life through the diary of Maria Carolina de Jesus of São Paulo whose book, published in 1960, created a literary sensation. But it is also true that newspaper stories bolster the attitudes of Rio de Janiero's middle class which tends to stereotype "the *favelado*" with many of the qualities of the dangerous, poverty-stricken, infectious, antisocial person. And indeed, for some *favelados*, the slums or deteriorated housing in marginal neighborhoods do provide shelter and a certain anonymity which shields their petty criminal activities from the eyes of the police. As indicated earlier however, and as more extensively documented by Pearse (1958) and others, many *favela* families are well integrated, regularly employed, and possess conventional standards of behavior. This is particularly true for the older and more established *favelas* such as Jacarezinho. In this last, for example, identifiable as an entity for 35 years, there are now about 75,000 people, and many houses which began as shanties have over the years acquired outer walls of brick or tile, coats of stucco and paint, electric wiring, and water pipes. Some of these latter are still attachments to public mains, occasionally purchased through entrepreneurs who have established the initial taps, but the end result is light and running water. This process of gradually attaining the amenities of urban life is apparent in the uneven development of individual homes in all the older *favelas,* indicating that people do not necessarily rush to leave the *favelas* as their economic status improves. This is partly due to the inflated rent and cost of real estate elsewhere but it is also a consequence of the sense of personal control over their dwellings which many *favelados* have and would not find in conventional apartments, of the security which comes from a network of acquaintances, and the possibility of obtaining credit in the overpriced *favela* stores, and above all, of the convenience of the *favela* to the city and to jobs.

Despite the tendency of so many settlers to remain in the familiar surroundings, there is a certain amount of mobility within the slum neighborhoods themselves. In Jacarezinho, the poorest, least educated, and most recently arrived inhabitants live in the most deteriorated shacks on the muddy border of a sewage-filled stream, the Rio Jacaré (Crocodile River) forming one of its boundaries. They are squeezed down by the more affluent, concentrated midway up the hill and moving in both directions as their fortunes improved. More dark-skinned people, too, can be seen in the riverside neighborhood, which, with its thieves, prostitutes, and high rates of disease, used to be called the *"outro lado da vida,"* the "other side of life." While there is some uncertainty about the *favelas'* exact racial composition, it is generally agreed that they are heterogeneous, with roughly equal numbers of whites and browns and a slight preponderance of blacks. The information on hand suggests, however, that most of the relatively low percentage of blacks in the total Rio population do reside in *favela* neighborhoods.

ATTITUDES OF SLUM DWELLERS

Kahl (1965), as noted earlier, compared the attitudes of a group of *favelados* with those of factory operatives and managers. The three groups were not differentiable by an index of national identification—a way of quantifying feelings of solidarity and of meaningful participation in the national society. Similarly, all three groups placed a unanimously high value on education, rating free education above the right to an effective political voice, a minimum wage, and access to state social services. In keeping with this last, managers and operatives favor universal higher education because of its collective benefits to the national community rather than as an expression of individual rights. The *favelados*, revealing the more traditional dependent attitude toward a paternalistic boss, tend simply to reaffirm the government's obligations toward citizens.

Other features characterizing *favelados* were: more negative attitudes toward immigrants who might appear as intruders with unfair advantages in the labor market; a strong dislike (among 40 per cent) of competition; a belief—apparently as an act of faith since they rated their economic conditions as unchanged or worse in the past five years—that industrialization was producing benefits for people like themselves; an agreement with the operatives more than the managers, that the church is a positive force in national development and that religion is a personal aid. Unexpectedly, 15 per cent of the *favelados,* more than in either of the other groups, had recently worked actively for a political party or candidate. This last finding fits the impression gained during the period of psychiatric data-gathering for the present project as well as in traveling throughout Brazil: The *favela* dweller in his search for a new *patrão* is ready to relate to the local equivalent of the precinct captain or neighborhood boss who, in return for political compliance (understanding the large number disenfranchised because of illiteracy), may deliver jobs, food, firewood, or other favors.

Another recent study of *favelados* is that of Bonilla (1961). Although half his sample of 150 men and 50 women said their economic status had worsened during the preceding five years (one of Brazil's most sustained periods of economic growth), 67 per cent of the men and 42 per cent of the women agreed that the new industries were improving the lives of others like themselves. Negative about the sincerity of help offered to them by influential national groups as well as the state and federal governments, they rarely credited police or teachers with doing anything beyond their assigned duties to help the *favela.* In contrast to the interview responses of articulate *favelado* patients in the present study, and to the reports of Carolina de Jesus and other observers, however, the persons of whom Bonilla wrote were conscious of receiving a fair amount of social support from those surrounding them within the *favela.* Seventy-two per cent of the men and 66 per cent of the women believed *favelados* to be very, or more or less, united. As Bonilla noted, "it is vis-à-vis the world outside the *favela* that he feels bypassed, forgotten and excluded" (p. 3). It is probable that the *favelados* who become psychiatric patients are among the more socially isolated within their own area and feel themselves excluded, victimized, or at least unsupported.

COLLECTIVE ACTION AMONG SLUM DWELLERS

Associations of *Favelados* have sprung up in different communities, but none have developed institutional stability. Nonetheless, there were enough with shared interests so that by the summer of

1968 a federation of local associations, A Federação das Associações dos Favelados do Estado, could list 80 representatives from 97 associations. The Federation's deliberative council met in that summer to discuss its relations with private and government agencies which might help them. Even so, the viability of the Federation remained in doubt because it could not count on the concrete and financial support of any public or private group.

Collective action arises when squatters and slum dwellers, through threats against their homes, are confronted with the fact that they at least share enough interests so that they can be threatened in common. Similarly, they may unite in order to acquire water, sewers, electricity, gutters, and paving. Inhabitants of the Ilha das Dragas, a small island in the Lagoa Roderigo Freitas in the upper-class district of Leblon near Ipanema, organized themselves to oppose eviction threatened by a projected new road. The island slum, Favela de Vila Operatio Cristo Redentor, is composed of 418 homes, mainly shanties or *barracos*, sheltering 1,987 persons. The vice president of the organization was quoted in the Jornal do Brasil (August 30, 1968), when evictions were being rumored, as saying, "we cannot remain here if the state says no," but asserting at the same time that there existed "understanding" between his society and CHISAM (Comissão Habitacional de Integração Social da Area Metropolitana). This was the agency charged with arranging new housing and preserving the interests and social integrity of those threatened by relocation or unable to obtain proper municipal services for their homes. The "understandings" were that no evictions would take place until after the construction of public low-cost housing to which the *favelados* would be moved.

In the summer of 1968, CHISAM announced its plan to construct no less than 33,000 low-cost residential units over a period of two and a half years in various neighborhoods of Rio and in the municipios of Duque de Caxias, Niteroi, São Gonçalo, Nova Iguaçu, and São Joao de Meriti. Its guiding philosophy was to be the location of homes as close as possible to the inhabitants' places of work. CHISAM was also studying plans for rehabilitating several *favelas,* by substituting houses for shanties. As these plans became known, residents of various favelas in the Zona Sul sought contact with the CHISAM administration asking that their slums be included in the project. *Favelados* of Bras de Pinã, containing 3,500 persons, or between four and five to a *barraco*, were especially active in seeking implementation of "works of urbanization" which had been promised to them months earlier. One year before, in fact, the Governor of Guanabara had presided at a ceremony transferring the area of Bras de Pinã from the jurisdication of COHAB, a state controlled construction agency, to CODESCO (Companhia de Desenvolvimento de Comunidades or Company for Community Development), another agency working on contract from the government and concerned with social research and development as well as building. The final date for beginning the urbanization project was to have been January 1968, but at the time of a major protest from the *favelados* in August 1968 nothing had yet been started. The board of directors of their association (Union for Defense and Betterment of *Favela* de Pinã) did not blame CODESCO directly, preferring to designate a bureaucratic machine which has the power to provide all financing for homes as the problem. At the same time, they expressed gratitude for four new *bicas,* or water outlets in the *favela* which made it possible for them to retain some faith in the government's promises.

In the Barra da Tijúca and the Baixada de Jacarepagua, site of some of the finest beaches in the Greater Rio area, disorderly unplanned construction is proceding apace, along with the erection of future clubs, hotels, and a spate of *boates* and *inferninhos,* tiny dark nightclubs for weekending visitors. The expected completion, in the early 1970's of tunnels and roads integrating these areas with the Zona Sul makes the probability of a rapidly increasing population density almost inevitable; slum development is already in progress and *grilheiros* have begun to appear. A *grilheiro,* or landgrabber, is named after the *grillo* or cricket, perhaps because he works at night. It is very often the *grilheiro* rather than the squatter himself who first takes possession of the unclaimed land. He divides it into tiny *loteamentos* which he will number with signs and then rent to newcomers who will put up their own shacks. Or he may even begin the process of shanty building, and illegally tap water and electric supplies and rent bootleg lines to the shanty dwellers at inflated prices. Sometimes an enterprising small householder already living in an area will, for a fee, permit *favelados* to tap into his lines.

Near the elegant Clube Canaveral, for example, are the homes of its waiters, cooks, porters, and other hotel, bar, and restaurant helpers, as well as construction workers, and drivers. Their shanties lack light and running water; the Marapendi Canal serves as their sewer. They constitute the Favela da Restinga and feel themselves threatened not only by *grilheiros* and others who claim ownership of the land upon which they live (which they say belongs to the state), but also by members of the Clube Canaveral who would like to have the unsightly slum removed as quickly as possible. As in the case of older *favelas,* they are trying to organize an association of inhabitants in order to press claims for what they do not have, the appurtenances of urbanization plus materials, so that they might build homes of masonry—*casas de alvenaria.* Various authorities have been consulted about what to do. The Professor of Social Organization of Cities, in the post graduate course on Urbanism at the Federal University of Rio de Janeiro had one remedy: Destroy everything already built and start completely anew.

Low-costing housing for former *favelados* has so far been little and uncertain—the crisis faced by residents of the Conjunto Residencial de Irajá in an urban zone of Rio is but one example. This huge curving apartment house sheltered hundreds of ex-*favelados,* most of whom found there their first experience with conventional housing, paved walks, and inside faucets and toilets. Some had arrived after the floods of January 1966 under the Plano de Calamidade of COPEG, another housing agency. The crisis was occasioned by reevaluation of the New Cruzeiro and changes in the cost of living, which, in accord with earlier agreements, required the tenants to pay higher monthly installments toward eventual purchase. In most cases these were completely beyond their means, so, accepting fate, they sadly made preparations to return to their former hovels. Many also lost their apartments in the Conjunto Residencial da Marquis de São Vicente in Gavea. It was only in the Cidade de Deus in Jacarepagua that the crisis was avoided because the payment, spread over 144 months, was based on a percentage of the minimum wage, alterable only with increases in salary.

FAVELA REHABILITATIONS CENTERS

These centers require attention in the present volume because they are part of the supportive network which helps protect potentially vulnerable people from the decompensation which might lead to hospital admission. For some, already disturbed, they constitute an alternative to the hospital and hence drain off persons who might otherwise become mental hospital statistics.

As of mid-1968, the Fundação Lea XIII operated seven Centros Sociais with the purpose of developing occupational skills in *favelados* and other marginal people, and a less explicit aim of helping them develop some awareness of what they might accomplish collectively. Community organization efforts, meeting with only occasional modest success, are aimed at combating the *favelados'* and marginals' traditional dependent passivity which is encouraged by the paternalistic charity of the church. Among the most viable *favela* groups are sport clubs. An eighth center was sponsored by the Banco da Providencia, a private church-sponsored group. Jacarezinho, the site of the largest center sponsored by the Fundação, concentrates on operating an extensive machine shop offering sophisticated training to men and youths, many of whom come from other *favelas*. An old single-storied building with concrete floors, located near the top of a hill, houses the machine and other shop and craft areas; a paved street makes it possible for materials to be delivered by truck. The dun-colored building is surrounded by dusty, open space. The center's community development activities were hard to evaluate in August 1968 because the young social worker in charge had only been on the job for three months and was herself in the process of adapting to the *favela* people and environment. Her dedication was clear, but her class-related problems in communicating with the people around her were apparent. In beehive hairdo and miniskirt, her appearance as well as her attitude bespoke a patroness dispensing favors rather than someone helping the *favelados* to learn to help themselves. She felt that their main desire was for "a piece of ground," and that given that, they could "adapt to anything."

The center of the Banco da Providencia is located high on a hill in the *favela* of Euclides da Rocha in the Santa Clara area of Copacabana. This is an example of a highly organized and stable slum. Its 650 dwellings include 2,500 people. It may be approached by path from a street at the end of the Tunel Velho or by a dirt alley extending from an ancient brick road, the Ladeiro Tabajara, named after an Indian tribe. The brick road winds its way up the hill from a point near the exit of the Tunel. The alley was probably constructed many years ago to provide access to a few middle-class homes built on the hill by some Portuguese small businessmen. It then allowed easy access to the unused land by *grilheiros* or by invaders who settled directly on it.

From the street one may look up and see the *favela* of Euclides da Rocha extending on three sides, with the area over the tunnel forming the center of an inverted "U." Like other slums, at a distance it seems a patchwork of weathered board fronts and sheet or corrugated tin roofs, creating a jagged profile due to individual variations in the height of the shacks. No space is visible between the houses. Only one side can be reached by the path, and this begins behind a billboard standing almost on the sidewalk of the street below. Behind the billboard, hidden from the street, is a precipitous, narrow dirt-and rock-strewn path with a few tufts of green grass growing here and there amidst occasional bits of garbage and broken glass. The path is eroded, for it acts as a waterway during heavy rains. The people who traverse it at this lower level are, however, well dressed for they are coming "down" and have prepared for the descent "down into the town." One may encounter, picking their way down the steep irregular incline, a woman with carefully coiffed hair and high heels, a man in a clean shirt and trousers with shined shoes, and young girls dressed in the familiar school uniform of white shirt and navy blue miniskirt. About a quarter way up the hill are the shanties, many with laundry hanging from their windows, and women (very few men are apparent) working or standing nearby. The muddy walkways between the homes are narrow, with activities in one shanty audible and often visible to those next door. Through the open doors one sees an occasional refrigerator sometimes standing on a dirt floor. Furniture is usually limited to plain deal, or in some cases, enameled tables, one or two straight chairs, and metal bedsteads, occasionally double-decked. Mattresses and bedclothing are worn and soiled. Old upholstered chairs or sofas are occasionally seen; they are in poor repair and have been gifts from employers (of the women as *empregados*) or picked up as they were being discarded. A number of metal pots and pans, enameled basins and, almost always, a metal washtub are present. But within *favelas* there are always exceptions and some shacks, expanded and developed into conventional small homes over the years, are more adequately furnished. There are more television aerials than usual, for this *favela* has its own official electric power line. Another several hundred yards up, below the dirt alley, the path emerges onto a flat surface which has been graded to provide a meeting place or an area for dances. A raised stand of scrap lumber at one end is large enough to accommodate three or four men with instruments. Another steep climb of about two hundred feet, between shanties, leads to the alley. It is rutted with heaps of garbage. Several dogs are in evidence and two pigs lazily root in the refuse. Nearby is one of the three communal wells which serve Euclides da Rocha, in use as always.

At the end of a steep path one sees the white buildings of the center. Plantings around its three buildings and access path give evidence of attempts at beautification. A long two-storied whitewashed stucco structure with blue shutters contain stalls for training in shoemaking, cooking, sewing, and craft work. Nearby are a low white stuccoed chapel and a faded yellow building with red poinsettas blooming near the door. This is the home of a nurse, a French nun, who was brought here five years ago by the local parish to operate a dispensary for the *favelados*. When the center was established in mid-1966 she had already been accepted by the *favela* dwellers and was an invaluable aid in gaining their acceptance of it. The *favela* men had built the chapel and the nurse's residence, and then, with donated materials and supervision, they constructed the training building. Of even greater importance, the parish had been conducting small group discussions over the two years preceding the establishment of the center with the general aim of promoting self-help. While they did not anticipate the center's arrival as such, they gave the population a feeling of participation in its development, and when it did come there was no overt resistance at all. The final decision to go ahead with establishing the center was made in January 1966 at the time of the most disastrous floods in Rio's history. It was then that Banco da Providencia workers, engaging in relief operations in the *favela,* were thrown into greater contact with the parish operations and with the people themselves. Because of the age and relative stability of this *favela*, many of its inhabitants impressed the volunteers as having values more akin to those of the middleclass living "below" than they had found in other slums. This suggested Euclides da Rocha as a good place in which to start their first center.

The center's 11 shops or "stalls" contain 119 people, all in training. A training course usually occupies about five months with individual progress treated flexibly. During the day the groups are composed of largely women and adolescents. The men, who are working elsewhere during the day (usually at odd jobs, for only a few work regularly in factories, though several are taxi drivers), come at night. Each shop is in the charge of a volunteer or a local person who receives a small salary. Before a new shop group is started, market needs are surveyed; a need for seamstresses, cooks, or shoemakers is discovered, for example, and this determines the direction of the next training group. The craft shops make cheerful covers for stools, produce leather belts, coasters for glasses, clothing, and shoes, much of which is sold at the annual Feira da Providencia. The shops have acquired a reputation for good dressmaking, and some customers come directly to the *favela* to make a purchase. Cooking-class products are also sold to people living in the *favela*. In addition to these service-and product-oriented programs, the center places a high priority on reading and writing classes for adults.

The part-time volunteer social worker and psychologist reported that most of the adolescents did not seem to have very high levels of aspiration, that they did not observe symptoms of a conflict between such aspirations and awareness of the impossibility of achieving them. Many youngsters thought vaguely about becoming mechanics or drivers, but their motivation to act was low; sometimes the social worker showed them newspaper ads just to prove that people were indeed looking for employees. Many adolescents dreamed of becoming *futebol* stars. Others were limited to a fantasy of "driving things" or "fixing motors." Most have dropped out after one or two years of primary school; education is not highly valued by them or their families. Although they do play soccer down "below" from time to time, it is doubtful whether the *favela* boys have much meaningful contact with those in town. There is less doubt about the girls; they have practically no associations with those below.

THE PATIENT SAMPLE

The housing and neighborhood characteristics of the patient sample should be viewed in light of the homes and living areas of the Rio de Janeiro population at large. The data in this section indicate the relative crowding and inadequacy of patient homes. They also show the proportionately large contribution to the sample of working-class suburbs, including areas of Rio State on the outer perimeter of the metropolis. *Favelados,* are underrepresented in the sample despite the prevalence of inadequate housing. This most probably reflects the major contribution of Casa Eiras to the population studied. The patients' living areas were almost evenly divided, as indicated in Table 125, between urban and suburban districts, with an additional seven per cent in rural parts of Greater Rio in immediately adjacent Rio State. As noted in Chapter IV, a few individuals who had come for treatment under INPS auspices (while their parents or spouses stayed temporarily with relatives in the city) described their mainly rural or small town neighborhoods and homes as their place of origin. These were in Petropolis or Teresopolis or other Rio State points outside of Guanabara but still within the region regarded by city planners as Greater Rio. All these places, contributing approximately three per cent of the total sample, were close enough to be within the metropolitan sphere of influence. An additional four per cent of the patients had come expressly for Casa Eiras hospitalization from more distant places, including the states of São Paulo, Minas Gerais, Matto Grosso, and Espirito Santo. Again, in every instance, at least one relative took up temporary residence in the city. These were uniformly employed and financially stable people.

The clear preponderance of all of the patients or their accompanying relatives (42 per cent of the total sample) lived in suburban areas associated with the relatively stable working class, both skilled and unskilled. The less homogeneous urban regions included central, peripheral, and residential as well as slum sec-

tions. The first has both high-rent apartment buildings and deteriorated structures or shanties. Peripheral urban zones include
fewer apartment houses and more inexpensive single-family dwellings, although in certain areas such as Tijúca some large old
houses remain and new apartments are being erected. The residential sections, of which Urca is an example, contain larger
one-family homes, but even here single deteriorated or subdivided
residences may be encountered.

As shown in Table 126, only nine per cent of the patients occupied *barracos* or homemade shanties, with an additional three per
cent in unfinished or unclassified structures. At the same time,
approximately one-fourth of the patients lived in dwellings which
did not have both or any electricity and running water. While
exact comparative data are not available, it appears probable
that the housing of the patient group is representative of that of
the urban Guanabara population at large. The bulk of the patients
occupied separate houses. Fourteen per cent were in *vilas*, living
units contained in a single low building along an alley or around
a courtyard with separate entrances for individual habitations, or
in separate small houses, usually so close together as to be almost
touching, arranged in a cluster around a common courtyard. The
remainder were divided between the somewhat more affluent, residing in apartment houses and the predominantly unmarried or
temporarily separated because of migration, who occupied rented
rooms. These last were occasionally in the homes of relatives.
Apartment buildings represent the most expensive housing in the
sample; because of the high cost of apartments in the central
zones, the apartment-dwellers in the patient sample resided
mainly in the peripheral urban zones. Many variations in living
or sleeping arrangements were described. A man who built his
own *barraco* in an urban *favela*, separated the sleeping space for his
three children from that of his wife and himself by an improvised
curtain. Another, whose housing seemed adequate by most
criteria—essential services, separate rooms with kitchen and bath
in a single dwelling in a residential neighborhood—revealed its
inadequacy when he reported that he, his wife, and six children
all shared a single sleeping room. Some dwellings without both
services were more spacious. A patient living in a home given him
by the Department of Justice as part of his salary had no running

water but ample space, allowing himself and his wife a room to themselves. Other illustrations in greater detail are given below.

Social Characteristics According to Area of Residence

For purposes of analysis, living areas were divided into those containing more stable and integrated as compared with less integrated neighborhoods. Rural zones were omitted, although in most instances these would probably have qualified as unintegrated in the sense of there being little communication with neighbors. The following and other examples of housing conditions in rural areas illustrate the difficulty in arriving at clear classifications that do not overlap.

A 30-year-old white married Protestant (Evangélico) housewife and unskilled agricultural laborer ("with the hoe") lives with her husband, an unskilled factory worker, and eight children in a "clay" house in a rural area of Rio State. A wooden floor covers part of the house, but most of the floor is earth. They obtain water from a well and use a kerosene lamp for light. There are no sanitary facilities—they use the woods for excretion. She and her husband occupy separate beds, the younger children sleeping with her.

A 20-year-old brown unmarried Protestant (Pentecostal) agricultural laborer was brought to the city by his father for treatment. They live in a sharecropper's cottage owned by a *fazendeiro* in Marapé in Espirito Santo. They use a kerosene lamp for lighting and transport water to an outside trough by a bamboo pipe from a spring. They, too, use the woods for excretion. At his own insistence, the patient sleeps alone; his five brothers are in another room and his parents and two sisters in a third. In addition to sharecropping, his father ordinarily sells some of his produce as a vendor in a street market. Other family members will handle this task, however, and his father will stay with a relative in a nearby rural zone of Rio State while his son is hospitalized.

Designated as Area I were the more stable areas with fewer transients, higher rates of regular employment, and a more socioeconomically homogenous population with greater membership in social and occupational organizations. These include the residential, suburban, and peripheral urban zones; 65 per cent of the patients lived in these neighborhoods.

The following are some examples of living circumstances in these areas.

A 25-year-old white unmarried Protestant (Assembléia de Deus), an unskilled sewing helper, lives with her mother, brother, and father (a gardener for Petrobras) in a single house owned by the company in an industrial zone (near the oil refinery) in Petropolis, a resort city an hour's drive away from the city center but considered part of Greater Rio de Janeiro. They use a kerosene lamp for lighting, obtain their water in pots and tins from a neighbor's house, and have improvised a wooden outhouse. The patient has a bedroom for herself. Before moving from rural Minas Gerais 10 years earlier, all members of the family worked as sharecroppers. Communication with neighbors is limited: the patient's mother said "we have neither friends or enemies."

A 45-year-old white Catholic housewife, resident of the same suburb for 31 years, has lived in a main floor apartment with all services for seven years. She shares it with her husband (a typographer), a married daughter and son-in-law, and three grandchildren. The patient and her husband have one sleeping room, the daughter and husband another, and the three grandchildren another. Her only close friend is a sister who lives nearby; she has no intimates and little relationship with her neighbors.

A 33-year-old black Catholic unskilled government *funcionário*, born in São Joao de Meriti, lives in a house divided between two families in a residential neighborhood in nearby Nilopolis in Rio State. Light comes from a kerosene lamp, water from an outside well. There is, however, a bathroom. He and his wife share their bedroom with two younger children; two older ones have a sleeping room for themselves. Although he has always been seclusive, he does have one or two friends in the neighborhood with whom he can talk.

A 30-year-old white Catholic, a skilled manual railroad worker, lives with his wife and three children in Pavuna in the suburban area of Anchieta. Their rented house has all facilities, but is so small that the entire family sleeps in the same bedroom. He is highly thought of by his neighbors and has intimate friends, whom his wife, an informant, considers "pernicious. . . a bad influence." The patient was brought to Rio by his family from Juiz de Fora, a town in Minas Gerais, before he was six years old.

A 42-year-old white married Catholic taxi driver and mechanic who works on the side as a *biscateiro*, lives in a single house in a residential neighborhood of Tijúca where he was born. It has all services. He shares it with his wife, who sleeps with him in one bedroom, and two daughters who occupy another room. He has many close friends in the neighborhood.

A 17-year-old brown Protestant (Assembléia de Deus) unmarried *biscateiro*, a stonemason's helper and sometime paid agricultural laborer, lives with his mother and two brothers in suburban Caxias in Rio State. His only friends are "church brothers," some of whom live in the neighborhood. He has worked since age 10 shining shoes and occasionally going out begging with his father, dead for two years. His mother is a laundress. The house has electricity, and they obtain water from a collective faucet in the courtyard, "a *bica* on the Nile." The two brothers share a bedroom. The patient sleeps with his mother in her bed.

Area II includes the central urban, deteriorated, and slum neighborhoods, home for 21 per cent of the patients. The central urban areas include both slum and high-rent apartment houses. A few of the patients in the Sanatorio Botafogo occupied this latter type of housing. Some in Casa Eiras were in lower rent apartments, but the majority occupied single dwellings. The absence of purely homogeneous neighborhoods in Rio de Janeiro accounts for the failure of a division of the patient population along residential lines to yield the consistent differences obtained with classification, for example, according to literacy or occupation. Another factor is the scarcity of reasonably priced housing. Because of this, families with regularly employed and sometimes moderately well-educated breadwinners may remain in slum areas or in overcrowded quarters without adequate basic services. Finally, many *favelados* and those in substandard housing, but not residing in officially defined *favelas*, were reluctant to move when either private opportunities or public housing became available to them. Among the reasons given were feelings of independence; some spoke with feeling of the fact that they "owned" the shanties which they had built themselves. Economic considerations were cited as major reasons for not moving. These included the need to pay higher rent or in some cases any rent at all, to pay for electricity which they had habitually obtained by tapping powerlines, the need to travel long distances to jobs, for the women and *biscateiros* the problem of finding work with nearby well-to-do people, and the ability to rely on credit from the tiny slum grocery stores. Helping neighbors and local friendships were only occasionally mentioned.

A 55-year-old brown Catholic housewife lives in a *vila* with all services in the urban area of Irajá, along with her husband and four children. All the males in the family share one sleeping room, the females, the other. She and her husband came from Alagoas six years earlier in order to be with their children. They had worked on their own small farm and also as paid agricultural laborers. Now she cares for the house while her husband, a manual unskilled leather-cutter in a suitcase factory, contributes to the family earnings.

A 22-year-old brown unmarried Catholic port laborer, rents a room along with his brother in his aunt's house in the port area. It has all utilities. Other occupants of the house include his uncle and aunt, their 12 children, and a cousin. The patient and his brother left their home in rural Minas Gerais because their father had been converted to Protestantism and tried to force them to do likewise.

Table 127 shows the overlap which exists between the two housing groups. Almost a fifth of the more stable Area I dwellers (those in residential, peripheral urban, and suburban areas, exclusive of identified suburban slums or *favelas*) do not have both electricity and running water in their homes, and almost seven per cent live in shanties. Many indices of sociocultural status showed no or only small differences in favor of Area I dwellers including such major items as education and occupation. The only indices registering a greater than 10 per cent difference between inhabitants of Area I and II are those listed in Table 127. These show more (though not significantly so) of the former are fully literate (fitting the impression noted earlier that literacy is a more functional index of status than is education), read newspapers and magazines as well as books, and own television sets. Significantly more in the central urban Area II had migrated within five years and had four or more children. The relative stability and status-desirability of the two areas is also suggested by the fact that twice as many fathers of Area II as Area I dwellers had been illiterate. This may reflect the function of the central urban zone as a staging and integrating area for migrants from the country.

In summary, even with the heterogeneity and overlap noted above, division of the study population on the basis of area of residence divides it to some extent on the basis of indices of stability, integration, modern values reflected in smaller families, and capacity to participate in the social information network.

Table 128 shows statistically significant differences in the interpersonal network according to area of residence. Area I dwellers, knew less about their immediate neighbors but had more close friends than did Area II dwellers. They also had more contact with welfare workers (as was true for more affluent patients generally). Area II dwellers, in contrast had more and friendlier contact with the clergy, (as was true for recent migrants and less affluent patients). There were no differences in availability of relatives in the same neighborhood, although this, too, has been shown to vary with recency of migration. The pattern of participation in dances and spectator sports, while not revealing statistically significant differences between the residential groups, also followed the pattern noted according to recency of migration and economic status; proportionately more of the inhabitants of less stable and lower status Area II were game watchers and dancers.

SOCIAL CHARACTERISTICS ACCORDING TO QUALITY OF HOUSING

Basic housing quality was determined by the presence or absence in the dwelling of electricity and running water. As noted above, approximately one-fourth of the patients lived in homes with neither or only one of these essential services. This was between three and four times the number living in shanties, and about four times that in urban or suburban *favelas*. Many without essential services, not living in shanties or *favelas,* belong to the seven per cent of the total living in rural areas of Greater Rio de Janeiro. The substandard nature of housing in the rural perimeter is in part due to the tendency for migrants from more remote regions to use these neighborhoods as an initial stopping point, erecting transitory homes after their accustomed models in the interior, or utilizing abandoned structures left by other migrants.

The data presented below make it clear that differentiating the patients on the basis of housing quality results in more marked differences in social and behavioral characteristics than a division on the basis of area of residence. Those living in dwellings with neither electricity nor running water or with only one of these services include many, although not all, of those who are illiterate, uneducated, recently migrant, black or brown, and in the lowest occupational status. But other elements are present which may be obscured by data-pooling. Many who live in *favelas* feel some security-giving ties to their subcommunity. Others, with more education and higher occupational status, remain because of inertia or are frustrated by the unavailability of housing more suited to their social position. Among those who are indeed at the bottom of the socioeconomic ladder, other low-grade dwellings with basic services are available if one searches for them so that remaining in homes without both essential services may well imply a certain passivity or resignation. It is necessary to scrutinize the actual data on housing in relation to other factors in order to discover its meaning for individual behavior.

SOCIOECONOMIC INDICATORS

As shown in Table 129, higher percentages of patients occupying quarters without both essential services had little or no education, were illiterate or only partly literate, were in the lowest occupational category, and lived in *favelas, barracos,* and homes with little room. A higher proportion also shared their sleeping quarters with family members other than a mate. A division of the patient population on the basis of this last criterion did not, however, reveal the same segregating power with regard to other social or psychiatric characteristics as the presence or absence of essential services. Beyond these findings, it may be noted that 15 per cent of the homes without services were located in urban areas other than slums, leaving (after including the 21 per cent in urban slums) almost two-thirds in the surburban and rural zones. Further, while the number was very low, a few homes without services were occupied by Class III and IV workers and approximately a third of such homes were occupied by Class V artisans. In other words, regularly employed skilled workers do occupy housing without basic services. The question of what if any psychological characteristics differentiate them from those of similar status who have moved into more adequate homes, is unanswered.

Finally, it is not surprising to note that more of those in less adequate housing feel their socioeconomic status to have dropped during the preceding year, and that those with essential services feel their status to be better than their fathers. At the same time, more than a third without services regard themselves as in better circumstances than their fathers, indicating that this group also contains many who are upwardly mobile from a previously lower (usually rural) economic status.

DEMOGRAPHIC CHARACTERISTICS

The only data revealing statistically significant differences between the populations divided according to housing are those concerned with marital and color status. The other differences listed in Table 130 are, however, consistent. Table 130 indicates that slightly more of those living in dwellings without essential services are under 25 and that fewer are more than 41 years old. Along with the tendency for occupants of inadequate housing to be younger, more are unmarried and fewer have had children. This weighting of younger, unmarried, childless people in the less adequate housing group reduces the relative proportion of the poor who have been unable to advance up the socioeconomic ladder. That is, occupancy of substandard housing is for a variable proportion of the population a transitory state, hopefully on the way to something better. Others are young people from rural areas brought by their parents to Rio for treatment.

Only six per cent of those in homes with both running water and electricity were black—between a third and a fourth of the percentage occupying homes without essential services. Fewer patients in this category were brown, also, and the percentage of whites with services far exceeded those without them. Thus the relationship of housing to behavior is associated in part with the high proportions of occupants of poor housing who are nonwhites. Finally, more inadequate housing was occupied by patients coming from large families (presumably from more traditional rural lower-class origins). This was true for fewer of those with small families of their own (who presumably had embraced more modern values).

There were no differences between the groups in regard to religious affiliation or observance.

CHILDHOOD INFLUENCES

No differences existed between the groups with regard to indices of early family stability, modes of discipline, age of earning money, and father's age at death. As indicated in Table 131, however, almost three times as many occupants of inadequate housing had illiterate fathers, and almost half as many of them as the others had literate mothers. In other words, despite the variable characteristics of those in substandard dwellings, more came from families which were less socioculturally advanced. Presumably, this family background would be predictive of either an inability to move into better housing due to economic circumstances, or a lack of strong motivation to move because of familiarity with, and high tolerance for, substandard living conditions. As noted in preceding chapters, illiterate fathers were also characteristic of illiterate and occupational Class VI patients. Thus the mobility-blocked population of low SES, based in part on lack of childhood advantages, is overrepresented in the substandard housing group.

INFORMATION AND SOCIAL PARTICIPATION

As indicated in Table 132, fewer of the occupants of substandard housing owned or utilized newspapers, magazines, books, television or radio, or went to the movies. At the same time, 28 per cent of those who did have essential services used the radio as their only medium of general information, 39 per cent never attended movies, and only half read or watched television. As noted in earlier chapters, fewer of the less advantaged people had contact with welfare workers or used welfare organizations but more watched soccer games. Housing quality unlike area of residence, does not differentiate people with respect to relations with the clergy or to participation in dances.

MIGRATORY STATUS

Table 133 confirms earlier impressions that more of the poorly housed patients were born outside of Greater Rio de Janeiro, that more had lived for shorter times in their current homes and, among the migrant, that more had come from rural areas. There were no significant differences, however, between housing groups regarding recent migratory status either at the 10-year or five-year level. While the most inadequately housed group is more residentially mobile than the better housed and includes more who originated outside Rio, especially in rural areas, it does not, unlike the central urban group, include a significantly larger proportion of recently migrant patients.

HOSPITALIZATION AND FAMILY DIAGNOSIS

Table 134 shows that more than a third of those without essential services were seen in the Pronto Socorro in contrast to 11 per cent of the others. This fits the additional, though not statistically significant, difference between the 52 per cent of those in more adequate housing as compared to 38 per cent of the others who had had previous psychiatric contact. The only difference in reason for admission between the two groups was in the prevalence of paranoid behavior which motivated the families of those with less adequate housing to bring the patient to the hospital almost twice as frequently as the others. This difference, while congruent with those based on other low SES indices, was small and did not reach significance. Family diagnosis fitted that reported in other samplings of the less advantaged families. The poorly housed, just as the less educated, less literate, and less occupationally skilled, diagnosed more mental illness or religiously inspired behavior, and the more adequately housed diagnosed relatively more strange or bad behavior or response to life stress.

PRIVACY OF SLEEPING QUARTERS

As noted in Table 126, 51 per cent of the patients slept in a room alone or with their mate or spouse, while 43 per cent shared their sleeping rooms with children or other family members. The remaining six per cent had other arrangements, sometimes involving strangers, or were undetermined. Those sleeping alone or with a mate and those sharing quarters with children or other family members were not significantly different in respect to sociocultural or to most behavioral-psychiatric variables.

Table 135 presents the few items on which differences of more than 10 per cent were noted between groups defined on the basis of sleeping privacy. Lack of sleeping privacy is correlated neither with low general socioeconomic status, nor with a higher frequency of particular psychiatric complaints. On the contrary, proportionately more of those with the greatest sleeping privacy complained of some form of anxiety, tension, and fatigue. It is possible that the findings are obscured by pooling data. The pattern of minimal differences may reflect, on the one hand, the increased social support available to married patients with families (who in the normal course of events might share sleeping areas with children), and on the other, the greater social isolation of the unmarried, including proportionately more men, who, along with younger or more affluent married couples, have more sleeping privacy. In at least one recorded and possibly in other instances, sleeping alone was a consequence of emotional disturbance. If lack of sleeping privacy is an indicator of home-crowding such crowding is not associated with a higher incidence of complaints.

Psychiatric and Behavioral Characteristics

TENSION, ANXIETY, SENSITIVITY, AND FRUSTRATION

Table 136 lists the psychiatrists' ratings of their own responses during interviews with the less adequately housed group as more remote, apprehensive, and hostile, and less empathic, interested, and cheerful than with those in more adequate housing. Similarly, this latter group of patients was rated as more cooperative and more comfortable with fewer showing unusual speech content or perspiring palms. In this respect, findings for the less adequately housed resemble those for the less advantaged and more recently migrant. More of the patients with essential services revealed themselves as preoccupied with one or two themes, dramatic and attention-seeking, and actively advice-seeking. This last contrasts with the more frequently encountered statements of unsatisfied wishes to be cared for among the less adequately housed.

Table 137 shows that more of those in substandard housing also exhibited situational worries and interference with speech and thinking due to tension while more of those with essential services feared that they would lose control of themselves, or reported constant diffuse, nonsituational anxiety which was not revealed in direct behavior. Again, the differences fit those commonly encountered according to SES level.

SOMATIC COMPLAINTS

Complaints about body function, including fatigue, weakness, and diarrhea (which might be due to infection, malnutrition, or overwork) were consistently expressed by more of those without essential services. The greater prevalence of certain psychophysiological complaints among the more literate, better educated, and nonmigrant patients, however, does not appear with the patient sample segregated on the basis of housing quality. There were no differences between the groups concerning the expression of hostility or impulsive behavior.

DEPRESSIVE INDICATORS

Table 138 shows that depressive feelings were significantly more frequent in patients with essential services than among those in less adequate or substandard housing. This finding does not fit the reports of more depressive symptoms among the lower SES patients described in preceding chapters. Differences between groups with respect to depressive mood indicators are in the opposite direction and are more significant, however, when the sample is divided according to area of residence. The inhabitants of less desirable locations in the central urban districts and *favelas* more consistently show depressive behavior, including frequent affective displays. They are more frequently guilt-ridden, especially over achievement failures, weighed down by self-critical and inferiority feelings, and suicidal. These apparent depressive concomitants of poverty, life failure, and blocked mobility as indicated by area of residence are not congruent with the greater sadness and depressive display among the better housed, or the more frequent appearance of depressive symptoms in the more occupationally skilled. As suggested in Chapter 132, some of the apparent contradictions may be due to the differing social determinants of particular depressive symptoms. It is not known how many of the depressed patients with adequate housing lived in undesirable or deteriorated areas. A characteristic of these areas, perhaps relevant to the prevalence of depressive symptoms in residents who became patients, is their use as temporary lodgings for transient or recently migrant populations. Life in such an area, with a poorly integrated interpersonal network and without the opportunity to move on, may have greater emotional significance than the quality of housing per se.

THE BREAK WITH REALITY

Table 139 is congruent with previous comparisons of the less and more advantaged segments of the patient population. The patients occupying substandard housing more frequently complained about their treatment from others and were more often suspicious and distrustful; they more often experienced auditory and visual hallucinations, illusions, and misinterpretations; they more often insisted on the reality of their experience and planned specific action based upon it; and they more frequently suffered from disorientation in time and place. As shown in Table 140, similar differences were present according to area of residence.

SEXUAL BEHAVIOR

There were no differences between the groups. In this respect housing did not divide the population in the same way as did literacy, education, color, or occupation.

Past Psychiatric History

The only items differentiating the two groups in a consistent manner were those concerned with a past history of loss of consciousness. As seen in Table 141, the less adequately housed more frequently reported previous histories of lapses or fainting spells, head injuries with loss of consciousness, seizures, and fevers with altered consciousness. In no instance did the difference reach 10 per cent, or statistical significance, and they are reported here only because of their consistency.

DISCUSSION

In certain but not all respects, symptom-pattern differences between housing groups resemble those encountered when the population is divided on the basis of other SES related factors. Thus, more occupants of substandard housing exhibited situational worries, interference with speech and thinking due to tension, and somatic complaints which might have realistic bases. In contrast, however, to findings for such overlapping groups as the less educated and unskilled, feelings of guilt over achievement failure, inferiority and self-criticism are no more frequent in the poorly than the adequately housed, and feelings of sadness and weeping are significantly more frequent among those with better housing. These depressive indicators appear rather as concomitants of poverty, life failure, and blocked mobility as indicated by areas of residence. In this last instance, neighborhood, with its connotations of integration into a social group and the possibility of interpersonal support, seems more important than housing quality as such. The relative withdrawal and affective flatness of the overrepresented unmarried (noted in the next chapter) also contributes to the lower proportion of depressive symptoms among the inadequately housed.

Division both according to area of residence (not related to age, color, or marital status) and housing quality yielded similar results with respect to indicators of impaired reality-testing. These findings are completely congruent with previous comparisons of the less and more advantaged segments of the patient population. There is no evidence that patients living in Rio substandard housing have been downwardly mobile as a result of psychosis or alcoholism, although the *favelas* have been traditionally regarded as refuges for such downward drifters. Occupants of substandard housing and poorly integrated neighborhoods tend to come from illiterate families; rather than having been downwardly mobile, these patients have remained in the depressed social class in which they were reared. A certain proportion of migrants among the patients moved to the city from rural areas because of their psychiatric disturbance, and their presence may also contribute to the high rate of psychopathology and impaired reality-testing among those in Area I. The relationship of these findings to the reports of such investigators as Burgess (1955), Faris and Dunham (1960), Leighton and colleagues (1963), and others, is problematical, for they all suggest that areas characterized by social disorganization or a failure in integration produce more psychiatric casualties, especially those with impaired reality testing (schizophrenic behavior). It seems probable that among other factors, social isolation and separation from accustomed human relationships, as well as the absence of other aspects of the supportive social network, are more prominent in the more anomic Area II than Area I. The assumption that these features are related to a high yield of hospitalized patients is supported by the work of Levy and Rowitz (1970), based on the pioneering findings of Faris and Dunham in Chicago in the 1930's. They found, like Faris and Dunham, that schizophrenic admissions were generally higher from the low income areas, although, unlike the early findings, this was not true for first admissions. Levy and Rowitz suggest a drift hypothesis to explain their findings: as schizophrenics proceed through their subsequent admissions they may be aggregating in the poor city center which, in 1961 when their data were gathered, was the same locus of poverty and social disorganization as it was in the twenties and thirties. The Greater Rio data indicate that both disorganized, low income neighborhoods and substandard homes (sometimes from other neighborhoods) yield the highest proportions of patients with impaired reality testing (schizophrenic behavior) in this population of first-time admissions to mental hospitals. Like Chicago in the 20's and 30's, Rio de Janeiro in the late 1960's had no general hospital psychiatric units or alternatives to the public or INPS hospitals for the lowest-class mentally ill, so that all of their first admissions went to these units while those from the small middle and upper classes were more often seen in private sanitoria.

The observations on psychiatric patients in Rio are compatible with those of others regarding nonpatient inhabitants of other

Latin American slum areas. Information about another group often reluctant to leave undesirable living arrangements is provided by Back's (1962) data on housing aspirations of Puerto Rican slum dwellers. While 70 per cent of this sample said that they would prefer to move, 68 per cent said that they had never actually looked for another place. Asked what they would want in the "ideal house," 88 per cent listed "closeness to work," 87 per cent "schooling facilities," 79 per cent "known stores," 57 per cent "quiet, no bars or jukeboxes," and 53 per cent "good neighbors." Most of the other questions, aside from "sanitary services" (45 per cent), and "three or more bedrooms" (43 per cent), elicited a considerably lower number of positive responses. Neighbors were de-emphasized as either push or pull factors in moving, with only 14 per cent wishing to remain because they liked their neighbors and five per cent saying that they wished to leave because they disliked them. One of the most interesting features of Back's data is the suggestion that self-identification as a slum dweller has positive identity value. Such persons appear more resistant to moving to public housing projects than those in substandard housing conditions who do not accept the name of slum for their home.

Similar resistance to housing change, either in nature or location, has been noted elsewhere in Latin America. Holmberg and Whyte (1956), for example, in the Vicos Community of the Peruvian Sierra, observed that changes in community organization, planting, work arrangements, and health care came long before even the smallest change in household construction techniques. Reichel-Dalmatoff (1953, in Dietz et al., 1965) regarded the windowless shacks of rural Magdalena in Colombia as owing to the occupants' limited knowledge of health and disease prevention. The emphasis on ability to tightly lock the house may as plausibly, however, be linked to the suspiciousness and fear of robbery of the slum dwellers, reported by many, including Peattie (1968) in Venezuela and Rogler and Hollingshead (1965) in Puerto Rico. Patch (1958, in Dietz et al., 1965) reported that workers in Peru offered company housing were suspicious of cold concrete floors after years of wooden housing. The propensity of the slum dwellers to establish tiny businesses on their own was also reflected in their wish to convert parts of the houses to canteens dispensing corn beer.

Rogler and Hollingshead describe the lack of trust slum dwellers of San Juan, Puerto Rico have for each other, their lack of mutual respect and readiness to accuse or to feel persecuted or attacked. Peattie, in a lower-class neighborhood in a small town in Venezuela, noted the difficulties when living under such circumstances in following the ideal of being a family "of respect" which "doesn't get involved" in fights. Here she is describing adaptive or security maneuvers rather than the direct expression of anger or projective defenses against hostile impulses. The practice of using children as intermediaries to ask for favors or loans "seems to be a way of avoiding either an embarrassing refusal or direct hostility." Aside from this, "there is a strong and explicit reluctance to say anything to a neighbor who may be carrying on some annoying activity" (p. 58).

Rotondo's (1961) study of the inhabitants of a *barriada,* the *favela* equivalent in Lima, is focused on symptomatic behavior and, therefore, more immediately relevant to the present study. Significant differences were found between these people, mainly unskilled migrants from the coastal highlands and the inhabitants of a nearby rural village. The slum dwellers scarcely knew each other, preferring to associate with relatives and a few rural friends residing in other neighborhoods. They typically had poor opinions of each other, and could not be interested in systematic community activities. More of them than the villagers were anxious during questioning, became confused under stress, exhibited depressive symptoms, were easily offended, lost their tempers easily, and distrusted others. Rotondo was impressed by the few attempted suicides (all in Lima natives, not migrants) in contrast to the high incidence of pessimistic attitudes and depressive symptoms, suggesting that this might be due to "a streak of passivity." He also concluded that "the symptoms observed are not of a manic-depressive type, but of the reactive, circumstantial type" (p. 254). Feelings of being misunderstood and general anxiety symptoms of various kinds occurred with approximately equal frequency in inhabitants both of the slum and the village. Within the slum, attitudes of marked distrust were considerably greater among migrants from the highlands than the coast or the Lima natives, suggesting a carryover into the city of certain characteristics of the rural mountain dwellers.

In the end, both housing- and neighborhood-based data point to a possible relationship between overt psychotic behavior and the adaptive requirements of lowest-class Rio life. Contributing elements are powerlessness and lack of hope for the future, continuing reminders of one's low self-esteem and lack of worth in respect to the power-holders, and the problems of maintaining some personal separateness and boundaries when living at such close quarters with others. Added to them are the fatigue, indignity, social isolation, and vulnerability to illness and exploitation associated with life in substandard housing and disintegrated neighborhoods without public services or civic organization. These factors lead to guilt about failure to meet expectations, social isolation, anxiety about the motives of others, defensive denial or anger which cannot be expressed, and inability to find a sense of purpose and meaning in life. All of these elements are reflected in behavior clinically described as depressive or paranoid, but more realistically as suspicious, beaten, worn-out, and hopeless.

CHAPTER 9

GENDER STATUS, THE FEMALE ROLE, AND MARRIAGE

THE EMANCIPATION OF WOMEN

No thoroughgoing studies of the role of women in modern Brazil exist, but most observers agree that in the colonial period, and long thereafter, women were secluded, permitted little or no participation in community life outside the home, and in the great majority of instances were cast into a role akin to that of a slave. In the 1960's role and freedom seem to vary both with social class and geography; a young woman of middle-class family in Salvador do Bahia may still be expected at the age of 25 to ask her father's permission before attending an evening function with a man she has known for years. Professional colleagues from Bahia and elsewhere report that upper-class girls are concerned with protecting the family name, are often grateful for what their families—particularly their fathers—have done for them and want to show their appreciation. Some who feel themselves caught in the press of changing traditions may consult a psychiatrist rather than a priest; in these instances they appear less anxious about relations with their families than with the inner significance of their own romantic attachments. Chaperonage is still practiced to an important degree, especially for younger women in the Northern and interior tradition-bound parts of the country. At the same time, unchaperoned dating, usually in a group and often including relatives, is customary in the metropolitan areas of Rio de Janeiro and São Paulo. These cities, especially Rio, differ from the others in that they shelter young people who have come to attend educational institutions, to work in government or other offices, or to participate in the artistic and cultural life of the city. Of course, by the very fact of their parents having permitted them to leave home, these late adolescents and young adults may be regarded as "liberated" or at least as participants in modern rather than traditional value systems. Their presence and— because of the inaccessibility and cost of adequate living quarters —their use of cafes as places to meet, talk, and sometimes even to work, has stimulated much recent discussion of the revival of Rio "bar-life" as an "extension of the living room."

The young women who form part of Rio's cultural life are hardly represented in our patient population, but their existence, embodies an ideal of feminine freedom, not yet generally attained in Brazil, which others are rapidly moving toward. Thus, Wagley (1963) noted that in 1961 over 70,000 young women (as compared to 2,400 men) were attending normal schools or teacher-training colleges. These institutions function both as agents of upward social mobility and of social liberation for women. A tolerant attitude among middle- and upper-class men toward educated professional women, and the relative openness of professional schools in this respect have also contributed to a gradual increase in the number of female physicians, lawyers, psychologists, and others whose influence is beginning to be felt in national life. Perhaps it is their influence which has contributed to the increasing involvement of nonprofessional upper-class women, through church-related and other organizations, in social welfare work in the *favelas*. Upper-class women, members of the so-called *alta sociedad* (high society), may become influential in local government through personal contacts and contributions of money for "good causes." This seems to be an aspect of the slow awakening of the national conscience to the overwhelming social inequities of the country. Nonetheless, in the 1960's black women in the *alta sociedad* were a rarity and while an entire lower-class family may vote as a bloc in return for material support, its women simply do not participate in political life.

Women's suffrage in Brazil was not legalized until the electoral code of 1932, and the first participation in the vote was in 1933. While this was significant for the educated class, the most important stimulus freeing large masses of Brazilian women from the home was probably the second World War and the vastly expanded labor market of the 1940's associated with it. Yet, the true extent of women's participation in the labor force remains uncertain; Blay (1967) observed that women frequently work at home and don't want to be registered because they do not want to contribute to a retirement fund. This probably accounted for the fact that between 1949 and 1963 the Institutos de Aposentadoria, concerned with social security coverage for retirement, noted an absolute increase in the number of women registered, but a decrease proportional to the number of men. Blay believes that in the São Paulo area most women remain in the traditional weaving and spinning industries, and that relatively few are employed in newer industries such as automobile manufacturing. Other observers have reported that the majority of lowest-class women work outside the home at least part time, as maids or laundresses. Ponte (1966) believes that two-thirds of the women of Guanabara may still be regarded as culturally marginal or in the process of modernization. He studied a stratified, representative sample of 2,431 women between the ages of 20 and 50 in 1964, scoring each on an index of modernity. This involved attitudes toward participation in politics and equal work opportunities with men. Education was the most important factor associated with a high index of modernity, with high scores reported for 50 per cent of the women with at least a secondary education. Social origin was also a determinant, however, and 37 per cent of women of high social-status origins who had had no schooling yielded high indices in contrast to 20 per cent of those with low social-status origins. The find that 50 per cent of the women who had attended high school or gone further did not share "modern" aspirations suggests the persisting value of male dominance. Age has an interesting significance; in Ponte's sample, the middle-aged group (between 40 and 50 years of age) with secondary education includes the largest number of persons with high modernity scores. As he notes, these are the people who experienced the populism of Getulio Vargas and Juscelino Kubitschek while the younger age group probably were not directly exposed to such stimulating and rapid social change.

THE MASCULINE PREROGATIVES

Perhaps the most obvious difference in male and female role with a reflection in psychiatric symptomatology is related to sexual behavior. It is true that the Brazilian male is not *"macho"* —obsessively concerned with his masculinity—to the degree reported for his Hispanic American counterparts, particularly those in Mexico; but it is also true that the Brazilian youth, in sharp contrast to his sisters, is expected to be a bit wild. "Playboys" (the popular term for idle, well-to-do young men), supported by their fathers and devoting their energies to sexual conquest, are regarded with tolerance. Maintaining a mistress, a second family, or a "little house" is more difficult for their fathers' generation than it was in the past, for financial reasons, but the practice is still sufficiently institutionalized to make it acceptable to a wide range of people. A major element militating against its indefinite continuance, aside from economics, may be the increasing self-assertiveness of the educated wife. In the lower classes, the concept of sexual submission as a form of wifely duty for which pleasure is not necessarily expected is widespread. The tendency, reported by Harris (1956), for the small-town occupant of the interior to regard his wife as a sexual object rather than a person with reciprocal feelings is still regularly encountered.

Prostitution is less prominent than in the past, and—especially with advancing Protestantism—has come to be regarded by some as morally reprehensible. Prostitutes are accepted as a realistic necessity, however, with many fathers encouraging their sons to seek them out and very few actually discouraging them from doing so. Lower-class girls, and sometimes middle-class girls who have acquired a "reputation" because of an unfortunate affair and are therefore unable to find husbands, are a ready source of part-time prostitutes. This is also true for lower-class girls whose common-law husbands have abandoned them after fathering a child or two.

Homosexual jokes are circulated at least as prominently in Brazil as in the United States, and perhaps even more so, but in some respects Brazil shows a more general acceptance of the homosexual role: Witness the fete of transvestites held around carnival time with photographic coverage in major magazines. This does not, however, seem to reflect general security regarding sexual identity. A number of psychiatrists and psychologists have noted in private communications that despite the relatively low intensity of the *macho* phenomenon in Brazil, there still exists considerable pressure to behave "as a man," i.e., to engage in frequent and complete sexual intercourse and to capitalize on any potential opportunity in this respect whenever it arises. This implies a need to be anxiously aware of one's sexual functioning, and perhaps to overestimate the seriousness of lack of sexual interest or temporary impotence which might be regarded in other cultures as a natural refractory period or the result of fatigue. Newspapers regularly carry advertisements by genito-urinary specialists and others, offering relief for problems of impotence and related difficulties. Similar advertising aimed at the cure of frigidity in the female was not noted.

Some light on the early development of a sense of masculine identity is shed by Rosen's (1962) work on achievement motivation. His data indicate that socialization practices among the middle class in Brazil, as reported by mothers and perceived by their sons, are determined by the authoritarian, father-dominated families. The only way of dealing with severely authoritarian fathers is through revolt or submission—and submission in the form of ingratiation and obedience was the dominant adjustment. Since aggression against the father is "perhaps the most heinous sin in the Brazilian family," the children often learn to avoid even the appearance of aggressiveness which competition suggests. The mother, who herself is expected to be submissive and deferential in the role of wife, does not interpose herself between father and son, but, rather, is authoritarian to the boy in her own right and at the same time, excessively protective and indulgent. Rosen regards this "combination of authoritarianism, excessive protectiveness, and early indulgence, which boys experience in a type of structure very common in Brazil—the authoritarian father-dominated family" as . . . "partly responsible for the finding that Brazilian boys, on the average, have markedly low achievement motivation when compared with their American peers" (pp 623–624).

MARITAL STATUS

Divorce is not legal in Brazil, but those who wish to may become *desquitado* or separated. Members of the educated classes who wish divorce or remarriage generally accomplish this outside of the country. There is some reason to believe that the relative ease of maintaining a permanent relationship with a mistress or lover, because it allows some personal gratification or sense of fulfillment for spouses no longer interested in each other, reduces the pressure for divorce and permits the continued integrity of families. Aside from the conventional state of marriage, or the legally recognized one of *desquite,* the major category of relationship is the common-law or companionate marriage. This is practiced largely in the lowest socioeconomic stratum and is due to the economic obstacles to marriage as well as the man's unwillingness to give up his sense of personal freedom. Many, if not the greater number of such unions, are reported to be as stable as those solemnized through legal or religious means, but in some instances they are contracted by women who, having lost their virginity, are not considered desirable marriage partners. The relationship may then be less valued by the man and therefore less stable. Frazier (1942), Herskovits (1943), and Ribeiro (1945) have contributed to the literature on the common-law or *amaziado* relationship, particularly among blacks, as it has existed in Bahia and Recife.

Despite the possibly diminishing intensity of family ties for the urban middle class, marriage must still be viewed within a familial context. The network of relatives remains as a source of friends, protectors, and contacts which result in favors of many kinds. Personal observations and discussion with professional colleagues suggest that in spite of social change this pattern continues to be important as an emotionally reinforced system of reciprocal and expected assistance, and that the acceptance of a new addition to the group by marriage is a very important matter. This impression is supported by the fact that approximately 15 per cent of the patients in the present study who said they had "intimate friends" or friends with whom they "could talk," volunteered the information that these "friends" were, in fact, relatives. It became clear in discussions with many of the patients' relatives, especially during home visits when they were more inclined to talk about such matters, that while they live at considerable distances from one another, in times of unusual stress, e.g., the mental hospitalization of a disturbed spouse or child, at least one available family member would consider it an obligation to assist. For much of the time however—in contrast to observations of traditional rural and small town Brazil—their most significant mutally reciprocal interactions were with friends. An upper-class informant, discussing the *pistolão* (pull or pressure exerted in one's favor, usually within the government), made a similar point. He noted that such favors may be done for people on political grounds or as part of building up an expectation of mutual help; while kinship added to such factors may be the deciding element, kinship alone is rarely the crucial point: "Friendship probably counts for more . . . some people nowadays are even proud because they haven't obtained positions for their relatives—this really is a change from the past!"

Lycia de Mendonca's work is the richest source of recent statistical information about marriage in Rio de Janeiro. Most of what follows is taken from this source. De Mendonca's data come from the same group of almost 2,500 women between the ages of 20 and 50 studied in 1963 by Ponte. The proportion of ever-married (not including common-law marriages or consensual unions) in this group was similar to that reported in highly industrialized countries, and was higher than that reported for the Brazilian general population in 1950. Thus, the 1950 census indicated percentages of 51, 75, and 82 as ever married in the age ranges, 20–29, 30–39, 40–49 respectively, while the 1963 sample showed percentages for these ages of 62, 90 and 95. The UN Demographic Yearbook listed 85 per cent of the United States female population in 1960 between ages 25 and 34 as married in comparison with only 74 per cent of Brazilian women of the same age. The age of marriage is also comparable with that in the United States. Forty-one per cent of the sample were married at age 19 or younger and an additional 42 per cent between ages 20 and 24. Education was a major variable in this respect. Of those who had no education at all or had not gone beyond primary school, 85 per cent were married before their 20th birthday. This dropped to 73 per cent for those who had had some or had completed secondary school, and to 56 per cent for those with some or completed university education. The average age at marriage for female university graduates (excluding those who did not get married at all) was 22.3 years. Considerably fewer women of the upper class than the others in Mendonca's sample were married, implying that marriage is no longer the only objective of the middle- and upper-class woman. This suggests another cultural modification as well, since a woman's right to education has traditionally been secondary to that of sons in the family. Thirty per cent of the daughters of men in Class I occupations were unmarried. This was true for 17 per cent of those from Class II and 25 per cent from Class III. A break occurred after this, with only 18 per cent of daughters of men in Classes IV, V, and VI remaining single.

A more continuous progression was noted in regard to education. Of those who had not gone beyond primary school, 15 per cent were unmarried; secondary school students and graduates included 27.5 per cent unmarried; and university students and graduates averaged 44 per cent unmarried. While this last figure was undoubtedly weighted by considerable numbers of those still studying who were awaiting graduation in order to be married, it suggests a possible conflict between the expectations which one sex might have of the other. There are no data on the feelings of middle-or upper-class Brazilian men about having educated women as wives, but much unsystematic observation suggests that if education were seen as synonymous with a wish for independence or a tendency to dominate, it would not be regarded with pleasure. Similarly many Brazilian professional women have been heard to say that they would prefer to remain unmarried rather than conform to the submissive role of a traditional wife.

Being black was associated with a slightly lower likelihood of marriage. While 80.5 per cent of whites and browns were ever married, this was true for only 76 per cent of blacks. There was no association between marriage and religious or rural-urban status. Consensual or common-law unions were found mainly but not exclusively among those with little or no education; most but not all of the male partners were in Class V and VI occupations. There was also an association between color and formal marital status. Within the black group, 47 per cent were legally married, in contrast to 15 per cent in consensual unions; comparable figures for browns were 55 and nine per cent, and for whites 70 and 2.5 per cent. As noted earlier, these unions often carry mutual responsibilities and may be quite stable. In some cases they become legalized with the advent of children, but in others, the family may be more accurately characterized as "partial" with only the mother as the central element. Some households consist of an old mother, one or more daughters, and their children. The grandmother will take care of the children while the younger women work outside in order to support the household. Frazier (1942) wrote similarly about the matrifocal character of many black families in Bahia 30 years ago, speculating about the African cultural as well as the socioeconomic roots of the situation.

Approximately equal numbers of those with legal and consensual unions in the Rio study were Catholic. Twenty-three per cent of the legal, in contrast to only nine per cent of the consensual unions were Protestant, fitting the prevailing ethic of this religion in Brazil (see Chapter XI.) Fifty-four per cent of the consensual unions in Mendonca's sample were contracted below the age of 20, in contrast to 38 per cent of the legal marriages. Thirty-eight per cent of the female partners in consensual unions engaged in paid work outside the home, in contrast to 28 per cent of those legally married. In general, the figures suggest that the formation of consensual unions is associated more closely with economic deprivation than any other single factor. This fits the Brazilian saying: *"pobre não casa, junta"* ("poor people don't marry, they just get together").

Among the 2,500 women there were 108 broken marriages, 17.5 per cent of which were legalized in the form of *desquite*. The women in these last were almost all urban, educated, and between the ages of 40 and 49, and the legalization of the separated state was probably associated with a need to provide for their children. Approximately six per cent of the sample were widowed, with their average age being 43. Sixty per cent of these had been born outside of Rio de Janeiro and a third of them had arrived at age 40 or more, looking for employment. Thirty-six per cent of the widows were employed as *empregadas domésticas,* 29 per cent in other capacities outside of the home, and 35 per cent remained in their own homes.

The question of marriage in relation to skin color has been explored by Hutchinson (1965). He found in two small-town populations that 86 per cent of husbands and wives (including both legal and consensual unions) were of similar color, with seven per cent of the men marrying lighter wives and the same percentage marrying darker ones. Within the group of black husbands, 25 per cent had lighter skinned wives, while 17 per cent of the black women had lighter skinned husbands. Of 811 marriages, only three per cent could be called mixed in the sense that one partner was clearly black and the other clearly white. Hutchinson's (1959) analysis of the same population studied by Ponte and by Mendonca suggests that upward social mobility may be achieved more frequently through marriage by black or brown women than by whites. Two-thirds of the black and three-fourths of the brown wives in the four upper status categories (based on occupational levels) had arrived there from lower status levels, in contrast to a third of the white wives, i.e., their husbands' statuses were higher than those of their fathers. In the two lowest status categories, a fourth of the white wives had arrived through lost status (i.e., from fathers' levels) as compared with five to 10 per cent of the browns and blacks. In this study Hutchinson also investigated the frequently expressed idea that Negro women bear fewer children —a proposition which has been advanced as the reason for the progressive "whitening" of the skin which is supposed to be taking place in Brazil. He was able to conclude that ". . . the color of a mother's skin does not override a general tendency for fertility to decline with rising social status" (unpaged).

In this respect, Kahl's (1967) data are relevant. He interviewed a sample of 627 men in Rio de Janeiro in 1960 about their preference for family size. Contrary to general expectation and to findings from Mexico, the Brazilian sample clearly favored the small family ideal. The key predictor was urban location. Kahl felt that once urbanization begins, certain aspects of Brazilian culture predispose to a rapid move toward this ideal. These are (in contrast to Mexico), more confidence in non family ties, less dependence on relatives, and less emphasis on male dominance, all leading to a conjugal family structure approximating the modern urban mode.

THE SAMPLE

The patient population was predominantly male (65 versus 35 per cent female), reflecting the greater tendency to protect the female in the home and the fact that incapacity in the males who are the breadwinners requires more prompt and drastic attention. The sex ratios among the patients in all three of the hospitals utilized for the study were similar. Of the total patient group, 32 per cent had never been married or had a consistent mate, and seven per cent had had consensual unions or common-law marriages. Thirty-nine per cent had been married only once with both civil and religious ceremonies, and an additional 20 per cent reported civil ceremonies alone. The remaining two per cent constituted two individuals who had had religious ceremonies only, a single individual who had been married twice, one married in another country, and two of undetermined marital status. Four per cent of the once-married were separated (including a single individual who was *desquitado*) and three per cent were widowed. These separated and widowed persons were divided almost equally between the civil-religious and civil ceremony only groups.

The significance of having a religious as well as a civil ceremony was alluded to on a number of occasions by patients and relatives during the interviews. While the details of the explanations varied according to sex and socioeconomic status, the messages were always similar. The *ginásio* educated mother of one young patient reflected on the subject at length during a leisurely home visit: "I lost interest in the Catholic church after my father died, even though my mother went to mass regularly and had many priests among her friends. Then I met my husband-to-be who was a Protestant, and I decided to get married in his church. It would have been difficult to get married in the Catholic church because of so many silly requirements. Anyway I wasn't religiously involved. It's just that socially it's required, you know, something to do with virginity. If you don't get married in church, people will think you aren't a virgin, like you have to get married. If you and your bridegroom go through with the religious ceremony everybody knows things are all right, and the two of you together are doing things the way people want you to do them."

A female patient, also expressing the general wish to do what the family wants, said, "I wasn't intending to have a religious ceremony because it didn't have any special value for me, but my mother insisted so much that I decided to do it."

A 40-year-old, white, primary-school-educated mechanic de-

scribed his pre- and extramarital relationships: "I always preferred *mulatas*. The best of all was an old *mulata* woman I know.
She wasn't the best looking, but there wasn't anything she didn't
know how to do." When asked about his wife, however, he said,
"I wouldn't marry anybody you could have before marriage. My
bride had to be able to wear a crown of orange blossoms in the
church."

The relatively high proportion of unmarried persons in the
sample reflects the preponderance of males who are under less
pressure for marriage than females, as well as the fact that this is
a population of psychiatric patients, i.e., persons with difficulties
in relating to others. Seventy-one per cent of the unmarried individuals, or slightly more than the proportion in the total patient
group, were male.

In order to develop groups sufficiently large for comparative
purposes, and of contrasting sociocultural status, data tabulation according to marital status was limited to two groups: the 32
per cent of the total with no spouses or consistent mates, and the
39 per cent having first marriages with both civil and religious
ceremonies. Since the omission of a religious ceremony may also
reflect economic incapacity as well as loss of virginity or lack of
participation in the dominant value system, it is clear that in this
comparison the "married" group is weighted on the side of social
participation and conformity as well as economic achievement.

Social Characteristics of Male and Female Patients

SOCIOECONOMIC INDICATORS

Table 142 lists those socioeconomic indicators revealing some
differences, usually at least 10 per cent, between the male and
female members of the patient population. Education is included,
since the small, though not significant difference in favor of the
women is compatible with other status differences. A slightly
lower but significantly different proportion of female patients or
their nonpatient husbands, than of male patients, is employed in
occupational Class VI. A considerable number of those in the
upper occupational categories are school teachers or high level

secretarial and clerical workers. Less than a fifth of this patient population are *empregadas domésticas*. Aside from the fact that more men are in the unskilled manual category, the economic differences in favor of the female patients, which might be expected because of their husbands' occupations are slight and not significant. Nonetheless, significant differences do exist in subjective estimates of upward socioeconomic mobility, in favor of the females. Hutchinson's (1959) observations, noted earlier, suggest that some of this mobility may be the result of having married men of higher social status than their fathers'. (Although data on fathers' occupations were collected, they are too uneven to offer conclusions.) Greater mobility for females may also be associated with the availability of normal schools for teacher training.

SOCIOCULTURAL PARTICIPATION, FAMILY, AND BACKGROUND FEATURES

The majority of items in these categories revealed no differences according to sex. Table 143 lists all items with at least a 10 per cent difference between the sexes and a few others which seem relevant. Contact with the clergy and church membership and attendance are much more frequently reported by women than men, a finding congruent with the greater support given the Catholic churches by women. It is interesting to note that this difference extends to participation in Spiritist or Afro-Brazilian groups. While there were no differences in the general amount of reading, television watching, or radio listening, more women than men reported owning one or more books. This difference is congruent with the suggestion that female patients do tend to be of higher social class than the males. Many more men than women attended soccer games, and in keeping with their greater freedom and mobility, more regularly attended movies. Most of the female patients and their relatives indicated that, in contrast to the men, the lower-class married woman has only a domestic and work life and that her civic and social participation is negligible or nonexistent.

Some differences in backgrounds between males and females also fit the general cultural context of greater protection, restriction, and sanctioned dependency for females. Slightly fewer females were disciplined by beatings or were independent prior to age 14. The males were less connected with families, more than twice as many as the females having migrated alone. Considerably more males arrived as adults, i.e., after age 21, presumably with members of conjugal rather than families of origin.

Hospitalization and Family Diagnoses of Male and Female Patients

Table 144 shows that more females had had previous outpatient psychiatric contact before hospital admission. This suggests either a longer illness or reluctance on the part of the family to hospitalize them. A few more males than females were described as having had relatively brief illnesses before admission. The only difference in reasons for admission involved assaultive behavior. This was listed as a reason for hospitalization in four times as many males as females, a finding congruent with those for most societies, but the absolute numbers are very low.

There were no differences according to sex in the family diagnoses.

Psychiatric and Behavioral Characteristics of Male and Female Patients

TENSION, ANXIETY, SENSITIVITY, AND FRUSTRATION

The data in Table 144 suggest that the female patients were more disturbed in general than the males, although many items did not reveal a sufficient difference to be listed. Men were more conventional, friendly, and cooperative in the interviews and seemed less anxious. The women were not only more anxious and less cooperative, they wept more and seemed to be more dependent and attention seeking. The single item differentiating the interviewer's responses according to sex was that concerning his feeling of being liked by the patient; almost five times as many of the males as the females evoked this report by the psychiatrist. It remains uncertain whether this was a consequence of the greater initial anxiety and tension of the females, whether this last itself reflected a certain culturally based distrust of the doctor by the female patient, or whether there were other determinants of mutally negative interaction.

Table 145 shows that in addition to showing more disturbed behavior in the interview situation, the females described more anxiety symptoms and interference with function than the males. These do not include the complete gamut of such symptoms but among those showing at least a 10 per cent difference between the sexes, there is complete consistency. Males, as might be expected, exhibited more evidence of hostile tension and impulsivity. Although the differences are slight and not statistically significant, they are consistent.

DEPRESSION

Table 146 lists the depressive indicators with at least a 10 per cent difference in occurrence between the sexes, plus a few others which are closely related. Significantly more females weep and appear sad and express themselves as being sad, depressed, suicidal, inferior, or suffering from intensely unpleasant or dulled feelings. The single item of guilt concerns failure as a parent. There are no differences between the sexes in terms of feelings of inadequacy and incompetence.

THE BREAK WITH REALITY

Differences between the sexes in this respect, limited to Table 147, are very few. More females, though not significantly so, seem inclined to be grandiose, perhaps reflecting their real-life secondary status, and more regard other people as untrustworthy—again a possibly realistic perception by members of a discriminated-against group. Females do, however, show significantly higher incidences of temporal and spatial disorientation. The fact that almost no females were admitted with histories of excessive alcohol intake supports the assumption that the greater frequency of impaired reality testing and disorientation among the lowest SES groups is not a function of excessive alcohol intake.

SOMATIC AND SEXUAL PROBLEMS

As indicated in Table 148, the picture is mixed with reference to somatic complaints. More women than men complained of fatigue, anorexia, dizziness or faintness, dyspnea, slowed motions, and something strange inside the body. More men complained of weakness, headaches, and sweating or hot flashes. More women complained of lack of sexual satisfaction and diminished sex drive. The men in contrast more often said that their sexual impulses were overly intense, and more than a quarter of them, as compared to no women at all, described their usual sexual relationship as casual or transitory. This last may have been related to the more frequent report among the actively seeking men than among the passively accepting women, that sex was a source of anxiety, guilt, or shame.

Past Psychiatric History of Male and Female Patients

No significant or consistent differences were noted in this respect.

Social Characteristics of Married and Single Patients

As noted earlier, these comparisons are between the unmarried and those married with both legal and religious ceremonies. Persons with consensual unions, who constitute a small fraction of the total group, and the somewhat larger number married with civil but not religious ceremonies, are not included in the comparisons. The following individual examples, mainly of young unmarried males, provide a background against which to view the statistical data. Some relevant examples have already been described in preceding chapters, particularly that on housing, and others are noted in the Chapter X, concerned with age status.

A 27-year-old unmarried white *biscateiro*, a primary school graduate who might have been expected to achieve more, was born in the suburb of Meier. For two years he has rented a room, which he has to himself, in a married sister's apartment in a converted tenement in the urban center of Rio. Other inhabitants of the apartment include the sister and her husband and their four children. Previously, he had lived for two years in the home of one of his brothers, and prior to that he was with his parents. According to his sister, at the age of 18 he abandoned the Catholic church to become an *Umbandista*. (See Chapter XI). The patient says that his real reason for going to the Umbanda center is to look for women and that he always finds one after every service. During recent months, however, he has lost interest in this as well as in work. Admission was precipitated by his having attacked his sister.

A 28-year-old unmarried white primary school graduate lives with his parents, a brother (with whom he shares a room), and four sisters in a single house with all utilities, in a residential area of Corumba, a small town in Matto Grosso. He would like to work but has never been employed, and his father, a government employee, prefers to keep him at home. His major regular activity has been accompanying his parents to Catholic mass each Sunday. His parents, the principal informants besides himself, note that for some years he has easily forgotten what he learns, has trouble explaining what he has read, and, although he listens to the radio, seems disinterested. Formerly "mad about" football and the cinema, he hasn't attended for three or four years, and his father has forbidden him to go to dances. The neighbors recently threatened police action because the patient was "molesting and persecuting" neighborhood children. Finally, his mother and father brought the patient to Rio where they remained for three months, living with a maternal aunt in a residential neighborhood, before his behavior convinced them that hospitalization could no longer be delayed. His father will return to Matto Grosso, but his mother is prepared to remain in Rio for several months if necessary. They believe that an "epileptic condition" will be discovered to be the basis of their son's disturbance.

A 24-year-old unmarried white man, born in the urban district of Irajá and educated to the third year of ginásio, has lived most of his life in the suburb of Madureira, sharing a room with a brother in a single house with all utilities. Other occupants are his parents, a paternal grandfather, two nephews, two sisters, and two other brothers, a total of 11 people. He works in a secretarial capacity (Class IV) for a major electric power company. While professing no religion, according to his father, a principal informant, he frequently attends Macumba sessions. (The father who was briefly hospitalized years earlier because of a nervous breakdown "from overwork," is a Kardecista Spiritist who changed from Catholicism when he was 18 years old.) The patient does not attend dances, soccer, or the beach, but goes to the movies approximately once monthly. He has been drinking more heavily during the approximately one year of mounting tension, insomnia, irritability, and seclusiveness culminating in hospitalization. While accepting the need for hospitalization, his parents do not regard him as mentally ill, but only as having changed his behavior.

A 28-year-old unmarried white secretarial worker in a federal prison (Class IV), was born in Itapéruna in Rio state and has lived with his family in the largely urbanized *favela* of Jacarezinho in suburban Meier for 18 years. They own their home, which has electricity but no water. Five siblings now live elsewhere. For a time, the patient and his parents shared a sleeping room, but later they constructed another one as an annex to the house which he and his father share. A good student, the patient was admitted to a seminary upon the intervention of a public school teacher, but after the second year of *ginásio* there he was asked to leave because of erratic behavior. While professing nominal Catholicism, he does not attend mass. He has supported himself since the age of 18 but he has had many jobs. He left some because he felt "tired of working" and he was discharged from others because of absenteeism, coming late, or repeated minor altercations with fellow employees. There have been occasional crises during which he behaves peculiarly and does bizarre things. On one such occasion, six months prior to hospitalization, he was arrested for "disrespect for a policeman" after refusing to be taken off the streets. Nonetheless, he has a devoted group of friends who like him very much and take him home when they find him behaving strangely. People in the *favela* also turn to him for help in preparing and typing petitions and writing letters. His parents regard him as mentally ill and brought him to the hospital because they are concerned about his future economic effectiveness.

A 25-year-old unmarried white, third grade educated, unskilled housecleaner, was born in Conservatória in Rio State and migrated to the city with his mother and a brother when he was 12 years old to look for work. They had been abandoned by their brutal father when the patient was eight. The brother now lives elsewhere. The patient and his mother share a single rented room without electricity or water in a *barraco* located in a *favela* in Vincente de Carvalho, in the urban zone of Irajá. A Catholic, he attends mass on occasional feast days and has also visited some Macumba sessions. He engages in no amusements, "living only at work and at home." He has been passive, withdrawn, and suspicious for years. Shortly before admission he threatened to attack a neighbor for some fancied persecution. His mother and an uncle's wife who accompanied him to the hospital have regarded him as mentally ill for several years.

An example of a person living in a companionate or consensual marriage, or a state of *amigado,* is a 33-year-old white man who arrived at the hospital accompanied by his mother and his *companheira.* He still lives in Madureira where he was born, inhabiting a single house with electricity and an irregular water supply, with his mate and their three children, the youngest of whom shares their bedroom. Although he finished the first year of *ginásio,* he is an unskilled bus washer (Class VI). He regards the work as tiresome, preferring a previous job as assistant in an automobile repair shop. He says that he "believes in God but has never had a religion." (His father, separated from his mother for eight years, and a heavy drinker, was also unaffiliated.) His chief amusements are going to movies and playing cards. Although he attends the movies at least once weekly, he never takes his mate with him, nor does she participate in his card games with his male friends. He was brought to the hospital because of bizarre behavior associated with unwillingness to work. The family admits that he should be hospitalized, but while feeling that he "needs a rest," does not regard him as mentally ill.

Several examples of unmarried females have been noted in earlier chapters. Another, somewhat older one is a 38-year-old brown third grade graduate, a skilled *operária* on a factory nightshift who works secondarily as a seamstress. Born in Oswaldo Cruz in Madureira, she now lives in the same suburban zone in Rocha Miranda in a single house with electricity but no piped water, owned by her widowed sister (who accompanied her to the hospital) with the latter and her two daughters. The entire family sleeps in one room. She has no religious affiliation although she "believes in God and in the Christian Spiritist truth." (Neither her father nor mother adhered to any formal religion, although the former had studied for a short time in a "priest's school" and "liked to read the gospel.") The patient "is not a friendly person," according to her sister, who is her only intimate. She has been increasingly withdrawn, depressed, slowed up, and preoccupied, and has not gone to work for four months. The sister considers her behavior "strange" rather than mentally ill, but regards hospitalization as necessary and believes that the "rest" will be good for her.

SOCIOECONOMIC INDICATORS

Table 149 shows that more of the married are literate, presumably reflecting greater adequacy, social competence, and conformity and drive. While a few more of the single, in keeping with their younger age, have completed or gone beyond the primary years of education, this finding is not statistically significant. The married patients have more occupational achievement and security. Similar proportions of the married and unmarried are in Classes I–IV but considerably more of the former are in the stable Class V, and fewer are in the lowest Class VI. Differences in housing quality also suggest more advanced economic status for the married. More of the married live in the relatively stable suburban-industrial areas, while the single tend more frequently to live in the town centers (including small towns in Greater Rio) or in outlying parts of Greater Rio de Janeiro. This last may again be associated with youth and the possibility that some live with their parents, as well as with less economic achievement, and recent mobility.

Socioeconomic mobility figures are mixed, with the married patients having more often achieved higher status than their fathers, but more frequently also having declined during the preceding year. This last may be associated with family responsibilities and the possible advent of additional children, or physical illness which, coupled with progressive psychiatric impairment, can result in a rapid economic decline. Single patients, who have achieved less and bear less responsibility for others, are less vulnerable to loss of status or goods with increasing psychiatrically based impairment.

DEMOGRAPHIC CHARACTERISTICS

Table 152 indicates, as expected, that the married patients are older than the unmarried. More are white, with proportionately more browns among the unmarried; and a few more claim a formal religious affiliation. In other words, the married as compared with the unmarried group have more of the characteristics of social stability and relatedness.

The migration picture is inconclusive and, logically, appears to be a function of age. A few, but not significantly more, of the single—as might be expected on the basis of their relative youth and dependence on parents—were born and reared in Greater Rio. Nonetheless, a quarter of them, approximately twice the proportion of the married, had come into the area within the preceding five years (again, because of the variability within the group, the difference in mobility according to marital status is only suggestive, but not statistically significant). Some of these latter had moved with their families into Rio (there were no differences according to marital status in the number migrating alone), and difficulties in adapting to the new situation were probably added to those pre-existing. This group also includes almost all the patients who were brought to Rio by family members for the express purpose of hospitalization.

The married migrants, as expected, include the largest proportion who were more than 21 years old at the time they moved into Greater Rio. The majority of them, in accordance with data on older migrants reported in Chapter IV, were already burdened with conjugal family responsibilities at the time of their move and, therefore, more socioeconomically vulnerable. Their somewhat better economic status, however, coupled with the fact that almost a quarter of them changed occupations after the move, suggests that at the same time that they were vulnerable, they were relatively active copers with the new environment and that their responsibilities, coupled with the experience of prior achievement, stimulated them to greater compensatory effort.

INFORMATION AND SOCIAL PARTICIPATION

More of the married than the single, as noted in Table 151, owned the major informational appliances, i.e., radio and television sets. More of the younger singles, however, owned books, read, and were frequent movie-goers. In keeping with earlier findings, and undoubtedly determined by family need as well, the married patients had more frequent and friendly contact with welfare workers. It may indicate something about the closed nature of the family as a need-supplying system, that almost a third of the married, significantly more than the unmarried, knew nothing about their neighbors and over a half never attended movies. This last, as well as their low attendance at dances in contrast to the unmarried, may, of course, reflect their need to use money for other purposes. Many of the patients specifically noted that they had stopped going to dances after marriage, suggesting both the increased need to conserve friends and a diminished need to engage in the kind of social and sexual exploration preliminary to marriage.

Hospital, Family, and Childhood Factors in Married and Unmarried Patients

The items showing a 10 per cent difference or more in these respects are listed in Tables 152 and 153, but the data are inconclusive though suggestive. A few more of the married patients appear to have come from more stable homes. Although the significance of differences is slight or nonexistent, they report being reared, disciplined, and having had siblings by both parents, and a lower incidence of homes "broken" by early parental death, divorce, or desertion. At the same time, more (but less than half) of the singles report their parents to have been literate. This may reflect their relative youth, or even some bias in the nature of the younger people who are admitted to psychiatric hospitals, mainly upon the initiative of their parents, i.e., these are the more responsible parents who have not allowed their mentally ill children to become vagrants.

Hospitalization of the married was almost never at the Pronto Socorro (only three per cent), reflecting the protective value of the family system as well as the fact that more were regularly employed. Twenty-nine per cent of the singles were seen in this emergency facility, even though fewer reported a relatively short illness (six months or less). This may have been, in part, because of the higher proportion than the married admitted because of assaultive behavior (almost a quarter of the singles.) The longer, untreated illnesses coupled with being younger, unmarried, and less employed also suggest that the single population included more chronically schizophrenic or schizoid persons with an illness dating from the developmental years, who were brought to the hospital during an acute episode by parents who had given up trying to shield them. In these instances, the fact that they did not have more previous outpatient contact than the married may be plausibly attributed to their continued residence under family supervision until hospitalization could no longer be avoided. A significantly higher proportion of the married, in contrast, were admitted because of depressed or suicidal behavior, and over half had had previous contact with a psychiatrist.

Over twice as many of the families of single patients, including parents and siblings, as those of the married, diagnosed their disturbed behavior as due to a mental illness. The families of married patients, in contrast, including most often spouses and sometimes parents and siblings, were more inclined (although these perceptions were reported by only 27 and 21 per cent respectively) to regard them as behaving strangely or in response to life stress. These may reflect the perceptions of people accustomed to seeing the patients as competent adults, in contrast to those who had reared them and were accustomed to having them dependent and to caring for their fluctuating health.

Psychiatric and Behavioral Characteristics of Married and Unmarried Patients

TENSION, ANXIETY, SENSITIVITY, AND FRUSTRATION

As indicated in Table 154, the married patients behaved in a more conventional manner, seemed less disturbed, and evoked less discomfort in the interviewers. The psychiatrists felt both more pity and hostility for the single patients, and were more cheerful and optimistic in the presence of those who were married— although the percentages were low in all instances. The disturbed interview behavior of single patients was not markedly anxious, tense, or depressed. It was, rather, less cooperative, emotionally inappropriate, and communicatively unclear. They were more distractible, silly, hostile, fearful, or apathetic, and expressed unsatisfied wishes to be cared for. These observations are consistent with those in Table 155, indicating the unmarried patients to be more sensitive and vigilant to other peoples' feelings about them, concerned with their own failure to have achieved what they wanted, impulsive, and suffering from greater interference with thinking and decision-making. Few anxiety items showed a statistically significant difference between the two groups. These, including worries about relatives, were more frequently reported by the married than the single.

DEPRESSION

Table 156 presents a picture congruent with the observations noted above. Weeping, sadness, and suicidal attempts were more frequently observed among the married. The depressive behaviors more frequently encountered in single patients were, in contrast, those associated with muted or absent affect, a sense of isolation, emotional detachment, or status-sensitivity in relation to others. This last included guilt about role inadequacy, including failure of filial performance.

THE BREAK WITH REALITY

As indicated in Table 157, the single patients markedly more often than the married, expressed paranoid feelings and thoughts, complaining of persecution and misjudgement in a variety of ways. Similarly, they more frequently reported auditory and visual hallucinations (although no more visual hallucinations of people), the reality and importance of which were greater for them. Proportionately more were disoriented and reported illusions and misinterpretations. Again the clinical findings suggest, in general, that the unmarried more often than the married patients suffered from impaired reality-testing, high sensitivity to the opinions of others about them, social isolation, personal detachment, and affective flattening.

SOMATIC AND SEXUAL COMPLAINTS OF MARRIED AND UNMARRIED PATIENTS

Table 158 shows that the married patients complained more often than the unmarried about psychophysiological disturbances.

They also complained more often of impotence or frigidity, sexual functioning impaired by worries, and proportionately more regarded their sexual lives as influenced by their present illness. This may simply reflect the fact that they lived with a person of the opposite sex and that a certain standard of sexual activity was expected of them. The single patients, younger, more socially isolated, and less consistently in close contact with the opposite sex, more often noted sex to be a source of anxiety, guilt, or shame; they also more frequently complained of their sexual impulses as being too strong or too weak. Approximately a fifth of the single, in contrast to none of the married, said that masturbation was their only form of sexual activity. This again is probably a function of youth and lack both of initiative and opportunity for anxiety-free heterosexual relationships.

PAST PSYCHIATRIC HISTORY OF MARRIED AND SINGLE PATIENTS

Data recorded in Table 159 show that more single patients reported school and work adjustment problems, difficulties in learning to relate to others, and childhood temper tantrums during their developmental period. Marital status is the single independent variable on the basis of which statistically significant differences in past history have been identified. The findings are congruent both with the relative youth of the single patients, who consequently had more vivid memories, and with their character and psychopathology—of a socially withdrawn, affectively detached nature. The suggestion is strong that the differences noted reflect the long insidious development of chronic psychiatric disorder among those who were single at the time of hospitalization.

DISCUSSION

Although there have been marked changes, survey evidence suggests that approximately two-thirds of Guanabara women may still be regarded as culturally marginal or in the process of modernization. Education and social status both contribute to positive attitudes toward women's participation in politics or occupations on a status equal with that of men. At the lowest level, where the majority work outside the home in menial, unskilled, or house-keeping tasks, at least on a part-time basis, the complex of ideas and attitudes around the concept of "modernization" is still abstract and remote from the realities of daily survival. The female role also exists in a complementary position to that of the male, as reflected in accepted masculine prerogatives.

The linkage of depression to female status has been observed in other cultures, and this, as well as their dependent, attention-seeking, and to a lesser degree grandiose behavior, is congruent with their minority status. Compared with men, they have less personal freedom, and are more dependent for social and economic survival upon their expressive qualities as these influence others. Somatic and psychophysiological complaints were mixed, and apart from the females' more frequent complaint of something strange inside their bodies, it is difficult to explain the symptom differences according to gender status.

Sexual complaints were distributed in the expected fashion. The more frequent lack of sexual satisfaction and interest among women fits the traditional, culturally approved, stereotype of the religious women. Sexual complaints may also be a consequence of the male's emphasis on using sex as a continuing proof of his own virility. A greater degree of conflict in the males, associated with their inability to deny the life significance of sex (as the women more frequently appeared to do), is suggested by their more frequent description of sex impulses as overly intense and the source of anxiety, guilt, or shame.

Because divorce is not legal in Brazil, and varied forms of legal separation are not widely used except among the more affluent educated classes, most partners joined in civil and religious ceremonies tend to stay together despite personal incompatibilities. Marriage as an institution and family integrity may be facilitated by the establishment of long-term extramarital arrangements for personal, emotional, and sexual gratification. Since these arrangements are most often between husband and an unmarried or unattached woman, the wife's adjustment may more frequently involve denial of sexual interests, relegation of her marital relationship to the status of an obligation, and an increased focus of her interests on children, extended family, religion, or social activities. The network of relatives, which still provides the major context for marriage in spite of the diminishing intensity of family ties for the urban middle-class, continues to be an important system of reciprocal and expected assistance and friendship. Marriage, as in the United States, is less frequent and occurs at a later age for upper-class university educated women. Data on consensual or companionate unions confirm the general supposition that they are more frequent in Rio de Janeiro among the poorest, the illiterate, least educated, least affluent, and nonwhite. Unions of this type constituted only seven per cent of the total patient sample. The limited data suggest that mixed, clearly interracial marriages are rare, and that when they do occur, may be a source of upward social mobility for nonwhite females.

These features are congruent with the general features of married as contrasted to single people in most Western cultures where marriage is one aspect of socially approved achievement. These are people who grew up in contexts where religiously sanctioned marriage was valued; they have been more capable of getting along with others, coping with the social system, and assuming some degree of responsibility. They have also grown up with somewhat greater degrees of social (white) and familial support. The picture is mixed because some of the single patients are younger and, like members of their generation, tend to be better educated, read more, and go more frequently to movies as well as dances.

The protective value of the conjugal family and the degree of premorbid achievement of the married who became patients, as well as their smaller tendency to assaultiveness, are reflected in the fact that almost none of them were seen at the Pronto Socorro. Single patients were most often hospitalized because of assaultive behavior, and married ones because of depressed or suicidal behavior. This may plausibly be related to the alloplastic tendencies of the unmarried and the internalizing tendencies and problems in meeting self-imposed responsibilities of the married. Most significantly, the reasons for hospital admission reflect the evaluation of families of origin (in the case of the unmarried) or conjugal families, and the fact that for a few of the unmarried hospitalization was initiated by public authorities as a consequence of public disturbance. The marrieds, many more of whom had been maintained as outpatients prior to hospitalization, were more fre-

quently diagnosed by their families (as were the more socioeconomically advantaged in general) as behaving strangely or in
response to life stress. The unmarrieds, fewer of whom had previously seen psychiatrists, and whose behavior precipitating admission was more violent and intolerable, were more frequently
diagnosed by their families of origin, with whom they had been
living, as mentally ill.

Psychiatric differences between the two groups fit the pattern
expected on the basis of social differences. The married patients,
more conventional and less disturbed, evoked less discomfort in
the interviewing psychiatrists. They were more cooperative, emotionally appropriate, communicatively effective, and less distractible, silly, hostile, fearful, apathetic, or dependent. They complained less of aspiration/achievement discrepancy, feelings of
inferiority, interference with thinking and decision-making and
reported less impulsive behavior. Their depressed behavior was
more often intensely expressive-emotional in contrast with that of
the unmarried, who were more detached, exhibited muted
affectivity, and were sensitive to their status vis-à-vis others.

The married patients complained more of various forms of
somatic disturbance, including impotence or frigidity, and more
regarded their sex lives as influenced by their present illness.
More of the unmarried noted masturbation to be their only form
of sexual activity, complained of the variable strength of their
sexual impulses, and described sex as a source of inner conflict.
The likelihood seems high that their sexual problems were of
life-long duration and were part of the constellation of problems
resulting in their remaining unmarried.

In general, the symptom pictures and interview behavior of the
single patients may be regarded as reflecting their general lack of
interpersonal interest and skills, emotional withdrawal, and lack
of premorbid achievement. The difference from the married is
most marked in respect to paranoid feelings, auditory and visual
hallucinations, illusions, and disorientation. Their more frequently impaired reality testing combined with the symptoms
and behavior noted above form a general syndrome consistent with
various forms of schizophrenic behavior.

Evidence supporting the supposition that the single, in contrast
to the married patients, suffer from life-long difficulties—under-

standable in terms of incomplete or distorted development as much as or more than of crisis, failure, and regression—is seen in the comparative life-history as well as psychiatric illness data. More of the singles reported school and work adjustment problems, difficulties in learning to relate to others, and childhood temper tantrums. These differences between married and single patient groups in Brazil are similar to those reported in the United States.

CHAPTER 10

AGE AND PATIENT BEHAVIOR
IN A YOUTHFUL POPULATION

THERE ARE no systematic studies of age role in modern Brazil. Adolescents receive sporadic attention, especially insofar as they are involved in violence directed against the universities, and some of their problems have been touched upon in the chapters on education and housing. While a special role for the elderly may be assumed in a country where families are of such central importance, this assumption has not been validated. A survey of Brazilian families would undoubtedly reveal many to be sheltering aged parents or unmarried female relatives, some of whom might be mental-hospital or nursing-home patients in other societies. There is no evidence, however, that the opinions of older people carry special weight or that such individuals are objects of particular respect.

AGE DISTRIBUTION IN GUANABARA

A salient feature of the Brazilian population which may account for the lack of investigative attention paid to the elderly is its youth. The relatively short life span, hardly reaching 50 in the less advantaged areas of the interior, has already been noted. This, coupled with the high birth rate, has resulted in the often quoted estimate that half the population is 18 years of age or less. Guanabara, with its predominantly urban population and relatively available food and medical care, has a life expectancy approaching that of the developed nations. Table 160 shows, however, that even here almost a third of the population in 1960 was 14 years of age or younger, while only between six and seven per cent had attained 60 or more. This compares with overall national figures for 1960 of 42.3 per cent less than 15 years of age, and 2.7 per cent of 65 and over. (In the United States, 1960 national census data show 31.1 per cent of the population to be less than 15, and 15.8 per cent to be 65 or older.) The *favela* population within Guanabara, i.e., those at the bottom of the socioeconomic ladder, showed an even more marked concentration of children and a tiny number who might be considered elderly. This may reflect the larger families of *favela* dwellers; it does not necessarily indicate a shorter life span, since there is some evidence that with increasing economic security a number of *favelados* move out into more adequate surroundings. In any event, *favelas* do not seem to be places of refuge for significant numbers of the elderly poor who have been unable to support themselves with advancing age.

The data in Table 161 may give a more accurate picture of family size and longevity. These show that while few Guanabara males survive past 60, the numbers of blacks and browns of this age or older are proportionately half that of the whites. Since the majority of the darkest skinned people of any age do live in *favelas,* this may account for the fact that only three per cent of Guanabara *favelados* had reached the age of 60. The higher proportions of blacks and browns of age 14 or younger may reflect both the shrunken numbers of older people and the tendency of nonwhites to have larger families than whites.

LOWER-CLASS ADOLESCENTS

The childhood and youth of the lower-class child, who more often than not has dropped out of school by the age of nine or 10, is by middle-class North American standards, severely truncated. In rural areas every child is another potential field hand; in cities or small towns he may soon be helping his parents in home industries or acting as an informal apprentice to his father, in addition to doing the usual chores and errands; and urban slum children, almost as soon as they can walk, begin to participate in the scavenging and begging that are a necessary part of existence. The average lower-class child thus makes an abrupt and rapid transition into adulthood and must look forward to full-time employment, if available, by the time he is 14 or 15 years old. His motivation as well as his skills, however, may be deficient to help him obtain and sustain steady work. Rosen (1962) notes that while a boy in this situation, with little protection or help, may receive much training in self-reliance, self-reliance usually means self-care and does not include the notion of competition with standards of excellence. The psychologist and social worker at the Favela Euclides da Rocha (described in Chapter VIII) confirmed that the adolescents with whom they were in contact lacked both clear-cut goals and knowledge of alternatives. "Draw a person tests," which they administered to an unselected sample, aged 14 to 17, at the Banco da Providencia rehabilitation center, produced results which seemed primitive and undeveloped. The psychologist said this was partly because the children had had no previous opportunities and were unaccustomed to drawing and to using paper and pencil in general. She also felt that for many, lack of mental activity had not permitted a full development of their innate capacities. Since they had "not learned how to think," even the smallest problem posed great difficulties. In her opinion, part of the problem also stemmed from the lack of any regular pattern for living: "There is no regular hour for getting up or going to bed or eating meals. They are just loose during the days . . . although the girls are a little more tied up because they have more duties around the shacks. Many of the families have only mothers and children, and when there are fathers, they are usually away doing odd jobs and hardly ever participate in the care of the children . . . most of the parents never went to school so they don't stimulate their children along these lines. . . ." In this rehabilitation center, between 20 and 30 adolescent boys were attached to training shops. Both the psychologist and social worker conducted periodic discussion groups, usually composed of the boys in the shops, where they talked about occupations and attempted to encourage them to think about their own futures in more or less realistic terms.

MIDDLE- AND UPPER-CLASS ADOLESCENTS

The tiny fraction of the total population made up of the young of the wealthy and the educated shows itself in Rio de Janeiro's discotheques, beaches, and restaurants; at museums and art galleries it is slightly enlarged by others with education and talent, though less money. While some enjoy their prolonged financial dependence and make a career of pursuing pleasure, others are intensely political, involved in "rebellion" against the "establishment"—in the person of the university administrations, and are deeply troubled by the authoritarian aspects of Brazil's military government since the *golpe* of 1964. And yet, even after prolonged conversation, it is difficult at times to be sure of just what these young people do want and of the precise nature of their values. Their ambiguity and the fluctuations of their political expressions which seem to mirror fashions in ideas, have led to many of them being known as *esquerdistas festiva,* or "good-time leftists." A Negro student from the United States, visiting in the summer of 1968, was especially bitter in his condemnation of what he regarded as the essentially frivolous nature of the Brazilian youths' political concerns; he noted that while they were concerned with "imperialistic" actions of various governments, they were untouched by and uninterested in the poverty in their own backyards. He also saw their blindness to the existence of racial prejudice in Brazil as an aspect of their lack of sensitivity to basic socioeconomic inequity. (University youth, almost without exception, are white as are most of those in secondary schools. While tuition is free, books and clothing are not, so economic discrimination—though hidden—is important.) Despite ambiguity and problems in definition, many Brazilian observers feel the activities of the educated young represent a kind of "awakening" for them; at least they no longer confine themselves to cultivating hedonistic interests but become members of some well-intentioned group. Others who simply play, or just go to school and conform are "still sleeping."

The values of relatively well-to-do youth as measured by questionnaire suggest basically authoritarian attitudes, despite professions to the contrary. Five hundred and two white Pôrto Alegre secondary school students were divided into groups of approximately equal size as upper-middle, middle-middle and lower-middle class on the basis of their father's rankings on a scale of occupational prestige. They were tested with a series of multiple-choice questions related to feelings about authority and dominance. Approximately half of those in all groups, and slightly more in the lowest category, admitted to some feeling of fear toward their parents. More than three-quarters in all groups, with the highest proportion among the middle and lower, stated that they accepted their fathers' authority without argument (although 56 and 59 per cent in the latter two groups identified mother as the dominant parent.) Negative feelings toward those with dark skin color were frequent and most so in the lowest class. Only 41 per cent of these, in contrast to 60 and 57 per cent of the upper and middle groups agreed that "most of my friends welcome colored people since they are at my social level." Similar proportions in all groups, however, 33 per cent of the upper, 36 per cent of the middle, and 42 per cent of the lower, agreed with the statement, "I do not care if there is color or race discrimination in my city so long as I am not personally involved." Despite their evident respect for authority and conformity to established values, the majority, and especially the lowest group, seemed to regard the social structure as potentially open to change and were hopeful about their own possibilities. Sixty-eight per cent of the lower group, 59 per cent of the middle, and 52 per cent of the upper believed that laws might be interpreted according to their own personal viewpoints. Only 13 per cent of the lower as compared to 24 per cent of the middle and 39 per cent of the upper group saw the social system as allowing possibility of upward mobility.

In general, it appears that while from a third to a half of the upper middle-class high school students, more than those of lower middle-class families, exhibited attitudes which might be regarded as conservative and uninterested in changing their social environment, their basic values, just as in the United States, are more egalitarian than those in the lower middle class. Concern about physical health was more frequently expressed (perhaps realistically so) in the middle and lower groups, and expressions of independence were more often noted among the upper middle than the lower middle classes. The value of independence, however, as based on the questionnaire, concerned freedom of individual decision-making and liberty from parental domination rather than the espousal of causes with which others did not agree.

ADOLESCENTS IN MENTAL HEALTH FACILITIES

Adolescents are not significantly represented in Brazilian mental hospital populations, as they are in the United States. Those who are encountered in the Pronto Socorro or in the large mental hospitals are apt to suffer from epilepsy, brain damage, mental retardation, or the most severe bizarre schizophrenic behavior. The concept of "adolescent turmoil," or of a more or less transient "borderline state" in pubertal children is not generally recognized. While there are no systematic surveys of the general population, it seems likely that large numbers of disturbed adolescents who would be hospitalized or in clinics in the United States are tolerated in their homes or have joined the population of floating homeless in Brazil.

The main point of outpatient assistance for adolescents in Rio de Janeiro is the Centro de Orientação Juvenil, a unit of the Federal Department of Children. There is a clinic for adolescents at the Catholic University, but the Center is the only public resource under governmental auspices. Here the psychodynamic orientation is even stronger than with the primary school mental health staff described in Chapter VI; the staff makes a point of saying that the focus of the Center is not psychiatric but psychoanalytic. Clients considered psychotic are not accepted for further guidance, although some attempt is made to advise their parents of possible disposition. The director is a psychologist, and the staff, all part-time, includes other psychologists, social workers, and psychiatrists. In addition, a variable number of students of nursing and of social work spend time there collecting material for their dissertations. The Center is a federal installation and referrals may come from all over the country, but most are students in the Guanabara schools referred by their teachers, physicians, or families. Beyond referrals, information about it is spread by word-of-mouth, as is the case for the clinics associated with the Guanabara school system. The clients are more often than not middle class, and many people who could afford private consultation come here because they think in terms of guidance and counseling rather than psychiatric assistance. The typical intervention is relatively brief and psychoanalytically oriented, i.e., uncovering and interpretive face-to-face psychotherapy. The therapists spoke of the importance of a warm, supporting attitude, saying that an impersonal or "classically analytic" stance would cause the youth being treated to complain of being persecuted and not understood. At any given time, there are apt to be from 40 to 50 people in therapy, which typically consists of weekly interviews for one or two months. In some instances, depending on the personal involvement of the therapist, treatment may continue for one or two years. The psychotherapeutic emphasis of the Center makes a waiting list inevitable, but they manage to conduct five or six evaluative interviews weekly in addition to therapy.

The most common reason for referral is family concern with the child who is not getting ahead, not performing well, or repeating a grade. The concern often seems less with learning ability per se than with passing, since graduation is a key to mobility, a better job, and improved social status. The staff, also regarding this as a pressing issue, describes it with the informal descriptive diagnosis of *vida parada*, "being stuck" or having the expected life progress stopped.

Antisocial or aggressive behavior is rarely a cause for referral. More commonly, parents of sons become concerned with the opposite: with passivity regarded as incipiently homosexual in character, although there is usually little of an overt nature to justify their anxiety. In these instances they may describe the boy as not being aggressive enough, staying home too much, or preferring the company of his mother to that of his father. The fathers may often have been "self-made men" who lived in tough neighborhoods during childhood and had to fight to survive. Upon being interviewed, they characteristically reveal some concern that their sons are not as strong or resilient as they, and may not be capable of maintaining or improving the family position gained with such effort. While similar concern with masculinity is encountered among fathers of emotionally disturbed or underachieving sons in the United States, it does not as a rule define an important segment of referrals. The concern with family status appears unequivocally more prominent in this Center than in United States school guidance clinics.

Other specific common complaints were difficult to identify. Many problems seemed to center around the rapid social changes occurring in the city. A girl presenting a school problem, for example, revealed much guilty resentment against the uncle with whom she was living stemming from his restrictions against party-going. Ventilation of this issue led to some clarification of her entire dependency-independency conflict. As a rule, though, the staff felt that the parents, more than the adolescents experienced difficulties and needed guidance in dealing with the changes in social customs. Some of these were handled during group sessions attended by teachers and principals as well as by Center staff and family members.

Middle-class Brazilian adolescents, for these are the ones with whom they mainly deal, are regarded by the Center staff as having strong affective ties with each other. Problems of social isolation or the feeling that no one understands them, so often encountered in the United States, do not seem important here. Except with psychotics, the staff rarely encounters complaints of lack of feeling or purpose in life, or lack of certainty about personal aims and identity. These features are attributed to the "super-protection" of the family, and, the absence of independence as a strong value as in the United States, (this in spite of the problems surrounding the general loosening of parental restrictions). It is thus possible for the adolescent to remain comfortably dependent until marriage, or until he himself is ready to move away from home. For their part, the parents were raised in the tradition of children remaining at home until they are ready to establish a new conjugal household of their own. One member of the staff who had visited many United States treatment centers, felt that, in general, interpersonal communication is much better and more meaningful in Brazil than in the United States. She related these factors to the apparently low suicide rate in the Rio de Janeiro secondary school population. When suicides do occur, however, they often tend to be hidden because of religious or social reasons.

Many Rio de Janeiro families, just as in the traditional towns of the North and the interior, still require their daughters to be accompanied by chaperones when out with a man in the evening. This practice is declining, however, and is rare for unmarried women by the time they reach their mid-twenties. Increasing freedom from parental supervision, more frequent contacts with contemporaries who have left their homes in other cities to live in

Rio, and the greater conversational boldness of escorts are noted by staff members as growing sources of conflict for adolescent girls. In many instances the basic problem is an absolute lack of elementary sexual information. Students who come to Rio from other cities and are no longer surrounded by their families find considerable sexual freedom. The group of fellow students is felt to be a family substitute to which they transfer their dependency, and sexual relations may be an aspect of the attempt to reestablish intimate ties at a new level with a different group. In general, sexual and social freedom among Rio de Janeiro youth are regarded as being more immediately related to educational level than to any other single factor.

THE SAMPLE

The patient population consisted mainly of young adults. Those between 21 and 45 years of age included 79 per cent of the total group; six per cent were under 21; only seven per cent were over 50, and none had passed 60. In order to arrive at reasonably sized groups for comparison, the patients from 15 to 25 were placed together as the youngest group; those from 26 to 45 made up the middle group; with the oldest group comprising those from ages 46 to 60. The youngest group included 22 per cent of the total population; the middle group, 63 per cent; and the oldest, 15 per cent. Within the youngest group, the largest number were aged 21 to 25, constituting 74 per cent of the subsample. Those in the middle group were almost equally distributed, with a peak of 32 per cent between ages 31 and 35. Of the oldest group, 52 per cent were between 46 and 50, 34 per cent between 51 and 55, and 14 per cent between 56 and 60.

Some of the psychosocial characteristics of individual patients according to age, particularly those under 21 and still living with parents, have been indicated in earlier chapters. Several in the youngest group were brought from other parts of the country specifically for hospitalization. Many had been kept at home in spite of long periods of clear psychiatric disturbance until socially disruptive behavior, often evoking hostile responses in others, made it impossible to further delay hospital admission. Additional examples follow.

A 20-year-old unmarried white unemployed primary school graduate, was accompanied to the Pronto Socorro by his mother, a principal informant. He has lived for three years in a single-roomed shanty with electricity but no water, built against the home of a married sister in the peripheral urban district of Braz de Pinã. He depends for financial support upon his mother's consensual partner of three years, a mattress-maker. The patient was raised by his mother until he was 10, and was then in a residential school for seven years. He was "always" a behavior problem, and she dealt with him by force, stating: "I would take his clothes off and beat him with a strap. I used to lock him up in a dark room." She felt part of the problem was marijuana; he once sold a radio to get money to buy the drug. For a while he worked in a pharmacy, but he has not worked since age 15 and is not interested in looking for a job. His mother stated: "He has no shame, he is interested only in his companions and a lot of them are Negroes. The blacker they are the worse for him, because it only makes him more shameless. His only friends are some bare-faces just like him. He steals from his relatives to get marijuana. For the past three years he has been smoking daily. If I tell the police what they do, they will kill me. They have already threatened to do it." Hospital admission was precipitated by assaultive behavior combined with paranoid accusations. On an earlier occasion his mother had him arrested, and he spent three days in jail after having attacked his sister with a piece of broken glass. His mother said: "I suspect he is sick in his mind." The patient practices no religion, although he has attended an occasional Catholic service when forced to do so by his mother. She also notes that although he has phimosis, he has never agreed to an operation: "He has a discharge like a female."

An 18-year-old white unmarried telegraph messenger with some high school, was brought to the hospital by his mother, a principal informant. He had migrated with his mother, now 47, and two older sisters, one of whom had been briefly hospitalized for nervous symptoms, from Alagoas, 11 years earlier, after the family was deserted by his alcoholic "irresponsible" father. They live in a *vila* with light and water in suburban Madureira. The entire family sleeps in the same room, the mother and daughters in one bed and the patient in another. The patient is a Catholic but attends mass only on special feast days. He attends *futebol* games regularly and goes to the movies approximately once monthly, but has no apparent interest in girls or dances. He was brought by his mother to the Casa Eiras because of bizarre (nonaggressive) behavior. She believes him to be mentally ill, attributing it to "too much exposure to the sun while working."

A 17-year-old white unmarried girl, a primary school graduate, was brought to the hospital by her father, a 52-year-old taxi-driver born in Barra de Tijúca in suburban Rio. She was born and reared in the same house in Copacabana. The house has essential services and a patio, and she still lives there with her parents, three brothers, and two sisters. She and her sisters share a sleeping room. She has worked since age 14 in a factory where she is now a skilled operative. A religious Catholic, she attends mass at least once weekly. She also, because of her father's wishes, accompanies him to *futebol* matches almost weekly, in addition to regular attendance at movies, the beach, and every month or two, at dances. Admission was precipitated by her mother, a 46-year-old *mulata* taxi driver, after finding the patient drunk. The father said that he didn't know what the trouble was, the patient denied having a drinking problem, and neither felt that hospitalization was necessary. Anxious about the possibility that something might be wrong, and confessing to the social worker that he had never been able to punish his daughter, the father decided to go ahead with admission, especially since it was covered by the INPS.

A 20-year-old white housewife, a primary school graduate, was brought to the Casa Eiras by her 27-year-old husband of five years, a truck driver. They live with their three children in a house with essential services in the suburb of Madureira where she was born. She is an indifferent Catholic, attending mass only on feast days. Aside from rare attendance at the movies, she participates in no organized amusements, although she liked to go to the beach before becoming ill. She has not felt well since her last pregnancy and has been increasingly apathetic and withdrawn with periods of occasional marked tension and suspiciousness since giving birth to her last son, five months before admission. Her husband is not able to offer a diagnosis, but believes that she needs hospitalization.

An 18-year-old white *biscateiro* with a fourth grade education was brought by his mother to the Pronto Socorro. The family had previously lived as sharecroppers on a *fazenda* in Rio State, where the patient had worked intermittently "clearing the land." All of them, including the patient's three sisters and a brother, had moved, a few months before admission, to a house with electricity and a nearby well on a small property they owned in Sepetiba, a suburban area of Greater Rio in Rio State, with the aim of having him admitted to the hospital if it seemed inevitable. First, however, they had hoped that the experience of attending school would be helpful. When he would not remain in school in spite of his father's threats and curses (he never struck him), the family decided there was no point in further delay. At the Pronto Socorro the mother asked if outpatient treatment would be possible, but upon being told that admission was necessary, she acquiesced. She believes that his peculiar behavior, developing over approximately 18 months and including occasional hallucinations and delusional beliefs, is due to mental illness caused by "syphilis." The father and an older brother, however, believe the patient to be "*encosto*" or possessed. His father, who had considered himself a "scientific Spiritist," took the patient to a Spiritist Center for treatment on several occasions, but it was ineffective, and he is now disillusioned. The mother had not wanted her son subjected to the treatment, although she mentioned one of his sisters who, "when nervous used to fall asleep for several hours," and was cured after going to a "center." His mother notes the boy is Catholic and used to go to mass on feast days. "Before becoming ill" he liked to watch *futebol* and went to the beach at least every week and frequently more often.

A 19-year-old brown man (he considers himself *prêto*) who is unmarried and has a fourth grade education, was brought to the Pronto Socorro by two older brothers who had acted as heads of the family since the father had died when the patient was 12. His father had been a heavy drinker who tried to commit suicide by setting himself on fire but, after joining the Protestant (Evangélico) church, he had stopped drinking and eventually died of tuberculosis. The patient, his 54-year-old mother, and five of nine siblings (the patient was the eighth to be born) live in a rented house without electricity or water in the suburban com-

munity of Nilopolis in nearby Rio State. The patient was learning to do metal work and earned money as a shoemaker, but for
the year prior to admission he did not work and lived on his
brothers' and his mother's earnings; the latter is a laundress. The
patient feels himself disliked because he is ugly; he feels inferior,
speaks of his wish to die, and has been assaultive "because of the
injustice my mother did me by allowing me to be born." Driven
by a delusion-based need to defend himself, he stole money from
his brothers in order to buy a revolver. Although the patient himself had no religious affiliation (his mother became Protestent after being widowed), he was taken by his family to the Evangelical
church to be exorcised of evil spirits which they felt had possessed
him. After this, however, he developed "such an exaggerated
kindness" that he still seemed possessed, so they brought him to
the hospital. While the entire family considers his disturbance religiously inspired, i.e., by spirits, the oldest brother said that it
reflects a "diabolic temptation taking advantage of the mental
weakness brought on by syphilis." He, speaking for the family,
believed hospitalization to be necessary since "after God, the resource is the doctor."

An 18-year-old brown unmarried *biscateiro* was brought to the
Pronto Socorro by his mother, a 46-year-old *empregada doméstica*.
He was born in Teresopolis, his father dying when he was two,
and he spent the next five years with an aunt. In the meantime,
his mother remarried and he went back to live with her and his
step-father, but he was unhappy because the latter drank heavily
and when drunk, threatened to beat him. At this point his
mother put him in school. After three years he had not succeeded
in passing the first grade, was frequently truant, and was finally
withdrawn. For the past two years, the patient, his mother,
step-father, and one of his six siblings have been living in a
one-room rented *barraco*, without water or electricity, in a *favela* in
the urban zone of Bomsucesso. (Because Teresopolis is considered
part of Greater Rio, the patient was not classed with the migrants.) The mother has regarded the boy as mentally sick since
puberty on the basis of his lack of involvement in work or school
activities and his increasingly bizarre behavior. He has visited
Spiritist centers of several varieties in recent years, apparently
searching for some sense of personal meaning. In spite of this, and

the fact that he was baptized as a Catholic, he states that he has no religious affiliation.

More of the youngest patients were admitted because of paranoid behavior and on an emergency basis. Their complaints more often reflected sensitivity, feelings of lack of achievement, and impulsive tendencies, and a few more suffered from sexual guilt and anxiety. In general, more of the youngest exhibited symptoms of an acute psychotic nature. They were more dramatic, showed more impairment of thought, were more often paranoid (though there were no differences in frequency of hallucinations), and more than the others, were detached or apathetic. The differences are less marked, however, and involve fewer indices of paranoid behavior or impaired reality testing than for the most socially and economically deprived segment of the patient population. The most parsimonious interpretation of the greater behavioral disorganization of this group is that their mental hospitalization reflects the culmination of a disorder begun early in life coupled with a failure to mature. They have not had the opportunity of the others to become fully enculturated, to acquire the full range of coping skills, or to achieve outside of school.

Some illustrations of patients over 50 were given in previous chapters. Those which follow indicate the range of backgrounds as well as some similarities.

A 60-year-old black unmarried woman, illiterate and without schooling, was brought to the Pronto Socorro by her nephew who supports her from his earnings as a stonemason's helper while she keeps house for him. They live in a house with light and water in the suburban area of Nova Iguaçu in nearby Rio State. She grew up in Paraiba and spent most of her young adult life doing agricultural labor on a *fazenda*. At age 48 deciding to see more of the world, she came to Rio where she had a number of relatives in order to "work and make money." Until the onset of the present illness she was an *empregada*. In the past year she has become argumentative, suspicious of the neighbors, seclusive, and apparently attentive to inner stimuli. At the same time, she continues to get along well with her nephew who, with other members of the family, considers her to be "possessed." Nonetheless, they believe hospitalization to be necessary because, even though the "centro espirita" has been efficient in her care, "the doctor is the one who

knows whether it is illness or possession." Attendance at the centro
was not viewed as incompatible with her church membership or
the fact that, according to the nephew, "she is very Catholic and
talks about nothing but priests."

A white 57-year-old housewife with three years of schooling was
brought to the Casa Eiras by her 67-year-old husband of 40 years,
a retired house painter living on a pension. They have lived for
37 years in a house with two bedrooms and all services in Pena in
Irajá, the district in which she was born. She sees much of a
married daughter who lives in an adjoining house and has a television set. Another married son and daughter, the last suffering
from "nervousness," live not far away. A religious Catholic, she
used to participate in all the celebrations and attend mass at least
once weekly, but now complains that her difficulties no longer
permit this. She is civic minded, supports an organization for the
care of the blind, and is "loved by everyone in the neighborhood." For the past year she has shown signs of an increasingly
intense depression, and now her family, who regard her as mentally ill, believe hospitalization to be necessary.

A 52-year-old white, third grade educated, married boilermaker
from the naval arsenal was brought to the Casa Eiras by his
50-year-old wife of 28 years. He was born in Bomsucceso where he
still lives, but much of his early childhood was spent in Portugal
where he was sent to be with relatives following his mother's
death. He came back to Rio at age 12 to be with his father and
stepmother, but because of the former's severe beatings he ran
away at age 14 and has been financially independent ever since.
The patient, his wife, and three children, now ranging in age
from 14 to 28, had their own home with all services for many
years. Because of his progressive incapacity, less than a month
before admission they and their youngest child moved in with a
brother and sister-in-law. He feels sad, weak, tired, without energy, and can't stand the noise of the shop where he works. His wife
says that "he is not going crazy." She doesn't know what is happening, but she agrees that he should be in the hospital to "rest
and fortify himself." She is apprehensive because this is the first
time in their married life that they have been separated. Both are
Catholic, but at his initiative they have attended Macumba ceremonies several times in the past five or six years.

A 52-year-old black streetsweeper, a primary school graduate, was brought to the Casa Eiras by his 40-year-old wife of 20 years. Born in Botafogo, he has lived for 16 years with her and a daughter in a *vila* with essential services in São Joao de Meriti in Rio State. He has not worked for two years, feeling put upon, depressed, occasionally responding with anger, and complaining of a variety of physical problems. His wife regards him as mentally ill and believes hospitalization to be necessary.

A 51-year-old brown unmarried *biscateiro*, an itinerant radio repairmen with three years of schooling, was brought to the Pronto Socorro by his sister. This was four days after his arrival from Areia Branca in Rio Grande do Norte to stay at her home. His sister and her husband and seven children live in a house with electricity and water in the *favela* of Céu Azul in Engenho Novo in the suburban district of Meier. Eleven months earlier, the woman with whom he had lived for three years had died, not long after the death of their six-month-old baby, his only child. He became depressed, suspicious, and argumentative and resisted his landlord's demands that he move out. Finally, in response to continued pressure, he threatened the landlord and was placed in jail for a week. Upon being released, he decided to move to Rio (his stated reason for moving was to find work) and migrated alone by coastal steamer. Almost immediately after his arrival, his sister and brother-in-law concluded that he was mentally ill and needed hospitalization. The patient had been born "on the shore" of the Solimões River in Amazonaus where his father was a fisherman and *seringueiro* or rubber gatherer. When the patient was 10 his father decided to move the family, including nine children, back to Areia Branca where he had been born. He died when the patient was 33 but the patient's mother, aged 71, still resides there. The patient was a poor student and a disciplinary problem in childhood: "They beat me badly because I was very stubborn and nervous." He worked as a sailor and a farmer, but didn't "like to receive orders" so he finally decided to become self-employed. While brown-skinned with Negroid features, he refers to himself as "mixed Portuguese and Indian." He denies any religious affiliation. He drinks moderately and never attends movies, soccer games, or the beach, but he gambles every day, "even when there is no money."

SOCIAL CHARACTERISTICS ACCORDING TO AGE LEVEL

SOCIOECONOMIC INDICATORS

Table 162 shows that a slightly higher, but not statistically significant, proportion of the youngest patients had completed or gone beyond primary school. This is attributable to the increasing availability of educational facilities during the past 20 years, and to the fact that more of the youngest were born in Rio de Janeiro which has one of the greatest concentrations of schools in the country. Proportionately more of the older patients had electricity and running water, and their dwellings were less crowded. These findings reflect the time required to achieve some economic security, the unmarried status of the youngest, and the likelihood that some children of the oldest group had already left home. Reports of having bettered the father's socioeconomic status which accompanied increasing age also suggest the time required to achieve relative economic security.

DEMOGRAPHIC CHARACTERISTICS

Those items showing at least a 10 per cent spread between age groups are shown in Table 163, but most differences are not statistically significant. Almost two-thirds of those under 25 are unmarried. This figure drops rapidly and changes little after 40. Numbers of children increase rapidly with parental age, again with little change after 40. The youngest patient group includes slightly more who were born in Greater Rio de Janeiro, and only 13 per cent, as might be expected in view of its age range, who had arrived after age 21. Similar proportions of the three age groups, between a quarter and a third, had moved into the city within the five years preceding hospitalization. There were no differences in color, literacy, or other related factors according to the age groupings.

CHILDHOOD INFLUENCES

Table 164 reveals that the proportion of patients with literate parents diminished slightly with increasing age. This may be attributed both to the development of educational facilities in recent years and the number of parents of younger patients living in Rio de Janeiro. Since the youngest patients were most frequently brought to the hospital by their parents, the literacy figures may also be regarded as concomitants of concern, responsibility, and some knowledge of community resources. Data on the parents of these younger patients were therefore, also more frequently available. The lack of statistical significance of the findings is due largely to the number of unknowns regarding the parents of older patients.

A few more of the younger patients had siblings by both parents, were disciplined by scoldings rather than beatings (in contrast to the older, for whom beatings had been predominant), and fewer had been financially independent prior to age 14. These factors suggest a generally higher degree of parental support for the younger age groups, and reflect urban-rural differences in childhood experience as well.

INFORMATION AND SOCIAL PARTICIPATION

Fewer patients in the middle age-groups, as shown in Table 165, were friendly with their close neighbors, and more knew nothing about their neighbors than the patients in the other two groups. They also had less contact with and fewer were more friendly with the clergy. This suggests less need for other people than among the youngest and the oldest patients, and a greater degree of self-sufficiency, or perhaps of preoccupation, among the middle age-group. They had slightly more contact with welfare workers, perhaps because they had more family responsibilities and knew how to get help, but they were not more friendly with them. More of the youngest danced and more of the oldest watched soccer. More of the youngest who had had some education and presumably greater curiosity watched television, read newspapers, magazines, and books and attended the movies. The middle age-group, apparently more closed in and preoccupied, were least frequently involved in these informational activities.

HOSPITALIZATION AND THE FAMILY ACCORDING TO AGE

As noted in Table 166, slightly more than a quarter of the youngest patients, proportionately twice as many as the others, were seen in the Pronto Socorro, even though their parents were in general covered by the INPS. The proportionately higher frequency of paranoid behavior precipitating extrusion from the family and the decision to hospitalize during a crisis—even with a long history of illness—contributed to their use of the emergency facility. Proportionately more of those in the middle age-range were patients at Casa Eiras. More of these middle range patients, too, were admitted because of depressive symptoms and had had previous psychiatric contact. In other words, while there were no differences in duration of the episode leading to the present hospitalization, more of the middle range adults, presumably bearing the greatest economic burdens, had had symptoms demanding previous consultation. Depressive symptoms in these responsible persons were taken so seriously by the family that, in significantly greater proportion than for the other age groups, they resulted in admission. This was so despite the findings in Table 169 that this group did not reveal more depressive symptoms upon psychiatric examination, once hospitalization had occurred. The oldest age-group did not have a similar history of earlier dealings with psychiatrists. This can be attributed, at least in part, to variations in available mental health facilities according to region and time.

Family diagnosis may have been another factor contributing to the choice of institution. The oldest patients most frequently were considered by their families to be suffering from life stress rather than illness. This, associated with relatively infrequent symptoms of a bizarre or striking nature, may account for a low level of urgency in expelling them from the home. Their relatively low use of the Pronto Socorro may also reflect their low incidence of aggressive or threatening behavior in comparison to the younger patients, as well as reluctance to hospitalize a spouse or parent.

PSYCHIATRIC AND BEHAVIORAL CHARACTERISTICS ACCORDING TO AGE

TENSION, ANXIETY, SENSITIVITY, AND FRUSTRATION

Interview behavior and the psychiatrists' responses are noted in Table 167. The interviewers least often reported that they liked the middle range patients, felt pity for them or found the interview interesting, and most often reported a feeling of remoteness.

This is evidently not a consequence of generally disturbed behavior but rather of the patients' relative lack of dependent, clearly needful, or ingratiating behaviors. In fact, proportionately more in the middle group were described as showing an actively cooperative approach and being respectful, courteous or friendly, while proportionately fewer, in comparison with the other groups, were silly, hostile, fearful, apathetic, dramatic or attention seeking, or actively advice-seeking. The youngest group was most disturbed and least cooperative.

Anxiety symptoms are listed in Table 168. Constant diffuse anxiety is most prominent in the middle group. Fear of loss of control decreases progressively with age. The most consistent pattern of anxiety concerns the body. Somatic anxiety, insomnia, and the frequency with which worries interfere with work ability, show proportionate increases with advancing age. Thought process changes are evidently not associated with the organic problems of aging, but rather with the acute impairments of reality-testing in the young, since they diminish in frequency with age. Anger and impulsivity are reported least frequently by those over 40. Feelings of tension, isolation, frustration, and being deprecated are proportionately more frequent in the under-25 group.

DEPRESSION

Table 169 shows two clear patterns of depressive indicators associated with age. Feelings of sadness, weeping, and high intensity feelings as well as feelings of body weakness or inferiority were most often encountered in the oldest group. In contrast, detached, apathetic, dulled feelings, and a sense of inadequacy and of guilt about role performance were most often seen among the youngest patients.

THE BREAK WITH REALITY

Table 170 shows that the two younger patient-groups, in contrast to those over 40, most often felt persecuted or badly treated. Feelings of being regarded as mentally or physically inferior were most prominent among the very youngest, under 25. Data regarding hallucinations show no consistent significant differences according to age.

SOMATIC AND SEXUAL PROBLEMS

Table 171 reveals a clear progression with age in the frequency with which psychophysiological complaints are reported. The only exception, seemingly of a psychotic nature, is the statement of having something strange inside the body, most frequently heard among the youngest patients (and, as noted in Chapter IX, among females). Impotence or frigidity, and absent or weak sexual impulses are most frequently reported by the oldest group. The older patients also more frequently described their sexual pattern as being part of the present illness. Casual or transitory sexual contacts, sex limited to masturbation, and sex as a source of anxiety, guilt, or shame were most often described by the youngest patients.

Past Psychiatric History According to Age

Childhood and adolescent problems for which differences were reported, (Table 172) appear to have occurred most frequently in the younger groups. This may be owing to the diminishing importance and increased forgetting of these events with time, or they may be associated with the character and psychopathology of those whose first mental hospitalization occurred in youth rather than middle age—especially their difficulties in impulse control, relating to others, and maintaining reality contact.

CHAPTER 11

RELIGION: SOCIAL SUPPORT,
THERAPY, AND PATIENT BEHAVIOR

PROMINENT in the Brazilian cultural context are a series of inter-twined religious-magical belief systems which in varying quality and degree influence the world view of almost all members of the society. These systems, Roman Catholicism and various Protestant sects, may be observed in relatively pure historical form. The less solidly institutionalized groups of African, Amerindian, or Spiritist (Allan Kardec) descent appear to be in a phase of continuing syncretistic evolution. More significantly, they constitute an ever present backdrop, an only reluctantly identified alternative for the "officially" Catholic population. Cult and Spiritist centers are consulted by large numbers of persons who eventually become psychiatric patients, although the majority of devotees do not. For those not seeking help for particular problems, they clearly pro-vide a source of social support, a feeling of belonging, and a sense of connection with powerful and esteemed figures with potency far exceeding those of the earthly powers who ignore or reject them in their daily mundane lives.

Roman Catholicism as a fundamental social institution is upheld by other Brazilian institutions controlling the greatest wealth, and by individual upholders of tradition and establish-ment power. As Willems (1967) put it, " . . . the owners of the big landed estates constitute the bulwark of the traditional social order and its symbols. Catholicism, if only in name, is one of these symbolic values to which this class, perhaps more than any other, appears to be deeply committed" (p. 99). The attachments with greatest meaning for the minds and hearts of the less power-

ful are perhaps more accurately indicated by the phrase, "Father-
land of the Gospels," in the title of a book by Francisco Candido
Xavier (1938), a leading Spiritist medium. "The Gospel" is used
in the sense of the "true word," of an answer containing both
spiritual and material solutions to their sufferings for which the
people search. And they seem susceptible in a striking way to
those answers and promises which are made them by a host of
alternatives to the establishment religion.

Willems suggests that this state of affairs may be a function of
an anomic society. He identifies two major characteristics of
anomie in the process of departure from traditional forms of religious organization: "(1) The proliferation of [Protestant] sects
exhibiting structural and sometimes doctrinal discrepancies, all
competing with one another, the Roman Catholic church, and, in
Brazil, with Spiritualism and Umbanda. (2) A floundering mass
of followers drifting between religious experiences of various kinds
without ever developing a lasting allegiance to any particular sect
or faith." He goes on to note that anomic conditions, or those of
social and cultural disorganization, are favorable to the emergence
and dissemination of innovations—religious and otherwise. By the
same token, he recognizes that, "if schismatic movements experience little difficulty in attracting large followings, it may prove
considerably more difficult to hold the fickle crowds and to convert them into a hard core of loyal adherents" (pp. 259–260).

Official figures concerning religious membership have only recently been collected in a systematic manner and are still subject
to interpretation. During 1965, for example, there were, according
to the Anuário Estatistíco for 1967, almost two million Catholic
baptisms of newborn infants. In the same period, only about
60,000 Protestant children (of unstated age) were baptized. During the same year, however, the defection or death of approximately 260,000 members not withstanding, there was an increase
of almost 300,000 in the total number of identified Protestants to
a total of approximately 2,500,000 as of December 31, 1965. This
is much below Damboriena's (1963) figure of 4,071,643 Brazilian
Protestants in 1961.

In this country of approximately 80,000,000 people, there were
just 9,320 priests listed at the end of 1965. At the time of Pope

Paul's visit to Bogota in 1968, the Jornal do Brasil (Aug. 19, 1968) compared an estimate of one priest (of any type, in any post) per 6,855 Brazilians in 1965, with one per 571 in Belgium, one per 827 in France, and one per 1,570 in Portugal. The failure of the church to respond to the daily religious needs of the people was linked to the size of some rural parishes, which include from 20,000 to 35,000 persons and are from 200 to 2,000 square kilometers in area. Finally, as another editorialist put it: "Yesterday the transmission of the religious message was easily accomplished with the support of the family, the school and the parish which reinforced the doctrine taught in the pulpits. Today the intermediate groups such as the school, the high schools, and the family are often in contradiction, opposing themselves to the ideas transmitted to them by the church (Op. cit p. 2). These figures and the editorialist's comments suggest just how tenuous the connections are between the traditional religious organization and the great masses. All observers agree that the scarcity and personal unavailability of priests, especially in the vast hinterland, are major contributors to the church's inability to maintain control over those who might otherwise be its parishioners.

Figures on Spiritist and Umbanda membership are even less representative of the true activities and emotional ties of the people. The Anuário Estatístico for 1967 lists a total of almost 733,000 Kardecista Spiritists as of December 31, 1965, a net gain of almost 20,000 during the preceding year from a turnover of approximately 175,000. Naive professions of Catholicism, however, and sincere insistence that they are fervent Catholics, are commonplace among people of all social classes who regularly attend Spiritist or Umbanda sessions. The total number of Umbandistas, probably a fraction of the true figure, was listed as approximately 106,000, a gain of almost 12,000 members over the preceding year. Exact data on numbers or demographic characteristics of members of Umbanda or Spiritist groups have so far not been obtained and would be difficult to gather.

According to the official sources noted above, about four per cent of Brazil's Protestants lived in Guanabara at the end of 1965 and about five per cent of childhood baptisms took place there. This compares with 11 per cent of the Kardecista Spiritists and almost 37 per cent of the Umbandistas. If to these last are added those in Rio State, the proportion of the total formal adherents of Ubanda living in the entire region reaches 61 per cent. These figures fit other impressions that the alternatives to conventional Western religion attract more adherents in urban than rural settings, and that Rio de Janeiro is the major urban center of Umbanda and its variants.

The 1960 census reports that of approximately 3.3 million inhabitants of Guanabara, 88 per cent were officially classified as Roman Catholic. Protestants and Spiritists included four per cent of the population each, with about 8,000 more of the latter. *Umbandistas* were not included in the survey, but approximately two per cent claimed to subscribe to "other" religions, to be "without" religion, or made no statement at all. Of the remaining two per cent, about half (30,000) were Jews, with the others divided between Buddhism, Islam, and the Greek Orthodox church.

The 1960 census of Guanabara *favelas* yielded virtually the same results. Ninety per cent were Catholic, six per cent were Protestant, and approximately two per cent each admitted to Spiritist, "other," "no," or "undetermined" religions. The additional major faiths represented too small a number to achieve statistical representation; *favela* populations included 45 Jews, 25 Buddhists, 21 of Greek Orthodox faith, and 15 Mohammedans.

Other factors make it highly improbable that the census data provide an accurate picture of the Spiritist and Umbanda groups in Guanabara. One is many people's reluctance to identify themselves as practitioners, particularly of Umbanda or Macumba. This carries the unfavorable connotations of black magic for some and for others it may also be a source of shame or embarrassment because of its lower-class connotations. A second source of census error is the fact that so many people who consider themselves members of the Catholic church also attend Afro-Brazilian or Spiritist sessions. This dual attendance is facilitated by the syncretistic nature of the practices, both of which invoke the names of Catholic saints and prayers.

ROMAN CATHOLICISM AND BEHAVIOR

Smith (1963), Wagley (1963), and others have reviewed the literature on the role of Catholicism in the life of the individual

Brazilian, as well as its history. There seems to be agreement that despite the overwhelming proportion of the population regarding itself as Catholic, a relatively small number, perhaps no more than 10 per cent, regularly attend services. Ribeiro (1945) reported that 91.7 per cent of 948 representative families in Recife, studied in 1939, defined themselves as Catholic. In only 22 per cent of these families, however, in a more traditional area than Rio de Janeiro, did the members declare that they practiced their religion with any degree of regularity.

In general, most of those who are active practitioners of the faith are women. The men stand apart, even though they may have been baptized, married, and expect to die with appropriate religious ritual. As Willems (1967) notes, the nominal Latin American Catholic male "refuses to be 'pushed around by priests' and on the rare occasions when he decides to participate in some religious activity he does so without assuming future commitments of any kind." He has also described the church as an agent of social control which, while defining certain directions which behavior might take, also stimulates certain resistances. "Inherent in the structure of the Catholic church there is a persistent demand for indoctrination and regimentation, unquestioning acceptance of priestly authority, and submission to church law. And this demand for unconditional surrender to the church (or any other institution, be it secular or sacred) sharply contrasts with one of the most deeply ingrained traits of the Latin American way of life—the right to question abstract rules meant to cover a wide range of personal situation or events" (p. 43).

The anti clericalism stemming from the traditional authoritarianism of the churches and the association of the clergy with the holders of power and wealth are compounded by the Brazilian man's attitude toward sex. He finds it hard to believe that any male who is not homosexual would voluntarily embrace a life of celibacy and suspects that the priest is as much on the lookout for sexual liaisons as himself. This attitude is regularly reinforced by commonly shared jokes and stories, many of which involve nuns as well.

All of these elements help sustain a type of Catholicism called "soft" or "relaxed," (sometimes attributed to the nature of the Portuguese in contrast to the Spanish) which may be compared with the "hard" Catholicism of Europe or the United States. They also contribute to a type of hostility easily ready to emerge should the occasion present itself. There are few countries in the modern world in which one might hear, as the author did in Salvador do Bahia in 1962, two men talking in this way about another. The first said, "He certainly is fat isn't he?" His friend replied, "Yes, he's probably a priest in disguise."

This historical legacy of attitudes, while still justified to some degree, is completely inappropriate to the emerging group of liberal priests deeply dedicated to the socioeconomic improvement of the poor. The younger among this small group may work in villages or slums, stimulating the development of cottage industries and the formation of marketing cooperatives. Among the older ones, Dom Helder Camara has been perhaps the most outstanding in his fight for the development of adequate housing for urban slum dwellers. He, Eugenio Sales, and others, as noted by Mutchler (1965), are the first bishops of humble origin to represent a poverty-stricken people since the seventeenth century. The Brazilian Church, as Vallier (in Mutchler, 1965) has described it, is "moving away from its former emphasis on hierarchy, priestly control and passive ritualism towards a communal, lay-dominated activism that is aimed at evangelizing the lower and working classes, and through them, influencing the social-political process" (p. 104). This represents political and social rather than religious action; religion is considered divorced from the solution of worldly problems by most of Brazil's nominal Catholics according to Mutchler. He notes Callado's comment in 1964 that even the 200,000 reached by the rural Catholic unions of Pernambuco "will follow anyone who will lead them to immediate and practical objectives like the organization of unions or the demand for higher pay. The peasants demand one thing of a leader whether he is a priest or a communist, and that is a better standard of living" (p. 48). The charitable and rehabilitative activities of the Banco da Providencia and similar organizations described in earlier chapters are not so much regarded by those who benefit from them as direct churchly functions as they are accepted as familiar aspects of a Catholic culture.

Aside from attitudes toward priests and organized religion, Catholicism forms the most prominent and durable aspect of the matrices of everyday life. At the crisis points of life such as birth, death, baptism, and marriage, the institutionalized behavior of the largest part of the population is that which involves the church. Crucifixes and Christ figures are regularly encountered in public buildings and in the offices of leaders, including university professors. Before a new building is opened to the public, for example, it is blessed, and a figure of Christ is *entronizado* (enthroned) on a wall. The major Catholic holidays are apt to be public holidays. It is accepted as a matter of course that church institutions and projects of all kinds will receive financial support from national and local government sources. And the church has so far been able to prevent the legalization of divorce. These are among the factors which have resulted in Brazil's often being called "the most Catholic country in the world." As Wagley (1963) has put it " . . . Catholicism permeates Brazilian national culture, not so much as an active religious system but as a way of life—a fundamental national institution" (p. 251).

The split attitude toward Catholicism, then, may be summarized in terms of the automatic incorporation of much of its form into the daily culture, on the one hand, and the rejection of its role as a valid source of spiritual power, on the other. This is a consequence of its long local history, of insufficient numbers of religious personnel, and of a possible failure in the church's adaptation in the evolving needs of the people.

Folk Catholicism

Small-town dwellers of the interior, rural farmers, and share-croppers practice a form of Catholicism which depends in large measure upon relationships with local and particular saints who are regarded as capable of delivering concrete rewards and punishments. They play their role in response to promises of various fulfilling acts by the supplicants. Many local saints are traditionally concerned with such fundamental matters as crops, the weather, fertility, issues and problems which the individual feels he cannot control without the aid of supernatural forces. As one Jesuit priest, quoted by Willems (1967), has written, " . . . here also lies the explanation of a certain passivity, and a perpetual supplication for miracles, the liberating intervention" (p. 36).

Their practices are liberally influenced by magical beliefs imported from Portugal and their other European countries of origin, and mixed with those derived from the African slaves and Brazilian Indians. A vivid, day-to-day picture of the importance of this admixture of ritual and dependence on supernatural forces and Catholic heritage in making most of life's small decisions is provided in Marvin Harris' (1956) account of small town and rural life in the Bahian interior in the mid-1940's. Da Costa Eduardo (1948) also furnishes details of religious practice among the majority of Maranhão blacks who, while professing Catholicism, may also hold beliefs of African origin. The villagers, representative of broad segments of the national population, have no church and only occasionally go to a town for a particular festival; this, and the town priest's once or twice yearly visits to officiate at baptisms and weddings, constitute their contacts with the "official" religion. Some, however, keep sanctuaries with images of saints in their homes where people regularly come together to recite prayers and sing hymns, to thank the saints for their personal protection or intervention in crises or to petition them for favors. Such *ladainhas,* as they are called, are sometimes followed by social gatherings or dances. Processions to ask for rain constitute another form of observance.

As viewed by Wagley (1963), these practices are more closely akin to the Catholicism of the 17th century than the 20th. Their most spectacular manifestations are the pilgrimages to the numerous shrines scattered throughout rural Brazil. Some pilgrims travel several hundred miles on foot, resting in towns along the way and begging for food, to fulfill a vow in payment for a wish come true (such as a sick child's escape from death), or to seek supernatural help. Willems (1966) describes folk Catholicism as flexible and, in spite of occasional outbreaks of fanaticism, basically tolerant and receptive to innovations. The most frequent source of change within this framework is probably the miracle. A vision of a saint, Christ, or the Virgin, appears to a person involved a thaumaturge or new saint: "Folk Catholicism stresses the belief in mystical experiences, in possessions, and in charismatic leadership" (p. 211). Queiroz (1952) also emphasized the emergence of *beatos,* "saints" and miracle workers in rural areas. As Lanternari (1963) has summarized his observations: "In short, the picture is dominated by persons endowed with great prestige who play a role very similar to that of Shaman or prophet, despite the Catholic setting in which they operate" (p. 190). Lanternari regards the occasional messianic movements arising within the framework of folk Catholicism as having a close historical continuity with the Brazilian Indian movements of the 16th to the 19th centuries; these had an express belief in an earthly paradise and in a messiah coming to bring salvation. As Metraux (1931, in Lanternari, 1963) has indicated, these movements and their associated cults frequently focused on the goal of liberation from the white man's rule, and nuclei of antiwhite resistance formed around their prophets. In modern Brazil, deprived, culturally isolated farmers and villagers, especially in areas where they were subject to landowners' feudal domination have, under the spell of striking and demanding leaders, been most vulnerable to such movements. This seems thoroughly congruent with these powerless peoples' vulnerability to magic beliefs which has culminated at times in the murder of adults, children, or animals suspected of harboring the devil within them. One such incident investigated by anthropologist Carlo Castaldi (1956, in Wagley, 1963), took place as recently as Easter Week of 1955 in a village of small farmers in the interior of Minas Gerais. On that occasion, four children accused of being possessed by the devil were sacrificed by community leaders. In the absence of church supervision the villagers had become converted to Adventism *(adventismo de promessa)* but they were actually rural Catholics who had no teacher or leader in their new religion any more than they had in their old. It seems likely that similar incidents, although not so extreme, occur in isolated communities more frequently than reports suggest. In the summer of 1968 the Brazil Herald, the English-language newspaper of Guanabara, carried a story which may be regarded as typical. In the nearby village of Vassouras in the State of Rio, a wild boar called Josino was said to have been the devil. For two years his depredations resulted in loss of stock and inspired the people with fear; he was reputed to have eaten the town drunk who disappeared into the jungle. Once the local priest tried to exorcise the devil from the boar, but after eight hours, he emerged scratched and bleeding from the jungle, saying that Satan had attacked him. Finally, attracted by live chickens hung near a local shop, Josino entered the village and was killed by a group of 50 men armed with guns and knives. He was shot and stabbed repeatedly and just before death, according to the story, uttered a piercing human-like cry, interpreted by the people as "the devil's death rattle."

These issues are dwelt on here for two reasons. First, the urban working class which consists so largely of relatively recent rural migrants may have had its dependence upon folk Catholicism and its associated magical beliefs weakened, but complete abandonment seems unlikely. And it seems just as unlikely that, even with the forsaking of specific beliefs and practices, deeply ingrained styles of thinking and perceiving, vulnerability to magical ways of handling crises, and the passive expectation of liberating intervention by powers beyond them (possibly now transferred to secular forces), will have been completely lost. Second, the development of folk religion, including sporadic messianic movements outside of the formal Catholic organization, has general psychosocial significance. This has been expressed by Willems (1967): ". . . the marginal masses demonstrated their ability to organize themselves in their own fashion and thus to defy the tutelary aspects of the established social order, particularly the salvation monopoly of the Catholic church and the privileged status of its clergy . . . " (p. 33). Lanternari (1963), also noted that the messianic movements which professed adherence to Catholic doctrine and the papacy were in practice opposed both to official Christianity and to the oppressive local political leaders and landholders. Many of these movements, originating in the isolated Brazilian backlands, culminated in a "holy war" against government institutions and the founding of new "holy cities" by local prophets. Bastide (1961), reviewing the conflicting but complementary Marxist concepts, sees messianism as allowing exploited groups in an agricultural economy to become aware for the first time of their exploiters, although at the same time it diverted energies from the material and class struggle to preoccupation with religious myths. Bastide sympathizes with the former idea, seeing it as a first manifestation of a refusal to accept colonialism; he refers to Balandier's (1951) view that the religious channel is used to express opposition to the colonial power when political resistance is blocked.

Protestantism and Behavior

Willems, in his major study (1967), regards folk Catholicism as in some ways a transition to certain forms of Protestantism in Brazil. It shares with the subvarieties of the Pentecostal faith, an emphasis on possession, miracles, communication with divine spirits, and other mystical experiences. For both groups, religion is an emotionally vital process with significance for everyday life and both seem to share a capacity for change and innovation.

The largest Pentecostal sects in Brazil are the *Assembléia de Deus* (Assembly of God) and the *Congregaçao Cristão do Brasil* (Christian Congregation of Brazil); a separate group related to the former is the *Assembléia de Deus Cruzada de Fé* (Assembly of God, Crusade of Faith). Other sects are primarily concerned with divine healing, and they are continuously dividing, subdividing, and changing their names. Many are personalistic movements with leaders who are both charismatic and messianic. Most of these leaders meet in revival tents, have their own radio programs, and preach the gospel of immediate salvation—Jesus saves here and now in this world. Many attract crowds of people because of their reputations as miracle healers. As Willems suggests, the size of its membership and its proselytic zeal indicate that Pentecostalism has been more adaptable to the needs and aspirations of the masses than any other form of Protestantism. He analyzes its organizational patterns, in a manner similar to the descriptions above, as expressing " . . . a protest against the Catholic church and its ally the ruling class . . . by pointedly stressing egalitarianism within the sect and by opposing the Catholic principle of an ecclesiastical hierarchy and a highly specialized priesthood . . . " (p. 249). In addition to its democratic nature and the opportunity afforded to every man to be a "priest," Pentecostalism seems to offer "a solution to various personality problems manifest in the practice of 'vices'." The convert who substitutes conventional socially approved behavior for drinking, fornication, or stealing " . . . cleanses himself of social stigma and becomes respectable in the eyes of the in group and the society at large." Willems goes on to point out that folk Catholicism no longer functions for the migrant to the city as it did in the traditional rural society, and that new solutions are necessary. Protestantism

provides a new solution, and within Protestantism, Pentecostalism
has special appeal because it "continues the ancient tradition of
messianism in a new and more exciting way by promising the
coming of the deity here and now to the individual believer . . .
the gifts or powers of the Spirit . . . make essentially powerless
people feel strong beyond natural limits . . . [and provide] . . . a
temporary escape from the hopeless squalor of life to the thrills of
intense emotional experiences" (p. 249). Finally, the believer finds
within the social structure of the sect an opportunity to develop
his personal community and to attain some psychological and
economic security.

Protestant missionaries have found receptive audiences in the
mobile populations of new frontier communities. The evidence
suggests that it is just among those classes, whose chances of upward mobility were increased by industrialization, that the largest
number of converts has been made. The areas of highest Protestant concentration are those which have received the largest
numbers of rural-urban migrants, i.e., those most exposed to culture change.

It is not valid, however, to think of all Brazilian Protestantism
in terms of the active possession sects. Unlike the rural contexts of
folk Catholicism, the largest Protestant populations, subscribing
to more traditional forms, are concentrated in the most urbanized
and industrial areas. While the Pentecostal sects are essentially
class organizations, with membership predominantly among the
lower classes, the historical churches are not. To the extent that
they include members of the middle and upper classes, they accept traditional values, including occupational achievement,
wealth, and political power. In the past, and now to a decreasing
degree, being a Protestant (usually Baptist, Methodist, or Pres-
byterian) meant being regarded as dependable, honest, and
efficient beyond the limits normally expected in Brazilian society.
This itself brought commercial benefits to church members. As
Willems put it, "The practice of the Protestant virtues is conveniently rewarded by an emerging industrial civilization that promises a higher level of living to the thrifty, sober, industrious and
well educated . . . Protestant asceticism frees part of one's income
for the acquisition of things that symbolize a higher level of living." There has been and still exists " . . . an acute awareness of
and belief in economic advancement" among Protestants, particu-

larly among members of the historical churches (p. 251).

But the influence of Protestantism has gone far beyond supply-
ing personal rewards to its adherents and, through its fostering
of economic advancement and upward social mobility, loosening the class structure. It has even had an impact upon that bas-
tion of the Brazilian social order, the family, and upon the most
traditional of masculine sexual prerogatives. Willems has expressed this concisely:

> An autonomous congregational structure is obviously incompatible with
> the primacy of family and kinship prevalent in the traditional social
> order. Thus the Protestant family has to accept a subordinate position
> within the congregation. Furthermore, the web of social relationships
> within the immediate family had to conform to the basic norms of
> the Protestant ethic, a requirement which resulted in the deletion of
> male sex prerogatives and thus led to more egalitarian relationships
> between male and female members (p. 250).

In summary, the rise of Protestantism in Brazil appears to represent the emergence of a new institution following the disruption
of the old order in consequence of industrialization, migration,
and modernization. As formal and folk Catholicism became less
useful and functional, the new institution grew stronger and developed its own subvariants. It offered solutions to the problems
experienced by individuals caught up in the process of social
change. It brought people together into new forms of organization. Perhaps the greatest strength of the new organizational
forms has been their ability to simultaneously supply individual
emotional gratification and a sense of spiritual purpose to their
members at the same time that they facilitated their economic
advancement and eventual upward social mobility, and gave
them a sense of community and group identification.

Afro-Brazilian Cults: Candomblé, Macumba, and Umbanda

The most active and rapidly growing folk religion in Rio de
Janeiro, and one which figures prominently in the histories of
many psychiatric patients, is Umbanda. A syncretistic set of be-
liefs and practices, it incorporates elements from Catholicism,
European-born Spiritism, religions coming from the Yoruba,
Dahomey, and Banta people of Africa, and from the Brazilian

Indians, particularly those of the Amazon basin. An impressive feature of Umbanda is its variability and flexibility. Each center is an independent organization. While all share certain elements of ritual and belief, actual practice varies with the inclinations of individual leaders and with the developmental history of the particular center.

An understanding of Umbanda requires some grasp of the African and Amerindian elements which are part of its structure, as well as of Macumba which—continuing—still shares aspects of its belief system. African cult forms represent adaptations from elements brought to Brazil by slaves. As Ribeiro (1952) following Herskovits (1937), has pointed out, these may be understood in part as expressions of an "acculturative process." Rather than the imposition of one culture upon another, they are the consequence of a continuing permutation and fusion of cultural elements which retain their vigor as they remain functionally useful for individual and group survival. The atmosphere in which this fusion took place was suggested by Herskovits (1937). He noted the efforts throughout the New World to convert the slaves to Christianity, and the continuing influence of Catholicism as the official state religion on the life of the people. The powerful position of the state religion, coupled with the Europeans' constant fear that the African cults might offer a focus for revolt, contributed to the cults' inferior social position and made it necessary for rituals to be conducted in secret. Ribeiro (1969) also emphasized the role of the dominant culture and its associated prestigious religion in repressing and demoralizing the religions of slaves or others in a minority status, such as colonized peoples. This stimulated a phase of clandestine practice and accommodative reorganization incorporating elements from the more powerful church. It can lead, too, as suggested in the section on folk Catholicism, to attempts at religious reaffirmation through messianic movements or the increased use of magic. As a final phase, the new syncretistic beliefs and practices become restructured into new churches and cults and whatever magic persists is incorporated into the new rites and theology.

Bastide (1961) wrote in somewhat similar terms that " . . . messianic or milleniarian movements are not so much movements of retreat and escape into the imaginary as they are bonafide attempts at a rational solution for problems posed by contact with the whites" (p. 470). "In order to extricate oneself from the horrible chaos into which white men had plunged the traditional social order, what better way . . . than by appealing to the very ones who had formerly created this traditional order: Ancestors and Cultural Heroes?" (p. 474).

CANDOMBLÉ

The most widely studied Afro-Brazilian cults have been Candomblé in Bahia, Xangô in Recife, and Macumba in Guanabara, in Rio de Janeiro State as well as, to a lesser degree, in São Paulo. In the far South, in Rio Grande do Sul, the cults were known as *batuques* (also the name of a dance preceding the development of the *samba*), and in the Amazon region, in the cities of Belèm and Manaus, they were the *batuque* and the *babaçue. Catimbó*, based on the indigenous Amerindian cult of *jurema* (an intoxicant and hallucinogen extracted from the bark of the mimosaceae tree), was described by Bastide (1959) as a major native cult spreading from Pará and Maranhão as far south as Recife. With its own elements of Spiritism, it too has become mixed and fused, depending upon particular localities, with beliefs in Christian saints and African gods. Unlike the African religions, the precursors of *Catimbó* had no dances. They were practiced in closed rooms with the aid of magic herbs (especially tobacco, the use of which it contributed to *macumba*) and the *"princesa"* Jurema. With time, however, *Centros de Catimbó* as well as *de Caboclos* (also referring to aboriginal spirits) became so syncretistic that some, according to Ribeiro (1952), have been transformed into "houses of Angola", following the line of differentiation which in Rio de Janeiro resulted in *macumba*. Its priests received multiple spirits, including the old Negro "masters": *mestre* Joaquim, *mestre* Antonio de Lima and others who, occupying or possessing the priest or medium during successive trances, would produce appropriate modifications in his behavior.

The opportunity to build quarters devoted to the practice of an African religion was impossible on the plantations. Therefore, the *terreiros* or meeting places of the Candomblé—the group which historically appears to have been the major precursor of the others—were customarily located in relatively isolated suburbs or rural settings and were usually almost inaccessible. Macumba, in contrast, is mainly an urban phenomenon; it was only in this setting that financial support and protection from possible police persecution could be found. The major *terreiros* now can be reached by bus or private automobile, and a number of Macumba and Candomblé Centers have been open to tourism for years.

There are no thoroughgoing accounts in English of the history, present function, and operations of Candomblé and its derivatives, although some of its aspects, particularly the drumming, have been described by Herskovits (1944). The cult and its subvariants have been studied and documented by several anthropologists, of whom the pioneers were Nina Rodrigues (1901), Etienne Ignace (1908) and Artur Ramos (1934). The comparative account of greatest interest to social and behavioral scientists is probably Ribeiro's (1952) who has identified the common features of the Afro-Brazilian cults of Recife and discussed them in terms of social structure and function. Brief but informative and relatively recent descriptions in Portuguese include those of Edison Carneiro (1948), himself a Bahiano, and the photographic work of José Medeiros (1957). Da Costa Eduardo's (1948) detailed description of religious beliefs and practices among the blacks of Maranhão reports that in the rural areas, only slight retentions of the elaborate religious and ritual complexes of Africa were found. These included ritualistic dances during which the participants were possessed and their own spirits "displaced" by a supernatural being. The dances, held at one or two month intervals, were attended by most villagers as participants or spectators, with beliefs concerning this aspect of life shared by all. In the capital city of São Luiz there were 20 cult houses in 1943–44. Established in the 1870's by groups of Dahomean ("Nina" or "Gege") and Yoruban ("Nagô") descent, they were known as *terreiros* or *casas de mina* (after the name given to blacks coming from these areas and the coast of Mina), and the dances held there were termed *tambor de mina* (literally *mina* drum). In all, the basic African pattern of possession and dancing accompanied by drums continued.

The story of the evolving Afro-Brazilian cults may begin with the fact that, for several historical reasons, there occurred a concentration of Nagô-speakers (mainly Yoruba) in Bahia in the late 18th century. Diegues, Jr. (1963) believed the Yoruba to have possessed the most advanced African culture brought to Brazil. Their religion and their divinities, according to Nina Rodrigues (1945, in Ribeiro, 1952), "already almost international," had given the basic pattern to the religions of neighboring people in Africa along with the help of the divinities of the Jejê, from the littoral of the Gulf of Guinea. The blacks of the African coast of Mina, for example, used religious dances, ceremonies, and organizational forms resembling those of Nigeria, Dahomey, and the Gold Coast (Herskovits, 1938). The Nagô-speakers of Bahia, therefore, constituted an elite and had little difficulty in imposing their language and religion upon the masses of other slaves. This religion, with some modifications based on interpretations of the official Catholicism of Brazil, became a model for the later development of the cults.

A possibly important contribution to the readiness of less socially integrated slave groups to accept the religious forms of a black elite is suggested by Ribeiro (1952). He notes that the dispersion of tribal groups by plantation owners fearful of rebellion resulted in new cultural contacts which reduced the differences between the groups, especially as they were all confronted with the common acculturative pressures of slavery. Under these circumstances, as Herskovits (1941) has noted, a strong "focal" culture, including a similarity with all cultures which had yielded slaves to the Americas, could have been a key to the development of new behavioral styles for blacks in the New World. In Ribeiro's opinion, too, the cults of the dead (e.g., Candomblé funerarios, primarily concerned with ancestors in present day Recife), possession as a key event in ceremonial observance, and the general religious conceptions of all New World Negroes were basically identical.

Many authors agree that Candomblé made its first appearance in about 1830, eight years after Brazil's independence. Candomblé itself was a word used to designate the location where the cult meetings of Bahia took place, and still do. This is usually a house or pavilion sheltering a floor of beaten earth, viz., terreiro, where the ceremonies, including dances, are held. The house was probably named after a dance popular among the coffee planta-

tion slaves, and this in turn appears to have taken its name from
the drums which accompanied the dance. Xangô in Recife did
not reach the degree of "splendor" of the Bahian Candomblé,
according to Ribeiro (1952), because repression by the police and
the Catholic Church and the hostility of the population (much
more Europeanized than in Bahia) required greater privacy and
smaller groups.

The principal figure of a Candomblé and of most of the other
Afro-Brazilian cults, is a *pai* or, more often in Brazil in contrast to
Africa, *mãe-de-santo,* i.e., a holy or sainted father or mother. The
pai may also be referred to by the Yoruba term for the priests of
Ifa (an ancient oracle or God of divination and prediction), as
babalão, derived from *baba* meaning father and *Awo* or secret.
Baba-li-Awo, later condensed to *babalão,* following Portuguese
word construction, meant father-who-has-the-secret. He may also
be designated by a related Nagô word for holy leader, *babalorixá,*
or if female, *ialorixá,* corresponding to the cult of Orixás. A sub-
stantial lexicon of priestly and oracular designations derived from
different parts of Africa, but mainly Nagô is used in a variable
manner by practitioners at different *terreiros.* The leader has
among his prime responsibilities that of deciding which should be
the special deity of particular initiates into the cult, and asking
the divinities for solutions to interpersonal, medical, or psychological problems presented by cult members. He presides over the
rituals, administers the organizational needs of the sect which
has a complex social structure, makes offerings to the gods, decides on the times of public and private ceremonies, engages in
ceremonial throwing of shells or nuts or other ways of divining,
and resolves problems of a ritual-religious or interpersonal nature
arising between members. He must also be concerned with the
financial support of his group—often a difficult problem since
members are drawn mainly from the poorer classes. If the leader
is male, his wife may be the *mãe-de-santo* or *ialorixá,* and she is apt
to be concerned with certain aspects of initiation ceremonies and
the discipline of female candidates and organization members of
lesser status. The *pai* or *mãe-de-santo* is the absolute authority of his
cult center. After him come a hierarchy of positions, each with its
functional and dominance status. Those who disagree with him
usually leave the group.

All the cults share a common characteristic derived from the Yoruba. That is, the believer is possessed by a divinity which uses him as an instrument in his communication with mortals. Possession is also a feature of spiritism and of *pajelancá* (the religious practices of Brazilian Indians led by a priest or *pajé*). In spiritism, however, it is the spirits of the dead rather than gods which are incorporated by believers. Among the Indians, it is the divinities of the rivers and forests, but they present themselves to and seize only the *pajé*, not the believers. It is thus not the phenomenon of possession itself which distinguishes the cults of African origin, but the circumstance of being possessed by or becoming the agent of one of a range of African deities who may enter members of the congregation as well as the cult leader.

Possession by the divinity occurs only for certain selected members of the cult. Among the Yoruba, these were often male, but in Brazil they are as often as not female—perhaps in consequence of the conditions of slavery. Even among the Yoruba, however, there are sex-linked differences in participation—according to cult. Prince (1966) observed that within the Sopono cult (of the smallpox gods) of the present-day Yoruba, it is the female members who undergo regular possession, whereas the male initiates perform other organizational functions.

The privilege of serving as the instrument (*cavalo* or horse) of a divinity or god is reserved for those who prepare themselves to receive it, or literally, to seat the saint *(assentar o santo)*. Preparation may involve such activities as passing through ritual baths, changes of clothing, hair shaving and in Candomblé, participating in sacrificial ceremonies. The progressive steps toward status as a holy son or daughter, *filho* or *filha-de-santo*, also involve complex learning. This includes acquiring the secrets of the sect, the words of songs and the steps of dances, as well as understanding and submitting onself to certain dietary and sexual taboos. The faithful are usually categorized on the basis of the time elapsed since their initiation, the various ritual steps through which they have passed, and the importance of the deities which have selected them as "horse." For the newcomer, status varies with where he was initiated and who had "prepared" him. According to the Herskovits (1943), "direction and participation [in Candomblé worship] are conceived as intellectual processes

opening the way to mystical perceptions and to an ultimate control of the supernatural world" (p. 271).

Preparatory rites also have a personal character, i.e., the individual becomes identified with and prepares himself in relation
to a single divinity; each *cavalo* is prepared to receive only his protective god and no other. This singularity is changing, however,
in that the same person may receive two or three, and in the
Macumba and Umbanda Centers of Rio, a succession of divinities. Nonetheless, the personal character remains. For example, the
Iemanjá (*mãe-d'água* or mother of waters) of one person cannot
manifest itself to another, even though his protector is also Iemanjá.

Following the African cult, the possessing divinity or god is
called an *orixá*. The *orixás* are intimately concerned with the daily
life of man, in contrast to the remote creator, identified as Olorum by cult leaders. Ribeiro's (1952) informants describe Olorum
as residing in the sky, not interested in terrestrial matters, neither
inducing possession nor requiring offerings. Having no cult dedicated to him, he can communicate with men only through the
orixás. His name is almost never heard in Brazilian cult centers. In
Brazil each *orixá* has become identified with a certain Catholic
saint and the *orixás* in toto are thought to command a vast number of spirits. Belief in phalanxes composed of hundreds of thousands of spirits of the dead (which has been incorporated into
Umbanda as described below) is derived from the Bantu cults
originated in Angola and the Congo.

The concept of a particular god who might possess and guide
the individual, or express himself through him, closely resembles
the familiar Catholic concept of the patron saint. Rituals of pla-
cation, vows and promises to repay the saint for wished-for solutions, tacking prayer papers to windows and door, for example,
are comparable with the obligations which might be imposed by
powerful *orixás* and thus facilitated the slaves' adoption of aspects
of Catholicism. Moreover, as Gilberto Freyre has pointed out in
various works, the slaves participated in the religious celebrations,
baptisms, feast days, special saints' days, and other similar events
at the house of the plantation master, all of which were celebrated with singing, dancing, banners, and flowers. The *padre*, often a son of the master, included the slaves in his teaching of

songs and prayers and introduced them to many saints, particularly the patron saint of the establishment. In this way, the African and his descendants in Brazil developed his own religious mixture and a pantheon including Yoruba gods and Catholic saints as equals to be treated as identities (Freyre, 1964). Herskovits (1937) interprets the differing identifications between African god and Catholic saint found in Brazil, Cuba, and Haiti as evidence that ". . . the inner logic of the aboriginal African cultures of the Negroes, when brought in contact with foreign traditions, worked out to achieve an end that, despite the handicaps of slavery, has been relatively the same wherever the forces making for change have been comparable" (p. 643). These factors probably also contribute to the ease with which African ways co-exist with those of the modern world and the Catholic church: "The mother who takes her newly born baby to the hospital clinic for a regular checkup, and welcomes the visiting nurse, finds no contradiction in calling on her diviner to ascertain the 'guardian spirit' of the infant—the African deity who will watch over it during its life . . ." (Herskovits and Herskovitz 1943, p. 264).

The relative positions of the gods in the Afro-Brazilian pantheon is indicated by their saintly equivalents and thus varies at times from that in Africa. Each major *orixá* is believed to direct one of seven "lines" or legions of spirits sharing certain affinities. Belief in this pantheon and its general organization is shared to varying degrees by members of most Candomblé, Macumba and, in a more diluted way, Umbanda organizations. The lines are subdivided again into the phalanxes noted above. Each line has its own color, number, type of food, chant, symbol, and so on, and descriptions of different groups are marked by many disagreements and inconsistencies of detail. The following list is made up from the writings of Herskovits (1937), Rene Ribeiro (1952, 1959), Carneiro (1967), Bastide (1959), and others, as well as from the author's personal observations. These names accord with information about Rio de Janeiro. Occasional variations are found in Bahia or Recife.

> *Oxalá*, known in Africa as Orixalá, the King of Purity, is the leader of the other gods. He is often equated with Jesus Christ, or a figure with some similar significance, such as Nosso Senhor de Bomfim.

Iemanjá, the water-mother or *mãe-d'água* of all *orixás,* has as her Catholic counterpart, Mary, mother of Christ and may also be known as
Our Lady of Piety or Our Lady of the Rosary. The flowers washed
up by the early morning tides on Rio's beaches have most often been
part of a sacrifice to Iemanjá, and it is to her that supplicants wading
into the surf at dusk pray. Hundreds of thousands may bring gifts
ranging from champagne and flowers to beer and cigars on New
Years' Eve. It was estimated that on December 31, 1964, a million
people crowded Rio's beaches to pay homage to Iemanjá.

Ogum, the Yoruba god of iron and war, is identified with St. George.
St. George on horseback, represented either in painting or in figure,
sometimes confronting the dragon, is one of the most popular figures
found in lower- and even middle-class Carioca homes or on automobile dashboards. He is popular as a warrior who can protect one in
difficult situations. In Bahia, Ogum is sometimes equated with St.
Anthony.

Oxossí, who took over the tasks of the god of hunting and owner of
the forests from Ogum, is the counterpart of St. Sebastian in Rio, and
usually of St. George in Bahia.

Xangô, the god of lightning and thunder is St. Michael the Archangel;

Oxum is the goddess of the river of the same name who has represented both St. Catherine and the Virgin Mary; and

Omolu (St. Lazarus or St. Bento), direct the other three lines.

The messenger between men and the divinities is Exu who knows
the tongues of men as well as the gods. He has been equated with
the Christian devil, but evidently did not have this significance
among the Yoruba, who considered him mischievous, a prankster.
There are many *exus* with the most diverse names and functions
depending upon geographical location, the particular *orixá* involved, the particular function he may be called upon to play,
and the particular *terreiro* to which the supplicant belongs or
which he has consulted. A leading female *exu,* for example, is
known as Pomba-Gira. While this may be literally translated from
the Portuguese as a gyrating or turning dove, the exact
significance of the name is unclear. Exu Caveira, another example, is regarded by many Cariocas as having been created by
Omolu and given the task of protecting cemeteries, especially that
of Irajá in Rio City. One occasionally even hears of the ancient
powerful association, Ifa-Exu. All ceremonies aimed at transmit-
ting wishes to the gods must begin with homage or gifts to Exu, a

despacho or *ebo,* and he may receive the first song and first steps of a dance as well; once he is thus placated, the ceremonies can begin.

Ribeiro's (1952) summary of the theology of Afro-Brazilian cults in Recife provides a generally relevant basis for understanding all the present-day Brazilian folk religions which invoke African gods. This theology includes:

> . . . belief in a creator, distant and little interested in earthly patterns; a variable number of mandatory deities, hierarchically classified, belonging to a mythological family, and interested in the life of the faithful to the point of inducing possession or applying sanctions to minor deviations of conduct; the existence of an ambivalent deity, a "trickster," a messenger of the gods with an important role in bringing auguries and revelations of destiny, with magical effects and actions; the influence of the spirits of ancestors able to influence for good or bad the lives of currently existing persons; the existence of personal divinities, minor entities and spirits inhabiting space; the possibility of controlling destiny and its revelation by means of divinatory practices with a conviction in the efficiency and power of magic [p. 141].

POSSESSION

As noted above, it is possible to be significant and powerful in the cult hierarchy without having been possessed, or with only a single episode at the time of initiation. Possession is, after all, but one element in the complex pattern of submission to the will of gods. Prince (1966) points out that the modern Yoruba do not regard spirit-possession as necessarily more therapeutic than other forms of involvement, and that whatever therapeutic effect does occur may be spread to the help-seeker's lineage and entire community. In the eyes of one elderly priestess of the Sopono cult in Abeokuta, Nigeria, for example, the major factor in the recovery of good health is the sick person's general conformity to the dictates of the *orixá.* Even so, as Ribeiro (1959) has so clearly stated, possession is a key event in the complex of rituals which integrate an individual with his cult group and sanction his participation in it. A dramatic highpoint of the public ceremonies is achieved when the gods are called on to play their part through the media of the faithful. Ribeiro perceives the histrionic quality of the pos-

session state as facilitating crystallization of the initates' new social roles. While he believes possession trances provide an opportunity for some individuals to relieve psychological tensions, he
follows Herskovits (1937) in emphasizing the need to interpret the
phenomena on the basis of established norms of conduct in the
societies in which they occur; the stylized nature of Afro-Brazilian
cult trance behavior, conforming to culturally transmitted knowledge about the nature of the possessing deity supports this view.
If possessed by such warlike gods as Ogum or Xangô, the possessed may adopt a ferocious facial expression accompanied by
brusque and energetic movements, for example, or he may be
provocative and coquettish if possessed by a water goddess such
as Oxum.

Initiates' trance behavior in early phases of their training vary
in detail from the timing of induction to the capacity to perfectly
express or "speak" the gods' desires. They may exhibit lapses from
approved style because of physical circumstances, e.g., menstrua-
tion, infringement of sexual or alimentary taboos, or what is understood by the cult leader as residual resistance to being possessed. The stylized or stereotyped nature of the phenomenon
encompasses all phases of the episode. Ribeiro (1959) reports that,
in his presence, a cult leader decided the initiate had been simu-
lating possession because he did not adequately respond to ritual
gestures made to *retirar el santo,* i.e., begin the process of departure
of the possessing divinity—although up to the final moment he
had accepted as valid the entire sequence of events. If the signs of
possession by the expected divinity are slow in appearing, the
leader or other member of the cult hierarchy, or even one of the
faithful, may request a special song for the god they wish to descend; they place hands on the head of the initiate, making him
twirl for a few moments, or they may play one of the ritual instruments, such as a *maraca* in the case of Xangô. Social reinforce-
ment and participation is present in other ways. During the brief
pauses in violent dance periods in the center of the area, the possessed may greet or salute the drummers, priests and other cult
leaders, important visitors, and friends. They are usually accompanied by other members of the faithful who are not possessed
but who assist them in achieving the trance, and who make sure
they do not fall or hurt themselves. The Herskovitses (1943) have

described in detail the strict etiquette, hierarchical order, and values exhibited by Bahia Candomblé cult members, on and off the dance ground. As one cult head said, justifying the long and arduous training, "What can anyone learn in a few . . . months? . . . It's a complete training for life and for success in life" (p. 275). Herskovits (1944) has also provided a thorough description of the "power" of drums, the role of drumming, and the training and presence of drummers in Candomblé.

It is difficult to delineate the interplay of personal psychological and social status and role factors in those who seek or who are capable of possession. Bastide (1960) believed possession to offer an escape from social restrictions. Ribeiro (1959) notes, more broadly, that cult participation offers its adherents new value systems and types of interpersonal relations which facilitate tension reduction without forcing them to renounce other values and norms of the Luso-Brazilian culture. This is especially true for those whose status makes it difficult for them to achieve self-realization or some compromise between their ideals and the pressures of daily life. These opportunities appear most attractive to those in the less privileged classes for whom environmental control by magical means, coupled with the increased self esteem of belonging to a prestigeful group, and even the possibility of economic assistance, constitute powerful rewards. Rorschach results presented by Ribeiro (1959) suggest types of individual needs which may be resolved in part by trance behavior. They do not clearly indicate, however, individually specific motives or conflicts determining the choice of divinity or the frequency and intensity of possession. Perhaps social rather than intrapsychic factors are the key determinants of entrancement; perhaps cult dignitaries may rarely enter into trances in comparison with lower status members because they have other ways of satisfying their needs which make dissociation unnecessary.

MACUMBA AND BLACK MAGIC

The most complex ceremonial progression as well as the most complex organization structure of Afro-Brazilian groups is that of the Candomblé and closely related cults. The Macumba and Umbanda centers of Rio de Janeiro appear in general to share

less clearly defined and complexly differentiated rites and structures. This seems to reflect a gradual evolution away from their
African roots toward a not yet crystallized form, determined by
the broad needs of the officially Catholic anomic urban masses. In
the case of Macumba the evolution has involved less emphasis on
traditional theology and more on the practice of magic.

It is especially with regard to the activities of the *exus* and the
practice of harmful or black magic that Macumba *terreiros* continue to play a part in the lives of innumerable Rio de Janeiro
residents of all social classes. While *exus* themselves can do evil or
good, depending upon what they are asked, they are used by worshippers almost exclusively to do evil. Their activities are thought
to be generally involved with, complemented by, or circumscribed
in some way by the old magic numbers three and seven. The
practice of black or evil magic, in contrast to the "high" or
"white" magic of Umbanda, is now often referred to as Quimbanda, a word apparently having its origin in the Bantu designa-
tion of the priest-healer-sorcerer as Ki-mbanda. Originally no distinction was made between the two types of magical practice, and
they were all subsumed under the general heading of Macumba.
The term Macumba is still used by many to indicate all African-based practices in which any kind of magic is employed.

The most common element of currently practiced folk magic in
Rio is the *despacho*. *Despachar* is a Portuguese word meaning to
dispatch, to settle, or to render a decision on. The *despacho,* then,
is literally a decision, ruling, or transaction; in practice, it is a gift
including ingredients which the supplicants believe will mollify
the celestial messenger or keep him happy so that their wishes
will be carried out. In Candomblé ceremonies, gifts may range
from sacrifices of goats, black chickens or other animals, to dolls,
or foods of special significance, such as *farofa* (manioc meal) mixed
with dendê palm oil. In the city of Rio de Janeiro, the *despacho,*
accomplished as part of a macumba ritual, is most apt to include
open bottles of *cachaça* (sugar-cane rum), roasted chickens, red
wine or beer, cigars, and open boxes of matches. Throughout Rio,
outside of cult ceremonies, the *despacho* of Exu as a means of pla-
cating, undoing, or accomplishing a wish (sometimes destructive),
must be deposited at a crossroads, described by Carneiro (1967)
as, "uncontested dominion of the celestial messenger" (p. 27). *Des-*

pachos can be found all over the city and in bottles, holding a clove of garlic and other items which may be washed up on the beaches; the favorite times for placing them in the water are on Mondays and Fridays at midnight.

McGregor (1966) has observed that ". . . it is among public servants and people with a medium college type of education, especially women, that black magic is rampant. With the natural rivalries, jealousies and petty enmities that persist in the multivarious sections of Brazil's mammoth ministries . . . the *coisa feita* [evil thing done by black magic] is a godsend to those nursing grievances . . . all these make a 'work' [the word *trabalho* is the regularly employed term] against the objects of their displeasure and sometimes vice versa, which means in turn that hundreds of Macumba or Quimbanda associations are kept financially well-fed" (p. 191). The operators of Macumba *terreiros* in contrast to those of Umbanda, will accept and sometimes demand payment for their consultations and, according to reports from many observers, are not beyond threatening their "clients" with bad luck if payment is not forthcoming. They may also advise a client that his "enemy" has made a *coisa feita* against him and that he must effect a *trabalho* in return, or perhaps *desmanchar*, i.e., undo the harm through the use of white magic. In any event, the Macumba counselor may strongly recommend that the help-seeker buy a certain things (possibly from him) and give him money as well if he doesn't wish his life ruined by Exu and a great phalanx of following spirits.

Close scrutiny of the daily press, particularly those newspapers specializing in more sensational news, usually reveals, at least once or twice a month, stories about crimes or sexual or violent acts committed in relation to a *terreiro* or to some type of Macumba practice. Such stories, often of doubtful validity, reflect continuing fear and prejudice directed against the cults. McGregor (1966) has reported several instances occurring in the middle 1960's. In one, a young girl was murdered by her mother because the latter had received a revelation at a Macumba seance that the girl was pregnant by her own father. (Autopsy indicated that she was, in fact, virgin.) In another case, a *pai-de-santo* stabbed his enemy to death but declared his innocence because at the time of the crime he was under control of Exu Seven Crossroads, who was responsible. In another center, a soldier pulled out a gun, killed the *pai-de-santo*, and wounded several others, shouting, "Caboclo Arruda is with me. Nobody is stronger than I!" Many of these seem to be acts committed by psychotic or disturbed persons, and, as discussed below, many of the patients in the present study attributed features of their illness to Macumba or other supernatural forces.

It was partly for these reasons, partly because Macumba *terreiros* were said to have served as regular refuges for criminals, and partly perhaps because they were made up almost exclusively of the uneducated, the black, and the lower strata, that they were subjected, to periodic police prosecution. Under the Vargas regime everything associated with Macumba was automatically categorized as bad. Nonetheless, the upper classes continued to patronize the cults, contributing to their continued life, and by the 1960's all systematic harassment seemed to have stopped.

As indicated above, Freyre (1964) suggested how the interpenetration of upper-class Portuguese Catholic and lower-class African Negro religious-magical cultures, began with the plantation-owners' milk mothers, with their wives' servants, and with their own concubines. In a certain sense, this class and caste intercommunication on the basis of cult practices has continued to the present day. The nonwhite maid or cook often seems to act as intermediary between her master or mistress and the *terreiro*. The degree to which awareness of if not actual involvement in Macumba-related magical practices is imbedded in the culture is reflected in the universal understanding of terms which refer to them. Although the author often encountered reluctance to discuss them and, among the affluent educated classes, some occasional embarrassment at admitting knowledge of them, he found no resident of Rio de Janeiro without such knowledge. Even professional colleagues can tell stories of well-educated friends using *despachos* as well as participating in other Macumba practices, and a total series of Macumba-related expressions are clearly understood by all. *Encosto*, for example, is derived from *encostar*—to lean against—and refers to the pressure or influence of a hostile spirit, such as a dead relative; nervous tension and difficulty in thinking clearly may be explained in terms of an *encosto*. *Caminhos abertos* or *fechados* signify open or closed paths. Any failure in life may occur because a pathway is closed. In order to open the way to success, a *despacho* may be recommended so that some *exu* will lead away the hindering phalanx of spirits, or the advice of an Indian spirit or *caboclo* may be suggested which will require bringing food or candles to a special place in the forest, a waterfall, or a riverbank.

Corpo aberto or *fechado* means body open or closed to evil. If one is a *corpo aberto*, vulnerable to black magic, or a *coisa feita*, a visit to a *terreiro* may provide a ritual means of becoming safe or closed. Amarrar is a Portuguese word meaning to tie or to bind; a person may be *amarrado*—tied—as a form of *coisa feita*, usually by some-one of the opposite sex who wants him as a lover. *Desamarrar* means to untie or free the target of the magic.

UMBANDA

This is perhaps the most rapidly growing folk cult in Brazil, with most of its adherents in Rio de Janeiro. Willems (1966) de-scribed it as ". . . the Afro-Catholic tradition of the Macumba [to which] were added some of the essentials of Spiritualism to make it more palatable to the slowly rising urban masses and their yearning for middle-class symbols" (p. 213). As indicated be-low, it is still in a state of evolution with many variations from one center to another. While the Afro-Brazilian pantheon is prominent in its observances, possession seems to be most often by spirits of dead slaves or aboriginal Indians.

The organizing committee for the first Brazilian Congress of Umbanda, in 1941, identified the 1920's as the period when Umbanda emerged as a different way of "working with spirits." According to sources quoted by Bastide (1960) the separation of Umbanda from Macumba took place around 1930, but its iden-tity as a widespread religious movement is still in an early phase of growth and consolidation. A major source of confusion lies in the difficulty in separating Umbanda from Macumba and the pro-totypical Afro-Brazilian cults beginning with Candomblé on the one hand and from spiritism of the Kardec variety on the other. Depending upon the particular center, Umbandistas, continue aspects of the form of Macumba and Candomblé ceremonies, all the while deprecating the ritual. In varying degree they practice rhythmic dances, *ponto* singing and chanting, handclapping, drumming, cigar smoking, and *cachaça* drinking. A subtle gradation exists from one center to another according to social scale, with the "lowest" engaging in the most vigorous activities while among the "highest," meetings may closely resemble *Kardecista* Spiritist study groups. Drumming in particular is eschewed by many centers as an element of Macumba, and instead, the rhythmic beat of the dance is maintained by loud handclapping in unison. The "low" centers also pay more attention to the African gods. The distinction between "high" and "low," however, remains a relative matter with many exceptions and individual variations. Kardecism at the far end of the spectrum, away from the vigorous activities of the Afro-Brazilian cult centers, is often referred to as "table Spiritism" in contrast to the "*terreiro* Spiritism" of Umbanda. Among those who attend, the black and very poor no longer predominate, and it may be significant in this respect that most Umbanda centers refer to themselves as Spiritist. Another identity problem lies in the tremendous proliferation of local groups or associations known not only as *terreiros* following Macumba, but *centros*, as in the case of Spiritist groups, *tendas* (tents), or *cabanas* (huts). Each obeys only its own "spirit guide" who may be a *caboclo,* the spirit of a Brazilian Indian; a *prêto velho,* an "old black," as defined by Treitas and Pinto (1951): the spirit of a wise slave "whose work on earth is not yet done," usually addressed as Pai or Mãẽ; any of the African *orixás* or their derivatives; or even some spirit from the "Far East." Some of the spirits may never have been incarnated as human, i.e. are not the spirits of the dead.

The social range of Umbandista spirits differs markedly from those of *Kardecistas* who seek only the spirits of those who during their lifetime have achieved status or special distinction. The inclusion of the spirits of slaves, which often appear to have reached higher levels of perfection than those of their masters, and of the *caboclos*, may be viewed as adding a special element of egalitarianism, and even of social protest, to the Umbanda movement which is present in neither Macumba or Spiritist sessions. The spirits of Umbanda express themselves through the person of the President or Chief Guide of the particular group, who while he is possessed "incorporates" the spirit or as its "horse" is "ridden" by it. An Umbanda association may have one or more affiliated groups which also obey its spirit guide, but, despite congresses and various other attempts to form federations, they have not yet developed a doctrinal or structural coherence comparable to that based by the Spiritists upon the writings of Allan Kardec. Some of this is because of the lack of a single guiding philosopher or prophet, and some because of the nature of local Umbanda leadership itself. The medium or *Guia Chefe* (Chief Guide) who incorporates the dominant spirit of a particular center is the commanding presence of the session and, if not the formal administrative head of the center, the true power behind it. He calls for or dismisses the spirits, develops the group structure and ritual according to his own style, and is the primary source of advice for the considerable numbers of those attending in search of some type of healing. He is not, as a rule, inclined to abandon his personal power to a federation, although circumstances may occasionally force him into it. Umbanda leaders arrested by hostile local police on charges such as "practicing medicine without a license," for example, become aware of their need for organizational strength; a single Umbanda center is usually not able to raise the funds necessary to finance a wished-for medical or welfare organization; or other problems may contribute to a decision to ally oneself with others. The largest such organization may be the Spiritist Federation of Umbanda, which according to Camargo (1961), includes 260 groups in São Paulo alone. The exact number of Umbanda centers in the country is unknown, and any such figure may well include some groups which may be more accurately defined as *Macumbista* as well as others closer to the Spiritists. Bastide, in 1959, reported an estimate of approximately 30,000 Umbanda centers in the Guanabara-Rio State area now encompassed in Greater Rio de Janeiro. Madalena and colleagues (1968) identified 27,000 registered *terreiros de* Umbanda as of 1960. In 1968, the author heard estimates from various sources, including chiefs of Umbanda centers, ranging up to 50,000 centers or groups.

The Anuário Estatistico reports approximately 65,000 or 61 per cent of the country's *Umbandistas* as living in Guanabara and Rio State at the end of 1965. A considerably smaller number were reported from São Paulo, suggesting that Umbanda is not only an urban but, to an important degree, a Rio de Janeiro phenomenon. The same official report places the largest concentration of *Kardecista* Spiritists, approximately a third of the total, in São Paulo. The next largest concentration, 18 per cent of the total or approximately 135,000 people, was in Guanabara and Rio State combined. In other words, Spiritism is much more widely diffused, spread throughout the nation and strongly represented in some states, such as Rio Grande do Sul, where official records list no Umbandistas at all. Whether or not the Rio de Janeiro-São Paulo difference in proportions of *Umbandistas* and Spiritists reflects the generally greater wealth, education, and industrialization of the latter is unclear. The figures for Rio Grande do Sul, perhaps the leading state in statistical indices of socioeconomic advancement, tend to support this possibility.

The medical and psychiatric significance of this group is probably even greater than the total numbers indicate. Camargo (1961) found that more than 60 per cent of those coming to Umbanda or Spiritist centers were seeking relief from some ailment. Madalena, director of the Center for Studies of Casa Eiras, the hospital to which most of the patients in the present study were admitted, estimated that perhaps 50 per cent of the patients seen in his private practice of psychiatry, and 90 per cent of those supported by charity or social security, had consulted an Umbanda or Spiritist center on at least one occasion.

A more concrete picture of the institutional development of Umbanda centers in Rio de Janeiro is afforded through the religious news sections in the Sunday editions of the newspapers. The amount of coverage varies, but all contain announcements and ads. The Sunday, September 8, 1968 issue of *O Jornal,* for example, begins its regular section entitled *"Terreiros"* with an article on the *pontos*, special songs sung "in the law of Umbanda." Readers are reminded that the *pontos* should not be abused, for they represent the phalanxist forces coming to the *"Terreiros* or Centros" in order to help them with their works (*"trabalhos"*), whether these be of "magic, *descarga* [literally discharge, but referring here to energy discharge or activity as in special baths used as treatment], or the development of mediums." Under the heading of *"Saravando"* (literally, "hailing" as in "hail Mary") are listed eight organizations with their addresses, the names of their leaders and, in some cases, of their Chief Guides, and the hours and days of sessions open to the public. *"Saravá"* or "hail" Umbanda! is a characteristic outcry beginning a ritual for this type of group, and all readers know that centers listed under *Saravando* are, indeed, Umbanda. The names of the eight centers listed in the column offer an idea of their variety and general nature:

Centro Espirita Iemanjá. The *Guia Chefe* for this Centro, however, is not Iemanjá, but Oxossi Tupiara, probably a spirit combining African and Indian origins, cf, Tupi, a leading tribe of Brazilian Indians.

Tenda Espirita São Judas Tadeu

Centro Espirita Recanto do Pai Joaquim. Recanto in this context means retreat. Pai Joaquim, who is the same as Mestre Joaquim, described above as being important in the ritual of Catimbó, is one of the best known of the *prêto velhos.*

Tenda Espirita São Sebastião. Here there is no modification or qualification of the name of Saint Sebastian, Catholic equivalent in Guanabara of Oxóssi whose seven phalanxes, as noted below, are all headed by *Caboclo* spirits rooted in the Brazilian Indian tradition.

Cabana Espirita Oxum-Mare. Oxum-mare is one of the Nagô *orixás* representing the elementary forces of nature, in this case the rainbow. Its Catholic equivalent is Saint Bartholomew. Created by Xangô, god of tempests, thunder and lightning, it is represented by the Africans in the form of a serpent. This announcement carried the names both of the *cabana* leader and of a mãe *pequena* or little mother, the person who in Candomblé is the immediate substitute for the *mãe-de-santo.*

Tenda Espirita Estrêla do Oriente. This means Spiritist Tenda, Star of the East. *Linha do Oriente* is one of the seven "lines" of Umbanda, each of which is subdivided into seven phalanxes or legions of spirits. The line of *Oriente* is, in terms of its Catholic equivalent, spiritually led by St. John the Baptist. Six of its seven phalanxes include peoples who might in some ways be considered "Eastern." These are Hindus, Arabs and Moroccans, Japanese, Chinese, Mongolians and Eskimos, Egyptians, Aztecs and Incas, Mayas and Toltecs, Carribean Indians, Gauls, Romans and "ancient European peoples." The seventh phalanx is composed of "doctors and scientists."

Tenda Umbandista Caboclo Urabatão Velho. Caboclo Urubatão is the Chief Spirit of the first phalanx of the *Linha de Oxóssi,* all of whose phalanxes are headed by Caboclo spirits. As noted earlier, Oxóssi's Catholic equivalent in Rio de Janeiro and Guanabara is Saint Sebastian. In Bahia it is Saint George.

Tenda Espirita Cosme e Damião. Saints Cosme and Damion are the leaders of the second phalanx of the *Linha de Oxalá*—equivalent, as noted above, to Jesus Christ—otherwise known as the *Linha de Santo* or holy line.

In addition to those related to the names of the centers listed above, the major "lines," include those of Ogum and Africana. As might be expected, the *Linha Africana* is constituted of spirits which appear as *prêtos velhos*. They are said to be familiar with the *trabalhos* of Quimbanda or black magic and to infiltrate the *Terreiros da Quimbanda* in order to undo or annul them. The seven phalanxes of this line are named after the peoples of particular regions of Africa. Thus the first is the Phalanx of the People of the Coast. The other regions listed are Congo, Angola, Benguela, Mozambique, Luanda, and Guinea. In each instance, the phalanx chief spirit is called *Pai* or father, except for the last who is *Zum-Guiné*.

As we have seen, the divinities of Umbanda include three general groups: (1) the Nagô *orixás*, known in all Brazilian cults of African origin, (2) the *caboclos*, representing an abstract conception of the Brazilian aborigines, often fused with *orixás* of one kind or another, (there were, according to Carneiro [1967], 401 Nagô *orixás* in Africa, or with Angolese or Congolese entities and (3) the *prêtos velhos* or *velhos escravos*, old blacks or old slaves, rich in the wisdom of Africa and of suffering humanity in general. Of the three customarily advertised Umbanda services, two concern the "incorporation" of *caboclo* and *prêto velho* spirits. The third is for *desenvolvimentos* or developments, i.e., the development in new cult members of the qualities of being a medium. And overall is the explicit recognition of Jesus Christ as the great master and reigning spiritual leader, even though he may be called *Oxalá*.

The developing Umbanda emphasis (much spoken about though not as clearly evident from observation of actual practice) on Christian (Catholic) principles rather than the African cults, is said to have begun in the late 1920's (McGregor, 1966). At that time, a *Kardecista* medium named Zealiode Moraes, incorporated a spirit known as Caboclo of the Seven Crossroads. As a means of helping to "purify" Umbanda from its primarily African rites, the Circle of the Caboclo of the Seven Crossroads moved to a house especially purchased for the purpose, designated it the Tent of Our Lady of Piety, and the process was underway. Umbanda is still accepting and assimilating innumerable angels, saints, "peoples," mythological personages, and others who come from the hypothetical homeland of *Aruanda* and know "the law of Um-

banda." These are included in the infinitely expandable phalanxes and subphalanxes of spirits.

The doctrine is further complicated by variations set down
with great authority by a long list of authors who have produced
dozens of books and pamphlets on Umbanda, many of a
how-to-do-it nature. Most of these are contributions from Spiritism in its various forms, concerned in one way or another with
the phenomonon of *mediunidade,* the possibility of human beings
serving as intermediates between the "Invisible World" (of disincarnate spirits) and the "Visible World" (of incarnate spirits, the
world of man). One example of such a volume is Teixeira's (1967)
The Book of Mediums. Its author, in a not unusual manner, describes *Umbandismo* as part of the Spiritist Church. *Umbandismo*
"unites individuals who while they do not reject the teaching of Kardec . . . have as the fundamentals of their religious
point of view the marvelous, singular and humble most sincere
lessons of the *Caboclos* and *Prêtos Velhos*" (pp. 15–16). He then
divides the practitioners of *Umbandismo* into the Umbandistas
who practice Umbanda, or white magic, and the *Quimbandistas*
who practice Quimbanda, or black magic. The 213 pages of this
typical book include sections ranging from the classification of
spirits, through the lines of Quimbanda, the organization of *terreiros, orixás* and other entities, to "the influence of disincarnate spirits on our physical body and our life on earth." Like many others,
it also contains the personal requirements for becoming a medium
and most especially a *terreiro* leader or *pai-de-santo,* the requirements are the virtues familiar in all religions. The leaders are
admonished about the importance of leading an upright moral
life, absolute honesty, and freedom from vices.

Matta da Silva's (1964), *Segrêdos da Magia de Umbanda e Quimbanda* also emphasizes the Spiritist nature and the ancient mystic
origins of Umbanda. Firmly noting that Umbanda " . . . is not
and never was the African cult . . . called 'candomblé' " (p. 10),
it acknowledges only that "the primitive impulse of its reason for
being—here in Brazil" was to increase the growth and evolution
of this "immense community creeping (or dragging) itself among
the practices and conceptions connected with the confused and
degenerate aspects of the so-called African cults . . . mixed with
certain influences arising from the rites of our aborigines" (p. 19).

It traces magical practices inherent in the "astral current of Umbanda" to the *"Kabala Aria ou Nordica"* (Nordic or Aryan Cabal) hidden "since the famous Schism of Irshu occurring in India 5000 years ago" (p. 5). It also has chapters on prejudice and the role of Negroes in Umbanda. Umbanda possesses

> . . . a kind of mysterious force attracting people of all understandings . . . it is genuinely a religion of the 'poor people' because . . . it preaches absolute tolerance and absence of any color or racial prejudice . . . because of the variety of its rituals from *terreiro* to *terreiro*, each person can find his own degree of affinity with it. . . . Spiritism offers, with a cup of water in which fluids can be reflected, an alternative which given its simplicity endangers the divinatory shells of the Nagôs . . . *guides* and *brothers of space* are interested in doing charitable work, and disturbed people are unburdened through the uses of passes and concentrations. The contact with *ocultismo*, in great vogue since about 1930 gave to Umbanda the smoke-cures, baths, *trabalhos* of the greatest diversity (as to *desamarrar*, to "untie" oneself from another person), revived signs and encantations, exorcisms and flagellations, and complicated the offerings to Exu with its requirements to open the bottles of *cachaça* and boxes of matches, and to discriminate as to whether *despachos* are deposited on the cross or the T of crossroads, excluding those over which street car tracks pass because "the influence of iron or steel neutralizes the effect" (p. 168).

Umbanda, then, from one standpoint, has a remarkable universalistic reach, accepting adherents and believers regardless of ethnic status, social class, or formal religious membership. (One of Matta da Silva's footnotes formally recognizes the "thousands of Catholic-*Umbandistas*" [p. 20]. This is done on the assumption that the "astral law of Umbanda" and its teachings are more fundamental to man's relationship with the universe than any folk or traditional religious faith or cult, and that beside them, all ordinary interhuman phenomena pale into insignificance. Its universally accepting, democratic, and subtly anti-establishment features are easily appreciated. From the other standpoint, its open theological and magical structure, allowing for infinite variation, seems to demand of its adherents an unlimited credulity as well as the capacity to live simultaneously in the worlds of the occult and of modern science and technology. Its thickly peopled theogony and spirit world and magical and ceremonial practices appear so naive and at times disorderly, that it is hard to understand their uncritical acceptance by so many people of better than average education and intelligence.

The universalist nature of Umbanda as well as its emphasis on *caridade* (charity), taken from the Spiritists, are reflected in its organizational behavior. Umbanda centers never charge for their spiritual or healing ministrations, although supplicants may be asked to contribute to a social assistance fund or one to help maintain the center, or perhaps to buy certain substances or objects to be used in the necessary rituals. A network of orphan homes, social welfare organizations, and even medical stations, initiated by *Umbandistas* or depending to an important degree upon their support, is growing at a rate threatening to overtake those with Catholic or Protestant support. Most of these, however, are labeled Spiritist, rather than Umbanda, and it is difficult without detailed investigation of the internal structure of any single center to determine under which rubric it might most logically be classified.

At the time of the first Congress of Umbanda, Kardec's works were explicitly recognized as the fundamental basis for all Spiritist practice in Brazil, including Umbanda. Umbanda was defined as a special way of working in the Spiritist field which had appeared in the 1920's, and "primitive rites," including hair shaving and blood baths (part of the secret ceremonies of Candomblé), were excluded from Umbanda practice. Resolution VII of this congress recognized Jesus Christ as the "supreme spirit" of Umbanda. A second such congress, held in the Maracanãzinho (little Maracanã) Stadium in Rio de Janeiro in 1961, attracted 7,000 people. Two of the speakers had been elected to the national Chamber of Deputies in the preceding year on an *Umbandista* ticket. One of these operated a weekly two-hour radio program (still in existence in 1968) consisting of nothing but Umbanda chants and news. A particular manifest of the mixed roots, the social consciousness and the (perhaps deliberate) popular appeal of Umbanda was the celebration at Maracanãzinho Stadium on May 13, 1965 of the anniversary of the freeing of the slaves in Brazil. In spite of the emphasis on removal of Umbanda practices from those of Candomblé, members of more than 500 Umbanda centers honored the woman whom they had named as *mãe-de-santo* of 1965. She was the Ialorixá of the famous Bahian Candomblé, Apo Afonja.

The attitude of the official Catholic Church toward Umbanda and Macumba is one of concern. In 1964, when the Umbanda Spiritist Federation asked the government (which offered neither positive cooperation nor rejection) to pass enabling legislation so that Umbanda doctrine and priestly hierarchy might be codified, the matter came to public attention. Msgr. Francisco Bessa, a spokesman for the Church said that Catholics who repeatedly confessed to having attended ceremonies would be threatened with denial of the sacraments. Tancredo da Silva Pinto (1964), however, then president of the Federation was quoted in the New York Times as saying, "We are not Catholics. Our faith consists of nature. Our gods are of the wind, the sea, the sun, the rivers and the fields. They are not the spirits of dead saints; our spirits have never existed on earth."

THE SPIRITISM OF ALLAN KARDEC

The works of Allan Kardec have been consistent best sellers in all of Latin America throughout the 20th century. The remarkable and continuing hold of his doctrine upon these people is a palpable token of their uncritical hunger for religious healing systems which offer immediate release from the tedium and hopelessness of daily life.

Allan Kardec is the name from "another existence among the Druids" taken by a French physician, Hippolite Leon Denizart Rivail. He was born, or to use his own term, "reborn," in Lyon on October 3, 1804 in a Protestant milieu and died or was "disincarnated" on March 31, 1869. Although he was trained in medicine his studies were not followed by practice. Instead, he became interested in philosophy and in the various Christian sects. He earned his living as a teacher, engaging in research in a variety of basic scientific fields. Eventually he devoted increasing time to interests in hypnotism and magnetism, but it was not until his middle years, the time when Europe became interested in the phenomena of spiritual seances, that he himself began to study them. He concluded that there was no intelligent "effect" (human beings) without an intelligent "cause." The cause, he decided was the souls of the dead; these he called "spirits" and created the word "Spiritism" to signify the "doctrine of Spiritists" as a distinct aspect of spiritualism. A major difference between this doctrine and others calling themselves spiritualists rather than Spiritists was the Spiritist emphasis on reincarnation and on the idea that the nature of a man depends on the nature of the spirit incarnated in his body. The spirit must go through repeated incarnations in the world of matter, the *mundo visivel*, until it attains the requisite degree of moral perfection. Disincarnate spirits can communicate with man through the persons of mediums; the nature of the spirit answering a call of a medium will be determined by the latter's nature as well as his aim in trying to establish communication. Kardec classified and investigated the phenomena of message reception from the dead, using, as various publishers have summarized it, "rigorously scientific" criteria, and finally integrated his findings and ideas into Spiritism *(Espiritismo)*, a doctrine with scientific, philosophical, and religious aspects. It was not as a religion, however, that Spiritism found its final form under Kardec's direction. It was rather as a means of harmonizing the various religions derived from the diverse conditions of the social and political milieus which gave rise to them. He considered himself a kind of secretary-general to the myriads of spirits in constant communication with the eternal *mundo invisivel*, invisible world, as an intermediary or a medium of transmission to the human world.

Kardec's doctrine was almost immediately accepted by the entire Latin-American world, although it was badly received in most Anglo-Saxon areas. In Brazil it excited immediate interest and with the passage of years various study groups were formed. By 1853, Rio de Janeiro had a small group of students of spirit phenomena, including some members of the nobility. Several groups also existed in Bahia, and the first publications appeared in 1860. Full details of this history are available in many translations of Kardec's work, such as that issued by the Brazilian Spiritist Federation in 1946. The important sources for Kardecistas are the publication in Paris of his *The Book of Spirits* in April, 1857; the establishment of the Spiritist Society of Paris and its journal, the *Spiritist Review* in 1858; and publication of Kardec's *The Book of Mediums* in 1861. The first of these was circulated in Brazil in 1858. Some of the most notable new organizations were the "Confucius Group," formed in 1873, and the Society of Spiritist

Studies, "God, Christ and Charity," formed in 1876. The Brazilian Spiritist Federation, encompassing all the smaller groups was formed in 1884. It was active in publishing, giving courses and public conferences, developing social welfare, legal assistance and medical facilities, forming branch societies and working groups. It was in large part responsible for Kardecism in Brazil growing to a point unknown elsewhere in the world. The organizational development of Spiritism has continued unabated. Spiritist youth organizations began to appear in the early 1930's, and in 1949 the Youth Department of the Brazilian Spiritist Federation was established with indoctrination as its primary objective. By 1951 there were 21 Federations in different states, but they were not joined together. The social welfare and evangelization center maintained by the two largest regional federations in São Paulo are said by Camargo (1961) to receive almost 10,000 help-seekers weekly. Published data in the Anuário Estatistico indicate that Spiritist welfare, medical, and educational institutions in Brazil are approaching the number existing under Catholic auspices and are almost double the number of those sponsored by Protestant groups. (As noted above, some of these sponsoring groups may more accurately be classified as Umbanda rather than *Kardecista* Spiritists.) The legal formalities necessary for classification and inclusion in public surveys are usually not followed in interior towns, therefore, many more are probably not listed at all. Estimates listed by McGregor (1966) put the probable number at at least 1,000,000 Spiritist centers and over 4,000,000 individuals who regularly practice Kardec's system. There are about 34 Spiritist magazines with a combined readership of approximately 300,000, not including the columns and special articles found from time to time in the daily press or in other magazines.

Some of the advocacy flavor of Spiritist messages in the popular press may be gained from the religious page in *O Jornal* (1968) described above. One article notes that if two people cannot get along in the married state the solution should be not infidelity but " . . . separation of bodies as well as of souls." "Lamentably," it went on, "in Brazil in spite of the separation of church and state and the falsity of the census, which because of the deep-seated prejudices of the reporters indicates a number of Catholics much higher than in reality to the detriment of other religions . . . the half-heartedness of the legislatures before the pressures of the Church led them to the point of inscribing the indissolubility of matrimony in our constitution!" A marriage indissoluble by earthly fiat, it suggested,'might result in the moral degradation of both partners and make things still more difficult by increasing the number of unwanted children into which spirits will have to be reincarnated.

Francisco Candido Xavier, born in Pedro Leopoldo in the state of Minas Gerais in 1910, significantly influenced the growth of Kardecism in Brazil. Beginning in August 1931, the writings of this relatively uneducated man from the interior aroused nationwide and later worldwide publicity. Their style and content could not be reconciled with Xavier's apparent abilities and education, and he himself disclaimed responsibility, saying that he had only been the medium who had received and recorded the materials from the spirit world. An important aspect of Xavier's (1938) work, was his comparison between the intellectual or research nature of spiritualism in Europe and the way in which Kardec's teachings in Brazil "lifted souls to a renewal of their faith, resting on love and charity, under the guidance of Christ" (p. 1). This frank appeal to the people's need for emotional involvement and participation and to their special need for hope and a sense of purpose, attracted masses of ardent converts. Some are from the upper classes, and a considerable proportion of the educated group do indeed support and participate in Spiritism. The lower class, though, especially in the centers of *espiritismo baixo* (low-spiritism) which cannot be functionally differentiated from Umbanda, are the people who may derive a sense of power and achievement from their religious participation as from no other sphere of their lives. As Camargo (1961) has noted, a compensatory mechanism is put into motion when "meek public employees and humble domestic servants are suddenly transformed into vehicles of illuminated spirits, bearers of sublime message" (p. 125).

SOME ASPECTS OF CEREMONY AND ORGANIZATION IN SELECTED SPIRITIST AND UMBANDA CENTERS

A few *Centros Espiritas* (none with the word Umbanda in their names) were listed in the Rio de Janeiro telephone directory in the summer of 1968. It should have been easy to locate them. Hours of fruitless walking from one commercial building to another, however, indicated that the solidity implied by the directory listing was illusory. Conversation with elevator operators, *porteiros,* and occasional tenants revealed that the Centers which had tried to locate in business buildings in the central city area had had rent problems. In general, the informants were reticent, leaving the impression that other problems as well had been involved in one or another Center's decision to move, and that, in any event, they did not enjoy discussing the matter of Spiritism, especially with strangers.

This experience confirmed impressions from previous visits to Brazil as well as experience in visiting a Macumba ceremony in Rio de Janeiro and a Candomblé in Bahia, which suggested that even in places which were open enough and sufficiently large for a foreigner to be present without attracting undue attention, prior arrangement was valuable. One or two Macumba or Candomblé *terreiros* are on the tourist circuit both in Rio de Janeiro and Bahia and are regularly visited by groups from the hotels. These have become so "folklorized," to use a common expression, that little of professional or scientific value can be learned at them. Discussion with a *mãẽ-de-santo* after one such ritual attended by a group of visiting psychiatrists (mostly Brazilian) who had been attending a convention yielded the comment that none of the dancers had become possessed because they felt that they were just giving a show; it was not the boredom or, by inference, the resentment of the participants as such which led them consciously to hold back, but rather that under such circumstances they could not become suitable *cavalos* for the spirits. It was the spirits themselves which did not find appropriate conditions to "descend" and be "incorporated" or "ride" the *filhas-de-santo* (holy daughters). To rephrase it in Spiritist, including Umbanda, terms, their quality of being a medium, of *mediunidade,*(this expression is not usually used in Candomblé *terreiros*), was impaired by the circumstances.

With these considerations in mind it seemed best to find a relatively small group where there was no "audience" in the sense of detached spectators, and where detailed conversation with the chief would be possible. Eventually, through personal friends, invitations were received to visit two such groups. One designating itself an Umbanda center might be called, following the discussion above, an example of "*terreiro* spiritism." The other, a private group composed exclusively of the educated upper-middle and upper class closely following the teachings of Allan Kardec, might be called an example of "table spiritism." In addition, two visits without prior invitation were made to one of the largest centers in Rio de Janeiro and the entire nation. Including extensive social welfare and medical services within its purview, it represents an organizational model of what many Spiritist groups would like to become. Finally, through another personal contact, an invitation was received to visit the only Spiritist psychiatric hospital in Rio de Janeiro.

TENDA DE UMBANDA SÃO JUDAS TADEU—OBSERVATIONS OF RITUAL

This *Tenda* was not listed in the Sunday newspaper's page of religious announcements. Contact was made through a friend with a double connection, symbolizing the manner in which participation in African-related sects has always brought together members of social classes widely separated in other aspects of their lives. Both his aunt, a woman with some college-level education, and his maid were *socios* or members of the group. If asked, both would probably identify themselves as Catholic. Both were reluctant to have any personal contact with the investigator, apparently because of some uneasiness about the possible need to explain their religious interests. The *Tenda* is located high on a hill in Catumbí, a district in the North Zone of the city. It is housed in an old stone structure, approximately 50 feet long and 35 feet wide. The roof is thatch over a wooden framing. The Tenda is not easily seen from the streets below during the day because of thick fronds of banana palm covering part of the area. At night, looking up, nothing is visible but a dim light.

It was suggested that a Friday evening, when a regular weekly session of *prêto velhos* open to all comers is held, would be the best time for an initial visit. The area was reached through the *Tunel* Santa Barbara under the hill of Santa Teresa. Finally the taxi turned up a narrow road, faintly illuminated with a pale yellowish cast by widely spaced street lamps. The friend (who himself had not previously attended) was waiting at a gasoline station on a nearby corner. Following the directions given by his maid, and with some additional advice from a few men loitering in a small store nearby, an opening was discovered in an old concrete wall running along the sidewalk. The steep path was dark, and a few moments of accommodation were necessary before its general outlines could be seen in the pale moonlight. The visiting party, including the author, his wife and three teen-age children, the friend who had made the contact, and Drs. Penna and Bisker, strung out in single file maintaining touch contact with each other. (Previous discussions had suggested that a family group would be welcome at the session, if everyone were willing to come as a participant.) In time, it was possible to see that the path ran along the site of some old stairs. Chunks of concrete and stone were irregularly interspersed with weeds and occasional bits of litter along the way. Here and there men evidently relaxing in accustomed places sat silently in the shadows looking beyond the hillside. The view was pleasant. Scattered star like points of light marked houses and shacks on the far side of Santa Teresa (the front of which faced Botafogo); in the absence of light coming up from the street below, the stars were easily visible in the clear sky above. After about eight minutes of climbing, the path ended abruptly at a dark corner of the *Tenda*. Around the corner, however, was a lighted entrance from which it was possible to see a relatively intact flight of concrete stairs descending straight down to the street far below, and opening onto the sidewalk about half a block above the point where the path which had been taken began. None of the loiterers in the store had bothered to mention it.

The building consisted of a long low room with an unevenly chipped gray concrete floor and walls of grayish plaster. The ceiling, supported by two posts on either side wrapped in grayish white paper was entirely covered with spaced rows of strips of the same paper, giving an impression of thatch or fringe and creating a feeling of closeness. Curtained-off alcoves at the sides of the entry contained numbered wooden bins for herbs and other ritual materials, a few chairs and some empty bottles. To the left of the entryway was a counter partitioning off a small "office" space. On the wall behind it was a notice reminding *sócios* of a celebration of the feasts of Saint Damion and Saint Cosme in the coming week. Behind the counter stood one of the *Tenda* officials, a sandy-haired blue-eyed man in his mid-thirties, wearing the routine uniform of white coveralls, unadorned except for a red heart pierced by a blue arrow superimposed upon a yellow Star of David, embroidered on the left front pocket. After a few moments of explanation, he welcomed the group to the meeting, listed each arrival by first name in a registration book, and gave each a small plastic tag with a number. On the backs of several of the tags were the words, "*Pai* Cambina," the chief spirit guide of the group. Each person was politely informed that at the proper time his first name and number would be called and that he then should go up for his consultation. There was no surprise shown at the unusual nature of the visitors. It was clearly expected that no one would be coming to a session unless he wished to obtain advice or treatment from the spirits. Within this set of expectations, everyone was welcome.

A few feet into the room in a direct line with the door so that people entering would have to pass it was a small altar bearing colored ceramic replicas, about 10 inches high, of Cosme and Damion. The figures were surrounded with offerings of flowers, coconut sweets, and small dishes containing other foods. About halfway into the room three rows of backless wooden benches were separated by a center aisle. On the left wall *Senhoras* was written in black paint and on the right, *Homem.* As each woman entered and seated herself on the left, an elderly mulatto woman with stringy white hair handed her a piece of white cloth approximately 30 inches square with which to cover her knees. A white latticed fence topped by a painted blue railing several feet in front of the benches separated them from the ritual area. Above it, running its entire length, was a neon tube which gave off a bluish-white light when it was turned on at the beginning of the ceremony. The ritual area occupied the entire width of the room behind the lattice and about a third of its length. Covered with brown sand, its most striking feature was a large altar which supported about 20 large, brightly colored plaster or ceramic figures of saints.

The top row of the altar was occupied by the four largest figures, with no evident regard for their place in any particular hierarchy, although one represented the Virgin Mary. These were flanked on either side by smaller figures of St. George on horseback and St. Sebastian. Christ was at the apex of a vaguely pyramidal arrangement of smaller figures below. The bottom part of the altar, rising to a height of about three feet, was a cupboard. It and the shelves on which the figures were placed, were covered with drapes of a white satiny material which reflected the neon light. This altar was apparently a source of considerable pride for the group, and when at the end of the ceremony on another night, the author asked permission to photograph it, permission was granted with evident pleasure. At one side of the altar was a long table on which were figures of St. George, the Virgin Mary, and a kneeling American Indian in feathered head-dress, as well as three vases containing artificial flowers, three glasses of water arranged in a triangular pattern, and several other small objects.

From 7:30 until 8:15 when the ceremonies began, members of the congregation arrived. One by one, for the most part, they took their seats, until a total of 35 people were present. All entered quietly, and a hushed air of decorum prevailed. Several of the people appeared to know each other and exchanged greetings upon arrival. The congregation was predominantly white, with a few of "tan" or brown skin, and only two were black, a man and a woman. Most appeared to be *operários,* possibly machine operators or truck drivers, small clerks, or *funcionários.* No one was dirty, ragged, or barefoot. Most of the men wore the usual Rio garb of a sport shirt hanging outside the trousers, the women wore simple cotton dresses. Many, as is usual, wore open sandals without socks or stockings. There was one seemingly middle-class family, the father in jacket and sports shirt, the mother well dressed with stockings and high heels, and their son; later, when the director of the session asked the boy his age and discovered it to be less than 12, he was asked to wait for his parents outside.

Before the ceremony, the various assistants—*filhos* and *filhas-de-santo*—put on their white coveralls or their ankle-length, high-necked, long-sleeved white cotton dresses embroidered with the design described above and occasionally some variants. There were eight in all, and all were barefoot. Three of the four men were white; with their neatly combed, well-barbered hair, they could have passed for young executives. The fourth had very light skin but negroid features and tight curly hair. He seemed older than the others, all of whom appeared to be in their middle thirties. The women included one black, one mulatto, and two whites. All were stocky, somewhat obese, and not so well groomed as the men.

The session began with one of the women swinging a char-coal-filled censor about as she passed through the room. The incense-laden smoke quickly dissipated through the open windows and doors. At the same time, other staff members were setting out small, crudely constructed wooden chairs, only about a foot high, at the edges of the sand area. Near each, on a small box, were bowls, cigars, and glasses of water. This completed, the *filha-de-santo* with the censor stood at the entrance of the ritual area, and the others entered one by one. As each came in, he bent and passed the smoke over his face and neck. Then he prostrated himself on a stone before the altar, the women first spreading out a length of white cloth, the men lying face down directly on the sand. The prostration was rapid, and some of the men did it with a bounce as though it were a push-up. The women and at least one of the men donned ritual necklaces after their obeisance and then stood on the sand in a loose circle, women to the left and men to the right, and singing, led by one of the women, began. The songs were *pontos* with rhythms primarily of African origin directed to the various gods of the *orixá* pantheon. Songs replete with references to *Ogum, Oxalá* and others shifted without perceptible pause to songs using the names of Jesus Christ and God. After some 20 minutes of song beginning with exhortations to several Exus who might interfere with the ceremonies if not placated, the leader appeared.

The leader, whose official title was Director of Ritual of the *Tenda,* was the *pai-de-santo* of the group. He was also the person who incorporated or was the *cavalo* of the Chief Guide, *Pai Cambina.* As he explained at a later visit, there had never had been a real person of this name. *Pai Cambina* was a Tibetan spirit from the Himalayas, and this was perfectly appropriate to Umbanda as a religion with African roots combined with Christianity, and embodying influences from Islam, Buddism, and other undefined Eastern religions as well. He noted in passing that some religious procedures of a similar nature are presently practiced by Negroes in the United States.

During the day the leader is a foreman of a gang of tunnel builders. Aware of class differences, he believes that he probably has a better income than any of his assistants and thinks it quite probable that many of those who attend the ceremonies are of higher-class status and have more money than the *filhos* and *filhas-de-santo*. Short, rotund, and white-haired with a neatly clipped white mustache, he had a distinguished presence, barefeet and white coveralls not withstanding. He led the singing in a loud clear voice with a good sense of rhythm, interrupting it twice for chatty discourses to the assemblage in the manner of a small-town United States minister making his regular announcements from the pulpit. On these occasions he stood near the entrance to the sand area, leaning from time to time on the blue railing. He made note of the regular Wednesday evening sessions of *desenvolvimento*, "developing" people who were to become mediums, i.e., those with latent *mediunidade* which should be made overt. (Unfulfilled potential as a medium is regarded by Spiritists and *Umbandistas* as a major source of emotional disturbance.) He announced, also, that on the following Thursday there would be a meeting limited to members of the *Tenda*. He stressed the organization's need for money. The only reward the *Tenda* could give its members was to hold some sessions for them alone. Money was needed for ritual materials, rent, and electricity. Also, if enough was accumulated, they would like to build a new center elsewhere in a better location.

After the leader had finished, three of the white-robed women in the sand began to shuffle slowly as they sang. Swaying slowly, rythmically from side to side and shifting their weight from foot to foot, they began to waver and wobble, and then one by one spasmodically doubled over without falling. They seemed to be in the onset of a trance. They walked in the bent position or squatted with contorted painful faces, issuing clucking, grunting, guttural sounds caused by forceful expirations of breath as they were "mounted" and "ridden" by the descending spirits. Then they were helped by the male assistants to sit on the wooden stools. The assistants, male and female, helped them put cigars, already lit by the three women, in their mouths and poured a liquid later identified as muscatel wine into the bowls—called *cuia*—which were made from a gourdlike plant. These ministrations were to calm the incorporating spirit and help it to become "fixed" in its new temporary body. The *cavalos* sat on the stools, rolling their eyes, puffing steadily on the cigars and drinking from time to time. They were now under the influence of spirits of the *prêto velhos*, who had, in response to the *pontos* and under proper ritual circumstances facilitated by the dancing, descended into and been "incorporated" by them. Because these were the spirits of ancient blacks, often weak, decrepit, and unable to walk, the *filhas* themselves, moved little and appeared bent and feeble.

Suddenly the leader himself now became entranced. His face turned fiery red, the color accentuated by his white hair. His eyes rolled up, he fell to the ground with a strangled shout, he clucked and grunted even more loudly and forcefully than the women. His assistants quickly helped him up, half carried and seated him on a wooden chair immediately before the altar, gave him an already lit cigar, and placed a bowl of muscatel in his hands. He sat there facing the congregation, legs straight out before him, puffing, drinking, occasionally grunting, occasionally issuing a fragment of song, with his eyes rolling and at times seeming to search the faces of those on the benches. Then, carefully setting down his cigar and bowl, he lifted a large heavy rock from between his legs and deliberately brought it down twice with a dull thud on top of his head. The congregation watched intently. Some seemed to be themselves on the verge of a trance. The leader, following the self-inflicted blow, seemed more dazed than ever. The air was becoming cloudy with cigar smoke in spite of the open windows.

Now a neatly tonsured mulatto man in a clean sport shirt and well pressed trousers stood up in front of the railing and began in a low businesslike voice to read names and numbers from the registry. There was room for four consultations at any one time, one with each of the three women and one with the leader himself. Each person seeking consultation removed his shoes before entering the sandpit, the women from one side, the men from the other. First the help-seeker and the medium greeted each other in a ritualized way, one putting his hands on the other's shoulders, then moving their heads rapidly to either side as though touching cheeks without making actual contact. Finally, seated on a low stool in front of *Pai Cambina* or one of the *filhas,* the actual consultation began. The seekers all talked at length. Sometimes one of the assistants standing nearby would participate. In other cases the activity of the *filha* seemed to consist mainly of blowing smoke in the "client's" face, making passes by waving hands about his head and shoulders in circular motions, and snapping her fingers—all intended to facilitate the therapeutic or helpful action of spirits in solving the problem or healing the illness of which the supplicant complained. Sometimes the helpful spirits, aided by the medium's actions, were working to remove the influence of a *despacho* which had caused a harmful spirit to do something injurious to the client. The leader's wife, who was one of the *filhas,* consulted palms. The special technique of the leader himself was to *jogar buzio* or throw small shells (literally, to play the shells—the *cawries* still specially imported into Brazil from Africa for the purpose), making divinations from the pattern in which they fell. Consultation varied in duration from a few minutes to almost half an hour, although a certain standard amount of time had initially been allotted to each person in the interests of efficiency. There was no one present who was not seeking consultation, but it was possible to hear the words of only one, an attractive well-dressed mulatto woman who seemed concerned about an examination she was going to have to take.

Finally, the name and number was called of the author's friend who had acted as a contact with the *Tenda.* He had been assigned for consultation to the leader to whom he explained that some of the group could not speak Portuguese. To this came the reply: "The spirits can communicate in any language." When the friend explained that there was an American psychiatrist in his group, however, the leader said that all of those with him could come up for a simultaneous consultation during which he would answer questions about his work. The entire party then removed its shoes, entered the arena, and after making the proper gestures of greeting was seated on low stools around the leader. Two of the male assistants stood nearby, occasionally filling the gourd with wine and answering questions upon the invitation of the leader, who treated them with paternalistic pride much like a proud parent asking a child to recite.

The leader began by asking if the author would like to see him administer another blow to himself with the stone, inviting him to examine both the stone and his scalp. The stone was then lifted three or four inches above his head and brought down once more with a loud thud. His hair was thickly matted, and it was not possible to feel any bumps or swellings on the scalp beneath it. The stone itself was very heavy. In one place it had cracked and a small bit had been broken off. The leader said that he would remain alive and in control of his "spiritual" powers until the entire stone had crumbled and worn away. During this and later conversations, he continued to puff on his cigar and take small sips of wine. He offered some to the male members of the party including the author's two teen-aged sons, and seemed pleased when every one sipped it. The wine was indeed sweet muscatel. In response to a question, the leader said he did not use *cachaça* (sugar-cane rum) or drums in his rites because they were part of the "more primitive Candomblé" ritual which in any event was "folkloric and not religion." When asked if his flushed face (he continued from time to time to grunt and cluck) might have been in part a consequence of the smoking and drinking, he indicated that he himself neither drank nor smoked but that the cigars and wine were for *Pai Cambina*, the spirit in him, and that when the spirit departed all the tobacco and alcohol would leave his system.

By this time his involved style of speech had become clear. It was not he who was speaking but *Pai Cambina*. References to the leader himself were made when the spirit, speaking through his mouth, would say "this horse" or "my horse" or "this one who is my horse." The response to the question about smoking and drinking was: "This one who is my horse neither smokes nor drinks, and when I depart, there will be no more tobacco or alcohol in him." At the same time, it remained difficult on occasion to differentiate the comments of the spirit from those of the leader, his "horse": the leader said that striking himself on the head with the stone was one way in which he demonstrated both to himself and his followers that so long as he was inhabited by the spirit he was protected against all harm. He then took a lighted candle, held it against the palm of his hand until the horny callus was burned black, and asked the author to wash the spot and rub it with sand. He smiled triumphantly when after much scrubbing most of the sooty blackness was removed along with a layer of dead skin. He cited the absence of an underlying burn as additional evidence of the effectiveness of spirit protection of his body.

Finally he asked if the author had any problems about which he wanted consultation. Questioned about the health of an elderly female relative, he threw 13 small shells upon the sand and replied that she was in good health, would not die suddenly, but would first become ill so that there would be plenty of time for people to know about it. In reply to his question about her age, he was given one two years more than the actual figure. Again throwing the stones, he said that she was, in fact, a year older, explaining that he dates people from the moment of their conception. Then he said that he could see someone standing behind her, a person (of unnamed sex) taller than average, with white hair and green eyes and that this person was bothering the author (who could identify no such individual) from time to time. He asked if the elderly relative lived near a river, and upon being told that there was one about 30 miles from her home, said that 30 miles was indeed nearby. He appeared to take the figure as confirmation of his judgement. This visit lasted until approximately midnight, at which time a few people still awaited their consultations. The author and his party asked the leader's permission to leave so that he might be able to consult with some of the others who wished to see him rather than one of the *filhas*. He gave this permission with seeming reluctance, still in the trance state seated on the stool, and asked the group to return as soon as possible.

The next visit, almost three weeks later, again after preliminary arrangements had been made, was on Wednesday, the night of the regular *desenvolvimento* session. The benches were pushed back to the rear of the room, leaving a large open space of dirty scratched concrete visible between the congregation and the latticework barrier. Of the 40 people present, considerably more than before appeared to be of the middle class. One adolescent white girl wore a neat school uniform. She was with an older woman who seemed to be her mother. There were four or five blacks and 10 or 12 who were "tan" or mulatto. In contrast to the previous occasion, the men and women were not separated. A well-dressed and groomed white woman in her mid-thirties seated nearby initiated a conversation while waiting for the session to begin. She said her family had come to Brazil from Spain when she was a child. She had been to the *Tenda* several times before and had come tonight because she wanted to consult the leader about a personal problem. A woman in the row behind was overheard telling her companion, "When I walked in all I could think of was *Pai Cambina, Pai Cambina,* and I felt better already." The session opened at eight o'clock. The leader, smiling, said that two doctors, one an American professor (the other being Dr. Penna), were present and that he was going to fulfill his promise that anytime they returned he would devote his time to them. Wednesdays were the only nights on which the mediums could consult with him, so this broke the rhythm of the organization. However, he had already told them that tonight it would be impossible, and he hoped the members of the assemblage who had wished to consult with him personally would not be too angry and frustrated. In order not to deprive those who felt that they must see him, he would work until six in the morning. He could not remain longer, however, because he had to be at his regular job at seven. He also explained that consultation with his spirit *Pai Cambina* alone may not be so essential as some people suppose. It is true that some spirits do come down to possess their "horse," but other spirits remain "astral," forming a kind of *junta de guiais* (board of directors of spirit guides), so that when *Pai Cambina* is consulted through him, the guardian angel or spirit of the help-seeker is simultaneously consulting with the astral *junta.* He explained, too, that if people couldn't consult with him they might consult with his wife because her guide sits with his at the head of the table of this *junta.* He told the congregation that he personally had the authority to change the schedules if he deemed it necessary. The place has a Board of Directors in which he is Director of Ritual. He is not concerned with operations, whether the rent is paid, whether sufficient numbers of candles and cigars are purchased, unless asked for his opinion. But when it comes to the ritual and its scheduling, no one else can say anything: *"Eu sou chefe absoluto"* (I am the absolute chief). When he mentioned the presence of the two doctors the people looked toward the author and his Brazilian companion in a curious and friendly manner. Later reports indicated that they, as well as the

Tenda staff, were pleased and proud that a foreigner would have chosen their *Centro* for a visit.

Although in the past Wednesdays had been devoted just to *sessoēs de desenvolvimento*, so many people had been coming for consultation in recent weeks that it had been necessary to schedule two sessions. The initial phases of the development session were identical with those already described. The censor was swung, participants arranged themselves in a rough circle on the open concrete floor in front of the benches, and the *pontos* were sung. This was to be a *caboclo* session, and because *caboclos*, in contrast to *prêtos velhos*, can stand up and walk (or at least can motivate their "horses" to do so), the ritual was much more active and consultations were held in the standing position on the concrete rather than seated in the sand arena. Many more people, including several newly developing initiates, were involved, 12 in addition to the leader—eight women and four men. Among those on the floor were three women who had not been present at the previously attended ceremony. Two were white. One of these arrived in high heels, a stylishly short skirt, and a short haircut of the type regarded in the city as most up-to-date. The other, well dressed but not miniskirted, was the mother of the school girl. She remained seated on the bench, but after the ceremony began she responded to the urging of one of the *filhas* and retired to the curtained alcove in the rear of the room, whence she emerged a few moments later barefooted and white-gowned with her long hair loosened from its previous restraining pins and hanging down freely over her shoulders.

Eventually all the singing women began the sideways shuffling, then, after appearing momentarily to lose their balance, many began to pivot. By this time little of the circular arrangement was left, and the impression was more of an aggregate of individuals than an organized group. The older adepts first became possessed apparently at the moment of pivoting or just before, after which they often took the initiates by the hands, doing a sideways step or rhythmically and alternately flexing their knees. They, as well as the male assistants who did not become possessed and were also watching to see that none of the entranced fell or hurt themselves, placed their forefingers on the heads of the new initiates while these latter pivoted about. The leader explained later that when people start their development, one of the first things they learn is how to pivot or rotate their bodies "without becoming dizzy," and how to make the half-falling motion without actually falling to the ground. Then the leader and his wife, who were also singing and moving in rhythm, suddenly became red in the face, uttered brief guttural expirational sounds, and, as each emitted a shout (later identified as the name of their possessing spirit), ran into the sand area, jumped into a kneeling position before the altar, and returned to the concrete floor.

The degree of freedom for possession and dance behavior was high since each participant had a broader range of deities or spirits available to him and these were less traditionally circumscribed than in Candomblé or its equivalents. The two new white women required noticeably more time to become possessed than the other participants, who included a black man and woman who had not been present on the previous occasion. The man entered the trance with dramatic generalized shaking and jumping and repeated the dash of the leader and his wife to the sandpit. Once possession had occurred, however, the white woman with the up-to-date hair style was the most dramatic of the entire group. Her hair fell over her eyes, her mouth was screwed up into the *schnauzkrampf* of the chronic schizophrenic patients depicted in early German psychiatric texts, her right arm remained elevated with the hand at head level and the index finger pointing skyward, and she appeared to be vigorously hyperventilating. This phase, which was sustained for a prolonged period, was initiated by forward and backward shaking of her body with much head motion. As each participant became established or "settled down" (as the *chefe* described it) in the state of possession (i.e., when the particular spirit "incorporated" by or "riding" her was firmly ensconced) she would go systematically from one medium to another giving them the ritual greeting. Two elderly black women went down the lines of people seated on the benches placing their open palms first on their right, then on their left shoulders, and making the barest head motion toward the cheeks; the style of this greeting varied considerably between individuals. The leader was greeted by each possessed medium in a manner symbolizing absolute subservience. They knelt before him (i.e., before his possessing spirit), crawled to his feet and prostrated themselves. The women also knelt to two of the nonpossessed assistants, *chefes de terreiro* (members of the group used the words *tenda* and *terreiro* interchangeably), standing at either side of the leader. It was observed, however, that the possessed man did not do this, although he did prostrate himself before the leader. In this *Tenda*, the *chefe* later explained, more women become possessed and therefore *filhas-de-santo*, but men have higher organizational status and are entitled to respect according to position. The two *chefes* had been in the group for 15 and 17 years respectively, and each had experienced possession only once, near the beginning of his membership.

After the onset and greeting phases, many of the dancers accepted lit cigars from nonpossessed assistants and puffed them as they slowly shuffled or twirled. During this period a number of the watching assembly came for consultation. There had been no prior registration at this session, and no names were called out. Those who wished consultation sought out the medium they wanted. They stood before the mediums as they talked, occasionally being touched as well as having passes made over them, and sometimes participating in the dancing movements. Participation was most marked in two women who had shown some signs of becoming entranced while they were still sitting on the benches. One, white woman of middle age, wearing dark glasses, stockings, and heels of moderate height (in contrast to the flat soles or sandals worn by most of the others), seemed exceptionally tense. When the dancing started, she had begun to frown and grimace. She sat on the front bench close to the dancers. Finally, one of the dancing *filhas* stood before her, took her by the hands, and raised her to a standing position. She arose stiffly, with rigid musculature and tense, immobile, flushed face and slowly followed the *filha* onto the floor. She stood before the medium for several minutes, face close to hers, speaking in a low tone, receiving passes and moving slightly. She then went from medium to medium, giving each the ritual greeting (ignoring the males, including the leader) before returning to her seat. It was later learned that she was university educated and from a Jewish family. Various informants had indicated that a few Jews and Protestants, although these are a tiny fraction of those who are Catholic, regularly participate in Umbanda or Spiritist activities. A psychiatrist informant, however, doubts whether more than a handful of the approximately 200,000 Jews in Brazil, including around 40,000 in Greater Rio, participate in such rituals. These are believed to be physically ill as a rule, or psychiatrically disturbed, seeking help not available from the medical profession. Others have said it is impossible to be both a practicing Jew and to attend the cults, in the same way in which one may go to a mass in the morning and an Umbanda at night. Nonetheless, at least one practicing Jew, a member of a learned profession, is said to be a *pai-de-santo*.

The other obviously disturbed member of the congregation was a poorly dressed black woman who also sat in the front bench. During much of the ceremony her eyes were closed and her head bent with her forehead resting on the tips of her fingers. About midway in the proceedings she slowly walked to the floor and after some hesitation selected the leader's wife as her consultant. She remained standing before her, hardly moving and saying little for perhaps 15 minutes and then slowly returned to her seat.

During this session, the frequently encountered folk diagnosis of *espinhela caida* or "fallen thoracic cage" (*espinha* signifying spine or backbone) was made and treatment instituted. The patient was a slight, sallow well dressed young woman. She stood with her shoes off in the midst of the dancing mediums and advice-seekers while one of the *chefes de terreiro*, who worked during the day as a hospital orderly, made the crucial measurements. These include the distance from the extended forefingers to the elbows and from one shoulder to another. The diagnosis is made on the basis of too little distance between the shoulders. The usual symptoms leading people to suspect this problem are weakness, fatigue, and inability to gain weight (classical symptoms of tuberculosis, which is widespread among the Brazilian poor.) Traditional treatments include certain foods believed to be especially nourishing and the application of an *emplastro*, a very broad adhesive tape available in drug stores which may be applied vertically on either side of the sternum. In this instance the Center leader told the *chefe* to "exercise" the patient. The latter in turn directed one of the possessed women to pull the girl's arms behind her. The other medium grasped them and pulled her onto her back. The patient remained in this back to back position, as though stretched upon a rack, for several minutes while the first medium prayed and made passes over her. In later discussion the leader said that the prayer was only a ritual and that the effective treatment was the exercise. Treatment should continue he said, on a daily or weekly basis until the arm and back measurements are equal. As he demonstrated the method of measurement, it was clear that the lengths varied both with the posture of the patient and the points chosen to begin the measurement. When asked about this possible threat to accuracy, however, he discounted it as meaningless.

Ninety minutes after the beginning of the ritual, the few seeking help were dealt with and left the floor. The mediums, the other staff members, and the leader then joined in singing a new set of *pontos* aimed at encouraging the departure of the possessing spirits. (Thus, the leader was actually in the position of commander of the spirits as well as the *Tenda*, since he initiated activities aimed both at calling the spirits down and at sending them away.) As each spirit took its leave, the "horse" or medium just *desincorporado*, uttered a single shout or particularly vigorous grunt, shook his head, appeared dazed, and then gradually refocused on his surroundings as he was evidently freed from the trance. The leader then announced an *intervalo* before the next session, one of *prêto velhos*, began.

During the *intervalo* the leader came to greet the author, saying he was sorry that he hadn't had the opportunity to do so before. Although there had in fact been periodic verbal interchange with him during the first session, the leader indicated that the conversation had been with the *caboclo* spirit which had possessed him (not *Pai Cambina* on this occasion) rather than with himself. He commented that occasional "accidents" did occur in *terreiros* when the spirits did not leave the possessed medium. This had never happened to him because he trains his people carefully. They are early taught how to *desincorporar* as well as *incorporar* the spirits. Learning how to incorporate includes not only the use of *pontos*, dances, cigar smoking, and drinking, all accessory to acquiring the proper receptivity, but also learning the motions appropriate to various spirits. The mediums may move actively about when incorporating *caboclos*, but cannot when possessed by *prêtos velhos*. "Of course," he noted, the spirit has no human form, " . . . it is a source of light, is all brain," and these ritual activities are not really necessary for the sake of the spirits but for "the people who would not be able to understand a spirit without form." The spirits originated the ritual forms necessary for human participants' understanding. They determined that during the *prêto velho* sessions, for example the mediums should crouch, move slowly, and speak with strange cracked voices so that they and the congregation would understand the nature of the spirits possessing them. There are also certain special rules: a menstruating woman cannot "work" with the spirits because she is a *corpo aberto,* a body open to possible injury from harmful spirits of Exus. Even though menstruating, she might become impregnated and the developing egg would be harmed. As a practical matter, pregnant women in his *Tenda* are not allowed to work past the fifth month because since he does not assign assistants to hold those who are possessed they might fall and hurt themselves. He summarized his attitude by saying, "If you read about Umbanda you'll read different things in different books and you'll be confused. This is why I don't recommend that my people read. I teach them myself." He, however, does "a lot of reading . . . about everything." The way in which he later discussed medical and psychological problems, using such words as "erogenous zones," suggested that his reading included clinical psychiatric and medical works.

According to the leader, every human being is a potential medium and is capable of going through the process of development. For some, such development may not be necessary and they can perform their spiritual functions without it. It is during the process of development that the initiate and the leader try to decide together what might be the former's most important task in life and in the *Tenda.* Some such as the two *chefes,* are only possessed once. The man who works as an orderly, for example, is a good administrator and organizer, valuable to the *Tenda* for this as well as for his contacts, via the hospital, with sick people wanting help. A third man, about 40 years old and present at both sessions, although associated with the *Tenda* for 20 years, had never been possessed. He was nevertheless a valuable worker for Umbanda and for the organization. Others who have been possessed repeatedly for many years may lose the capacity without warning. A freshly shaved and barbered white man of middle-class appearance who was standing nearby said he had "worked in Umbanda for over 30 years" but had not received the spirit for 12 years. He could not associate this with any life change.

During this conversation, the other members of the assemblage had been milling about, speaking quietly to each other, and in general behaving like an audience at an intermission. Several stood outside the doors but no one smoked. The assistants were busy moving the benches forward and putting the stools, chairs, water glasses, bowls, and bottles of muscatel in the sand area. The ritual began as on the preceding occasion. The mediums, including the new initiates, became possessed, were helped by the assistants to sit, and were given lighted cigars to smoke. The leader, as before, was more noisily entranced than the others. On this occasion he remained where he fell to the sand and was lifted by two assistants, carried to his stool, and propped onto it with his back against the lower part of the altar. Again he smote himself on the head with the stone, and the consultations began with people's names being called. They were free to choose any guide except the leader, he devoted the entire period to the author who, with Dr. Penna, was now seated barefoot before him, as on the previous occasion. It was possible to note that although the new mediums were available, no one sought their assistance. The chic white woman who had again assumed the *schnauzkrampf* during the early moments of possession, smoked a short briar pipe in lieu of a cigar. Several people in the assemblage remained on the benches until one in the morning, when it finally became possible for them to consult with the leader himself. One or two late comers, upon being told by a white coveralled man at the door of the leader's unavailability that evening, did not remain.

During this consultation session which lasted for about two and a half hours, conversation was more difficult than at the previous encounter because, although the leader was possessed as before by *Pai Cambina,* it was explained that tonight the guide didn't speak very good Portuguese. The speech emerging from the leader was largely that of an uneducated person, with the accent on the wrong letters and syllables; he often substituted r's for l's—*maricia* instead of *malicia.* Two of the assistants, *chefes,* were always present and were sometimes required to translate the broken speech into understandable Portuguese. The leader's request to the author to ask the *chefes* for help if he could not understand meant that the latter were also required to pay special attention to what *Pai Cambina* was saying. Occasionally he would ask one of them, usually with a snap of the finger or a toss of the head, to tell their experience or to describe a case in order to illustrate a point. Once he asked a *filha* to give some information. She was unable to remember it, and he dismissed her with seeming impatience. From time to time he used neologisms which his assistants were able to understand: *gimbo* was used to designate money which in Portuguese is *dinheiro* or *moeda*. This style of speaking is frequently encountered during possession by *prêtos velhos,* and it seemed apparent that *Pai Cambina,* despite his Himalayan origin, was, as suggested by the word *Pai,* functionally related to if not a member of one of the *prêto velho* spirit phalanxes. The discussion during this long consultation was rambling, although much of it inevitably focused on the medical-psychiatric functions of the organization. The leader's wish to have the author "believe," and his repeated requests and demonstrations in this respect were impressive. He was especially interested in persuading the author to investigate a commonly obtainable nut as a cure for cancer. At one point he unbuttoned his coverall and with a seemingly sharp knife stabbed himself in the abdomen. The knife, held at a slant, bounced off, and this was offered as further evidence of the strength of his spirit "protection." He said that he was planning, although he didn't know quite how to accomplish it, to have a photograph taken of himself just before he died in order to show the spirit as it was disincarnated from his body.

ORGANIZATIONAL ASPECTS OF THE *TENDA*

The Center has three functions: guidance and counseling, treatment of illness, and "development" i.e., recruitment and training new members and mediums. In recent years it has begun to hold ceremonies for baptisms and weddings. It has had funerals, but only at the death of a chief. It is gradually becoming able to perform all the conventional functions of any religious organization. The general structure of the organization has already been indicated. Although a Board of Directors is chaired for different periods by one or another of the *chefes de terreiro,* there is little doubt that the leader of the sessions, the "Director of Ritual," and the "incorporator" of the Chief Guide is the dominant figure. He himself is quite aware of this, saying that obedience to him is the first rule of the Center. He can change the schedules regardless of the mediums' preferences, and even though they may feel angry, they cannot show it. During the almost 30 years of the Center's existence here and in its former location in Rio State, 120 mediums have been members. Now there are 15 *sócios* who are mediums, the others presumably having departed because of disagreements with the leader or in order to start their own centers. People are not permitted to attend ceremonies or become *sócios* before the age of 18; any younger and they are considered "unformed," not able to validly decide to "choose Umbanda." Another source of *sócio* turnover is an occasional display of deviant (sexual or aggressive) behavior when *encorporado*. In this case one of the *chefes* takes the member "to a separate place" and talks with the possessing spirit, telling him how people should behave; all explanations are in spiritist, not moral or behavioral terms. A *sócio* or would-be *sócio* is never told not to return, but is given the rules of expected behavior. Usually he stops coming of his own accord, but, problems of this kind are rare.

The leader estimates that there are 15,000 Umbanda *terreiros* in greater Rio de Janeiro, not counting those practicing Macumba or pure *Kardecista* Spiritism. Some have tried to organize into federations and eight or 10 have succeeded, but the threat of losing authority as well as individual differences in ritual have as yet prevented formation of a single strong federation. Police still occasionally visit Umbanda centers and threaten to close them. This is allegedly because some Macumba centers are said to have been centers for narcotic traffic, a possibility regarded as doubtful by informed respondents. There is a police certificate on the wall near the entry way of this *Tenda* dated 1956, licensing it as a legal place of amusement. It has no legal status as a church. The *Tenda* is not really part of the neighborhood; the *sócios* and the staff come from all over the city and have no special attachment to Catumbí. When it was established 15 years ago, the neighborhood people rejected it, fearing the noise of Macumba drumming all night long. They were also afraid the *Tenda* might house delinquents or thieves. Now, however, the *sócios* get an occasional assist from the community. This is partly because, in contrast to some Umbanda centers where there are Quimbanda practices with devils and fire, this one works only for good. And this is due to the leader, personally. It is important for a leader to be beyond reproach. It is also important for his spirit guide to be strong. His guide is very strong, more so than the others, including his wife's.

THE LEADER'S DEVELOPMENT

The leader's father, a Portuguese immigrant, was an atheist and he himself believed in nothing. When he was about seven years old, living in Campo Grande in Rio State, he had a serious illness. His father took him to a *Tenda* where he was not only cured, but where someone predicted that when he became 25 he was going to become a medium. At age 25 he was having economic difficulties, he didn't believe in the rites or the spirits, he thought it was all a joke, but at the suggestion of a friend he went anyway, "just to have a look." At the very first visit he became possessed. When he returned home he reported his experience to his father, and it was only then that he was told of the prediction. Upon reflection, he decided that the *Tenda chefe* had hypnotized him, so as a test, he went back prepared to resist hypnosis. But in spite of the *chefe's* absence on the second occasion he was again possessed, and shortly thereafter his financial fortunes improved. It was because of this that he joined the *Tenda* and became an apprentice of its *chefe*. It was an intellectual not an emotional decision. He had never experienced a revelation or a call to become a leader or medium. Finally the *chefe* died and his wife took over, and the future *Tenda* leader decided to move on, taking some of the *sócios* with him. He went to another *terreiro*, still in Rio State, preparing to join it under the leadership of its *chefe*. That *chefe*, or rather the Chief Guide, the spirit possessing him, however, had recently had a premonition that he would be replaced. Indeed, shortly after coming to the new *terreiro* the new arrival was possessed by a spirit who said, "I [the spirit] am the new Chief Guide of this place." As the leader said, he was not responsible for what descended into him or what it said. This information was duly related to the old *chefe*, who said it was a test. The leader responded by saying, "Raise that box and underneath will be a knife." This was done and repeated seven times, in each instance with the discovery of a knife. It turned out that the old *chefe* had, in fact, hidden the seven knives in the *Tenda*. Then the leader said that if he would look in another secret place there would be a flag of a certain color with a specific design embroidered on it. The flag was there, so the old *chefe* decided to retire in his favor. But after ten years in that location—he could not explain just why, except that the spirit directed him—the leader decided to move to his present location.

He experienced a crisis several years after moving to the city. He had always said that he would leave Umbanda if he ever had a son who was born blind, crippled, or crazy. Then he had a child who was "all of these." When the child was two months old, the doctors said that he would never walk and they could not guarantee his survival. The child then had a grand mal seizure. When his wife reported this to the doctor, he wouldn't believe it, so the parents, feeling hopeless, decided to talk with *Pai Cambina*. (This was done by the wife speaking to the spirit guide through the body of her husband, the leader.) *Pai Cambina* said the child was going to walk and should take phenobarbital. Since this could not be purchased without a prescription, the mother was told to ask the doctor for it. The doctor refused, but then the child had a seizure in his office, so, although the doctor said that he was too young, he gave it to him anyway. (This was regarded as a consequence of the spirit's influence on the doctor.) *Pai Cambina* also prescribed exercises so that when the child was 18 months old he began to walk. The phenobarbital was stopped after two years. The child is now seven years of age in a special school. His vision is poor, but he is not blind. He cannot read or write, but he does walk and talk. This experience has strengthened the leader's faith.

PSYCHIATRIC-MEDICAL FUNCTIONS OF THE *TENDA*

The leader said that mental illness, physical illness, and spiritual illness are all the same—all have their roots in the spirit. He estimated that the Center (i.e., the spirit guides of the mediums) handled about a hundred consultations monthly for difficulties which might be classified by physicians as illness, and that perhaps 40 per cent of the help-seekers at any given session are repeaters. The majority come to him personally. The total attendance at the *Tenda*, counting all of the sessions, is probably between 300 and 400 visits monthly, but no figures or other exact data are kept. Nor could he estimate his rate of success. Some people, he said, really don't want to get well. These are the most resistant. Others really have nothing wrong with them, although they believe they do. To those who really have nothing wrong he gives "suggestion", he uses the influence of personal authority. There was the case of a man who was *pondo sangue pela boca,* "putting blood out from the mouth," a common diagnosis to which there seemed to be no need to add further details. The patient was bedridden, but there was some question about whether he really did have blood coming from the mouth. *Pai Cambina* came down and said to the patient (through the leader), "You don't have anything. How old are you?" The patient answered, and *Pai Cambina* said, "Now I'm going to tell you the story of your life." He then gave the actual facts of his life until the age of 40, at which point the patient said, "Stop. I'm convinced that I don't have anything." This meant to the leader that the patient wished to keep *Pai Cambina* from talking further, from revealing something about his life after age 40 which he wanted hidden and which had resulted in his malingering. This interview had been in the patient's home. When people are bedridden the leader and sometimes all the mediums may go to their homes to perform the rites, determine what is wrong, and try to set it right. Sometimes these visits, made on request, are to other cities and even to other states of Brazil.

The leader estimated that about 40 per cent of the *Tenda* case load consisted of marital problems. About two-thirds of the marital problems center on sex. Frequently the woman will not reach an orgasm, "because man is one kind of animal and woman another . . . man is too fast." The people wouldn't "know anything," and he would instruct them, tell the man to "go slow." Sometimes he must use rough language to make his point and tells the man, "You son of a bitch, don't you know what you are doing?" Sometimes he will see one of the couple, sometimes both together or each individually. Often only one of the marital partners will come for help. He rarely encounters impotence, but does occasionally deal with homosexuality (only in males). He explained (and was obviously lecturing at the same time to three of the male assistants who were standing nearby) that there are three types of homosexuals: the congenital, who might have endocrine problems; boys who have been too close to their male friends and because of lack of guidance do not later transfer their interest to women; and a third category, "not really homosexual," who have had a problem with a woman—she traumatized him and left and then he became homosexual. Sometimes, he said, "stimulation of the erogenous zones such as the buttocks" might lead a boy to homosexuality. Most often these people have accepted their homosexuality and consult him for something else. Occasionally parents of adolescent boys may come seeking sexual guidance for their sons. Other problems in the marital category may be a consequence of physical illness in one partner.

A second category of cases includes people with "sentimental" problems. These mainly concern relations between fiancees or romantic attachments, including the problems of unrequited love. Another important category is alcoholics. He produces good results in 80 per cent of the cases who come to him. They are forced to drink salted wine for eight days, after which they have no more interest in alcohol. Adolescents make up another group of cases, although there are not too many of them. Most are boys in conflict with their fathers, and usually the parents come seeking help. It is sometimes difficult to get the boy to come. The occasional girl is more amenable. He prefers not to see parent and child together, but first one and then the other. He feels that each generation differs from the one before it, that they have different needs, and that conflicts will naturally and inevitably arise between them. He has organized a rock and roll band associated with the *Tenda* which includes his children and those of friends. (His 17-year-old son, a member of the band, appeared after midnight in order to accompany his parents home.) They use the *Tenda* as their headquarters. This has no religious meaning, but he did give them some *pontos* which they might convert into "pagan music," as he called the "ye, ye, ye" of rock and roll. "If you don't help young people to do something useful, they may become criminal. Music is one way to discharge energy." He may see an occasional mother or father whose child is stealing, but this is rare.

An important category includes physical illness, especially congenital problems or those of obscure etiology for which conventional medicine has no answer, or where the Spiritist intervention may result in more effective work by physicians. A little girl had some type of walking difficulty, for example, and her parents took her to an orthopedist who said that she had a residual of poliomyelitis. This upset them very much so they consulted *Pai Cambina*. He said, no, your child does not have poliomyelitis, and recommended a pediatrician, giving his name and address. They consulted the pediatrician who said that she had flat feet for which he successfully prescribed exercise and special shoes. Another child was going to have surgery which the doctor had explained was hazardous. The father, a Catholic, was very upset and discussed the matter with the child's godfather, an *Umbandista*. The latter came to consult *Pai Cambina*, who told him to go ahead and let the child be operated on and everything would be all right. The surgery was accomplished without problems, the child recovered rapidly, and the grateful father brought flowers to the *Tenda*. A patient was not doing well with medical treatment. He consulted *Pai Cambina* who thought he should take a certain medicine, but didn't tell that to the patient. He advised the patient only to go back to the doctor, saying, "I will influence the doctor." When the patient returned, the doctor opened his medicine cabinet and chose exactly the drug which *Pai Cambina* thought the patient had needed. (When the grateful patient came back to report that he had improved with the new medicine, he was confirmed in the belief that this was, indeed, the result of the spirit's influence upon the doctor.) A more dramatic case was that of a girl with congenital heart disease ("she had some kind of a hole in her heart, she was blue"). It was decided that hazardous reparative surgery should be done. The father, worried about the outcome of the operation to be done the next morning at 9 o'clock, came the night before to consult *Pai Cambina*. *Pai Cambina* told him to let the operation proceed, that he would try to help. Then he asked all the mediums to work with him to help get a special spirit to descend, that of an Arabian physician who had died almost two thousand years earlier, so that he might guide the surgeon's hands. Somehow the message got through that the spirit could not descend until 11 o'clock the next morning, two hours after the scheduled start of the operation. This was disturbing, but *Pai Cambina* didn't tell the father. He asked only that at 11 o'clock the next morning all the mediums (who would be engaged in their usual non-*Tenda* activities) should "think of this child as being their own." This formed a *corrente de Umbanda* (a chain or current, joining forces for a common purpose). At that time, the leader "received a message" or had a premonition that the surgeon would find a defect differing from that which had been diagnosed. Later they discovered that the operation had not, in fact, taken place until 11 o'clock, that a different defect had, indeed, been discovered, and that the operation had gone smoothly. In a week the girl was "outside playing." Everyone attributed the surgeon's success to the guidance he had received from the Arabian spirit. The grateful father joined the *Tenda* and was now in an early phase of development. A tall white man with an intelligent manner, who had not yet experienced possession, he was there to corroborate the leader's story.

CENTRO ESPIRITA CAMINHEIROS DA VERDADE—
ORGANIZATIONAL ASPECTS

This name is translatable as Walkers of Truth, although the usual Portuguese for walker is *caminhador.* The general connotation of travelers, seekers, or pilgrims may be assumed. The word is not completely familiar, though, and is occasionally misunderstood and misprinted, as in the case of the newspaper announcement listed above calling it *Companheiros,* i.e., companions, fellows, or friends of truth. Discussion with members of the Center staff suggests that the suffix *heiros* does indeed imply friendship or fellowship among the "walkers."

This Center with almost 10,000 members is probably the largest in Rio de Janeiro. Like other large Spiritist groups, it is in the North Zone. Located in Engenho de Dentro, one of the peripheral ring of urban districts, near its border with Cachambí, it may be reached by bus involving several changes, or by taxi, which requires approximately 45 minutes from the city center. This is a mixed neighborhood with many factories and homes of *operários* and *funcionários,* mainly separate small houses with an occasional multiple dwelling. The building is five stories high, the largest and most impressive on its narrow street, and the only one not a residence. At the second-story level a sign about two-feet high bearing its name, extends across its entire front. Information during a daytime visit in September 1968 was supplied by two informants. One was the Director of Mediums, who also referred to herself as *chefe do terreiro,* a short, stocky, white woman in her early fifties, poised, pleasant, and authoritative, she conducted the writer and Dr. Penna on a tour of the premises. She had been associated with the group since its inception and quite matter of factly noted there are always visitors, that they consider publicity to be good for them, and that films have been made of some of their activities by German, French, Japanese, and other foreigners. They had been the subject of a local television show in the early summer of 1968. The other informant, was a retired military officer, white, about 50-years-old, who, upon the invitation of the Center's Board of Directors (elected by all members for three-year terms) had been invited to organize the secretariat. He thought he would probably become a member of the next Board and could give it much time since he had a private income and didn't work (he was pale, with clubbed fingers, and appeared emphysematous). He was not a medium and had never belonged to a Spiritist organization before. A friend of one of the Board members suggested that he be invited because he lives nearby and would like to do something useful with his time. There is no salary for this work. The central figure of the organization is its President, who also bears the title of Spiritual Director. He is the only person actually residing in the Center aside from the directoress and the girls of the home for orphans contained in the building. He is a high-ranking retired military officer, white, unmarried at 64, whose "whole life is devoted" to the place. (The newspaper announcement described the Center as "under the command of brother Joaõ Carneiro.") He founded the organization 31 years ago, had the building erected, is president for life, and most of his income goes into the Center.

The building was constructed 16 years ago by the members themselves who were stonemasons, carpenters, plumbers, and so on. Those with no specialty mixed cement and carried bricks. The women fed the workers, contributing both food and time. Most of the present members, exactly 9,791 at the time of the visit, contribute small amounts to the Center on a monthly basis. Many are very poor, but there are well-educated people, engineers and lawyers among them. Although most are from Guanabara and close enough for relatively easy access, some live in São Paulo and even Rio Grande do Sul. These last do not participate actively but make regular contributions. A very few contribute up to the equivalent of $25 or $30 monthly; for most, the contribution is from a few pennies to a few dollars. The Center depends on material gifts wherever possible. The orphanage receives milk through the Alliance for Progress and there are periodic campaigns during which larger contributions are solicited. The Board determines the use of the money. Some goes for construction of the new orphanage being built for 800 children.

Among the *sócios* there are 1,800 mediums, including approximately 1,200 women and 600 men. The period of development is long. As beginners they remain for two or three years in the group called *"esoterismo"* during which time development continues, including consultation with the *caboclo* Tira Teima, spirit guide of the *terreiro chefe* and Director of Mediums. Promotion is determined by the Director (by her spirit guide) as the one in whom authority concerning matters of this kind is vested. She occupies the position equivalent to *mãe-de-santo* in the Afro-Brazilian Centers, although she did not use the term. Perhaps the most striking feature of the organization is its ecumenism. Although *caboclos* clearly predominate among the spirit guides, the building contains an area for the practice of pure Kardecism, with the participants sitting around a table; it has another room labeled Umbanda; and a special suite called the *Fonte de Siloé* (Fountain or Source of Siloé). It was not possible to determine if Siloé refers to a spirit or to Shiloh, a biblical town of the Ephraimites where the sanctuary of the Ark was once kept. Everywhere are crucifixes and large images of the Virgin and Catholic saints.

An auditorium with a capacity for 700 people occupies most of the first floor. The building also houses a theater area and a gallery for children, fitted with folding seats. In addition to special consulting rooms, the upper floors include dining rooms for adults and children and the orphanage. There is a physician's office in which a free outpatient clinic manned by two volunteers (who accept token payment for services) is operated for two to three hours, three days a week. Dental work, confined mainly to extractions and providing dentures, and routine medical consultations are available. Members pay for all the materials and half the professional fee; the Center pays the other half of the modest expenses. The orphanage accommodates 120 girls and includes sleeping quarters, a kitchen and dining room, storage areas, a classroom, play areas, and an infirmary staffed by a volunteer nurse. Located on the top two floors, it is clean, light, and airy, and the numerous women, all volunteer workers, appear to relate to the girls in a warm, supportive, cheerful way. The workers are predominantly white. There were several mulatto children and one black child visible. The younger ones are taught to read and write on the premises, after which they are enrolled in public school. Most are prepubescent, but a few are in secondary school, and a still smaller number are scattered in special courses throughout the city. Some, for example, attend the *Instituto Brasil Estados Unidos* in Copacabana to study English. Where tuition is required the Center has been successful in obtaining scholarships.

The members of the Center are concerned with the problems of justice and suffering, and an orphan epitomizes injustice. Why should a child have so much suffering? This is part of the general motivation of Spiritist groups for social action. The new home now under construction (to accommodate 400 girls and 400 boys) is named after a familiar Catholic saint so as not to exclude non-Spiritists, since religious discrimination of any kind is regarded as bad. This new home is a major feature of the July issue of *O Caminheiro*, the official newspaper of the Center which is published on an irregular basis. Work on the building appears to be progressing slowly although its financial basis seems to be becoming established in a systematic manner. The entire back page of the paper was devoted to an advertisement by a nonprofit auto-financing fund announcing that all profits on automobiles and trucks bought through the fund go to the construction project.

PSYCHIATRIC-MEDICAL FUNCTIONS OF CAMINHEIROS DA VERDADE

The main source of "clients" is a regular weekly session open to all comers without prior appointment. Beginning at about three in the afternoon on Thursdays and sometimes lasting until well past midnight, people come for personal consultation. Some go directly to rooms where particular mediums with their spirit guides can be seen. Others who don't feel that they know the nature of their problem consult the *caboclo* of the *chefe do terreiro*. The spirit, speaking through the *chefe*, tells them whether to seek a conventional medical specialist or directs them for further Spiritist consultation within the building. The great majority are not considered suitable for outside referral and are sent to the *Fonte de Siloé*.

The *Fonte de Siloé* has three rooms in which it accomplishes its aims through "chromotherapy and music therapy for all those with disturbances *de carater psiquico*." One room done completely in red is designed to produce a "negative shock" in order to "counteract negative aspects of the nervous system so the two shocks will annul each other." Another room has stations with lights of different colors. The client walks very slowly past and around the lights in a predetermined manner and, according to expectation, falls asleep for a time at the third light. A long "operating room" with highly polished floors, rich hangings, and statues of saints illuminated with colored lights, along the walls has 30 white pillows and sheets arranged neatly in rows on the floor. People come to lie on these for "spirit-operations" on their peptic ulcers, malfunctioning gall bladders, and other "diseased organs." Later they return for aftercare, *curativos*. Two or three hundred people were said to come to the *Fonte* each week. Three or four sleep sessions once a week in the chromotherapy rooms were said to effect a cure in most instances. The major disorder was reported as "depression and melancholia. They cry, their mood is low, they don't want to go out of the house." The "operating room" functions once weekly with two weekly *curativos*, for people with somatic complaints. Additional rooms in the Center are for other treatment modalities, especially the establishment of a *corrente*, i.e., holding hands around a table so that spirit vibrations might improve the depressed person. One of the most impressive is labeled *Estrêla do Oriente* (Star of the East.) It has rich hangings, upholstered furniture, tables set with water glasses in special patterns, and complex designs painted on the polished floor. It serves as a meditation room in which people communicating with spirits of the *Linha do Oriente* might gain strength.

Occasionally a noisily disturbed psychotic person appears on the scene. An agitated 17-year-old girl arrived in an ambulance, en route from the nearby Pronto Socorro to the chronic hospital,

Juliano Moreira in Jacarepaguá. The driver and the girl's parents had together decided to stop at the Center and ask the President to see her. He assented, told her parents to remove the cuffs which bound her, and walked with her into the auditorium where a session was in progress. They sat together in the front row where she prayed and sang. Later he took her to one of the upstairs rooms and "worked" with her until 1:30 A.M. She left with her parents, "cured".

A SESSION AT CAMINHEIROS DA VERDADE

The regular schedule carried announcements of eight *sessoẽs* weekly, in addition to *trabalhos especiais* (special works) in the smaller areas and consulting rooms as previously noted, and *trabalhos de mesa* or *Kardecista* sessions around the table. Two were under the personal direction of the President and Spiritual Director. Others were led by different *caboclos* and *chefes da secão* (one of whom was the *chefe do terreiro*.) A visit was made on a Friday night when the session would be led by the Spiritual Director himself. The taxi driver decided that it would be easiest to find the place in the dark, coming from Ipanema, by proceeding straight out the *Tunel* Novo toward the highway on the edge of town, and then turning back in at the Bom Sucesso exit. Arriving in Cachambi where he had once lived, however, he was unable to find the proper street without stopping at a lighted storefront for directions. The Center proved to be well known and nearby. The street was dark, but fluorescent lights on the front porch of the building cast a pale glow over the sidewalk. Three little mulatto girls in white shirts and short navy blue skirts stood at the door selling chances on a radio raffle at the equivalent of about 25 cents each to benefit the orphanage.

In the daylight the main auditorium had looked somewhat like a large, bare church. At night the resemblance was less notable; specific features were emphasized by the liberal use of fluorescent lighting tubes. A raised stage about 50 feet across and 30 feet deep extended the entire width of the room in front of the seats, except for space occupied by two shrines at either side with their interior lights just visible behind thick beaded curtains. One shrine contained figures of far Eastern sages, and in a facing

alcove was a seated statue of Confucius reading a manuscript. In
a similar alcove on the other side was a mounted St. George slay-
ing a dragon. An altar was centered against the two-story high
wall at the end of the room behind the stage. This was a simple
brown wooden cabinet topped by a painting of the Holy Family.
Above the altar was a large white neon cross, at the center of
which in red neon tubing were the letters JNRJ (*Jesus Nosso
Redentor Jesus*). To the left, red neon letters spelled out "He who
gives grace will receive it." In blue, at the center above the cross,
was the admonition, "Love one another", and right of it in green,
"Without charity there is no salvation." Below the lettering a
large lithograph of an American Indian (representing a *caboclo*
spirit) and a photograph of Allan Kardec were surrounded by
frames set with ordinary incandescent bulbs. On another wall
hung two more lithographs of similar Indians, one with colored
flashing lights around the frame, and a large handsomely
mounted photograph of the founder, President, and Spiritual
Director. Artificial flowers were in abundance—bouquets under
the lithographs and photographs, artificial white lilies of the valley attached to the posts of the railing separating the stage from
the rest of the auditorium.

The audience occupied only a fraction of the auditorium.
There were perhaps 35 people scattered throughout the seats,
women to the left and men to the right. Several women had small
children with them, and they talked with each other and walked
freely in and out during the ceremony. Other people entered from
time to time, walking down the side aisles to the shrines where
they meditated a moment, in some cases appeared to make the
sign of the cross, and departed. A slight mulatto woman of about
30 with uncombed hair wandered about the auditorium trying
with indifferent success to sell copies of *O Caminheiro*. She occasionally danced and twirled about to the music and often sang
along with the *pontos*. The audience appeared bored most of the
time, occasionally talking among themselves. They were predominantly mulatto, and all were poorly dressed. One or two elderly
men sitting alone dozed. There was no sense of congregation as
there had been in the *Tenda*. The only participation was during
a prayer about 30 minutes after the onset of the ceremony when
every one present was requested to stand.

The ceremony began with smoking censors. There was, however, no movement of the censor-bearers among the seated observers and none of the dramatic kneeling and prostration seen at the *Tenda*. Men gradually filed onto the stage until about 45 were present in two circles, an inner one of about 12 and an outer of about 33. Approximately two-thirds were white, four were black, and the rest mulatto. All wore white smocks of the kind associated with dentists in the United States, white trousers, and white tennis shoes. They held hands in a chain with arms crossed, and periodically more men would come onto the stage and join the inner circle. After several minutes of singing, as they began to shuffle in rhythm, one by one the clasped hands were dropped. First one, then several began to twitch and grunt and seemed to be entering the trance state. It was at this point that the proceedings were interrupted by prayers to Jesus and Mary. (Spiritist prayers are available in a number of publications by Serrana [1967] and others.) Following the prayer the singing became more rapid, the circle disintegrated completely, and the men began to dance as individuals with perhaps half obviously possessed, the others standing to the congregation's right, singing and only shuffling. Some of the singers and all of the dancers, excepting two or three with pipes, lit cigars which they puffed as they moved. No *cachaça* or wine was used. The dancing was highly individual, much freer than that in the *Tenda*, sometimes whirling and pirouetting, sometimes with a samba-like shuffle. When each song stopped the dancers stopped abrutly, only to begin again after the moment's silence. No drums or instruments were employed, but as time went on they began clapping their hands with great impact, the singing and dancing increased in tempo, and several uttered shrill cries, dropping to their knees. This had an apparently contagious effect for those nearest the man who fell would do likewise. Many squatted and walked bent double in the manner of the *prêtos velhos*. Some were instructing or helping others. Many made passes toward each other and snapped their fingers. Some waved green branches around their own heads and those of others. There was much posturing, almost catatonic in appearance, as the dancers represented the activities of particular spirit guides. Finally, after almost two hours, when a tremendous peak of activity and noise had been reached, with men in individual trances all over the stage and only a small nucleus of four or five remaining upright and singing, a signal was given by the leader, and all knelt wherever they happened to be. Another prayer, different from the first but also invoking God, Jesus and Mary, terminated this phase. The second and final phase of the ceremony devoted to *desenvolvimento* was a lecture. Two leaders stood while everyone else sat on the floor and discussed the art of mediumship and the importance of solicitude and personal virtue in attaining *mediunidade*.

A KARDECISTA GROUP—THE CRUZADA MILITAR

This private group, known as the Military Crusade, is confined to army officers and their families. It is led by a retired general in his sixties who became interested in Spiritism after having seen an apparition, "a bride" (apparently the Virgin Mary), about 15 years earlier. Other people present were said to have touched the "bride's" clothing. Characteristically, the person who arranged for the writer to visit the group did so only after considerable hesitation, not wishing to be thought a believer himself. He emphasized that he had not been present at the time of the apparition, but that the general—who now claimed to have passed through a minimum of 15 incarnations—was considered a reliable observer. He was held in sufficiently high esteem to have been asked to organize and be the leader of this group.

The session was held on a weekday afternoon in an old building in the Lapa district, one of the most deteriorated in the central city area. From the outside it looked like a warehouse with no identifying mark. At the first landing, after a flight of dusty wooden stairs, were several announcements, yellowed with age, which indicated the building had been used on a regular basis by several Spiritist groups. The general himself was waiting to offer his greetings at the top of the stairs. He regarded the visit of a psychiatrist, his first such encounter, as an opportunity for proselytizing, and spoke at great length about magnetism, the personal force which allows one person to communicate with another, and the importance of not confusing Spiritism with spiritualism. Much of what he said in this respect was reminiscent of the early writings of Anton Mesmer. He also sketched his general understanding of the view that the universe is inhabited by spirits in various stages of development and that in order to achieve increasing perfection they require contact with each other and with living human beings. There may thus be an influence of humans on spirits as well as the other way around. During sessions, mediums both become developed and help to develop the spirits as they call them down in order to be incorporated.

The meeting was held in a long narrow hall with a small stage at the end. The left wall carried a sign, "Men" and the right "Women," but the people present paid no attention to it. A portrait of Allan Kardec hung on one wall; a permanently fixed sign saying, "When you pray to God you are deepening and strengthening your spirit," on another. The general stood at the head of a long table on the stage and called people from the floor, one by one, to join him there. Sixteen came. Fourteen were women ranging in age from their early twenties to their late fifties, uniformly well dressed and of the middle or upper class. Two young men in their twenties, apparently junior officers, were dressed in sports clothes. Ten people remained in the audience, including two adolescents—children of one of the women at the table—and an elderly man, a retired general who years before had had a psychotic episode while serving in the Amazon region. The major content of the episode had revolved around bewitchment by Indian spirits, and after recovering he had become an ardent Spiritist. Before beginning the session the general introduced the writer and Dr. Penna as two physicians (not psychiatrists) who were studying Spiritism and had them sit near the stage so they could easily hear what occurred. He introduced each person around the table in terms of his special function as a medium: an incorporator, a seer, an automatic writer, and so on. Most were incorporators. He drew the shutters and had the lights turned off except for a single large dull white globe over the table. The people seated around the table clasped hands, and the general began with the Spiritist Prayer of Charity, invoking in its opening lines "God, our Father, who is all Power and Kindness" to give the supplicants the strength to deal with provocation, the light with which to find truth, and to put compassion and charity in their hearts. He went on with several other prayers, standing, his eyes closed all the while, until he was interrupted by a sudden break in his voice, a sharp inspiration and a noisy grunting expiration. The people at the table suddenly began to make passes with their right hands over their heads, snapping their fingers while waving their left hands back and forth by their left ears. They were bringing the spirits down. After perhaps 30 seconds, several made grunting noises and became rigid. Throughout, the general, obviously in command of the session, did most of the talking addressing himself to both the mediums and the spirits. Two of the women were clearly dominant in terms of the time they spent speaking and the emotion they expressed. They initiated the incorporated phase by alternately talking and weeping, interspersing this with occasional shrieks about seeing visions of hungry children. One spoke at length in a style which would probably have been impossible for her in the waking state because of its antigovernment connotations. She said she possessed great power over the masses which was going to be used to change the government and its military rulers. Finally, as her weeping began to seem out of control the general stood behind her, placed his left hand on her forehead, his right on the back of her neck, and said a prayer which appeared to calm her. He did this to others on four different occasions during the ninety minute session. Later he said that this was in order to keep the spirits from totally dominating the medium, from overpowering her, which would have interfered with the development of both spirit and medium. He also said that laying on hands in this way "reduced excitation in the hypothalamus."

Spiritists often regard physicians as doubters so it did not come as a surprise when, midway in the session, the woman who had first spoken began to attack the observers. Her main theme was they were not real doctors, because in order to know anything they required x-rays and blood tests; they were not concerned with peoples' souls. They were there looking for something in the guise of doctors. The general spoke to her sharply from across the table, saying that she should not be criticizing others but should look into herself (he was, technically, speaking to the spirit incorporated by the medium, not to the woman herself.) Later she incorporated a second spirit, that of a proud and arrogant person who descended as a kind of penance in the form of a *prêto velho* (i.e., one spirit acted as though it were another kind of spirit), speaking humbly and suggesting that doctors can help people and are worthwhile. The interchange of spirits was confusing at times, with a passage back and forth between mediums at the table and two spirits above waiting for a clear call as to which person they should descend into. One of the young men was silent throughout; the other erupted only once to say repeatedly "Very good, very good!" As people began to calm down, the general looked around the table as though to make sure that no one else wanted to speak. He then said a final prayer, gave an expiratory grunt, all participants snapped their fingers and made the passes again as the spirits left them, and the lights were turned on.

Afterwards there was an opportunity for conversation with the participants. Two of the women said that while they were at the table something came from deep inside them, shutting everything else out. One said she heard voices in her ear. The dominant one said that she always had visions when sitting at the table. None who came were there because of specific problems they wanted solved. About half were unable to recall the events of the session.

HOSPITAL ESPIRITA PEDRO DE ALCANTARA

A few of the approximately 14,000 physicians in Rio regularly advertise themselves as Spiritist in the press. Typically, an announcement might read, *"Medico Espirita"* (Spiritist physician) and indicate that the doctor engages in treatment both of the body and of the spirit, *"tratamento do corpo e do espirito."* The only Spiritist hospital of any kind in Rio is this one named after Peter the Second and operated by the *Associação Espirita Obreiros do Bem* (Spiritist Association of Workers of Good). It is a 90-bed psychiatric hospital for women located at the end of a quiet side street on the slope of a hill in one of the peripheral urban districts. Since the association does not have enough money to completely support the service, it admits patients referred by any doctor, who then has the privilege of caring for them, but the large majority are the patients of the physicians who work there. Most are paid for on contract by the national social security system, but a few are private. If the Association becomes wealthy enough it would like the hospital to be totally free and to conduct Spiritist sessions as does the Itapira hospital in São Paulo state. (These sessions are completely separate from the medical treatment.) The building itself, though old, is well-maintained and reasonably pleasant.

The staff includes three psychiatrists, an internist, and six, fifth-and sixth-year medical students, who obtain jobs there independently and receive no school credit for it. All the physicians, each of whom devotes approximately three hours daily to the hospital, have private offices and consult elsewhere as well. Two of the psychiatrists were present to receive the writer and Dr. Penna, arrangements having been made through a relative of one of the students. The doctors are not Spiritists, but are clearly sympathetic and believe that the phenomena deserve scientific study. (One, who had a personal interest in parapsychology, said he was more of a spiritualist that a Spiritist.) It is also necessary for them to allow the Spiritists to be involved in some respects. The Association must give its consent for any patient to be admitted free of charge. First the doctor, having seen the disturbed person in the Outpatient Clinic, must decide that hospitalization is indicated. Once he has made this decision, if the patient cannot pay or is not covered by social security, he must consult with one of the Spiritist mediums, i.e., the medium's *caboclo* guide. In addition, several may make a *corrente* and await spirit advice as to whether the patient should be admitted without charge. The *chefes do terreiro* have no interest in learning anything about medicine or psychiatry and in fact seem actually to ignore the possibility. No thought has been given to the possibility of arranging seminars or teaching sessions for them inasmuch as this kind of learning appears antithetical to their philosophy. Patients who have attended Spiritist sessions in the past often behave during their illness as though they are incorporated. The mediums themselves explain deviant behavior as reflecting an *obsessão* (literally, obsession or harassment) or the state of being *obsesso* (obsessed or haunted); this refers to the effect of a spirit being constantly close to a person, similar to being *encosto*. Or they explain the problem as due to a *trabalho* or a *coisa feita*.

The doctors noted that people who are already disturbed may become worse after attending a center. One such person went to a Macumba *terreiro* where he said that he had incorporated the *caboclo Pena Azul* (Blue Feather). Under the *caboclo's* influence he went home and broke the television set, resulting in his hospital admission. Nonetheless, they feel that patients who are Spiritists improve more rapidly here than in other hospitals because it is a supportive environment. All the patients know this is a Spiritist hospital, and if one wishes to attend the next door center while he is hospitalized, and if the family give permission, it is considered acceptable so long as the patient doesn't disrupt the ceremonies. A standard permission form is used which must be signed with the name and relationship of the responsible relative: "As the responsible relative of this patient I request permission for him to attend the Spiritist sessions of *'Obreiros do Bem'* if there are no medical contraindications." The relative also promises to escort the patient back and forth from the session. Originally there were joint sessions for patients and the public together. Now they are separate and, even so, permission is not given to those who are hypertensive, receiving insulin, agitated, or very depressed. The *chefe de terreiro* requires assurance that patients are functioning reasonably well before they come to a session. One of the psychiatrists and the internist, who is himself a Spiritist, often attend along with the patients. During a session the patient may talk with the spirit guide through the medium. A medium may also receive or incorporate the spirit which has been obsessing or harming the patient. When this happens, when the medium becomes the "horse" of the obsessing spirit, he, the horse, may reproduce some of the patient's behavior. The spirit guide explains things in Spiritist terms and almost never regards deviance as reflecting illness unless there is an obvious organic basis for it. Sometimes if a chronic schizophrenic appears at hospital for whom nothing can be done, the psychiatrists may, in a somewhat sarcastic vein, refer him to the Center. According to the doctors, nothing therapeutic is ever accomplished with such patients through consultation with the guides; even when less chronically disturbed patients do, as occasionally happens, benefit after sessions, there is no way of knowing what really caused the improvement because so many treatments have already been given. They would like to try the effect of Spiritist consultation on the patients without having already given them drugs, but it seems difficult to arrange. All patients receive drugs, mainly tranquillizers and energizers, from the first day of admission. ECT as well as insulin are administered, but fear of ECT among the patients is a significant problem. No patient receives formal psychotherapy although they are free to discuss specific issues with the doctors as they arise. The proportion of patients who are Spiritist is not known. Most would identify themselves as Catholic, in any case, and others would say that Spiritism is not a religion but a philosophy. None are Protestant or Jewish. Many of those with illness who attend the center have first had repeated visits to doctors without relief. For example, a woman suffering from back pain went to a session and was informed by the guide that she had a problem in her spinal column. She then consulted an orthopedist who diagnosed something else. Not long thereafter she did, in fact, develop a spinal problem. It was then that her husband, an engineer, began to believe in spirits.

CLINICAL PSYCHIATRIC ASPECTS OF SPIRITISM, UMBANDA, AND MACUMBA

Participants in the sessions of *centros espiritas* or *terreiros* seem to fall into two general categories. First are those who regularly attend, the majority of whom evidently derive much social support from participation in the life of their particular centers and construct personal communities around them. Those who become mediums may well, as Camargo (1961) indicated, find some compensation for their humble daytime lives as at night they become "transformed" into vehicles for "sublime messages." The sense of personal power, meaningfulness, and belonging so obtained can conceivably have preventive value, reducing vulnerability to disabling psychiatric illness. The opportunity to periodically relinquish one's hold on reality under controlled conditions may also afford prophylaxis against a major irretrievable break. This issue has not, however, been systematically investigated, and it is equally plausible to suggest that regular participation in ceremonies focusing on the supernatural may weaken a person's hold on reality and make him more vulnerable to psychotic or at least dissociative episodes which will interfere with adaptation.

Among the regular attendants there are undoubtedly a number who are chronically but quietly psychotic or severely neurotic and the support obtained from regular attendance probably facilitates their ability to survive outside of mental hospitals. No systematic study has been made, but one knowledgeable psychiatrist estimates that at least 10 to 20 per cent of the regular *frequentadores* have diagnosable psychiatric illness. Personal observation suggests that investigation would not show the staff and leaders of established centers to be psychotic or seriously neurotic and might well show that their high intelligence and superior organizational ability would counteract the possible maladaptive consequences of psychiatric illness.

The second category of participants includes those who attend only occasionally or do so under the stress of current physical or social-psychological problems. Many have been to physicians without being helped, while for others, the visit to a *terreiro* or center is the first step on the path which finally brings them to a medical institution. As noted previously, the Director of the Center for Studies of the Casa Eiras Hospital estimated that over 50 per cent of his private patients have been to *terreiros* or Spiritist centers before consulting him, and that this is true of perhaps 90 per cent of the less educated and affluent whose care is supported by charity or the social security system. Many of the occasional visitors, who while not subscribing to the faith are desperately searching for help, are quite ready to believe if the wished-for miracle occurs. Most are referred by friends or neighbors who have their favorite *terreiros* and their stories about someone whose cancer was improved or whose child was saved by the spirit guide. The incidence of physical and psychiatric illness is probably higher in this group than in the first.

As suggested by the foregoing descriptions of particular centers, there is a considerable overlap between groups in their systems of diagnosis and treatment. Depending upon the individual center, mental or emotional discomfort, situational difficulties, and sometimes organic malfunction are attributed, to: (1) acts of black magic, when someone has done a *trabalho* against the victim or caused a *coisa feita*, (2) failure to fulfill an "obligation" to an *orixá* which may result in retaliative punishment by the offended divinity and, (3) failure to develop one's latent capacities as a medium which may be followed by a number of consequences, e.g., the person may be *encosto* by a spirit which wishes incarnation or incorporation but cannot achieve it because the person's *mediunidade* is not sufficiently developed.

Treatment includes counseling, specific "spirit operations," a variety of undoing rituals, and participating in ceremonies of *de-*

senvolvimento. The effect of the milieu and the social support and catharsis it offers is self-evident, but not explicitly identified by most center practitioners. Most Macumba and Umbanda healers, (i.e., their spirit guides) recommend medicinal plants from time to time and even write prescriptions which can be filled in special stores. Each district has at least one such shop, and there are several in Copacabana and Ipanema. They stock everything necessary for rituals, sometimes including materials and books used by Kardec Spiritists as well. In some small interior towns pharmacists fill ordinary prescriptions written by Spiritists.

HISTORICAL PSYCHIATRIC VIEWS OF SPIRITISM IN RELATION
TO BEHAVIORAL DISTURBANCE IN BRAZIL

The first scientific reference to the problem in Brazil was a report published in Paris by Rodrigues (1901) about an episode occurring in 1885. A lawyer and his family, in Taubate in São Paulo state, began at dawn on the 13th of October in that year, following a three days long Spiritist session, to celebrate a ceremony which they called "the construction of Noah's ark" in preparation for a world catastrophe. They paraded, singing, to the town square, where they were joined "both by slaves and people of good family." The women were described as half-dressed and disheveled; many had not eaten for three days, and their accompanying children "looked like corpses." One person who seemed resigned to his fate and knew what was going to happen was sacrificed and his blood drunk by the group. Others were tortured and beaten to force evil spirits out of their bodies. Finally, the rituals were stopped by aroused onlookers, some of the participants were placed in a hospital and others in prison where, agitated and "maniacal," they destroyed part of the prison wall. Although this episode was described as a "collective psychosis" beginning "during a Spiritist session," it appears to have had much in common with some of the extreme behavior associated with messianic movements, the belief in witchcraft and possession by the devil, so much a part of folk Catholicism.

Another episode occurring in Campina Grande in the state of Paraiba, probably around 1920, was also described by an unidentified author as a case of collective psychosis (*Brasil-*

Medico, 1923). A woman with some psychiatric symptoms was said by a local cultist to be possessed by a bad spirit. Cure required, he said, that she be transformed into a toad, which should then be killed; resurrection in the healthy state would occur within 24 hours. At nightfall, members of the family beat the patient to death believing that they were killing the toad. When resurrection did not occur after several days, they finally threw the mutilated body on a garbage dump.

A major figure in this field was Henrique de Brito Belford Roxo, who as professor and department chairman initiated courses in psychiatry at the Faculty of Medicine of Rio de Janeiro in 1918. At the inaugural session of these courses he remarked, as reported by Ribeiro and Campos (1931): "The cases of mental illness provoked by Spiritism are increasing markedly in recent times and it is a rare day when I don't see at least one . . . syphilis, alcoholism, and Spiritism are factors which occur in 90 per cent of mental cases" (p. 61). Roxo (1918) exhibited the ambivalence still characteristic of many professionally trained observers in Brazil. On the one hand, in his major textbook of psychiatry, he strongly advocated that "nonscientific" spiritist sessions should be banned, especially "among Negroes who because of their lack of culture, suggestibility and tendency to mysticism" are vulnerable to mental illness. On the other, he felt the "Spiritism practiced by crudite men which promotes adjustment should be studied. It should not be ridiculed. Many times, that which today is not explicable and not admissable represents the great truth of tomorrow" (pp. 468-476). Roxo felt especially strongly about "the Spiritism of Candomblé," which, he said, should be "condemned as a source of madness." He noted the frequency of ideas of persecution among Spiritists (without systematic supporting data), and the occasional case of murder committed on command of spirits, the victim being regarded as the personification of a bad spirit. Following the Brazilian tradition, he supported his view with reference to French authorities. In the final edition of his book in 1938 he remarked that Professor Levi-Valensi of the Paris Faculty had regarded Spiritism as the "antechamber of madness" and listed attempts to outlaw these and other magical practices as public health measures in Paris, Vienna, and Bucharest. In this respect his attitudes still live in a number of physicians currently working in Africa. In July 1968 the present author heard, in the ancient Medical Faculty of Salvador do Bahia in Northern Brazil, an impassioned plea by a psychiatrist from Portuguese Angola for the eradication of witch doctors and their practices which he regarded as clearly productive of mental illness.

In a more technical vein, Roxo (1918) discussed both the social context of Spiritist practices and their specific psychopathology. He described the syndrome he called *delírio espirita episódico* as an "atypical form of psychopathic personality," with repeated short-term hallucinatory states following the emotional shock experienced in Spiritist sessions. These occur mainly in uneducated, gullible people, often burdened by

> physical or moral suffering, who instead of seeking cure from a doctor or priest go to a Spiritist session . . . [where they deal] with an astute man who exploits the poor. There is an intermediary, a medium, frequently an hysteric or with some form of psychopathy. She tries to convince people that she can cure their problems through the actions of a dead person transformed into a spirit which will come into their body . . . other times the spirit will come to their side . . . what is called an *encosto* . . . the pseudo-healer says that the patient has annoyed some person now dead who takes vengeance against him [pp. 741–742].

Roxo described the Spiritist session as follows:

> Many people gather in a little room. The medium is the middle, the *chefe* at his side. The chief says that they will seek a known spirit. The medium begins to tremble, utters cries, and jumps around, becomes agitated. One sees frequently what one sees at the movies in the dances of Negroes with extravagant movements, contortions and gestures. Now he is questioned by the clients, each telling about his problem . . . the spirit only gives prescriptions for homeopathic remedies . . . to be bought in a pharmacy . . . which pays the pseudo healer. Often he says there is a moral cause [of the client's problem] and he finds a good spirit which can destroy the bad one . . . the sessions almost always end with nervous crises and a general state of excitement . . . when the sick person returns to his house he has been much impressed. He thinks much about what has happened. Later, usually in the middle of the night, he begins to hear the voices of the dead people insulting or threatening him. He feels . . . disturbances within him [*da sensibilidade interna*] which he is convinced are caused by spirits. He can no longer sleep. He develops intense fear. His agita-

tion progresses to shouts and movements. There are always auditory and synesthetic hallucinations" [p. 742].

Roxo emphasized that the people described in the above manner were not mentally sick before the session. He regarded their hallucinations as corresponding to what the French call *bouffée delirante,* noting that they seemed contagious, were more common in Brazil than Europe, and most often occurred in Negroes,". . . in part because of their African heritages with its beliefs and easy suggestibility." The *delírio* rarely involved a confusional state. Occasionally there was some sadness, but without self-accusations as in the case of classical depression.

Ribeiro and Campos in 1931 also considered that delirious or psychotic states might develop in consequence of Spiritist sessions. (The Portuguese word *delirante* is sometimes translatable as psychotic.) They noted, however, the importance of predisposition:

> Among those who frequent sessions are many whose mental equilibrium cannot cope with such an atmosphere of mystery. They are mainly those with an hereditary disposition to mental illness. Psychologically weak in face of the difficulties of life they adopt Spiritism as a religion. Their faith is intense and stable but their low intellectual level does not permit them to be critical of what is happening, and, therefore, easy prey to anxiety, they develop *delirante* states with reference to desincarnate spirits as the central theme [p. 63].

They also considered Spiritism a way in which people of "schizoid constitution who easily lose contact with reality" might escape from close contact with others; they noted the possibilities for gratification of "hysterics, mainly females, [who] spontaneously show themselves as mediums in the most varied and exhibitionistic ways"; and (without specifying it) implied that the belief may be used as a form of defensive rationalization when the patient who has a "bad thought which must be followed by a bad act" doesn't regard the thought as his own and attributes it to spirits (p. 71).

CASE HISTORIES OF PSYCHIATRIC PATIENTS WITH PREVIOUS MACUMBA OR SPIRITIST CONTACT

It was often difficult during interviews to find out exactly what type of center had been consulted by the person seeking help.

People generally prefer the label *centro espirita* to any other because Macumba, and to a lesser degree Umbanda, has connotations of intoxication, marihuana and lower-class status. This experience has been reported by many workers in other settings.
Class is always in the forefront of consciousness. Possibly for this
reason, some centers which are indistinguishable from Macumba
are known as Spiritist; a center in the *favela* Euclides da Rocha
from which the noise of drumming and singing emanates every
Thursday night is such a one. A social worker from the Banco da
Previdencia went to the center to make an announcement about
the rehabilitation services being developed in the *favela*, but she
left before the ritual began "because I am a Catholic."

As noted above, almost everyone has as least one friend who
has consulted a center of some kind because of physical or emotional problems. Psychiatrists also have such friends who do not
seem to be inhibited in their search for cultist help by the professional expertise so close at hand. One such deserves mention because he has consulted so many *terreiros,* in the manner of a man
"shopping" among physicians that he is something of an expert
on what they have to offer. Originally looking for assistance because of nervousness and occasional crying spells, he has been
able to avoid becoming a psychiatrist's "patient" up to the time
of this writing. When a new spell or phase in the cycle becomes
imminent he looks for a new *terreiro.* In general, those which prescribe the most complex ameliorative procedures have been most
effective. Two which stand out are having to obtain an ox heart
from a slaughterhouse, and a particularly complicated *despacho.*
For this latter, he, accompanied by a friend and the latter's nine-
months-pregnant wife, was required to go to seven very busy crossroads and light a candle and break a bottle of *cachaça* at each.
This procedure, which occupied most of the time between midnight and five in the morning because the crossroads were so far
apart and difficult to locate, made him feel very good, and by late
afternoon, after having slept most of the day, he felt quite recovered.

The following cases, collected during July 1968 by Dr. Jayme
Bisker, illustrate the nature of contact with centers by low-income
patients seen in a psychiatric clinic under INPS contract.

A 22-year-old unmarried white man was diagnosed as schizophrenic. He was grandiose, thought that he was the "Chief of Bra-

zil," and that people were trying to kill him. This was an exacerbation of what had apparently been a chronic but not dramatic illness. During an earlier period of hospitalization he had had ECT. Now he was receiving thorazine and was being seen in the follow-up clinic for 10 minutes every other week. His mother thought that the spirit of her sister who had died shortly before the exacerbation was influencing her son, i.e., that he had an *encosto*. She believed that when her sister died, her spirit tried to *apanhar* (catch up with, seize, or enter) another body and that the boy, since he lived in the same house, was most easily available. The patient refused to go to the *terreiro*, fearing that he would be killed there, and at the same time refused to eat. The mother then threatened to return him to the hospital for more ECT, and this was sufficient to make him start eating again.

A 45-year-old married mulatto *funcionário* in the Ministry of Agriculture had been depressed, but improved with an antidepressant drug. When the doctor inquired if he had ever attended a spirit center, he was surprised, asking how he had guessed because he no longer believed in Macumba. He had regularly attended between the ages of 17 and 31, mainly to find women for sexual relations, but also because he developed a social group with others who went. He became secretary of the *terreiro* and *cambono*, or first minister, of the *pai-de-santo*, bringing candles and *cachaça* for the rituals. He stopped going soon after his marriage.

A 45-year-old white married kitchen helper in the Air Ministry who lived in a Tijúca *favela*, was brought to the clinic by her son three days after being discharged from a private psychiatric hospital, Santa Juliana located in the suburb of Meier, which had a contract with INPS. She had been hospitalized for incipient delirium tremens, feeling persecuted, and hearing voices. (According to the interviewing psychiatrist, this is rarely a cause for hospitalization among the lower classes.) Her son said everyone in the family drank heavily and got along well together, but that his mother's ability to handle 10 bottles of beer daily was apparently failing. Before going to the hospital, she had been taken to a Spiritist center on four separate occasions by the mother of her son's wife. There she was told that she had to *trabalhar* (work) in order to develop herself spiritually, but as she went to the center against her will, she did not improve.

Ten years before his visit to the clinic, a 37-year-old white mar-

ried small-boat pilot on Guanabara Bay, had developed hallucinations and delusions that people were trying to kill him. He had
improved after treatment in a state mental hospital. Five years
ago he became "nervous" and went to a *terreiro* looking for help.
He wanted to believe, but couldn't bring himself to do so and
gradually became worse. Now he came voluntarily to the clinic
hoping that drug treatment would be effective.

The above were four of six consecutive patients seen on a single
day who had been asked about Spiritist center contact. The other
two, both depressed, one an assistant guard at the Federal Psychiatric Center, became irritated and angry at the question, saying
that they didn't believe in that kind of thing.

Of 20 randomly selected patients, 10 male and 10 female, resident on the wards of the Psychiatric Institute of the Federal
University of Rio de Janeiro, the following 14 (90 per cent of the
women and 50 per cent of the men) proved to have had at least
brief prior contact with a center or *terreiro*. These patients were
interviewed during July, 1968, by Dr. Manoel Wilson Penna.

An 18-year-old unemployed, unmarried, lightskinned girl with
negroid features, who had completed 10 years of schooling, was
diagnosed as a manic-depressive psychotic in a manic phase.
Short and thin, with hair dyed almost red, she was miniskirted
and very active. She said that her problems were due to *Pomba
Gira* (Turning Dove), a *caboclo* who likes her very much and sings
and laughs. As a child she frequently accompanied her mother to
a *centro espirita*, but remembers little about it. Two years before
admission she began to feel weak, confused, didn't know what she
wanted to do, and had not found herself (*não me encontrei* is a frequently heard statement). Suddenly she saw candles walking,
began to weep, and had premonitions (*"começou adivinhar as coisas,"*
i.e., "I began to guess or predict things"). Once, for example,
sleeping at a cousin's house, she felt that her mother was not well.
The next morning when she returned home, her mother said that
she felt cold. She left school, began visiting bars, and felt that it
was she whom her sister's boy friend really loved. Finally, after
many months with mixed symptoms of elation and depression,
she was taken by her mother and some friends to a *centro espirita*.
It had a dirt floor and the people wore white and were barefooted. A woman there "received the spirit," who was gay and

joking. This spirit diagnosed the patient's problem as due to *Pomba Gira,* saying that she, the patient, was a medium, and that if she wished to resolve her difficulties she should develop her *mediunidade* and join the center. In other words, the *caboclo* spirit was influencing her because she was not fulfilling her destiny as a medium. (Following a frequent formula, if a person is born to be a medium and doesn't become one, the spirit which needs him so that it may come down and be incorporated becomes frustrated and upset and begins to bother him.) At the center she was given a necklace to protect her "from all evil" and was sent home. She soon became more agitated, however, and the Pronto Socorro at Hospital Pinel sent an ambulance to her home. After a brief examination there she was transferred immediately to the Psychiatric Institute. At the time of the interview she had been hospitalized for two months and treated with tranquillizers. Much improved and in charge of the ward bulletin board, she felt the isolation and rest provided by the hospital had been helpful. She did not regard herself or any of the other patients as mentally ill, however, but rather as spiritually disturbed, complicated in some instances by physical fatigue. At the same time, her mother, with a history of mental hospitalization many years earlier, seemed to her to be sick as well as *atrasada* or backward, i.e., she would never advance herself mentally or socially.

A 20-year-old single white school teacher with three years of normal school (special teachers training at the high school level), was diagnosed as schizophrenic. This was her third admission in 18 months. The first two were at the Casa Eiras for a few weeks, each paid for by the INPS, after which she had just stopped working without warning and begun to wander aimlessly about. On the present occasion she had started to feel anxious, irritable, suffer from general malaise, *mal estar* (literally, the opposite of well-being), and heard a voice but would not define it. She was taken to a *centro espirita* by her father and several siblings. There her difficulties were diagnosed as due to the spirit of her mother, dead for several years. A thin, quiet person, she was ardently interested in astrology and the personality characteristics of people born under different signs of the zodiac. She was a Bull, but when ill, believed that she was a Lion and acted more assertively and authoritatively. When this happened, after the experience at the

center, she was taken to a doctor who recommended hospitalization. This time, because the family had a friend working in the
medical school, she was brought to the Psychiatric Institute rather
than back to Casa Eiras. She says she has "sickness of the soul,"
because she feels guilty about everything, especially about sexual
fantasies involving her father who, she says, molested her when
she was young.

A 28-year-old married white former beauty operator who is a
primary school graduate with two children aged two and three
was diagnosed as having a postpartum depression. After the birth
of her first child she was hospitalized for eight months; she was
now in her third month of hospitalization for the second episode.
She had become nervous, irritable, and weak, finally leaving her
husband because, she said, he spanked her. She went to her
mother's home, and from there was brought to the Institute
where she had been before (referred from the Pronto Socorro in
Engenho de Dentro as an interesting teaching case) by her
brother. At first she considered herself to be suffering from "broken defenses" because she didn't rest and watch her diet after giving birth, but a kitchen helper in the Institute told her that this
diagnosis is no longer used and that she has a case of
aborrecimento—a poorly defined word meaning angry, harrassed,
sad, gloomy, or fed up. She felt this way mainly around her husband because he was not treating her well. She said that if you
don't explode and keep it inside it bothers you. When living in
Espirito Santo where she was born she had been Pentecostal but
never devout. Even though she was not Catholic, she said, "Catholicism was created by God, while Protestantism was created by
man." Since coming to Rio eight years earlier she hasn't been in
a church. Soon after her first child was born but before she became sick, she went to a Spiritist center "just to look." She didn't
explain the nature of the interest which brought her there, but
decided not to join it because "they work for evil as well as for
good."

A 21-year-old, white, unmarried, seven months pregnant
woman with no schooling had been admitted because of a suicidal attempt. She was reared as a foster child in a lower-class
home in the same tiny village with her family who were too poor
to keep her. A year ago she had come to Rio to work as a maid,

soon becoming pregnant by the owner of the house. Her first suicidal try by taking a handful of pills produced no results. Two
months ago, after hitting herself on the head with a hammer, she
was brought to the Institute. Actually she had been anxious before becoming pregnant because she is able to make predictions,
posso adivinhar coisas. She would casually think that small things
were going to happen, and then they did happen. She has attended several different *centros espiritas* both in her home village
and in Rio. In the village this was motivated by her wish to forget a married man with whom she was and still is in love. In Rio,
having spoken of this problem to her *patrão,* the lady of house, the
latter took her to her own favorite center. She had a consultation
with a spirit through a medium whom she liked very much.
While incorporated, the medium gave her passes to purify, protect, and strengthen her personality and suggested that she should
forget the married man and look for someone else. She also told
her to be patient with her family whom she hated for having had
her live elsewhere. When the doctor asked why she didn't go back
to the medium upon discovering her pregnancy, she said that she
was afraid she would realize who the father was and tell the *patrão.*

An 18-year-old single mulatto secondary school student who
lived with her parents in a rural area one and one-half hours by
train from Rio had been admitted because of anorexia, weakness,
constipation, headaches, insomnia, and anxiety. She had been
taking anticonvulsants since first having a grand mal seizure at
age 12. A friend of one of her teachers happened to know a doctor on the Institute staff, so she was admitted two months ago.
She felt better almost immediately and now wishes to leave. Before hospitalization her mother took her to a *centro espirita* several
times. She doesn't believe in Spiritism and while acquiescing reluctantly to the visits doesn't think that she was helped by the
passes which she received there. Nonetheless she can understand
why people go: *"a gente tenta tudo"* ("people try everything").

A 34-year-old white housewife with four years of schooling,
who had separated from her husband, was admitted to the Institute for the third time in an acute paranoid state. In 1959 she
had been hospitalized for seven months, in 1965 for two years,
and this time for two months. Now she complained of headache

and backache. Earlier she had felt apathetic, would do nothing at home, and was suspicious of her brothers and husband. Her self-diagnosis was *"espiritismo"* i.e., something to do with spirits. She said that she was a medium, but hasn't been interested in developing herself as such. "Not developing has a bad effect on the organ, the organ of eating, of everything." She has attended Spiritist centers for years, and feels that she is in trouble because she didn't become a medium. She still hears voices occasionally telling her that she is *"Media de Evangelho,"* the Medium of the Gospel. Last week she went out from the hospital to visit the center of *Caminheiros da Verdade.* There she was told that she should defer complete counseling until after her discharge from the hospital. Nonetheless they advised her, she said, to leave Rio and go to live with her mother in Rio Grande do Norte, which she had left to come to Rio when she was 18. (She was clearly very homesick, especially for the regional food of the north.)

A 23-year-old unmarried black illiterate domestic worker who had migrated one year earlier was admitted because of feelings of depression, anorexia, preoccupation with past failures, insomnia, left upper quadrant pain without apparent organic basis, and occasional auditory hallucinations, usually of her parents saying that she was no good and ungrateful. Her father deserted the family when she was an infant, and her mother had had a series of lovers including one who had sexual relations with the patient when she was 14. Later she went to live with her real father who soon impregnated her with twins who were aborted. She felt victimized, angry, disgusted, and guilty, that she should be among married women instead of girls, and dreamt of marriage and white garments. As she grew older and remained unmarried she grew more depressed and finally decided to come to Rio, where she felt even worse. When a physical examination failed to reveal a basis for her abdominal pain, she was referred to the Institute. She says that she has a "nervous disease" due to all the bad things she has experienced. In childhood she regularly attended Macumba with her mother. In Rio, her *patrão*, also from Bahia, took her to a Macumba even though she didn't want to go. At the Macumba they diagnosed that she had an *encosto* and also that someone had done something to her, a *trabalho*, which had to be undone. "A treatment was made" for her; they danced and made a small *trabalho*. The *mãe-de-santo* when *incorporada* gave her a complex prescription with many items to get from a Macumba shop, but she didn't follow it because she didn't believe.

A 38-year-old white married housewife, mother of two adolescent sons, who had completed seven years of schooling, was admitted to the Institute because of barbiturate intoxication. For the four months preceding this she had rarely gotten out of bed and didn't care for her home. She said that she frequently attended a *centro espirita*, and believed in Spiritism but refused to give further details.

A 43-year-old black single illiterate domestic worker was brought to the Pronto Socorro Pinel by her *patrão* and transferred from there to the Institute because she had become panicky, hearing the voices of animals which threatened to kill her. Although she had never attended a center or *terreiro*, she had gone to consult a *médico espirita*—a physician who was also a Spiritist. He had given her a prescription but she had never had it filled. She believed at the time of the interview that she had a "nervous disease," but also that animals were in fact talking with her.

A 28-year-old single black law student and typist was hospitalized for the third time with a diagnosis of paranoid schizophrenia. He came to the Institute through the intervention of a friend of a friend who knew the director. His first admission from December 1966 to March 1967 came when he felt that his friends were making "psychological warfare" against him for going out with a white girl, and he became increasingly anxious and suspicious. Later in 1967 he was rehospitalized for similar reasons. In March 1968, four months before the interview, he was admitted again, he said for "nervousness," but according to the hospital record, for acute paranoid behavior. The patient did not feel that color had interfered with his advancement. He had been uncomfortably aware, however, of being the only Negro in the school when studying English at the *Instituto Brasil Estados Unidos*. He has followed the civil rights movement in the United States since the events of Little Rock. He has attended Macumba ceremonies since childhood, and for several years was a drummer in a *terreiro*. He said, however, that he really didn't believe in the religious or magical aspects of the cult but was interested mainly in its musical and folkloric aspects. In support of this he was able to demonstrate his familiarity with much of the anthropological literature on Afro-Brazilian cults, including the writings of Nina Rodrigues, Artur Ramos, and René Ribeiro.

A 22-year-old white single unemployed resident of Niteroi was brought for admission two weeks earlier by his father because of a history of social isolation, obsessive doubting, and inability to choose a profession. He claims to be feeling well and wishes to leave. He has never had a close friend, spending much of his time reading Kafka, Sartre, and other philosophical writers. Because he owned a camera and enjoyed photography he considered publicity work as a profession, but rejected it as being "untruthful" and "harmful." He thinks of himself as Roman Catholic, although he never attends church. He has attended several Spiritist centers in his vague search for a purpose in life, but did not find them helpful and does not like them. His major complaint is that they are too "promiscuous," i.e., "everyone knows everyone elses' problems."

A 23-year-old white illiterate "*biscateiro*" was hospitalized two months earlier, having been brought by his relatives because he heard voices and said that people in the streets were talking about him. He has been preoccupied with a "foul smell" in his mouth for two or three years. After the onset of the "foul smell," he attended Macumba ceremonies on several occasions. "They talked" with him and prescribed several beverages made from roots, leaves, and other substances. Since he did not improve with them, he stopped going. He then went to a spiritist center, requesting an "invisible throat operation." He was refused and told that first he had to develop faith. One year ago he joined the Pentecostal church, *Assembléia de Deus,* and before admission attended services every Sunday night. His sister joined at the same time, although his mother continues as Catholic. One consequence, he said, is that he now masturbates, or as he put it, "practices evil" rarely, although he used to do so several times daily.

A 44-year-old white single restaurant owner, a Spanish immigrant in Brazil for 16 years, was first hospitalized in the Institute for 25 days in 1956 because of a "nervous breakdown" with depression, fatigue and feelings of confusion. The present admission was 18 days ago because of fatigue, insomnia, irritability, agitation following an argument with his partner, and feeling overwhelmed with his responsibilities. A friend had brought him to the Pronto Socorro Pinel from which he was transferred to the Institute. He had been reared as a Roman Catholic. When first depressed in 1956 he went to several "*terreiros* de Umbanda" for treatment, but they did not help. After discharge from the first hospitalization he continued looking into different *terreiros* and other centers, finally finding one specializing in "*espiritismo cientifíco.*" He liked their style of working around a table, felt their religious doctrines to be correct, and began to develop his "reasoning ability." Now he is being initiated by mail into the *Cristão Rosacruz* (Rosacrucian) organization with headquarters in Los Angeles.

A 44-year-old white automobile body painter, partly literate with a second grade education, a remarried widower with two sons, had migrated to Rio from Paraiba via two years in Recife 20 years earlier. He was admitted to the Institute upon the advice of a friend as he became progressively depressed following a series of arguments with an associate at work. He believes in *espiritismo*, but only the type in which people meet around the table. He regards *terreiros* whether of Umbanda or Macumba as "phony." He used to go to them but only to find girls with whom to have sexual relations. There were always many who were available, having come there for the same purpose, and these included a number of higher socioeconomic status.

THE SAMPLE

Fewer of the patients than the 88 per cent reported for the Guanabara population at large professed Roman Catholicism. This may have been a consequence of the context and style of interviewing or because this being a psychiatrically disturbed population, it was perhaps less certain of its religious identity. A clear majority of 70 per cent did, nonetheless, so classify themselves.

Fourteen per cent of the total, including a few who claimed "personal" convictions, were not affiliated with any religious faith or group. This again is considerably higher than the two per cent of 1960 census respondents reporting "other" or "none." The remainder was almost evenly divided between Protestants and those who listed themselves as Spiritist, Afro-Brazilian (i.e., Umbanda or Macumba) or "other." The Protestants included nine per cent of the total (as compared to four per cent of the general population), the Afro-Brazilians four per cent, the Spiritist one per cent (as compared to four per cent of the general population), and "other" or undetermined, two per cent. There were no Jews in the sample. In general, this psychiatric population appears to include an underrepresentation of Catholics and an overrepresentation of those without formal affiliation. An additional dimension was added when the practice of a religion in addition to the primary affiliation was included. Thus, nine per cent of the group admitted to continuing but not necessarily frequent attendance at some type of Spiritist center in addition to the previously claimed affiliations. Still another four per cent claimed an additional type of religious observance not included under any of the above headings.

Sixteen per cent of the group claimed attendance at their religious center at least once weekly, a figure compatible with reports for the population at large. Sixty per cent of the patients never attended any type of service or went only on occasional holidays or ceremonial occasions. Possibly reflecting the nature of people who become psychiatric patients, or the changing nature of the society, 37 per cent of the patients did not follow the religion of their parents. Three per cent of the total began their religious life in a different group; 13 per cent changed affiliation at approximately 18 years of age; 14 per cent, as previously noted, were unaffiliated; three per cent practiced other religions while simultaneously retaining the parental affiliation.

For purposes of analysis the following categories will be used: no affiliation; Catholic; Protestant; Afro-Spiritist. This last combines those who list Spiritism or Afro-Brazilian religions as their primary affiliation with the 18 per cent of Catholics, the 15 per cent of Protestants and the three per cent of unaffiliated who acknowledged occasional Afro-Spiritist attendance. Thus, they comprise 22 per cent of the sample. Even so it seems likely that the acknowledged proportion of Afro-Spiritist observers is considerably lower than the actual figure.

The reported frequency of actual church or ceremonial attendance according to affiliation is shown in Table 173. While three-fourths of the Protestants and somewhat under a half of the Spiritist or African-based cultists reported attendance at least once monthly, this was true for less than a quarter of the Catholics. These findings fit the impression among the nonhospitalized population of indifferent religious observance by the large majority of Catholics for whom church affiliation is more a matter of family and cultural tradition than of personal conviction or socioeconomic advantage. Conversely, for most of the Protestants, affiliation with their particular churches seem to have personal as well as status significance and to provide them with a new supportive context combining adaptive and ego-defensive advantages.

Similar proportions of Catholics and Protestants reported occasional attendance at Afro-Spiritist centers. While the proportion of the former, however, approximated that in regular attendance at the Catholic church itself, that for the latter was much smaller than the percentage in regular attendance at Protestant churches, suggesting that Protestant attendance, especially at Pentecostal services, probably satisfies the needs which motivate many Catholics to attend Afro-Spiritist centers. The largest proportion of those listed as Afro-Spiritist belong to Umbanda or Macumba centers; more than two-thirds of these, in keeping with a possible help-seeking attitude report occasional attendance at centers other than their own as well.

SOCIAL CHARACTERISTICS ACCORDING TO RELIGIOUS AFFILIATION AND ATTENDANCE

The demographic characteristics of the patients according to religious groupings are indicated in Table 174. In most instances the differences between percentages are not statistically significant. As expected from the general lack of religious involvement among men, a considerably larger proportion of the unaffiliated than of the other groups were male. The equal division between the sexes in the Protestant group give it the largest proportion of females. This may be associated with the Protestant ethic of sexual equality, in sharp contrast to the Latin tradition of a double standard favoring a variety of masculine prerogatives. A corollary of this may be a greater readiness among the less traditional Protestants to send behaviorally disturbed females to hospitals. Color differences between groups are small and not statistically significant. The only suggestive tendencies are a slightly higher proportion of blacks among the Afro-Spiritists and browns (defined in Chapter 4 as more socially marginal) among the Protestants. The relative social isolation of the unaffiliated is suggested by the significantly larger proportion of unmarried patients among them. This undoubtedly reflects the high proportion of males within this group, who, unlike females, must assume the initiative in order to become married.

Table 175 shows that proportionately more of the unaffiliated had declined in socioeconomic status during the year. Whether such a decline is corollary to relative isolation and a lack of social integration, or whether it is a consequence of the same factors, e.g., mental illness, antecedent to such isolation, is uncertain. It must be recalled, though, that all subjects in this sample were mentally ill to an extent precipitating hospital admission, suggesting that mental illness per se is less important in this equation than socioculturally determined differences in behavior (including sick behavior) between persons so diagnosed. The Afro-Spiritist and Catholic patients appear socioeconomically similar to each other. The Protestants, as indicated in Table 175, include the higher proportion of migrants and most frequently did not arrive in Rio City until adulthood. By the same token, more originated in rural settings and more reported improved socioeconomic status, evidently in partial consequence of migration, during the preceding year. The most residentially stable were the Afro-Spiritists, and, as shown in Table 176, they include the largest percentage born in Guanabara, over 10 times the proportion of Protestants. These findings support previous suggestions that Protestantism in the population at large tends to be associated with upward mobility, often associated with geographic mobility, while membership in the Afro-Spiritist groups tends to be an urban phenomenon not associated with mobility. Table 176 also shows that the Protestants, though mobile, came predominantly from Eastern states closer to Rio de Janeiro rather than the more distant North.

Table 177 shows that a somewhat larger though not statistically significant percentage of Protestants, like other in-migrants,

live in shanties or *favela*-type housing. They also suffer relatively
more from crowding. The Afro-Spiritist among the patients are
not significantly different from the Catholics on the basis of housing.

As indicated in Table 178, Protestants, like others of rural
background, are proportionately less educated and literate than
any of the other groups, proportionately more often than Catholics or Afro-Spiritist employed in Class VI, manual unskilled occupations, and less often than any group in occupational Class
I-IV. The unaffiliated, while not less literate, have the largest
proportion in the lowest occupational class. This may be another
reflection of their relative social isolation, lack of support from an
intact wage-earning mate, and lack of support from an institutional or interpersonal network. The proportionate predominance
of Afro-Spiritists in Class V occupations as compared with other
groups, supports the impression that these people—at least those
who have become patients in conventional facilities—are not at
the bottom of the socioeconomic ladder, and in fact, share more
traditional bourgeois characteristics with the Catholics than the
Protestants.

Differences in the use of informational media are shown in
Table 179. Despite their low literacy level, proportionately more
of the Protestants claim to read newspapers, magazines, and
books. This may reflect their religious habits which more frequently than the others involve reading or at least holding and
quoting religious tracts and the bible. Afro-Spiritists, whose ceremonies involve dancing and singing, least often claim to read.
Fewer Protestants attend movies (sometimes claiming religious
prohibition) or watch television, and, in respect to the former,
they resemble the Afro-Spiritists. The Afro-Spiritists, however,
along with Catholics own proportionately more television sets.
The most frequent movie-goers are the unaffiliated, with the
Catholics inbetween. This suggests that movie-going is negatively
associated with personal interest and participation in a religious
organization, and positively associated with lack of such interest
and belonging. Whether or not this is due to religious prohibi-
tions against attending certain films, or simply because church or
center participation satisfies affiliative needs and occupies the
time which might otherwise be devoted to movie-going is uncer-

tain. It may be relevant that, as seen in Table 180, less than a third the proportion of Protestants as compared to Catholics are frequent spectators at soccer games, although this is not true for dancing (more often engaged in by recent migrants). Somewhat fewer Afro-Spiritists than Catholics are frequent soccer watchers and more are sometime dancers. Soccer and movie attendance are both spectator activities in contrast to dancing, and both are paid entertainment attended by individuals. Soccer attendance, however, unlike solitary silent movie watching, is a group activity with much shared feeling and action. Dancing is even more active and very much part of collective social interaction; for the Afro-Spiritists this is associated with their religious observance as well. This may account for the observed differences between groups.

As noted in earlier chapters, the migrant poor had less contact than others with representatives of the welfare system, and more and friendlier contact with the clergy. This may account for the marked differences in these respects between Protestants and other groups. The fact that nine out of 10 Protestants reported contact with the clergy, and for approximately two-thirds—over three times the proportion of any other group—this contact was friendly, must also reflect the social structure and interaction patterns characteristic of the Protestant sects in contrast to the Catholic. The relative identity of percentages for Afro-Spiritists and Catholics in this respect is unexpected. It probably reflects the considerable number of the former who attend centers seeking help for specific problems, who thus limit their contact to consultation with one or another *filha* or *filho-de-santo* rather than the cult leader himself. It may also reflect some confusion about whom to identify as a member of the "clergy."

Hospitalization and Diagnosis According to Religious Affiliation

Table 181 shows no significant differences between groups in the proportion of patients admitted because of anxious-defensive or aggressive behavior. Proportionately more Protestants than members of other groups were admitted because of paranoid-persecutory statements (although fewer showed paranoid behavior in the hospital). More, especially in comparison with the unaffiliated and Afro-Spiritist, also had illnesses of 6-months duration or less. The tendency to a shorter period of prehospitalization disturbance may reflect their more intense involvement with their families who were more sensitive to behavior threatening the integrity of the family group. Paranoid statements, which usually appear before socially disturbing actions, were apparently least often regarded as legitimate and adaptive in the Protestant groups, even though paranoid behavior more often characterized rural migrant patients in general. For more non-Protestants than Protestants, hospitalization was precipitated by bizarre acts. Protestant families, who were least tolerant of paranoid behavior, most frequently, as indicated in Table 182, regarded the disturbed behavior as reflective of illness. Catholic families and those of unaffiliated patients, in contrast, most frequently regarded the disturbed behavior as strange or bad. It may be assumed that for the Catholics this reflects a rigid although not usually observed behavioral code. The families of the unaffiliated patients were also mainly Catholic, and the patients' failure to subscribe even nominally to the church may have already placed them, in their families' eyes, in the strange or bad category.

Past History and Family Background According to Religious Affiliation

Parental literacy, as seen in Table 183, was lowest for Protestants, while Catholics and Afro-Spiritists resembled each other in this respect. This fits the impressions noted above concerning the social backgrounds of the various groups. Proportionately fewest unaffiliated patients had illiterate parents. Whether or not greater exposure to a broader range of ideas in childhood may lead to lack of church affiliation in adulthood is a matter of speculation.

Broken homes during childhood, as seen in Table 184, were least frequently reported by Protestants and most often by Afro-Spiritists. This last may reflect the help-seeking motivation of many who join Afro-Spiritist centers. The Protestant characteristics, along with the greater proportion reared by both parents and married with children of their own, again suggest that persons of low socioeconomic status, predisposed to and capable of a sustained search for stability and improved status, may be more likely in this normally Catholic nation to join the Protestant church. The family backgrounds of the unaffiliated resembled those of the Catholics aside from differences in literacy noted above. Proportionately more of the unaffiliated than members of the other groups had produced no children of their own.

The past psychiatric history items noted in Table 185 are difficult to interpret. Despite other indications that Afro-Spiritists might well have had important problems motivating them to seek help through center affiliation, they consistently deny previous difficulties. The major differences in other groups are the proportionately higher incidence of rages in the unaffiliated and their relatively higher incidence of reported head injury with loss of consciousness, both expected in a preponderantly male group. The relationship of these reports to their failure to affiliate with a religious group is problematical, but they do suggest difficulties in interpersonal relations which might have interfered with such affiliation. Conversely, the lowest reported incidence of head injuries and lapsing or fainting episodes among Protestants fits the developing impression that members of this group who have become patients are more socially capable in spite of early socioeconomic disadvantages.

Psychiatric and Behavioral Characteristics According to Religious Affiliation

RELATIONAL BEHAVIOR

Table 186 lists the nature of interview behavior according to affiliation. It is clear that the psychiatrists had less positive feelings for the Afro-Spiritists and may, in turn, have evoked negative responses from them. The only respect in which they were most frequently rated negatively, however, was in alertness and wakefulness, i.e., they seemed less alert, at times drowsy, and more often attending inner stimuli. The common features of this state and trance or pre-trance behavior are apparent. While fewer appeared to the interviewer to be paying close attention to him, fewer were described as revealing anxiety in speech and autonomic nervous activity. Interview discomfort was more frequently identified among the unaffiliated, who were more often described as silly, hostile, fearful, or apathetic and were least often described as respectful, courteous or friendly, or as paying attention comfortably. This fits previous impressions of this group as personally isolated and suffering from relational difficulties. The Protestants appear to have made the most strenuous efforts to relate, being described as dramatic or attention-seeking, and actively advice-seeking. The Catholics were apparently somewhat more conforming than the others, with fewer saying that they did not want help.

TENSION, ANXIETY, SENSITIVITY, ANGER

Table 187 reveals findings generally congruent with those in Table 186. More Protestants are seen to be situation- and work-oriented; more express anxiety about their life circumstances, their jobs, and their relatives; more also express the fears of loss of control often encountered in obsessive, striving personalities. The Afro-Spiritists, in contrast, are least job-oriented, with fewest expressing job worries or complaining about interference with their work. Their significantly lower proportion of phobic fears suggests that special places and situations are generally less important as sources of anxiety for the Afro-Spiritist. The Catholics appear least obsessive with fewer concerned about loss of control.

Data reported in Table 188 are equally congruent. Anger is most frequently denied or not mentioned and least frequently felt and expressed by the Catholics and Afro-Spiritists, who also least frequently report attacks of rage or arguments. Again, these latter appear to maintain some distance or to utilize certain defensive or adaptive techniques as a buffer between themselves and frustrating or upsetting reality, i.e., persons and situations. The impression of Catholic patients as more conforming and less striving is supported by the finding, not statistically significant, that proportionately fewer complained of achievement/aspiration discrepancy. Protestants, in contrast, proportionately more often acknowledge their involvement with angry feelings. These are differentiated from impulsive acts more frequently occurring among the unaffiliated who, despite a past history of rages, did not describe or show anger in the interview.

Feelings of sadness, uncomfortable high-intensity feelings, self-accusations, feelings of impending doom, guilt about social role failure, and guilt about failure as a parent are, as shown in Table 189, proportionately most common among the Protestants. Conversely, they were least often flat and apathetic. These findings are congruent with their strivings and social aspirations. As noted above, however, these features were apparently not the most disturbing to relatives since they were not more often precipitants of hospitalization than for other groups. This relative predominance of depressive symptoms does not coexist with evidence of repressed or suppressed anger; on the contrary, as noted above, Protestants were overtly expressive of anger than other groups. Nor did depression among the Protestants include a higher proportionate incidence of suicidal threats or attempts. In general, depressive behavior seemed part of greater emotional expressiveness, commitment, and freedom in the interchange with interviewers, as well as of responsibility, concern with one's own capacity, and involvement with others. The Afro-Spiritists least often reported feelings of guilt, self-accusation, sadness or suicidal threats and, along with those who were unaffiliated, most frequently appeared to be affectively flat or apathetic—again, as suggested above, a possible reflection of greater concern with inner states reinforced by Spiritist experience.

THE BREAK WITH REALITY

Indices of impaired reality-testing are listed in Table 190. The Afro-Spiritists, although they commonly experience spirit-possession in their religious observances, least frequently reported what seemed to be auditory or visual hallucinations of people or religiously significant nonhuman figures. Readiness to experience spirit communication in an appropriate ceremonial context apparently does not increase vulnerability to hallucinations as part of a psychotic break with reality. This finding also suggests that within the Afro-Spiritist population hallucinations are a less frequent determinant of mental hospitalization. Hallucinations per se were not often a precipitant of admission for any patient subgrouping however, and there were no significant differences between groups in this respect. Feelings of being stared at or talked about and of thought control were most common among the religiously unaffiliated described by other social and psychiatric indices as most alienated from others. The most insistent about the reality of their experiences were the Protestants, already noted as the most generally intense and action oriented.

In keeping with the above findings, Table 191 shows the Afro-Spiritists least often suffer from problems in memory, decision making or temporal disorientation. Disorientation in time was proportionately more often reported by Protestants. The possible relationship of this to their time-determined striving is uncertain.

As suggested in the case histories described above, approximately two-thirds of the patient sample made some reference—usually brief—to magical, Spiritist, or cult beliefs during the interviews. There were no differences, however, in this respect between those who attended Afro-Spiritist centers and others. Indeed, as noted in the present section, Afro-Spiritists least frequently reported or exhibited hallucinatory phenomena of any kind. In contrast to the findings of Stainbrook (1952) in a public mental hospital in Salvador do Bahia in 1951, no acute psychotic behavior was characterized by the acting out of being possessed by an African deity as in the Candomblé. Nor, in the present population, in contrast to that of Bahia, did the majority of lower-class men and both lower- and middle-class women focus on the cultural religious institutions in their delusional thinking. This difference may be due to the greater sophistication of the Rio de Janeiro patients, most of whom were employed in the metropolitan area, as well as to the more pervasive influence of the African deities in Bahia. In only a negligible number of instances did families diagnose the behavior leading to hospitalization as due to Spiritist or divine influence. Most of the references were to attempts to seek help at cult centers, self-determined or at the request of relatives. Some patients did speak of suspecting "works" having been made against them, or spirits "leaning on" them, in the manner described in the case histories above. A woman, for example, who heard her mother's voice telling her that she had the "bones of a crazy one" in her womb, had been consulting the mid-wife who had delivered her children, and was also a

mãe-de-santo. A young man who had been walking into other people's houses was taken by his mother, against the wishes of other
relatives, to a *Macumba* center prior to hospitalization, because his
father, now dead, had killed a man under the influence of a
spirit. A man stated that he heard "a bird whistle," but after
looking around his house without seeing the bird realized that the
noise came from a spirit. He said that he personally did not believe in *Macumba* but that he "respected the beliefs of those who
did." In only rare instances were the Spiritist or cult-related experiences woven into a delusional system. They were most typically offered by patients in order to help explain their depression,
weakness, confusion, or anxiety.

SOMATIC AND SEXUAL COMPLAINTS

The Afro-Spiritists who least often exhibited symptoms of anxiety, depression, impaired reality-testing, memory defect, or disorientation most frequently, as indicated in Table 192, complained
of organ anxiety and palpitations. The tense, depressed, situation-
ally anxious Protestants who least frequently complained of
physical pain or discomfort were more often concerned with
something strange inside their bodies, slowed physical movements,
fatigue, dyspnea and anorexia, all of which may be regarded as
physical concomitants of depression, exhausting work, and the
health and nutritional consequences of poverty. Weakness as a
symptom was significantly least prominent among the unaffiliated
in comparison to the more religious patients.

The Protestants, as indicated in Table 193, were most often
basically monogamous; the unaffiliated with the largest proportion of casual sex contacts were least so. Proportionately fewer of
the Protestants complained of absent or weak sexual impulses
and, along with the Afro-Spiritists, of sex as a source of anxious
tension. Proportionately more, however, regarded their current
sexual pattern as part of the present illness in comparison with
the unaffiliated, relatively few of whom viewed their sexual behavior as part of a mental illness.

DISCUSSION

In an atmosphere of economic oppression, deprivation, cultural isolation, and lack of meaningful contact with the traditional church, mysticism and belief in the supernatural have flourished. In the small towns and rural areas of the interior this has taken the form of folk Catholicism, often with messianic overtones. In the cities, especially in Rio de Janeiro, Umbanda, and Macumba as well as Kardecism are popular to a degree so far not accurately estimated. Umbanda and Macumba reveal, through their rituals and concern with African divinities, their historical roots in already syncretistic Candomblé, though these cults have begun to include increasingly prominent Spiritist elements. Many devotecs of all of these still evolving religious forms are seeking help for physical, emotional, or social problems. An important percentage of psychiatric patients in Rio have sought help from Afro-Spiritist sources before coming to conventional medical establishments. This help has been gained through the general support of belonging to a group, but perhaps more from the specific sense of communication with the supernatural, i.e., with forces more powerful than those of everyday life. Although the data reported here do not refer to the possibility, it is plausible to assume that these forces are perceived as specifically more powerful than those of the dominant controllers of the social order. The experience of possession is perhaps the most intense form of such communication, which, in addition to affirming the initiate's status in the Spiritist or cult center's hierarchy, also has some personal psychological value. Ribeiro (1959) referred to the various forms of tension release permitted by trance behavior. Mischel and Mischel (1958) listed some specific features of all trance behavior which seem applicable to Macumba, Umbanda, and Kardecista as well as Candomblé and related possession states. These are the acting out of sexual and aggressive behavior, the reversal of sexual roles, and temporary freedom from responsibility for actions. It should be noted here, however, that the evidence at hand for Umbanda and *Kardecista* centers suggests that the sexual acting out which may occur during their trances states is not consciously recognized as such by observing cult members, or even retrospectively by the initiate himself. Perhaps it is too constraining to think solely of sexual or aggressive acting out. The capacity to be possessed in a group setting with a variety of symbolic expressions and exhibitionistic gratifications from socially rewarded histrionics must do much to give a sense of purpose and significance to otherwise mean and struggling lives. Aside from possession itself, however, the Yoruba opinion reported by Prince (1966) seems relevant for the poor people of Rio de Janeiro: ". . . from the healer's viewpoint it is the joining of the cult and the carrying out of ritual behavior . . . within the cult that is therapeutic . . . the Yoruba do not regard spirit-possession as more therapeutic than other non-cathartic forms of involvement" (p. 158). Joining of the cult itself is, after all, the key to a connection with the world of spirits and divinities as well as to the other humans who share the beliefs.

Membership in a cult or Spiritist center, as suggested above, provides social support for many. Whether or not, following the previously described interpretations of messianism, the cults reflect significant forces in the direction of a restructured social order seems debatable. To the contrary, the Candomblé houses and closely related cult centers of Northern Brazil appear through their rigidity and ritualization to provide a substitute or parallel social order to that of the dominant white social world. In this sense they may reduce the likelihood of their members trying to produce a significant change in that world. The *Kardecista* centers, with predominantly white middle-class adherents similarly appear to provide an escape from confrontation with social realities. It is in the urban Macumba and Umbanda centers that the greatest potential for social change and restructuring resides. The former have in the past given some identity and sense of power to the poorest social strata on the basis of which they may have developed greater negotiating leverage, with the power-holders, albeit as an agglomeration of individuals rather than a system. The fact that this leverage may have involved "black magic" or the encouragement of criminal tendencies need not invalidate this suggestion. The Umbanda groups have already moved in the direction of overt politicization with the election of federal deputies and the holding of national congresses. Most centers, however, because of their uniqueness and especially the tribalistic concentration of power in their own hierarchies, with leaders reluctant to band together with others, exert their impact at the local level. This impact is probably more significant in consequence of their social welfare activities, which now offer real alternatives to those of the Catholic church, than of overt political acts. Umbanda is more open to a broad spectrum of individuals than the other Afro-Spiritist groups since it offers a wider range of participatory alternatives to interested persons and has not yet reached the degree of stylization characterizing either Candomblé or Kardecism. Still in a state of evolution, it will probably have increasing appeal for disaffected Catholics of the lowest socioeconomic stratum who are not ready for the work-oriented, more ascetic Protestant ethic, even with its Pentecostalist gratifications.

As for the subcommunities, however, there can be little doubt regarding the integrative function of cult centers. While the creation of new and gratifying groups may reduce the likelihood of revolutionary change in the overall social system, it provides areas of integration and creates communities where none existed before. The cult-and Spiritist centers offer opportunities for the realization of the integrative experiences noted by Leighton et al. (1963): leadership and followership; participation in group decision-making; increased communication; and increased observance of the traditional (i.e., the opposite of increased secularization). Burgess (1955) had earlier laid the groundwork for this type of thinking. He wrote, for example, "When society is well organized, it provides through its institutions and groups the necessary roles to utilize the energies and to realize the wishes of its members . . . perhaps the most important single factor in mental disorders and disturbances, is the failure of society to provide adequately for the social roles essential for the mental health of its members" (p. 3). Again, he noted that ". . . a high degree of social organization is associated with good mental health. . . . Local community organization in areas where it is absent or feeble is therefore an essential way to mental health" (pp. 8–9). With this type of consideration in mind, Prince (1966) has suggested that an important function of possession cults is to ". . . provide a tightening of the social structure" (p. 161). Supporting this suggestion, he reports a series of events he has observed on a number of occasions among the Yoruba. These begin with an increase in social pathology in a village, the diviner's diagnosis of failure of the people to observe their traditional responsibilities and rituals, and his direct prescription to increase their religious behavior, which in turn results in an increase in social contact and a consolidation of lineage and other important relationships. The community-building function of Rio cult centers may be understood in similar terms.

Protestantism throughout the country has offered an egalitarian work-oriented social group appealing to those in search of upward mobility and escape from old ties. In this sense it may become a significant force modifying the old order through changes in value system, as well as the development of a new social base and an alternative to the Catholic church, historically associated with state and oligarchy. The Pentecostal sects, moreover, offer the joy of immediate salvation without waiting for the remote heaven promised to Catholics who suffer the present with resignation.

CHAPTER 12

PERSONALITY, DEPRIVATION, AND POWERLESSNESS: THE RESULTS OF PROJECTIVE TESTING*

THE LONG established techniques about which there is the greatest body of recorded information are the Rorschach and Thematic Apperception Tests. No attempt will be made here to review their potentialities or the hazards which arise in attempting to use their results for cross-cultural comparisons. There is almost general agreement, furthermore, that the statistical problems which they pose may never be solved, and that conclusions drawn from them are more a function of the competence and interests of the administering and interpreting clinician, than of any presumably objective method of scoring.

It was decided in the planning phase of the present study that projective material should be obtained in order to complement the data recorded in Sociocultural and Initial Interview Inventories. To this end, prior to the phase of retaining actual data, preliminary experience was gained in the testing situation with the Rorschach and TAT as well as with the Holtzman (1961) Inkblot Test with lower-class patients. In these preliminary testing situations, carried out by a Brazilian clinical psychologist sensitive to interpersonal cues and broadly experienced with the middle and

---

* This chapter is based on a report submitted by Professor Jurema Alcides Cunha. Professor Cunha selected the stimulus cards, devised and selected scoring methods, trained the other psychological test administrators, and made the test interpretations. She conducted all preliminary testing prior to the actual data gathering. Approximately one-third of the tests during the data-gathering period were given by each psychologist. Besides Professor Cunha, the other psychologists were Senhora Celmy Andrade Araripe Correa and Senhora Regina Maria Leme Carvalho. The conclusions in this chapter, as in the others, are the responsibility of the author.

upper classes, several problems quickly became apparent. Most
notable was the lack of productivity of the patients. Faced with a
card demonstrably evocative with similarly diagnosed patients of
more elevated social class, their responses were few, laconic, and
simple. The psychologist, accustomed to a different communicative situation and to a freer and richer descriptive flow from educated, relatively well-to-do psychiatric patients, described the responses of the study group in such terms as "unimaginative" and
"lacking creativity." After the performance period, sensitive,
non-demanding management of the inquiry was required to elicit
fantasy material. Part of the failure to respond appeared to rest in
the patient's feelings that the tasks were not meaningful. Some,
for example, remarked that the tests were childish, and that their
children might do better than they in such a situation. Whether
or not these were rationalizations to conceal discomfort in an
unfamiliar evaluative situation could not be determined. It was
clear, however, that psychological testing posed much greater
difficulties for the patients than the more familiar clinical interaction with a physician in which the traditional pattern of talking
about one's problems was reinforced.

The lack of concrete form did not produce greater difficulties
responding to the Rorschach than to the TAT cards. In fact,
TAT responses were more meager. When the HIT was used,
however, with more cards presented for shorter times and responses limited to the initial one, the protocols were more impoverished and less informative than for the standard Rorschach.
Time seemed necessary for the patient to become accustomed to
the card and the idea that one could have fantasies about it, and
beyond that, that one might communicate these to an expectantly
listening upper-class woman psychologist.

Once a base line of experience and expectations was achieved,
the psychologist, having discussed the problem with the project
psychiatrists, who agreed, decided to limit the TAT cards to
numbers 1, 2, 3, 4, 9BM, 10, 12M, and 13BM. This choice was
made on the basis of her unsystematic observations of their evocative quality with the preliminary sample of patients, and with her
own previous experience. She also felt that this selection provided
the most unambiguous cues and avoided repetition of themes.
The slowness and sparseness of patient response was another fac-

tor contributing to the decision to reduce the number of cards and, thereby, the duration of the testing process. All of the Rorschach cards were employed.

THE PATIENT SAMPLE

It was initially hoped that approximately half of the 254 study patients might be tested. The extreme difficulty in persuading hospital administrators to postpone initiation of ECT or drug therapy after psychiatric interviewing was completed made it impossible, however, to follow the original plan, which called for psychological testing on the day following the research interviews. Thus, the final sample included only 65, or approximately a quarter of the total study group. The initial 60 per cent of this group of 65 were selected on a random basis within the limits imposed by the rapid onset of behavior-modifying treatment. That is, they were those admitted consecutively to the various hospitals who were examined by the psychiatrists and whom the psychologists, as determined by their own schedules at other jobs, were able to see. The remainder of the 65 were deliberately selected from succeeding patients interviewed by the psychiatrists so as to produce a psychological test subsample socioculturally and demographically congruent with the total study population. Two factors, however, conspired to make this test sample somewhat more representative than the overall study group of the socially deprived and culturally excluded population of Rio de Janeiro. One was the refusal of doctors and patients in the private sanitorium to permit psychological testing to be carried out. This led to a few more patients being seen in the Pronto Socorro where new unattached cases were readily available. A second factor was the wish to obtain sufficient numbers of nonwhite and nonliterate patients so that comparisons involving these two groups might ultimately be carried out.

These considerations led to a psychological test group identical in age distribution, sex, and marital status with the overall population of 254. Age range was from 16 to 54. Sixty five per cent of the sample was male and 35 per cent female. Fifty four per cent were married (civil or companionate), 38 per cent single, and the remainder widowed or separated. Recent migrants (within five years) comprised 33 per cent, as compared with 28 per cent of the entire group. Twenty per cent had no schooling, as compared with 14 per cent of the entire group. The proportions completing primary school were similar—19 per cent of the test sample and 20 per cent of the entire group. Forty per cent of the test sample, however, as compared with 29 per cent of the entire group, were classed as nonliterate. Similar differences were observed in regard to occupation. Seventy three per cent of the total population of 254 were in skilled or unskilled manual occupations, with 43 per cent in the former and 20 per cent in the latter category. While a similar 80 per cent of the psychological test sample were engaged in manual occupations, they were evenly divided between skilled and unskilled categories. Color composition was similar to that of the total group. Forty per cent were nonwhite as compared with 35 per cent for the overall patient population. The percentages of black patients were identical in the test sample and the overall group, at 11 per cent.

In summary, this subsample is identical in age, sex, and marital status with the overall patient group. It contains slightly higher proportions of recent migrants, and patients who are unskilled manual workers, uneducated, nonliterate and nonwhite.

A breakdown of various psychological test scoring categories according to the various sociocultural subdivisions yielded too few numbers in each group for significant comparisons. The data will be considered, therefore, in toto as the responses of an uneducated, unskilled, barely literate, culturally deprived and socially excluded population. The degree to which their status as Brazilians or *cariocas* contributes to their responses is unclear except in their use of certain culturally recognizable ideas, particularly in the realm of religion.

Theoretical Background and Scoring

The interpretive Rorschach categories utilized by Professor Cunha were chosen on the basis of their potential yield of relatively objective information. They recognized the following general aspects of projective test responses:

1. *Sensitivity to unconscious or latent aspects of personality.* These include (a) ideational drive-representations: drives with libidinal aims, drives with

aggressive aims, and anxiety and guilt about drive expression, (b) affective drive representations, (c) display of anxiety: emotions and attitudes expressed or implied, symbolic responses and cultural stereotypes of fear, and (d) psychological derivatives of drives: dependent orientation, sado-masochistic orientation, authoritarian orientation, homosexual orientation.

2. *Multiplicity of responses permitted the subject.* These are limited only by the restrictions of his own language and psychological make-up.

3. *Multidimensionality of projective techniques.* These include (a) failure to take the test and/or difficulties in mastering the test situation, (b) intellectual factors in functioning, (c) evaluation of control, (d) evaluation of creative potentials, (e) the introversive-extratensive relationship, (f) organization of affectional need and ways of handling affectively toned situations, (g) self-image, self-concept and self-identification, (h) perception of other people, (i) thematic analysis based on content variables, (j) ego functioning—hypothesis of ego organization, and (k) qualitative aspects of thought and verbalization: perceptual and conceptual disturbances in thought processes.

4. *Lack of subject awareness of the purpose of the test.* In a clinical setting, the subject may have ideas about what the examiner is attempting to assess, although he knows nothing about the variables involved. Emphasis was given to the patient's ways of mastering the test situation and to the degree of involvement, as clues to underlying personal factors.

5. *The profusion and richness of the response data elicited by projective techniques.* A Rorschach Summary of Significant Findings was constructed by Professor Cunha (1969). This includes alternative interpretative hypotheses presented as a number of scales of several variables, or particular patterns or configurations.

A TAT summary of significant findings was also constructed as an attempt to quantify content analysis. Aside from Cunha's summaries, interpretive scoring significance assigned to various categories and their interrelationships was taken mainly from Klopfer et al. (1954, 1956, 1966). Originally, hypotheses extracted from Klopfer were presented as alternatives. An example is seen in scales of intellectual functioning. These include assessment of intellectual potentialities, estimate of general level of efficiency, strengths and weaknesses of intellectual functions, ability to accept conventional lines of thinking, ability to conceive original ideas and put them into action, range of interests, and manner of intellectual approach. Hunches or guesses available from other authors were added to provide additional clues for the personality assessment. Finally, traditional scoring or content Rorschach factors were included to permit comparisons with other cultural groups.

The number of responses necessary for confidence in the record or upon which to base the estimate of form-level to permit the assessment of intellectual potentialities and of mental efficiency remains uncertain. Cunha's (1969) Rorschach Summary of Significant Findings was designed to meet some of the reliability problems by making it possible to confirm hypotheses in future studies.

Pre-training and supervised practice of the examiners and scorers was conducted to the point of achieving agreement in both administering and scoring procedures. Frequent conferences with the preliminary scorers were necessary in order to avoid differences in scoring systems due to varied training and background experiences, and in order to create independence from examiner effects among the three psychologists. All records were eventually rescored and analyzed and the data were summarized by Professor Cunha.*

RORSCHACH FINDINGS

The testing situation

Testing was carried out on the psychiatric units in which the patients resided, within a day or two after psychiatric interviewing was completed. The exact schedule was dictated by the convenience of the subject and the psychologist's ability to return to the hospital. In every instance the psychologist was introduced as a member of the research-clinical team and every effort was made to maximize rapport. All tests were administered in private offices under similar conditions. Most of the patients were submissive, docile, and cooperative (54 per cent); a few (19 per cent) appeared doubtful, suspicious or afraid either of the test or of the situation. The remainder (27 per cent) displayed a variety of difficulties, such as the emergence of delusional or confusional behavior or signs of inhibition or excitement. These test behaviors closely resemble those noted in the psychiatric interviews.

* Psychologist Suely Pereira Lima collaborated in the task of scoring.

*Intellectual-cognitive functions, intellectual potentialities
and general level of efficiency*

Most of the patients were so narrow in their vocabulary and fund
of information that the testing situation was discouraging for
both patient and examiner. The findings in this respect are summarized in Table 194. Most patients appeared to function on a
lower level than was warranted by their hypothetical innate capacities. Thus the limit of capacity was low (not even 1 R of
form-level 2) in 60 per cent of the cases, and average or slightly
above average level (at least 1 R of form-level 2) in 29 per cent.
Only four per cent of the cases actually surpassed the average. It
was impossible to estimate the limit of capacity in the remainder.

An inferior level of intellectual-cognitive efficiency (average
weighted form-level below 1.0, or 1.0 to 1.4 with a large proportion of responses undifferentiated, vague and global) was estimated in 89 per cent of the cases; 11 per cent scored average or
above average (average weighted form-level from 1.0 to 1.4 or
over).

While 89 per cent, as noted above, showed unequivocal evidence of impaired intellectual-cognitive efficiency, almost the entire group, 93 per cent of the cases, revealed difficulties which
could potentially impair intellectual efficiency. These were associated with evidence of loosened ties to reality (minus form-level)
in 32 per cent. Limitation of intellectual efficiency through a nar-
rowed interest (high A percent and/or lack of flexibility, and rigid
succession) was found in 30 per cent. Emotional interference with
the mobilization of resources for ordinary functions was seen in 21
per cent. This was reflected in much scatter of form-level and
fewer original responses than should be given by a subject of high
capacity; in lack of M's; in large numbers of global responses or
undifferentiated wholes; and in paucity of main O's with many
additionals. In 12 per cent, weaknesses seemed due to difficulties
in integration and a failure of adequate adjustment to intellectual
limitations or to emotional or pathological conditions (descriptive
tendencies, loose or confused succession); the remaining five per
cent of the cases showed a variety of apparent causes.

In summary, almost the entire sample appeared to suffer, according to Rorschach criteria, from some degree of intellectual-

cognitive impairment. For almost two-thirds, the hypothesized level of innate intellectual efficiency was lower than the expected norm.

Ability to accept conventional lines of thinking

Fifty-two per cent of the cases appeared defective in capacity to see the world in the same terms as other people (less than the average number of popular responses). Approximately half of these, however, seemed to have resources for adopting the conventional view as indicated by their additional responses in the inquiry and their ready acceptance of suggestions.

Twenty-six per cent of the patients showed an unusually strong emphasis on seeing the world in terms of its obvious aspects, with occasional evidence of trivial thinking (an above average level of popular response). The remaining 22 per cent appeared to see the world as others see it, without an undue emphasis upon conventional views (5 P in an average record of 20 to 45 responses). Of the whole sample, 35 per cent evinced a weakness of ties with reality on the basis of few P's, unbalanced use of locations (especially a low D percent), and poor form-level. This last figure is virtually identical with that noted in the section above.

In summary, 78 per cent of the patients perceived the world in terms different from those regarded as average or conventional according to Rorschach norms. Approximately a third of these revealed a stereotyped or superconventional view of the world around them. This could reflect limited endowment, a depressive construction of perception or a way of defending against anxiety or threatened disorganization. The majority, though, did not respond in this way and reported more unique and fewer popular responses. This last group is similar in number to those indicated above as suspicious, fearful, delusional, confused, excited, or inhibited.

Ability to conceive original ideas

Seventy-five per cent of the sample showed no evidence of this ability. The remaining 25 per cent appeared not to be making full use of their capacity to conceive original ideas (paucity of O's and scatter in form-level rating, O's not in optimal relationship to

P's, additional O's). The O minus responses were conspicuous. In 40 per cent of the cases the response appeared to violate common-sense and did not match the stimulus. In 16 per cent there was a farfetched or queer approach, showing a disregard for reality, while still matching the stimuli.

In summary, according to Rorschach norms, the entire sample appeared to be defective in creative ideational ability. In three-quarters of the patients such ability was simply not evident, and in the remainder it was not fully utilized. While over half the patients violated commonsense in a significant number of prob-lem-solving responses, this was not clearly due to psychotic im-pairment.

Range of interests

A narrow range of interests, implying a stereotyped view of the world, was revealed in 52 per cent of the cases (A over 50 per cent or overemphasis on other content categories such as anatomy). Only 34 per cent of the cases demonstrated at least an average range of interests (A from 20 to 40 per cent, with at least 25 per cent of content being outside of H and A, spread out at least among three other content categories). The remaining 14 per cent did not cooperate fully or failed many cards, making it difficult to estimate their range of interests. These findings are congruent with those above, indicating diminished or absent ability to con-ceive original ideas. It is approximately twice the proportion, how-ever, of cases which appear to manage anxiety or deal with the threat of personal disorganization by adopting a superconven-tional world view or one involving excessive attention to detail (20 per cent of the sample). Narrowing of interests and stereotyp-ing may reflect the operation of defensive maneuvers compatible with conformity and obsessiveness; utilization of such defenses would be promoted by and would also contribute to the intellec-tual-cognitive impairment present to some degree in almost every patient.

Intellectual approach—Ways of dealing with practical problems

These subjects were unable to differentiate between the obvious facets of the world around them, either because of defective intellectual capacity or emotional interference (D below 45 per cent in 57 per cent of the cases and form-level generally low). In a few cases, although the subjects seemed unable to differentiate, their neglect of practical, commonsense issues did not seem deep or serious (where D was below 45 per cent, but the subjects could readily accept details when limits were tested). D percent exceeded 55 per cent in 20 per cent of the cases. Seventeen per cent of these seemed confined to a concrete, practical, commonsense view of the world because they were not capable of a more integrated view (form-level mediocre); the remaining three per cent showed some drive to seek relationships between the various facts of experience (form-level good). Only 23 per cent showed D within the average range. Thus, according to Rorschach criteria, approximately three-fourths of the patients showed difficulty in making obvious reality discriminations of a kind involved in daily coping activities. For most, the problems were those of being unable to accomplish the basic differentiations. Approximately a fourth of the impaired group adhered inappropriately to practical, commonsense views because they were incapable of more complex conceptualization.

Intellectual approach—Ability to conceptualize or engage in abstract mental activity

In 59 per cent of the cases W was greater than 30 per cent. Twenty-one per cent of the patients showed A W level of 20 to 30 per cent; the remaining 20 per cent of the patients had a W level under 20 per cent. These results suggest an effort at perceptual and conceptual organization in the majority of subjects. This effort may represent: (a) a compulsive need to intellectualize, (b) an attempt to superimpose generalizations upon the facts without regard to their fitness, (c) a manifestation of compensatory intellectual ambition or, (d) a lack of the necessary intellectual capacity or a consequence of emotional interference impairing ability to perceive at an integrated level. DW responses in almost 43 per cent of the sample suggest insufficient critical capacity to prevent erroneous conclusions on the basis of inadequate evidence. In some cases there seemed little interest in seeking relationships between the various facets of experience and thus achieving an organized view of the world. Only a small portion of the sample (21 per cent) showed clear ability to conceptualize or engage in abstract thinking. These findings are congruent with those immediately above. Most patients revealed some evidence of effort at conceptual organization but almost half showed impaired critical capacity and only a fifth demonstrated clear ability to conceptualize or think abstractly.

Interest in the minutiae of experience

Minimal or only average interest in the minutiae of experience was exhibited by 82 per cent of the cases. In the remaining 18 per cent there was some emphasis on accuracy, correctness, and exactness (d% > 15%). The ability to perceive unusual details was expressed by an overintellectual approach (Dd + S over 10 per cent at the expense only of D in 31 per cent of the cases). Another 15 per cent indicated a defense against insecurity by clinging to limited areas of certainty (Dd + S at the expenses only of W). Among the different kinds of unusual approaches was an emphasis on S in 26 per cent of the patients and on dr in 16 per cent. Most of the cases presenting some S responses were coarctated or coarctative, in terms of introversive-extratensive balance.

In summary, slightly less than a third of the patients demonstrated an overintellectual approach and almost half some emphasis on unusual detail. These figures are roughly similar to those noted in preceding sections as suggesting some defensive obsessiveness in the face of anxiety and threatened personal disorganization.

CONTROL, RELATIONAL, AND AFFECTIONAL FACTORS

Evaluation of control

The large majority of patients, 71 per cent, used few determinants other than form (F per cent over 50). In at least 25 per cent of the total, little affective energy seemed invested in emotional contact (F C=O O-1 M and F per cent over 50). Twenty per cent showed some capacity to avoid personal involvement as an aid to routine situational adjustment (F per cent within the normal range, 20 to 50 per cent). Only five per cent had introspective tendencies and affectional sensitivity sufficiently developed to soften constrictive tendencies (F per cent close to 50, FK + Fc between ¼ and ¾ of F and FK + F + Fc not exceeding 75 per cent). Finally, in three per cent there was too little emphasis on nonpersonal relationships with the world to maintain control (F per cent below 20). For 35 per cent of the sample, weakened ties to reality were related to inadequate control (F per cent over 50 and minus form-level responses; F per cent below 20 and few other control factors represented). In most cases, M responses were absent (44 per cent) or M and FM together were infrequent (38 per cent). Since M is considered indicative of the capacity to utilize inner resources for the constructive solution of everyday problems of living, the low number of M point to insufficient inner control and defective capacity for thought. They suggest ego weakness, especially when associated with poor form-level. Although the scarcity of M itself may be associated with a poor cultural environment and/or intellectual deficit, one would expect to encounter more frequently an average amount of M (3M for the average person and 5 for an introversive one). The relationship between M and FM, and M and FM + m is another interpretive factor. In many cases presenting O-1 M, FM surpassed M, up to a ratio of 6 FM to O M. This may be associated with a childish type of fantasy, preoccupation with the gratification of egocentric needs, or impulsive and immature behavior if associated with an emphasis on CF. This situation was found mainly with O M. In only three per cent of the cases yielding at least 1 M, was FM greater than 2 M. About 12 per cent of the sample were able to give 3 M or over, but half of them without satisfactory relationship with FM. The cases with at least 2 M presenting 2 FM amounted only to three per cent.

The picture is poor in terms of inner resources. Thirty-eight per cent of the cases revealed a deficiency of inner resources as a means of adjusting, despite the number of M. These showed a trend toward wish fulfilling or escapist fantasy—M involving A, (A) or (H)—or to intellectual reservations and self-criticism which could interfere with the use of inner resources—M involving Hd, (H) and (Hd). In an additional 16 per cent, imaginal processes served to distort reality (M-).

In terms of outer control, 16 per cent could be considered emotionally flat, with no apparent interest in others (FC = O and no achromatic responses). Forty per cent showed inadequate control of emotional expression (CF + C outnumbering FC). Only 21 per cent displayed signs of socialized control of emotional expression (FC outnumbering CF + C). The remaining 23 per cent maintained some emotional control through the use of security or defensive mechanisms, such as withdrawal from genuine involvement, or repression. These were shown by a greater number of achromatic than chromatic responses especially, with, in many instances, the achromatic outnumbering the chromatic responses by two to one. Other indicators were M outnumbering 2 Sum C and F per cent over 50.

A more detailed analysis of the chromatic area revealed 17 per cent of the cases to have a pathological lack of emotional control (crude C) and 22 per cent inadequate control with the possibility of acting out (minus form-level in color responses). The tendency to act out was also identified in an additional 22 per cent of the cases in which the achromatic responses were less than half of the chromatic, especially with CF + C outnumbering FC. The cases presenting severe signs of potential loss of control totaled 61 per cent of the test sample.

In summary, the majority of patients were not able to utilize even the limited inner resources (clearly deficient in over a third of them) available for the maintenance of personal control and ego integrity. Avoidance of interpersonal involvement was used as an aid for routine situational adjustment by approximately a fifth, while for another fifth, control was impaired by their inability to protect themselves from incoming emotional stimulation. Impaired reality testing contributed to inadequate control in approximately a third of the cases.

Some Rorschach indicators of inability to constructively utilize inner resources are those associated with sociocultural deprivation and intellectual deficit. Others, however, are more commonly related to immaturity, tendencies to immediate need gratification and childish fantasy. Deficient inner resources appear related both to escapist fantasies and self-censoring immobilizing processes. Signs of socialized control of interpersonal emotional expression were observed in only a fifth of the patients. An ap-

proximately equal number achieved some control through the use
of various inhibitory mechanisms. The majority exhibited either
inadequate outer control or, in 16 per cent, no apparent interest
in others. In almost two-thirds there was some evidence of potential loss of control, including the possibility of acting-out behavior.

Creative potentials

As noted earlier, on the basis of O responses 75 per cent of the
patients revealed no capacity to conceive original ideas and in the
remaining 25 per cent, the capacity was impaired. On the basis of
M responses, no indication of creative potential or imaginal resources were revealed in 25 per cent of the patients. Some potential sources of creativity were found in 41 per cent of the cases: M
responses were reluctantly conceded, involved intellectual reservations, a fantasy flavor, or were not in optimal relationship to FM.
In 21 per cent of the cases the presence of FM, considered to
reflect a basic source of creative energies, was identified. Only five
per cent revealed a good quality of M, suggesting more constructive use of imaginal resources for creative adjustment. The remaining patients showed some, although rudimentary, indications
of the existence of inner creative resources. Creative potential in
object relations in the form of some potential empathy was observed in 30 per cent of the cases. The remainder could be various-
ly classified: 16 per cent presented limited ability to use imaginal
resources in an empathic way (real human figures in action);
in another 16 per cent, there was some responsiveness to emotional
impact (color responsiveness in general); in 17 per cent it was impossible to find clues to assess this point. The remaining 21 per
cent of the cases presented either some ability to accept recipient
affectional needs (Fc) or an overdeveloped need for affection (emphasis of Fc) or at least an interest in relationships with other
people (FC responses).

In summary, only a few patients gave Rorschach responses suggesting a constructive use of creative resources for adjustment,
and a quarter of the group revealed no indication of any creative
potential. The remainder presented some evidence of limited or
potential resources. Similarly, a creative potential for relating to

others could be identified in less than a third of the patients, while responses were not sufficient to assess this capacity in slightly under a fifth of the cases. For the approximately half of the group remaining, creative resources usable for relating to others were present only in a limited or distorted form.

The introversive-extratensive relationship

In terms of primary orientation, 65 per cent of the subjects presented a coarctated balance (O:O; O:1; 1:1, in 44 per cent) or a coarctative balance (not outnumbering 3 in both sides, in 21 per cent). Twenty-five per cent presented an extratensive balance (emphasis on Sum C) contrasting with only eight per cent with an introversive balance (emphasis on M). Only two per cent revealed an extreme intratension. The low ration of M to color responses is considered evidence of a tendency to a less productive intelligence, emphasizing relations with the outer world. In terms of secondary orientation, 43 per cent of the cases potentially confirmed or strengthened the impression given by M : Sum C. In 40 per cent of the cases there were also coarctated or coarctative tendencies. Examination of general responsiveness to emotional environmental stimuli showed that 43 per cent fell within the normal range (20 to 40 per cent of responses to the last three cards. Forty-two per cent showed a loss of productivity under conditions of strong environmental impact or were basically lacking in responsiveness to such impact. Only 15 per cent seemed over stimulated by environmental impact, regardless of overt expression.

Organization of affectional need

These patients, very poor in terms of cultural level and experience, would not be expected to produce many achromatic responses, except for the most undifferentiated ones. It is, therefore, difficult to use alternative hypotheses for assessing the organization of affectional need and the ways of handling affectively toned situations. Nonetheless, it was possible to conclude that in 30 per cent of the patients affectional need was poorly integrated within the personality, to the point of serious maladjustment (undifferentiated shading responses—K, KF, k, kF, c and cF outnumbering the differentiated shading responses). Twenty-seven per cent presented response patterns suggesting a tendency to act out (achromatic responses were over 50 per cent of chromatic, and CF + C was greater than FC). The remaining cases did not present enough clues to evaluate this item. The same considerations apply to signs indicating affectional anxiety. K and k responses were practically absent in 63 per cent of the cases. Diffuse and free-floating anxiety, however, was apparent in 24 per cent (more than 3 K or KF, or undifferentiated shading responses exceeding differentiated ones). The remaining cases showed no clear indicators.

Many subjects failed to produce Fc responses. The absence of Fc, found in 49 per cent of the cases, may be associated with a lack of acceptance or awareness of affectional need. Where present, Fc was mostly of poor form-level. Thus, the serious distortion of perception occurring in 25 per cent of the cases could reflect a strong affectional need, poorly integrated within the total personality. An additional 13 per cent of the cases produced Fc, but without a good control system; this suggests some sensitivity in the sense of being easily hurt. Responses cF, hypothetically associated with a relatively crude continuation of affectional needs for emotional closeness, physical contact and infantile dependence on others were found in 11 per cent of the cases.

In summary, Rorschach responses indicated some problem in the expression, awareness, and integration of affectional needs in most of the patients. This difficulty assumed serious proportions or contributed to a tendency to act out in more than half the cases. The most prominent specific findings were absent signs of affectional anxiety and lack of acceptance of their own affectional need. In smaller proportions there was evidence of strong but poorly integrated needs, vulnerability to being easily hurt, or needs for infantile dependence.

PERCEPTIONS OF SELF AND OTHERS

Body image, self-concept, and self-identification

The body image component of self-concept was analyzed both in terms of level of differentiation and evidence of concern.

Forty-three percent of the cases perceived only schematic and undifferentiated images of human beings, sometimes presenting linear movements. Only 32 per cent of the patients were able to produce human responses in the form of more differentiated images and only occasionally did they exhibit more complex actions, suggesting a higher level of differentiation of body image. The remaining 25 per cent did not produce H responses, or where they did, they were not sufficiently productive to permit precise qualification of the response.

Forty-three per cent of the cases presented some evidence of concern about body image or some definite sign of disturbance in the body image. Some examples of these include:

"A human figure with woman's shoes . . . the feet are deformed."
"A monkey . . . dead, headless."
"A butterfly . . . without wings."
"A picture from the sea . . . like a person. Two crabs are eating it."
"Two persons . . . disfigured. Their teeth are falling out."
"A fish. It has no head, only a tail."
"A child's little dog. But it has no legs."
"Maybe a human body . . . breasts, navel, but no face or anything else."
"Two human bodies, mutilated. No head or arms or legs, only the torso."
"A man or an animal. A one-legged one."
"A broken branch."

Only 30 per cent of the cases were completely free of body-image disturbance. While an additional 20 per cent presented no definite or conventional signs of body-image distortion, some somatic preoccupation could be inferred. For the remainder, the item was undermined or ambiguous.

Self-concept clues should be found in M responses. These identify the ways in which an individual feels himself within his living space. Schachtel, as quoted by Lindzey (1961), suggests that "the movement response is important because it represents a projection of kinesthesic sensations, which, in turn, are involved in the person's most intimate and characteristic self-perceptions" (p. 143). In terms of the amount of movement in space, described or implied, in 38 per cent of the cases the tendency was to increase and in nine per cent, to decrease living space. Twenty-one per cent of the cases, however, produced M responses in which human beings were "merely alive." The remainder did not produce M, or the kind of movement was not easily identifiable. As noted earlier, 44 per cent produced no M's. This finding is connected with a lack of mature identification. Therefore, in only less than half of the sample was it possible to relate the individual's feeling about himself to his tendency to increase or decrease living space.

In 24 per cent of the cases there was no single instance of human beings or even of animals interacting. Twenty-two per cent showed some instances of living beings as together, but true interaction was not described or clearly implied. In only 31 per cent of the cases was interaction described or clearly implied for human beings; in 20 per cent it was described or implied mainly for animals. The remaining cases included both human beings and animals. Twenty-three per cent of the sample expressed a constructive, cooperative relationship with others. Nine per cent revealed hostile or aggressive tendencies between a subject and object. The remaining 19 per cent presented varied forms of interaction, not infrequently of an infantile kind.

For evaluating self-identification, concepts of remoteness, limitation in life, wholeness, level of reality, and type of approach were employed. These were in part from Holt and Havel (1961), especially for human content. The protocols were so poor in terms of qualification of contents, however, that it was difficult to develop a detailed analysis. Animal responses were very poor, including many without specification. Those which were relatively specified were distributed through so many categories that it was hard to identify particular trends. Of the 453 animal responses produced by the subsample only 12 per cent could be regarded as popular. Of the more than half which were nonpopular, the largest proportion, 41 per cent, were cold blooded. These consisted largely of butterflies, snakes, fish, crabs, insects, shrimp; bat was also included in this category. Such responses, taken together with the foregoing, support the impression of a low level of self-identification. Human figures were less remote in native than animal responses. Twenty-seven per cent of the patients, however, produced responses revealing some degree of reality remoteness (especially nonspecific fictional, supernatural, mythological or similar characters or contents from dreams, explicit fantasy, and culturally popular fantasy figures). Forty-one per cent presented some degree of reality limitation. Seventy-three per cent showed some limitation in their type of approach; most of these emphasized anatomical and the remainder, sex responses.

In summary, the patients, with few exceptions, produced poorly differentiated, impoverished, and poorly defined human percepts. Evidence of reality limitation was frequently encountered. Gross body-image disturbances were prominent and, along with indications of somatic preoccupation, were present in 70 per cent of the cases. Anatomical responses were given by almost half the sub sample. Depressive, disintegrative responses were common. Self-concept could be related to tendencies to expand or contract living space in less than half the sample, but, congruent with the above, a fifth of the patients produced responses in which human beings were "merely alive". Interactional perceptions were totally absent in approximately a fourth of the patients, and clearly present involving humans for less than a third.

Perceptions of others

The low productivity and poorly elaborated responses did not facilitate conclusions about how other people were perceived. Nonetheless, protocols from 22 per cent of the cases suggested a childlike flavor in interpersonal relationships (M involving A, [A] and [H] legendary or fairytale figures). Sixty per cent of the cases presented some evidence of unsatisfactory relationships with both or one of the parental figures. Most of these presented some evidence that they had had unsatisfactory relationships with both parents (no M, no human figures, signs of shock or disturbances on Cards I, IV, VII, and X). In half of the remaining cases the possibility of unsatisfactory relationships with the father was suggested by a tendency to lack adult male figures and disturbances on Card IV. The other half presented evidence suggesting poor relationships with the mother in early childhood. These subjects tended to see no adult female figures and presented disturbances in the perception of Cards I, VII, and X. Indications of a serious frustration of affectional need in early childhood (emergence of cF) were present in 11 per cent of the cases. The remainder were undetermined in respect to this item. Thus, for a total of 71 per cent, something could be said about the nature of the parental relationship.

THEMATIC ANALYSIS BASED ON RORSCHACH CONTENT VARIABLES

This method of scoring was derived from Holt and Havel (1961). Responses with explicit or clearly implied themes occurred in a number of patterns. Table 195 indicates the ideational representation in Rorschach responses of drives with libidinal themes. As might be expected in this deprived, dependent population, the only category in which one or more responses occurred in a significant percentage of patients was the oral. Phallic-genital themes, without clear anatomical reference, occurred in the next largest percentage—the low level constituting a possibly significant finding in a predominantly male sample from a culture placing high value on sexual aggressiveness. The next largest group, 21 per cent of the sample, revealed anal libidinal themes, but again without clear body channels of expression. Except for the 44 per cent showing one or more oral thematic responses, libidinal expressions involving bodily channels occurred in small and similar numbers for the other categories listed.

Table 196 indicates the nature of ideational representation in the Rorschach responses of dependent and sadomasochistic themes. These occurred with equal frequency. Aggressive dependency and sadistic drive reflections occurred more frequently than oral or receptive dependency and masochistic drive reflections. These findings suggest the presence of significant repressed or suppressed hostility underlying the apparent dependency and submissiveness in approximately a third of the cases.

In view of these findings it is interesting to note that in 86 per cent of the cases there was no indication of sadomasochistic emphases associated with modes of interpersonal relationships. Authoritarian themes imputing power to those of high social status were prominent in only six per cent of the cases, and themes of subjugation, associating submission with low social status, were prominent in only two per cent. These data are congruent with the analyses of drives with aggressive aims shown in Table 197. The lack of evidence of overt outwardly directed aggression or hostility is impressive.

Table 198 shows the homosexual themes for male and female subjects revealed in the Rorschach responses. For both sexual groups the proportion indicating significant gender-identity problems is low and equal, and is less than a clinician might expect, given the prominence in Rio de Janeiro of specialists for the cure of impotence, real or fancied. There were some suggestions of active suppression of conflictful responses in this category and others of high anxiety, stimulating changing percepts. For example, a male patient who initially saw symmetrical figures as a penis and a vagina soon denied his perception. On another occasion a blot was seen as representing both male and female sex organs, but at the time of inquiry the patient insisted that the two "sex orders" were identical. Signs of anxiety were more frequent than reflections of hostility, but less so than might have been expected. Nine out of 10 protocols showed no signs of expressed or implied anxiety-laden feelings or attitudes. Symbolic anxiety responses were present to a very limited degree in approximately a third and totally absent in two-thirds of the protocols. At least some cultural stereotypes of fear, however, were seen in 51 per cent of the protocols, with many or overwhelming responses in another four per cent. In other words, cultural forms rather than individual emotional or symbolic expressions were the chief vehicle for displaying anxiety elicited by the Rorschach stimuli.

HYPOTHESES OF EGO ORGANIZATION BASED ON RORSCHACH RESULTS

General ego functioning

Estimates of ego strength and intactness of reality testing are based on the average form-level, qualitative aspects of thought and verbalization, quality of F and M, quality of control factors and O, and assessment of the modes of intellectual approach and acceptance of conventional lines of thinking. Such a scheme may be represented by a continuum from flexible reality testing, with energies used in constructive rather than defensive efforts, to weakened reality testing followed by primitive attempts at mastering confusing reality (see Cunha and Maraninchi, 1968).

Among the findings are the predominance of a low per cent of D with inferior form-level, sometimes found with other indices justifying the classification of most of the patients at lower levels. The same is true for scarcity of P, followed by cases of negative form-level, confabulation, perseveration, autistic logic, and so on. Table 199 shows the general results. Evidence of ego malfunctioning included mainly inferior perceptual capacities. No record presented a high form-level, and disturbances of thought processes were conspicuous.

Emotional integration and ego defensiveness

Many patients (43 per cent) displayed signs of a complicated system of neurotic defenses and marked interference with the integrative process. Only three per cent did not show apparent signs of poor emotional integration. In 29 per cent the subjective discomfort had begun to vanish with the emergence of objective test disturbances, i.e., the neurotic systems of defenses was failing. Signs of regression to archaic modes of defense were prominent in eight per cent. Increased ego defensiveness with no other problem was found in eight per cent of the cases. The remainder did not present sufficient clues for interpretive hypotheses.

Self-realization

In most of the cases (73 per cent) it was difficult to find clues sufficient to assess self-realization. The degree of investment of vital energies in ego defenses, not always effective, apparently did not leave sufficient ego resources for the constructive functions of self-realization. The basic necessary conditions for the emergence of some degree of self-realization were found in only 21 per cent of the cases. Only in the remaining cases (six per cent) were some of the conditions for self-realization present, and even in some of these, self-realization did not match capacity.

Ego defenses

Extensive reliance on repression was identified in 24 per cent of the cases, in shattered form in 21 per cent, and was suggested only by a few specific signs in six per cent. Specific signs of projection were identified in 30 per cent and were found in shattered form only in 16 per cent. Projection was extensively relied upon in only six per cent of the cases.

Other readily identified defensive operations included reaction formation: extensive reliance on in 11 per cent, in shattered form only in 16 per cent, and only suggested by specific signs in 10 per cent. Denial was extensively relied upon by three per cent, present in shattered form only in two per cent, and suggested by specific signs in 11 per cent of the cases. Isolation was revealed by specific signs in 11 per cent; in only two per cent was it extensively relied upon and in another two per cent it was found in shattered form. While signs of other kinds of defense such as undoing, introjection, etc. were found, they were not conspicuous. Generally it was difficult to find clues permitting the identification of leading defense mechanisms in such poor protocols. In many instances conclusions were arrived at by the overweighting of single signs. The two identifiable leading mechanisms were projection (in some form in 52 per cent) and repression (in some form in 51 per cent). Of the two, repression was more often extensively relied upon.

Relative strengths and weaknesses of the defense system

In most cases the defense system did not appear to function well. Defenses were unstable, weak, and beginning to fail, or a combination of these in 61 per cent. Rorschach indicators of defensive collapse were present in 10 per cent. The remaining cases were: undetermined (14 per cent); signs pointing to a rigid defensive system (13 per cent); apparently flexible (two per cent). In several cases it was difficult to evaluate the relative strengths and weaknesses of the system of defenses because of an admixture of neurotic and organic signs. In a few cases psychological test data indicated impaired cognitive function on the basis of cerebral deficit, but the nature of the organic process was not defined nor was it identified by the examining physician.

Perceptual and conceptual disturbances of thought processes

The absolute number of perceptual disturbances was high, and many patients presented more than one type of disturbance. The larger disturbances were those associated with complete disregard for the characteristics of the blot, except for a single aspect. These, including confabulation, confabulatory composition, syllogistic and positional responses, occurred in 56 per cent of the cases. Forty-seven per cent revealed disturbances of appropriateness in using blot characteristics. These included fabulation, inaccurate, peculiar, queer, farfetched, selective or multiple and overlapping responses. A similar proportion of cases exhibited disturbances associated with complete disregard of the characteristics of the blot. Some of these were magic-wand perseveration, fixed-concept perseveration, and perseveration of the type sometimes associated with organic deficit. Disturbances associated with a misuse of the characteristics of the blot (transposition, contamination, or both) were found in 24 per cent. Incoherent, absurd, neologistic, or bizarre perception of the characteristics of the blot occurred in 17 per cent of the patients. These included visual representations not based on or reflecting the commonly used, culturally shared, sometimes stereotyped ways of using stimuli. Magical use of the characteristics of the blot (self-reference, fluid transformation of percept, delusional responses) was found in 15 per cent.

In summary, Rorschach responses suggested the presence of conceptual and perceptual difficulties in varying degree in virtually all of the subsample. The most widespread type of difficulty, encountered in 56 per cent of cases, involved complete disregard for the characteristics of the blot except for a single aspect. These patients focused on a single feature of the complex stimulus, a response congruent with other efforts at maintaining control through denial, repression, and narrowing of attention. Slightly smaller proportions of the group entirely disregarded the blot characteristics in formulating their responses, or responded inappropriately or approximately to the stimulus. In contrast to the first category, these suggest an abandonment of or incapacity for control, and behavior in accordance with an inner frame of reference rather than the demands of the outer world. Small percentages of patients reported bizarre, disorganized, transposed or contaminated perceptions of the blot or its special characteristics.

RORSCHACH DATA FOR CROSS-CULTURAL COMPARISONS

As previously indicated, the productivity of this group was very low. Thirty-two per cent of the patients produced 10 or fewer responses to the entire list of Rorschach cards, 37 per cent produced from 11 to 15, and only 12 per cent produced more than 25 responses. The most global statement possible in this regard is that the patients were not reacting freely to their environment. Low motivation does not appear to have been the major reason for this. The large majority, 79 per cent of the protocols, presented no or only a single rejection. Two rejections were present in nine per cent and three or more in 12 per cent. Furthermore, the low level of productivity differs markedly from Brazilian norms established by Augras (1967) in a population of 322 nonmental patients. Her finding of an average 24.75 responses per individual subject is comparable to Beck's (1945) medium category including 20 to 30 responses. If Hallowell's (1955) belief that the productivity of adult subjects of diverse cultures in widely separated regions is mainly in this medium category, the low productivity of the present group may more plausibly be attributed to psychiatric or social-class factors than to culture per se.

Other studies indicate that most responses, regardless of culture or country, fall in H or Hd and A or Ad categories. Several authors have found the responses of nonpatient subjects to occur within a characteristic range: 10 to 15 per cent H and 35 to 50 per cent A. Of the present sample, 24 per cent fell within the characteristic or expected range of animal responses. Thirty-eight per cent each fell below and above the average. Often the response was simply, "an animal," without further specification. Patients showing a predominance of animal categories with little content variability may be regarded as having a shallow, ineffective intellect along with neurotic trends. An emphasis on animal responses has also been interpreted as indicating emotionally immature preoccupations. Only 20 per cent of the patients showed the expected response range for human content. Thirty-four per cent were below and 46 per cent above this average. Fully 67 per cent of the patients produced responses varying only from 0 to 2 human responses. The apparent scarcity of resources for human relationships is remarkable.

The diagnostic significance of popular responses has been characterized in various ways as noted by Hertz (1951). These include intellectual adaptation to collective thought, cooperativeness, and both the ability and need to think and feel as part of a group. Adrados (1967) has noted further that the responses most frequently given by Brazilians closely resemble those considered as popular by workers in other countries. In this present subsample only 32 per cent of the patients fell within the average range for popular responses. Forty-eight per cent were below and 20 per cent above average. While these data should be compared with 0 per cent, the responses were generally so banal that they could only rarely be categorized as 0. The low productivity and scarcity of 0 suggest inability to devote energies to intellectual production. The above-average group is suggestive of trivial thinking. The percentages of the below-average group may be explained by psychological maladjustment. M responses were relatively infrequent in the sample, with 44 per cent producing none at all. Another 44 per cent yielded either one or two, and in only 12 per cent of the cases were three or more such responses observed. In other words, 88 per cent of the sample were unable to produce at least the average number of M. The production of M's is considered to depend upon mental capacity, the ability to build up a differentiated image of man, and the manner of dealing with impulse life. Lack of mature identification can be inferred in a large number of cases (O M), appearing as a possible determinant of the scarcity of production of H's (indicative of resources for human relationships). The type of M response which does appear is further suggestive. For instance, in several protocols, movement such as sitting, talking, or walking occurred only in skeleton figures. This suggests social and personal impotence and lack of inner vitality. Human interaction responses rarely occurred, and where interaction was present, it tended to be cooperative rather than hostile. This was congruent with testing behavior in which patients were usually passive and constricted. Movement or FM responses were also sparse and did not occur at all in 37 per cent of the cases. One or two such responses were produced by 45 per cent and three or more were observed in only 17 per cent.

In summary, the Rorschach responses from this patient group show a number of clear trends in comparison with data from nonpatients in a number of national settings, including modern urban Brazil. Their overall productivity was very low in spite of seemingly adequate motivation, i.e., they did not react freely to environmental stimuli. The relative predominance of animal responses with little specificity or content variability suggests shallow and ineffective intellect and emotional immaturity. Human response data suggest a remarkable scarcity of resources for relationships with others. Popular responses were limited and banal, suggesting both lack of energy for intellectual production and a world view determined by inner needs and problems. Markedly sparse M responses and the types which did occur suggest impaired ability to develop a differentiated image of man, lack of mature identification, lack of inner vitality, social and personal impotence, and a passive, constricted approach to others. For most, these data point to a tendency to suppression of impulse life rather than its integration with value systems. There are also implications of tension, inner conflict, and lack of spontaneity. A conspicuous use of F at the expense of color and movement areas confirms this hypothesis. Many cases showed excessive control over psychological life.

Do these findings point to a cultural suppression of aggressive impulses? Overt hostility is in fact discouraged within the Brazilian culture. Hallowell's (1955) comments on the Ojibwa culture have suggestive relevance: "On the surface these people present a picture of amiability and placidity. Nonetheless, aggressive impulses do find expression covertly. One mode of expression is malicious gossip. The other major mode is sorcery" (p. 501). Both of these expressive modes are prominent in Brazilian culture. The first mode is observed in an almost institutionalized form of gossip while the second is seen in the widespread African Brazilian cults and forms of Spiritism. Thus, while social class-linked factors associated with deprivation and exclusion seem most prominent as possible determinants of the Rorschach findings, certain elements of Brazilian culture in general may also shape the responses.

Thematic Apperception Test Findings

Prior to the actual testing, eight cards (numbers 1, 2, 3, 4, 9BM, 10, 12M, and 13BM) were selected so as to provide a range of relatively unambiguous stimulus content. The collective data, however, were so meager and poor that a systematic analysis of each individual card was possible in only a small number of cases. Instead, therefore, a global analysis of the entire set of cards was constructed for each patient. This made it possible to arrive at some estimate of the common traits of the central character or hero and his inner states and emotions as well as to identify certain culture-linked responses.

The testing situation

Almost three-quarters of the patients were actively or passively cooperative in the TAT test situation. Fifty-one per cent exhibited no apparent difficulties in taking the test, while another 21 per cent were conforming, though dull and relatively unresponsive. Beyond the passive or cooperative group, 14 per cent of the total sample were clearly suspicious and wary; nine per cent appeared tired, worried or bored, complaining of being cold, sleepy, or uncomfortable; the remaining five per cent displayed varied uncooperative behavior, such as asking to interrupt the test or noting that they had other things to do. Although all did not respond to every one of the eight cards presented, in only a single case was there a significant problem in communication due, apparently, to seriously impaired reality testing. No one exhibited difficulties related to lack of familiarity with this kind of self-revelatory task.

Responses indicating personal involvement

As indicated before, most of the patients had had little or no formal education. Their limited vocabulary and fund of information made it very difficult for them to produce rich or well organized stories. Twenty-seven per cent seemed unable to go beyond a poor descriptive level. The presentations were immature and poorly organized or short and sketchy, with little personal involvement. An additional 25 per cent produced content composed for the most part of impersonal or superficial elements with only occasional issues, feelings, and conflicts seemingly of great personal concern. A total of 30 per cent seemed significantly involved with stories revealing important aspects of themselves. Only eight per cent of the total sample, however, were involved to the point of introducing frequent explicit reference to their personal lives. Detachment was not possible for three per cent of the patients who referred to the central character in the card as "I" and "me." Only two per cent of the patients were able to objectively discuss personal life stresses of an embarrassing or socially unacceptable nature. A final 18 per cent of the total exhibited marked impairment of response capacity on cognitive or emotional grounds. This group included eight per cent of the total sample who showed sufficient repetitiveness or other interference with the stream of thought to make the personal content seem psychologically irrelevant. Six per cent were unproductive to the point that it was impossible to infer underlying personal elements; and four per cent appeared so confused, anxious, or depressive that patterns of thoughts, feelings, and behavior mainly reflected their affective or anxious states.

Thematic and content analysis

In order to assess the central character's attitudes or traits, inner states or emotions, and the environmental forces acting upon him, the criteria listed in Table 200 were used. The distributions of themes and contents for the entire test sample are shown in Tables 201 through 207.

The patterns revealed in Table 201 resemble those suggested by the Rorschach test. The main trend is one of passivity, succorance, and self-abasement. Sex is present as a theme but not prominently so. Aggression, minimally expressed, appears at least in part to be directed against the self. There is no evidence of clear-cut outwardly or inwardly directed destructive responses. The pattern shown in Table 202 is consistent with other findings. Dejection is a major theme in a third of the cases, closely followed by anxiety. The following is a typical story: "A kind of . . . is crying . . . I can't say anything else."

The most important forces of the hero's environment, as indicated in Table 203, appear to be emotional affiliation and nurturance. Whether significant dependency needs are more related to the strong family ties of the Brazilian cultural ideal or to poverty and minority status is uncertain. The virtual absence of aggression suggests repression of hostile wishes in consequence of fear of the loss of a loved person or important object. Inducement or seduction themes complete the picture of passivity, nonaggression, and dependency. Table 204 shows the frequency of specific interaction patterns in the stories. Here the predominance of engagement rather than of breakdown or impairment themes is not wholly congruent with attitudes of dejection or loss or with earlier Rorschach findings. They may be understood, however, as reflecting passive-succorant wishes. As a rule, the stories in Table 205 concerned single individuals and only very rarely a second character. When a second character was involved it was usually as one of a pair. As seen in Table 206, stories rarely involved identifiable values. Table 207 confirms the initial impression that the stories were for the most part very poor, short, and mainly descriptive. The small number going beyond such a level usually presented an ambivalent outcome or unhappy ending. Only a few stories ended in fairly realistic terms.

Perceptual difficulties—missed elements

The response of the 65 patients included 62 instances of missed human figures and 95 of missed objects. Missed figures are associated with the individual emphasis of most of the stories in which interaction was very rare. Frequently the stories started by describing only a single character, continuing in this way until the end, despite the fact that some pictures contained two or several figures. Among the missed objects, "revolver" was absent almost 40 times, representing over half of the sample. This may plausibly be associated with the possibility of repressed or suppressed aggression. "Bow" and "violin" were also missed several times but whether or not this can be associated with sociocultural deprivation is unclear. Other objects missed, though less frequently, were "seat" and "books."

Misperception of sex and age

Men were labeled as women in 37 instances and they were oc·casionally perceived as belonging to a different age grouping as well. Only once was a female figure labeled a male and then as a dead man. In one story there was a fluid transformation of the percept; the same figure was seen first as a male and then as female. In another case, a female body was seen with a male face while still another perceived a figure which was at the same time both male and female. Difficulty in perceiving the approximate age occurred 12 times. Except for one, all instances point to regressive trends: adult figures were seen as child figures, one was seen as a portrait of a child held by one of the characters, and one adult male figure was seen as newborn.

Misperception of color, human figures, and other signs of identity

Skin color was mentioned only once, and then was clearly associated with feelings of inferiority. Other identity signs were noted on 22 occasions. Many involved authoritarian parental figures, mainly with religious or aggressive implications, such as "priest," "saint," "God," "a person with God's power," "policeman," and "soldier." One woman perceived a figure as a psychoanalyst, adding, "The psychoanalyst is a bad person who displays his bad instincts and is unable to cure anybody. Freud was the most devil being who ever existed." There were also instances of "crippled beggars," "drunkards," several "next world ghosts," "a ghost face like an owl," "a mentally ill woman," "a man as a vampire." Human figures were twice identified as cats, a man's leg was identified as a cat face, a human head was seen as a dog head, and a young boy was identified as a crouched animal. In two instances whole figures were seen as headless ones. One human figure was seen as a self-portrait and the patient identified one character in a card as himself.

Introduction of human figures or objects which were not pictorially present in the picture

This feature did not occur frequently. The following figures or objects were added as if they were seen in the picture: "a church, two saints, and St. George's horse," "workers," "two people," "a bundle of clothes," "a river," "a carriage," "a snake," "a door," "a table," "a grave," "a nightmare projected outside," and "myself."

Misperceptions of objects

The TAT cards used were relatively unambiguous in content, and it was assumed the patients would be able to identify all the objects represented. Moreover, the cards did not include those in which some cultural groups have shown the greatest perceptual difficulties. Nevertheless, there were significant instances of misperceptions of objects. The object most frequently misperceived was the violin; in some cases it was perceived as such, immediately denied, and then perceived as a different object. Violin was seen twice as a "coffin," as a "book," a "harp" which immediately turned into a "pressure cooker," a "tray," a "table," a "gun," a "plate," a "toy," a "picture," and a "drawing." These misperceptions are not readily explicable on the basis of lack of experience.

The bow was seen as a "compass," a "belt," and as a "suitcase." Revolver and books were perceived as a "purse," and seat was seen as a "package" and as a "table."

Culturally linked patterns of content

Traditional customs could be exemplified mainly by "blessing." In several instances fathers were described as "blessing" their sons; others were portrayed as "praying for a dead person's soul." The instances of superhuman beings, personal tutelaries or guardian figures, and authoritarian religious figures which did appear have been in part already mentioned. The popular figures of the so-called "fathers" or "saint fathers" of Umbanda and Quimbanda cults were present in several stories, as were apparitions of souls. The main distinctive feature, however, was the part played by cult practices, especially in the form of ceremonials. There were 12 instances of passes of the hands, a Spiritist ceremonial. Praying with therapeutic purposes was present several times, and in one case the patient described the card in terms of a Spiritist ceremonial, "space surgical procedure." Themes from Macumba were present as were those from Catholic rituals, i.e., sign of the cross, commendation of the soul, and so on. One story contained intermingled notions of magic and scientific therapeutic procedures: "The man is sick because of an evil eye. He believes that he needs to undergo a religious ceremony to get better. However, he would do better by consulting a psychiatrist."

In summary, the TAT stories were generally characterized by poor performance, poor content, slowed thought and speech, though only rarely was any patient uncooperative. Most of the stories were sketchy and descriptive, of poor quality, short, superficial, and with little personal involvement. They did not, therefore, permit a complete psychological personality assessment. The themes were childish, with the occasional emergence of primitive interests and magical solutions associated with incapacity to realistically perceive the environment. An atmosphere of sadness, unhappiness, or impotence in the face of reality forces and the life struggle was a frequent characteristic. Other stories presented a high degree of naïvete and concreteness, revealing restricted imaginal resources. Besides this, most suggested strong wishes to be passive and dependent. Perceptual distortions were widespread and suggestive of impaired capacity to relate to others except via passive dependency. Evidence of suppressed or repressed hostility and identity uncertainty was marked.

DISCUSSION

The test findings suggest personalities which are constricted, uncreative, and intellectually unproductive. They describe people impaired in their capacities to relate to others, to perceive themselves and others in complex differentiated terms, and with defective capacities for ego and interpersonal control. They tend to be passive and dependent, searching futilely for succorance, ready to regress to magical solutions and primitive world views, dejected, uncertain as to their identities—including their masculine status—ready to see themselves as abased, ill, decaying, mutilated, alone, or "merely alive." They are immature, prone under stress to see themselves as children, emotionally shallow, engaging easily in escapist or occasionally self-censoring tendencies. They blot out or distort unfamiliar or unacceptable perceptions. Their worlds are peopled by religious and folkloric figures as well as by representatives of unremittingly harsh reality. They reveal no aggression or hostility except for that turned against themselves.

How much of this picture can be attributed to psychiatric illness per se, to culture, or to the complex of factors associated with depressed socioeconomic status, personal and political powerlessness, and lack of education and literacy? The data contain a few suggestions. They indicate that some of the narrowing of attention, stereotypy of perception and constrictive world view is probably defensive in nature. These processes reflect an automatic unconscious effort to deal by repression and related mechanisms with potentially overwhelming anxiety and threat of personality disorganization. In addition, they appear to reflect the operation of various forms of perceptual limitation, including denial—the automatic exclusion from conscious awareness of especially threatening information from the outside world. The threat seems inherent in complexity and variety of a sort requiring more frequent and active discriminations and decisions. Presumably, for those who see themselves as powerless and ineffective, each such decision carries the danger of serious environmental or adaptive error as well as of impulsive expression of drives or wishes. The threat also appears to rest significantly on a valid perception of the surrounding society as one which may unpredictably attempt to influence the patient in order to achieve its own ends. Such influence may be forceful-aggressive, seductive, or concealed, but is exerted without concern for the patient's personal needs and integrity. Nonetheless, the patient continues, though anxiously and with little hope, to scan the outside world for possibilities of dependent gratification. He can perceive himself relating to it only by passive impersonal submission or via a regressive childlike role, by establishing a passive-dependent relationship in which his own adult identity is surrendered. This behavior, including regressive and externalizing tendencies, can plausibly be attributed to the complex psychosocial factors associated with powerlessness and cultural exclusion, regardless of particular cultural context. In addition, these patients use specific culturally available religious-folkloric figures and concepts in the service of the defensive, adaptive, and coping needs.

In the case of aggression or of hostile impulses, the defensive operation may be reinforced by overall cultural as well as social-class related factors. Hostile expression within the Brazilian family, especially against the authoritative father, is unacceptable and carries with it the threat not only of active retaliation, but worse, of loss of love. This is true, though less clearly, outside the family where certain institutionalized forms of gossip and participation in religious, cultist, or Spiritist ceremonies may provide culturally acceptable outlets. It seems probable that for these passive, help seeking, powerless patients any awareness of outwardly directed hostile wishes carries significant danger of loss of support and even of human contact. This would mean not only inability to survive, but rejection confirming one's essential worthlessness and unlovability. As indicated in the test results, awareness even of affectional needs seems dangerous.

This last consideration leads back again to the question already answered in part: what does it mean to be at the bottom of the prestige hierarchy, without social power, lacking the education and symbolic equipment to fully participate in the surrounding socioculture or even to become fully oriented in it, blocked in terms of upward mobility, chronically struggling to keep oneself and family "merely alive," and constantly reminded of one's lack of dignity, worth, and effective power in the eyes of others? Does this have particular significance in a socioculture which historically has emphasized the importance of *dignidade* and masculine virility? How do these factors influence projective test results?

There are few studies from other settings which directly illuminate these issues. Riessman and Miller (1958) have, however, reviewed a body of United States literature which does establish that low social class and its corollaries can significantly influence projective test results. Haggard (1954) has shown that such factors as test-taking experience, rapport with the examiner, motivation, language used in the test items, reading ability, and required response speed can markedly limit the performance of the lower-class child and contaminate the resultant picture of his intelligence. Since Haggard's study a large number of investigators have reported data suggesting that conventional measures of intelligence are negatively influenced by early life in a slum environment. Some implicated elements have been lack of sufficiently varied and manageable intellectual and sensory stimulation, lack of consistent relationship with a rewarding parental figure, and excessive coping demands from concrete environmental stress. Auld (1952), noting that most personality tests indicate more maladjustment or neuroticism within the lower class, suggested that many responses leading to this conclusion are, in fact, simply accurate reports of the lower-class respondent's reality situation. This seems true to a significant degree in the present patient sample. Differences in social norms have been shown by Rosenberg (1949) to lead to higher neuroticism scores by lower-class subjects on the Bernreuter Inventory. Gough (1948) and others have found that middle-class subjects are more adept than the lower-class at giving the conventional "adjusted" responses.

Data more immediately relevant to the Rorschach responses reported above have also been presented by Auld. Findings on lower-class compared with middle-class United States patients, which resemble those reported above, included: fewer total responses, proportionately fewer color and movement responses, and proportionately equal animal and human movement in contrast to proportionately more human movement responses. According to the usual Rorschach criteria these data indicate that lower-class subjects are less responsive to their environment and lacking in emotional warmth.

Rorschach data from lower-class in comparison to middle-class children studied by Stone and Fiedler (1956) included the following findings which resemble those reported above: more animal responses, proportionately more animal than human movement, less color-form, fewer whole responses, and fewer small details. While contrary to other findings, Stone and Fiedler's lower-class children gave more responses and more form-color, a closely related study confirmed the previous findings. This was carried out by Carlson (1952) on eight-year-old children. Those in the lower-class group had significantly fewer form-color and color-form responses, and used far less color in general than the middle-class group. Riessman and Miller (1958) suggest that some of the above findings may reflect the greater stress experienced by lower-class than middle-class subjects in the test situation. Decreased color responses in stress situations have been reported by Eichler (1951), and by Kimble (1945) who also noted diminished movement responses. Klatskin's (1952) review of literature on the impact of the test situation on Rorschach data noted that color responses are most affected by stress.

An alternative to the stress hypothesis suggested by Riessman and Miller is that lower-class response patterns are due mainly to apathy and lack of interest. Lower-class children, for example, as pointed out by Davis (1948), try to finish intelligence tests as quickly as possible and, typically, are uninterested in the task. Riessman's own data suggest that working-class men find Rorschach test material particularly unstimulating. It does not fit their desire for structure and definiteness, and constitutes a kind of task which they do not find immediately meaningful. This fits the comments of many of the lower-class Brazilian respondents who, as noted above, characterized the test tasks as meaningless and childish. In this sense the most readily given responses, requiring the least personal involvement or interest, and most available in the presence of high anxiety are those reflecting form and animal perceptions. In support of this idea Riessman and Miller note the evidence of Douvan (1956), of Useem and collaborators (1942), and others, that personality patterns of United States working men when their studies were done were "built around a cooperative, solidaristic, outgoing, emotionally responsive orientation, hardly reflected in the Rorschach pattern, especially the lack of color responses" (p. 252).

The Thematic Apperception Test has stimulated fewer methodological questions as to its cross-cultural applicability than the Rorschach, perhaps because its pictures lend themselves more easily to appropriate modification. Riessman and Miller report two social-class comparisons. Mason and Ammons (1956) noted, for example, that in upper-class stories a burgular was clever and escaped but in lower-class stories he was caught. These stories, like those from the present study population, clearly reflect some of the powerless aspects of lower-class life. Korchin (1950) found that, compatible with the present study, lower-class subjects gave shorter stories than those from the middle-class. Aside from the relevance of TAT pictures to particular populations, the same type of testing and interactional problems would seem to occur in relation to a lower-class subject as with the Rorschach. Among these are the likelihood that few lower-class persons have had experience in making up stories from pictures, and that inhibitions developed in relation to teachers and other authority figures may further impair their ability to communicate with an examiner.

One reported study on a population which shares many of the features of the present test sample is that of Klein (1966) who administered the TAT to a group of Andean Indian peasants leading the life of serfs on a large mountain plantation in Peru. These people, who were not patients and not considered deviant in any way, were more abjectly powerless than the lowest-class Rio de Janeiro slum-dwellers. In contrast to Rio, they had to contend with the harshest of climatic variations and were surrounded by the most inhospitable physical environment. For generations their families had lived in inbred peasant villages under the control of administrators, usually acting for absentee landowners, who had not stopped at murder to maintain discipline. A combination of interview and modified TAT techniques yielded protocols dominated by themes of passivity, loneliness, death, defenselessness, and the capricious power of nature and of other people. The self-concept was one of impotence and ineffectuality in the face of a powerful and malevolent world. Klein interpreted his data mainly in defensive terms: the responses indicated a defensive avoidance of sensation, of mobility, of interaction with others (hostile and power oriented), and of communication (to avoid the danger of exposure) which was necessary only for manipulating others. Emotions were expressed only as fear of rage of others and of being alone. Fried (1962), who also studied this society, noted that beliefs in the inevitability of a cruel environment have been institutionalized, and that there is no pressure for members of the group to aspire to less brutal living conditions, or even to pretend to feel anything for each other. These uneducated Indians, leading harsher and more hopeless lives with less potential for self-determination than the lower-class Brazilian patients in the test sample, provide a type of control group composed of people whose subjective discomfort has not passed the level which they accept as customary or "normal." Their TAT stories were also colored by themes of hopelessness, dejection, and perceptions of themselves as less than human, fragile, and disintegrating. Their responses support the idea that many of the projective test responses of the Rio patients reflect their life conditions and the nature of their participation in a particular sociocultural context rather than just the nature of a neurotic or psychotic process. The degree to which Klein's results reflect the stress of an unfamiliar testing situation or the impact of a task with no significant personal meaning is uncertain.

The differences in the present sample between interview behavior with physicians and social workers in a familiar helping role and psychologists in an unfamiliar testing role suggest that the stress and meaning factors discussed above do have some importance. Although the patients' rejection rate was low on testing, their productivity was noticeably less than with the physicians to whom they related in a traditionally help-seeking, dependent way, and with whom the expected behavior was familiar and immediately relevant, i.e., telling about their problems. Having been already hospitalized and exposed to interviews and other procedures, it seems unlikely, however, that testing constituted a stress in the sense of a specific demand for self-revelation. A number of other possibilities are inherent in the situation. One possible source of stress was the unfamiliarity of the task, requiring effort to comprehend it. This is different from lack of meaningfulness which may produce apathy and disinterest—although withdrawal and apathy are frequently encountered as reflections of defensive efforts to deal with anxiety. A second possible source of stress was the sex of the tester. For the male patient, the challenge to demonstrate his masculinity is always there, and this challenge becomes especially hopeless when he is not only sick but of a lower class with less socioeconomic power than the woman. Under these circumstances his only solution may be the adoption of a dependent role in which he relates to her as a child to his mother. This element may account for some of the regressive, immature, passive-dependent responses in the data. The confrontation with a more powerful and unreachable female may also stimulate hostility in the man; this hostility, dangerously unacceptable because of the threat it poses to the potentially helpful relationship, must be dealt with by suppression and repression as well as by denial of the cues from the tester (or symbols of the tester) which sustain it.

Beyond these issues is the question of how early and current life experience, in the powerless, deprived, uneducated, tired, person who has become a psychiatric casualty influences personality, as revealed by projective testing. As noted above, some of the patients' responses simply reflected the realities of their lives. Depression and hopelessness are understandable concomitants of a predisposition stemming from childhood deprivation to which is added inability as an adult to achieve a better life for oneself and one's family. The patients are at the mercy of forces beyond their reach. They are dropouts whose adaptive and defensive mechanisms have failed. Failure is a function both of current stress and of initial resources as influenced by early life experience. Their developmental experiences have been mainly in slums or working the land on remote farms, unaided and unstimulated by continuing formal education, dependent upon parents themselves worn by an abrasive life with little energy to spend on their children. Under these circumstances innate intellectual-cognitive capacities have had little chance to flourish and grow. The demands upon them have been largely for concrete, survival-oriented thinking and perceiving. People outside the immediate family have been viewed primarily as competitors for the scarce available resources. This means that they could not be perceived as rich individual personalities but only in terms of leading characteristics and potential threats. In the classic psychoanalytic sense, adult experience, on the base of early life predispositions, has produced a state of chronic narcissistic frustration and low self-esteem. Impor-

tant figures holding out the possibility of nurturance or authoritative guidance are reacted to ambivalently, and whatever hostility
threatens to emerge is defensively repressed and turned against
the devalued self. Realistically, responsibility for one's life course
is external—determined by the plantation owner, the employer,
the policeman, the mayor, or governor. The tendency to externalize is reinforced by the thickly peopled spirit and folk Catholic
world of the rural areas and the Spiritism, Macumba, and Umbanda, as well as the Catholic and fundamentalist Protestant
churches of the city. The route to problem solving, then, is primarily through regression (primitive thinking, magical solutions,
childlike dependence upon outer forces), or projection (attributing
to other people or groups one's own unacceptable and unconscious wishes).

It seems plausible to conclude that the projective test results,
including the impact of situational stress and lack of personal relevance, do provide important clues to the psychological organization of these patients. While the data must be understood as produced by psychiatrically decompensated individuals, they appear
to be at least as reflective of the test sample's position at the bottom of the socioeconomic structure as of mental illness as such.
Aside from references to folkloric and religious figures, and perhaps some problems around the expression of hostile wishes, these
data seem to reflect factors transcending the boundaries of Brazilian culture and present in persons from the lowest socioeconomic
strata throughout the world.

CHAPTER 13

A TRANSCULTURAL VIEW
OF SYMPTOMATIC BEHAVIOR
AND SOCIAL ENVIRONMENT

THE PRECEDING chapters have been concerned largely with the behaviors of psychiatric patients according to particular sociocultural statuses. They have described migratory, color, occupational, educational, and other statuses arising as part of the Rio de Janeiro context, and dealt with the psychiatrically relevant behaviors of people occupying these statuses. Status and role have been considered indicators of participation in the social process, and thus of the nature of the individual's relationships with his environment or behavioral setting. The present chapter approaches the problem from the other end of the equation. It focuses first on the behavior itself. That is, it describes anxious, depressed, paranoid, hallucinatory, and other behaviors, and then deals with the sociocultural statuses which contribute to their occurrence. In the preceding chapters discussion centered on the behavioral concomitants of a particular sociocultural status; in this chapter discussion will center on the sociocultural concomitants of a particular type of symptomatic behavior.

The word transcultural is used in Wittkower's (1967) sense to designate behavior which transcends a particular socioculture—behavior which can be identified in a variety of sociocultural settings. While this volume has referred to specific aspects of Rio de Janeiro and Brazilian life, its implicit concerns are social-psychiatric universals. The realities, stresses, and supports which determine the selection of Brazilians to become mental hospital patients and influence the nature of their psychiatrically labeled behavior have their counterparts throughout the world, especially in developing nations. Geographic and social mobility, urbanization, and the tensions associated with ethnically pluralistic societies require major attention in almost all metropolitan centers. The frustrations associated with discrepant aspirations and achievements, the problems associated with the shifting significance of age and sex status, the influence of physical stress on subjective experience, and the search for tension reduction by means of religous or other affiliations affect symptomatic behavior throughout the world. Suspicious, depressed, or anxious symptoms and attitudes cannot be understood without reference to the social context in which they occur, and most social contexts contain the same behaviorally relevant elements.

The traditional psychodynamic approach based on Freud's (1926) early concepts of ego defenses can, with the addition of Hartmann's (1939) adaptational concepts, provide a convenient beginning for the scrutiny of symptomatic behavior in relation to its social context. All behavioral settings confront the individual and his family with special adaptational challenges, opportunities for personal support and realization, and threats and dangers. All tend to reinforce, perpetuate, or extinguish certain behaviors. Some of these behaviors can be understood as reflecting coping or adaptive processes; others reflect ego-defensive processes. The former are concerned with establishing and maintaining a more or less stable reciprocal relationship between the individual and his (usually interpersonal) environment and can involve changing the environment. The latter are concerned with the maintenance of a more or less stable intrapsychic equilibrium. This involves keeping anxiety, guilt, shame, or other forms of psychological tension at a manageable level by inhibiting the conscious awareness or active expression of disturbing impulses, feelings, or ideas. Inhibition or control of this type is accomplished by the operation of various automatically triggered defense mechanisms. These mechanisms, never totally effective, permit some tensional discharge or gratification of unacceptable impulses in disguised form. Such discharge or gratification is ego-syntonic rather than ego-alien, i.e., it is subjectively experienced as normal or usual (no matter what the opinion of other observers) rather than as a symptom or foreign body. The repertory of defense mechanisms available to a person, their patterning and probability of use, along with their related complement of adaptive and coping devices combine with the nature of his available equipment (e.g., intelligence, talent, motor capacities, acquired skills) to form what is generally known as character or personality. Thereby a type of steady-state equilibrium is achieved involving both intrapsychic and interpersonal regulatory mechanisms; it requires the monitoring of information from within (based mainly on early programming, i.e., genetic, developmental, and experiential aspects of past personal history) and from without (based mainly on current environmental circumstances, i.e., the nature of the behavioral setting).

The preceding chapters have stressed the probable interdependence of psychological phenomena and the social environments in which they occur. They have presented the Rio de Janeiro behavioral setting as one maintained and modified by the actors within it; they noted further that "environmental input" or meaningful stimuli, i.e., the information received by the inhabitants or actors, varies with the latters' social and related biobehavioral differences. The degree to which adult behavior defined as symptomatic or psychiatrically sick varies with environmental events cannot be precisely stated. Too many variables are unknown. As indicated above, these (including physical illness or accident) include not only items which may be retrieved through retrospective past histories, but also those requiring detailed genetic study or on-the-spot longitudinal observation during infancy and childhood. Nonetheless, certain regularities become apparent when patient populations are scrutinized with respect to both sociocultural and behavioral variables. The present chapter attempts such a scrutiny, focusing on the most frequently encountered symptomatic behaviors in the study population. It suggests that certain life circumstances associated with a person's place in his socioculture (as revealed by his sociocultural status) do increase the likelihood that particular symptomatic behavior patterns will appear. These circumstances include recurring events which maintain or reinforce ongoing behavior. The interaction between individual behavior and the recurrent reinforcements which it elicits from others is basic to the social process. Individual behavior, whether defined as adaptive or symptomatic, can thus be understood as participation in the social process. While life circumstances may have direct impact upon the adult, their influence is understood here as resulting from a combination of such impact with a developmental experience conditioned by sociocultural factors mediated through the family.

THE TOTAL PATIENT POPULATION

SOCIOCULTURAL CHARACTERISTICS

As indicated in Chapter II, the investigation was originally planned to include the entire spectrum of socioeconomic status-related variables within the study population. Resistance by relatives and physicians of patients within the private sanitorium chosen for study, however, resulted in only five per cent of the 254 person patient sample coming from this source. Problems in interviewing patients before they were treated with drugs or ECT limited the number from the Pronto Socorro—source of the poorest patients and those least connected with social institutions—to 19 per cent of the total sample. Seventy-six per cent, or approximately three-quarters of the patients, therefore, came from the social security hospital, and the total group was more homogeneous in several respects than had been originally anticipated. As described in Chapter IV, 66 per cent of the patient population, or approximately twice the proportion in the population at large, had migrated into Rio within the preceding 10 years even though the large majority had sufficiently stable employment histories to qualify for social security care. Ten per cent had been born in the area and moved away as children, or, coming from towns in Rio State, had grown up in the urban sphere of influence and did not consider themselves migrants. Still, 55 per cent of the patients, in contrast to approximately 40 per cent of the population at large, had been born elsewhere and considered themselves migrant. Of these, at least 83 per cent had been reared and spent most of their lives in rural-provincial settings before coming to Rio. Using a five-year criterion, residential stability was greater: only 28 per cent of all the patients designated as recently migrant had resided within Greater Rio de Janeiro for five years or less. Seventy-two per cent designated as settled had been there for more than five years. Of this settled group, 38 per cent were migrants and the rest native. In other words, although at least half the patients had

had rural or isolated small-town backgrounds, almost three-quarters (including both natives and migrants) had lived in the metropolitan area for at leat five years. They were presumably enculturated and had had the opportunity to become part of a relatively stable interpersonal network.

The patient sample was representative of the Guanabara population as a whole in respect to color. As described in Chapter V, 64 per cent were classed as white, 24 per cent as brown, and 12 per cent as black. The proportion of whites, however, was considerably larger than in the *favela* or slum population.

The patients were less educated and less literate than the Guanabara population at large. As described in Chapter VI, 57 per cent had not completed the primary grades, and 29 per cent were illiterate or only partly literate. They were, however, better educated and more literate than the *favela* dwellers at large. The largest number of patients, 43 per cent, were, as described in Chapter VII, in occupational Class V; skilled manual workers. This is congruent with their major location in the social security hospital. No comparable data are available for Guanabara at large, although 44 per cent were listed in 1966 as "industrial," including unskilled as well as skilled workers. The proportion of Class V patients, however, is clearly higher than that for the nation at large with its continuing large percentage of agricultural laborers. Twenty-nine per cent of the patients were in Class VI, unskilled manual labor, and 25 per cent were from Classes I through IV combined. These last included nonmanual workers ranging from blue-collar supervisors through white-collar and a few professional persons. Female patients with no primary occupation other than housewife were categorized according to the employment status of their husbands, or for the one per cent unemployed and unmarried, of their fathers.

Favelados, i.e., dwellers in identified slum neighborhoods, are underrepresented in the patient sample despite the prevalence of inadequate housing. As shown in Chapter VIII, 42 per cent of patients or their accompanying relatives (in the instances of patients being brought to Rio for psychiatric care) lived in suburban areas associated with the relatively stable, skilled or unskilled working class, and 40 per cent lived in central, residential, or peripheral urban neighborhoods. Only 70 per cent of the group, however, had both electricity and running water in their homes, and 45 per cent had no separate sleeping room or were limited to such a space plus a kitchen and bath area (with or without water and/or electricity). The housing level of the patients reflected that of the Rio population at large.

The sex ratio, as indicated in Chapter IX, was 65 per cent male and 35 per cent female. Thirty-two per cent had never been married or had a consistent mate; 71 per cent of these single persons were male. Thirty-nine per cent had been married only once with both civil and religious ceremonies, while an additional 20 per cent reported civil ceremonies alone. Negligible numbers had been separated, widowed, married more than once, or were of undetermined status. Available census data do not provide reliable information for comparison with the general population. Given the age range of the patients, however, it seems probable that the females were married (legal or companionate) approximately as often as nonpatients of similar social class. The males, as noted in other societies, were probably less frequently married than those in the nonpatient Rio population at large.

The patients were mainly young and early mid-life adults. As described in Chapter X, 79 per cent were between 21 and 45 years of age; 22 per cent were between ages 15 and 25; 63 per cent between 26 to 45; and 15 per cent between 46 to 60. No patient had passed his 60th birthday. While this group obviously excluded the approximately one-third of the Guanabara population 14 years of age or younger, it fits the finding that as of 1960, only between six and seven percent of the total had attained age 60 or more.

Other features applicable to the patients as individuals and to the behavioral context of which they were part reflect the Brazilian cultural heritage and current stirrings of social change. They also emphasize the extent to which behavior may be viewed as participation in an ongoing historical as well as current social process, i.e., a process of cultural evolution. This process is significant for increasing numbers of people in all developing countries, as well as for deprived and culturally excluded populations in highly industrialized and developed nations such as the United States. Thus, the traditional Brazilian lower-class attitudes of dependency and passivity in regard to fate and to upper-class patrons co-exist with their new aspirations and developing self-awareness as workers: a new collectivity with shared values and negotiating leverage of its own. The traditional acceptance of Catholicism as an unquestioned part of the culture co-exists with an increasingly intense search by growing numbers of people for new religious forms offering immediate gratifications and reinforcing an economically productive life style, rather than delayed heavenly salvation after a life of deprivation. A continuing high evaluation of an elitist education co-exists with increasing awareness that the educational system tends to impede rather than foster upward social mobility. The movement of large numbers of rural and small town migrants continues into metropolitan centers without the jobs, housing, sanitary, educational, and social services necessary to accommodate them; this co-exists with developing disillusionment about the opportunities offered by the city, and anger at government and social agencies for their failure to provide the needed basic services. The traditional institutionalization of "respectful" relationships between black and white is just at the beginning of change; it co-exists, however, with growing discontent and resentment among the browns, more sensitive than in the past to their marginal status and driven by newly acquired and still unachievable aspirations. In short, this patient population is part of a context of early but potentially massive social change. Most are just beginning to be caught up in the "revolution of rising expectations." Most may plausibly be described in terms used by Riessman and colleagues (1964) when discussing psychotherapy for the poor. For them, "self-determination" may be a necessary prerequisite to "self-realization."

Approximately two-thirds of the patient population were working, responsibly involved with others, and clearly part of the cultural evolutionary process as their behavior became increasingly identifiable as symptomatic. The other third had not become part of the socially productive and responsible population prior to the onset of symptoms. They include most of the unmarried and most of the 22 per cent between the ages of 15 and 25 (with almost all of the six per cent under age 21). These resembled patients diagnosed as schizophrenic in other countries; their disturbed behavior had begun for the most part while still living with their parents. Many had been kept at home despite long periods of clear psychiatric disturbance until socially disruptive behavior, often evoking hostile responses in others, made it impossible to further delay hospital admission. They included most who were brought to Rio from elsewhere in Brazil specifically for hospitalization.

BECOMING A PATIENT

Seventy-two per cent of the patients were brought to the hospital by members of their immediate families (parents, spouses, siblings, or children) or other relatives residing with them or nearby. Another four per cent arrived under police escort or in official ambulances which had been sent out to pick them up for having created a disturbance. The remaining 24 per cent came in the company of private physicians, friends, clergy, neighbors, social welfare workers, employers or other colleagues at work, or more remote relatives. The evidence of familial support is in impressive contrast to the number of those appearing alone at an Inner City clinic in Baltimore, as well as to the suggestions of family detachment in more chronically ill or socially unacceptable cases in Brazil. Ninety-four per cent of all patients had accessible relatives in the city who were able to contribute information about personal history, the present illness and reasons for admission. The nature of the information sought, however, required the primary source of overall data to be the patient, himself.

Approximately 10 per cent of the first-time admissions making up this sample came alone (by definition self-referred). Solitary arrival, however, characterized many not in the study group, who, having had previous admissions, sought help independently at the Pronto Socorro as they recognized the recurrence of symptoms in themselves.

Table 208, which shows the reasons given by the patients' families, friends, or the authorities for bringing them to the hospital, reveals that overtly deviant behavior in the presence of family members was a factor precipitating hospitalization for almost two-thirds of the patients. The specific events identified as crucial for the largest number (20 per cent) were statements of an anxious, depressed, or suicidal nature. It is clear that families were most disturbed by evidence of subjective pain or mental suffering in their relatives. The next most important stimuli for family concern, acts of a bizarre, aggressive, or paranoid variety, including self-destructive attempts—as was true also for refusal to work—did not necessarily include evidence of the patient's personal suffering. In these instances the patients's behavior was physically or economically threatening to the family, or grossly incompatible with their social roles.

As noted in previous chapters and summarized in Table 209, the circumstances leading to hospitalization usually varied to some degree with sociocultural status. Physical assaults or threats were primary reasons for admission for approximately a third of the blacks (almost three times the frequency for either whites or browns). Such behavior was also a proportionately more frequent reason for hospitalization among the less educated, nonliterate, male, and unmarried. These groups include many whose capacity for verbal symbolic representation and communication with others is limited. Beyond this, the relatively high degree of tolerance for deviant behavior within the most culturally excluded subcommunities, and the self-esteem gaining value of aggressiveness for the unmarried (young) male black and those without skills, increases the probable occurrence of dramatic aggressive behavior, evoking immediate fear in onlookers, as a cry for help and a means of self-expression.

Refusal or inability to work is another behavior imposing particular strain on economically depressed families. As expected, this was a more frequent reason for hospitalization (although in a small absolute percentage of patients) among the recently migrant, the nonliterate and the uneducated. More browns than blacks reported this as an issue; the sensitivity of brown families to this point is considered a reflection of their frustrated achievement strivings. Similarly, this was present for a few more of those in the youngest group. In this last instance their long developmental history of illness suggests that inability or refusal to work may be logically understood as inability to assume an expected social role once a certain age is reached. It is at this point that the family diagnosis of mental illness is confirmed and the decision to seek help crystallized.

Paranoid or grandiose behavior as a reason for hospitalization fits the same general pattern. The families moved to definitive action by such statements from their members included proportionately more of the nonwhite, the uneducated, the illiterate, the unskilled, and the poorly housed. While the decision to hospitalize can be understood as a response to intolerable and threatening deviance, comparable in some measure to assault, it also occurs in a context marked by mistrust. These subgroups constitute a realistically oppressed population within which suspiciousness and feelings of persecution directed against both societal powerholders and neighbors are evident so that such behavior must become especially intense and its targets clearly inappropriate in order to move families toward hospitalization.

Apart from these considerations paranoid behavior was a more frequent reason for hospitalization in the youngest group. This fits the general impression of this group as more chronically and pervasively ill than the older patients; as noted in Chapter IX, a high degree of deviance also appears necessary before parents will seek psychiatric care in a paternalistic socioculture reluctant to admit its inability to socialize and to label or hospitalize its adolescent members.

The category of other bizarre acts is confused. On the one hand it includes unusual behavior not conveniently classified as assaultive or paranoid; on the other it includes co-existing acts. The single striking finding is that approximately a third of the Protestants were admitted because of paranoid or grandiose behavior, while none where admitted because of other bizarre acts. The Protestants, somewhat older, more often female, more frequently married, and more recently migrant than the other religious groups were more closely integrated into families; they apparently met family needs and expectations for conformity in most respects until their suspiciousness and feelings of being persecuted threatened family solidarity. Their relatively prominent paranoid behavior also reflects the number of recent migrants among them as well as the interpersonal sensitivity and upward striving associated with having chosen Protestantism as a way of life as well as a religion.

Anxious, depressed, or suicidal behavior was relatively more frequent as a cause for admission among the whites, the married, and the settled. This distribution does not appear to reflect the operation of a general SES factor insofar as it was proportionately least common among the literates and more common among the

Class V skilled occupations than among the unskilled or the nonmanual. The mixture reflects in part the more frequent distribution of symptoms such as insomnia among the deprived, and of symptoms such as suicidal thoughts among the relatively advantaged having more apparent social responsibilities. Being white, married, and settled share with occupational Class V the features of relative social and interpersonal security. Families accustomed to mutual, reciprocally affective relations might be expected to show relatively high sensitivity to evidence of subjective pain and to seek help for relatives on this basis rather than awaiting the appearance of more dramatic and frighteningly disturbed behavior.

Family or community explanations for the behaviors leading to hospitalization are listed in Table 210. Mental or physical illness were each offered as diagnosis or explanation for almost a third of the patients. Ideas about the remaining third included various types of life stress, most prominently persecution, religious or cultist influence, and negative characterological value judgements. Ten per cent of respondents offered no opinion.

As summarized in Table 211, without exception, and in most cases significantly, higher proportions of the least advantaged and socially stable families labeled the patients as suffering from "mental illness." For the recently rural migrants, the black, the uneducated, illiterate, and poorly housed this diagnosis is assumed to be a recently learned way of labeling otherwise confusing behavior initially regarded as a reaction to stress or as susceptible to religious or cultist cure. These were families, which having finally sought help from conventional medical authorities, had probably, as customary for them, accepted the diagnostic opinion of the powerholders. The families of the young and the unmarried, including more parents and fewer spouses, had not been so accustomed as the others to seeing their sick relatives in socially competent roles; more habituated to perceiving them as chronically "different," the diagnosis of mental illness was not alien for them. In contrast, the more educated and socially secure families tended more often to adhere to their own opinions rather than accept the official medical classifications. Thus proportionately more of them regarded the patients' behavior as resulting from life stress or evaluated it in socially judgmental terms as strange or morally undesirable. The black, uneducated, illiterate, and poorly housed were least judgmental and more accepting of their relatives' disturbed behavior as something over which they had no control, just as they seemed to be less critical of the doctors' opinions. The less frequent judgmental attitude of Protestants and Afro-Spiritists may be attributed to their sense of connection with the supernatural and a consequently greater tolerance for behavioral deviation according to ordinary temporal-secular criteria.

In most instances help-seeking did not seem to begin with the idea of isolating the disturbed relative in a mental hospital. More than a third of the patients, as seen in Table 212, had exhibited behavior probably diagnosable as mental illness from one to 12 months prior to hospitalization; almost another third had shown such symptoms for one year or longer. Any description of behavior in terms recognizable by a professional as psychiatric illness must be at least a partial function of sociocultural circumstances. As expected, significantly more (between 50 and 60 per cent in each instance as compared to 35 to 41 per cent) nonmigrant, educated, literate, occupationally nonmanual, and better housed patients had had psychiatric contact before hospitalization. These findings probably reflect financial capacity as well as the physical availability of resources, information, and the presence of an integrated supporting family. Significantly more females than males and married than single patients also had such contact, again emphasizing the supportive value of the family in maintaining disturbed members outside of hospitals, with the aid of outpatient facilities. This finding is not immediately compatible with that of Rogler and Hollingshead (1965) which suggests less familial support for psychiatrically disturbed wives than husbands in a Puerto Rican slum population. The relatively high proportion of youthful patients among the single is relevant, since, as noted before, families seem to prefer to deal with their disturbed adolescent members themselves rather than enlist professional help.

The failure to find differences in this respect according to color is unexpected, especially since (as shown in Chapter V), a larger proportion of whites than nonwhites were hospitalized at the social security facility providing prior outpatient care. The significant differences in most respects are not between whites and blacks but in relation to browns, more of whom were seen in the emergency facility. This suggests that while nonwhites do indeed have longer periods of illness in relatively tolerant communities with some contact with nonmedical agencies of social control, this is more true for browns than blacks. As noted (in Chapter V), blacks have a significantly higher occurrence than browns or whites of apparent illness lasting one month or less. But given their more dramatic behavior precipitating hospitalization, it seems probable that behavior identified as illness in this instance includes only those assaultive or bizarre acts evoking immediate response from social controllers. The importance of such controllers as well as family members in achieving hospitalization for the blacks is revealed by the fact that none of them (as noted in Chapter V) arrived at the hospital alone. The relative acuteness of their disturbances leading to hospitalization, then, may be less due to the conventional filtering system leading to the hospital than to the religious filter, i.e., Afro-Spiritist centers, plus a socioculturally fostered tendency to express psychological problems in the form of acute, physically active, hallucinatory episodes with some clouding of the sensorium. Such "oneiroform psychoses," as discussed in Chapter VI, have been reported in a variety of preliterate settings. A detailed discussion of this phenomenon among the lowest-class Mapuche in Santiago de Chile is provided by Munoz et al. (1966).

Data are not available on those patients who first sought help from general physicians, but it appears that many invoked the healing functions of their religious groups. This was probably true for nine per cent of patients and their immediate families declaring an affiliation with Protestant sects. As noted above, people are often reluctant to acknowledge membership in or attendance at Spiritist, Umbanda, or Macumba centers. The prominent healing functions of these, however, may be assumed to have been important for at least the five per cent of patients acknowledging formal Afro-Brazilian or Spiritist membership. Table 173 shows that an additional three per cent of the unaffiliated, 18 per cent of the Catholic, and 15 per cent of the Protestant patients acknowledged occasional but continuing attendance at such ceremonies, contributing to a total of 22 per cent of the patients who were regularly involved in Afro-Spiritist observances. When to this is added the fact that two-thirds of the entire patient group made at least casual reference to the healing functions of Afro-Spiritist centers, the assumption is strongly supported that they were among the first sources of assistance to which these disturbed people or their families turned. This assumption is furthur supported by the report (noted in Chapter XI) that 90 per cent of INPS patients coming to Casa Eiras, the main source for the present study, and 50 per cent of private patients seen at the same institution had first consulted Afro-Spiritist practitioners. These data resemble those emerging from the small random sample of University Psychiatric Institute patients (described in Chapter XI); nine of 10 women and five of 10 men had had at least brief prior contact (not always overtly help seeking) with a center.

Because (as indicated in Chapter XI) most Afro-Spiritist and Protestant healing-sect leaders prefer not to diagnose "illness" in the Western sense except as a rationalization for their own failure to heal, the likelihood is high that the initial inclination of family and community was to explain the patients' subjective pain or strange behavior on religious, spiritual, or magical grounds. The diagnoses and explanations listed in Table 209 were elicited only when other methods of treatment had failed and hospitalization had come to be the only alternative. This involvement of religious and cultist groups in the social control and behavior labeling system is not found to the same degree in major United States urban centers. The striking exception is in Puerto Rico which shares many of the sociocultural features of "developing" countries everywhere, particularly those in Latin America. Here, as Rogler and Hollingshead (1965) have indicated: "Spiritualist groups do not withdraw from the mentally ill person; on the contrary, they encourage him to become an active member. The ideology of Spiritualism provides an acceptable meaning to symptoms which are otherwise stigmatized" (p. 412).

The observations of Brody et al. (1967) for lower-class Negro males in Baltimore do not implicate religious or similar groups as significant in delaying the identification of psychiatrically disturbed behavior. Rather, the overwhelming factor delaying hospital admission in the United States urban centers is repeated contact with the police who perceive unusual behavior as social deviance, to be dealt with punitively rather than therapeutically.

These formal behavioral controllers appear to grow in importance with the decline, in a highly industrialized and anonymous society, of the effectiveness of informal groups such as those of a quasi-religious nature. Industrialization and institutionalized racial prejudice have contributed to chronic unemployment of undereducated black males unable to maintain instrumental and leadership roles in their families. Under these circumstances the mothers' utilization of the police and the "judge" in their efforts to control and socialize their sons perpetuates an uneasy alliance of client and legal enforcer in the process of behavioral control. Families themselves also contribute to delayed identification of psychiatrically significant behavior by referring it to the police or by viewing it as adaptive, i.e., as reflecting a realistic adaptation to oppressive social forces. Both Negro females and whites are perceived and dealt with less punitively by families and police.

The importance of the police as the gateway to the mental hospital in the United States is not confined to black patients. Hollingshead and Redlich's (1958) study of an almost exclusively white New Haven population demonstrated this to be true for lowest social class patients first admitted with a diagnosis of psychotic behavior. Social agencies rather than the police, however, provided more important gateways for those diagnosed as neurotic. These findings underline another difference between lower class Brazilian and United States patients: the importance of the family in psychiatric referral. As indicated above, Brazilian family decisions pre-eminently determined the final move to the mental hospital for the large majority of patients. In contrast, the more developed United States is characterized by dependence upon members of the new occupations who man the social agencies; these have arisen to replace the declining socializing and social control functions of families and naturally occurring informal groups. In the United States upper and middle classes families, friends, and self-awareness of impending psychological crises continue to be primary determinants of hospitalization.

The approximately one-third of the Brazilian families who regarded their family members as suffering from "mental illness" suggests a considerable difference even from Hollingshead and Redlich's New Haven middle-class group, most of whom were "unable to accept a psychogenic explanation of their relative's difficulties" (p. 341). The differences from Classes IV and V, more socially comparable to the present group, are still greater since these last regarded mental illnesses mainly as "somatic diseases." Whether these differences between the *Cariocas* and New Haveners are the result of the more than 10 years of public education elapsing between the two studies, or, as suggested above, of the gradual shift in attitude of Brazilian relatives over months of unsuccessful work with religious healers, or of their more humanistic and person-oriented outlook, is uncertain. Yet, the more intense personal involvement of these lower-class Brazilians with their psychiatrically ill relatives suggests that a more personal orientation, with greater value placed upon affective contact, may indeed increase their receptivity to psychological explanations of disturbed behavior.

The past history events listed in Table 213 are another indication of the attitudes of patients and families toward their difficulties. Such remembered events serve as reference points around which to organize seemingly disparate phenomena and satisfy the need to discover causative external events to explain the troubling and mysterious. Expectedly, recent happenings were most widely implicated. Thus, almost half the patients or their families believed events occurring during adulthood to have had psychologically traumatic significance for them. Marital conflict was reported for 40 per cent of the cases. This fits Rogler and Hollinghead's (1965) findings for a Puerto Rican slum population, where extreme marital tension consequent to inability to fill the expected social roles of husband or wife was a prominent aspect of the year preceding the perceived onset of mental (schizophrenic) illness.

More remote psychic trauma occurring in childhood was reported less frequently for the present population. Awareness of developmental problems and of chronically pre-existing adaptational difficulties was, however, revealed in reports of rage episodes, school or work adjustment problems, and inability to achieve bladder control. Such difficulties (as indicated in Chapter X) were reported for significantly more of the youngest patient group. While this seems partly due to their relative recency, it probably also reflects the developmental history of pervasive behavior disorder in those people becoming patients in late adolesence or early adulthood. These problems were reported with significantly least frequency (as shown in Chapter XI) for the Afro-Spiritist patients, probably in consequence of their denial of the importance of conventional past historical experiences. The proportionately highest report of adult and adolescent rages for the unaffiliated (62 per cent) fits their generally higher level of agitation in comparison with the other religious subgroupings.

Fainting spells and/or lapses of consciousness were reported for a quarter of the patients and other episodes of altered consciousness for smaller numbers. Clear-cut signs of neurological disease were not observed, but seizures or fainting were most often reported, 33 per cent, for unskilled manual workers, Class VI. Head injuries with loss of consciousness were reported for 23 per cent of this group and 22 per cent of the religiously unaffiliated, significantly more than for their comparison groups. The other group with evidence suggesting similar involvement was the partially literate. High fevers with altered consciousness were reported for 31 per cent of these. These data, not accompanied by consistent findings for other sociocultural statuses, do not suggest a general SES-linked finding. Rather (as discussed in Chapter VI), they may identify the partly literate group as marginal because of minimal brain damage. While Class VI workers are indeed at the bottom of the socioeconomic scale, they are less dramatically so than the illiterate and share many features with the black, the poorly housed, the recently migrant, and the Protestant. The relative prominence of loss of consciousness and head injury for this group alone may, therefore, be more easily associated with the specific effort and hazards associated with occupational status than with low general SES.

The significance of seizures, head injuries, or other similar events indicating brain damage as contributory to a variety of psychiatric symptoms is widely accepted as probable, but is not established. Knobloch and Pasamanick (1966) for example, have estimated that interruption of the "cycle of reproductive insult" characterized by damage to the intrauterine infant during delivery or in the first few months of extrauterine life by illness, malnutrition, injury, or other poverty-related factors would result in a significant reduction of the United States institutionalized population. Pollin and Stabenau (1968) suggest a variety of damaging factors, especially those leading to intrauterine hypoxia, with associated "soft" neurological signs, as important for the final emergence of schizophrenic symptomatology in genetically loaded individuals. While such factors are undoubtedly significant in mentally hospitalized populations of developing countries with inadequate public health services, their relationship to specific symptom patterns and their frequency in comparison to the United States is not established. The extent of organically based behavior disorder leading to mental hospitalization in the United States is indicated by Kramer's (1967) estimate, based upon 1963 data, that more than 26 per cent of admissions to state and county mental hospitals are due to brain syndromes. This does not include the over 16 per cent diagnosed as alcoholic nor does it take into account the possible contribution of organic factors to disorders with other psychiatric labels. (It should be remembered that the present series, with its minimal approximation of 15 per cent having had a seizure, excluded all of those diagnosed as suffering from brain syndromes.)

In general, the process of becoming a patient appears to have been influenced by the changing social context in a variety of specific ways. "Social class" as a unitary concept, or SES alone, are not adequate to account for the pattern of appraisal by self or others (to use Hollingshead and Redlich's term), as sick or deviant and the progress through various social control filters to become a mental hospital patient. There are no data indicating the proportion of severely disturbed people in the general population at large, who becoming identified as ill are then admitted to a psychiatric institution and labeled as "patients." It seems likely that this proportion increases with industrialization, the demands placed upon individuals to function at a complex level (not increasing "stress" and therefore symptom incidence, but rather increasing social visibility of deviant persons), the reduced protective capabilities of families and other naturally occurring sources of support, and the increased availability of socially designated institutions into which nonfunctional persons can be extruded from society. The likelihood of hospitalization is also influenced by family attitudes and the community's system of labeling and monitoring the movements of its members. People who are highly visible within the social system are most apt upon exhibiting deviant behavior to be sent to hospitals by family members or the larger society's control agents. In most of South America, as in Brazil, persons may still move at random outside the system of recording; many in marginal, undemanding occupations are not under constant social scrutiny. Furthermore, families, especially in small towns and rural areas, are still apt to expel psychotic or alcoholic members. No one knows how many alcoholic, chronically psychotic, brain-damaged, or mentally defective people are part of the vast floating migrant hordes or exist anonymously in the slums of great South American cities. Data presented in Chapters IV and VII on people residing in the Migrant's Center, the Beggar's Service, and Emaus provide small samples of these populations. There are no figures on the number who die from accident or intercurrent infection without ever having been listed in the national mental health statistics.

As noted above, the available data suggest that in United States urban slums, poor and sometimes black persons must be more floridly and acutely ill than others in order to be identified as sick, rather than criminal, and admitted to mental hospitals. This appears to be true in Rio de Janeiro as well, and also for men not part of a conjugal family group, and for migrants. Related factors such as illiteracy and distance from sources of societal power reinforce the likelihood of dramatic, aggressive behavior by otherwise inarticulate but suffering people occurring as an unconscious attempt to force communication and gain assistance. The single residentially mobile male, exhibiting signs of alcoholism, unable to find work, and withdrawing passively rather than becoming actively excited, is more apt to remain one of the drifting homeless or to be picked up by a social service center than to be hospitalized. Such men are therefore underrepresented in the mental hospital population; those becoming patients have been obviously and frighteningly deviant in order to achieve that status. In these respects the saturation with mental hospital facilities and the intense social monitoring of more highly developed countries appear to produce a different picture. Kramer (1967), reviewing data from the United States, England and Wales, Norway, and Australia, demonstrated excessively high rates, per 100,000 general population, of first mental hospital admission for the never married and the separated, divorced, and widowed.

Male rates are considerably higher than those for females in the never-married category only. These are persons who, becoming ill in early life, have never achieved the degree of social competence necessary to establish a consistent relationship with a woman and to become an economically productive family head. For the widowed, separated, and divorced female, rates are higher. Among migrant families in Rio the economic burden of a sick relative may result in his being taken to a hospital. Here, as among the poor Baltimore blacks, paranoid symptoms may be regarded as adaptive and justifiable, thus delaying hospitalization.

Overall, women appear to be underrepresented in comparison with the population at large and to be sicker than the men in the hospital population. In this instance family tolerance and ability to sustain a quietly psychotic female who still fulfills certain sexual and homemaking roles seem important. By the time the woman is sent to a hospital and assumes the patient role, she, like the migrant and the black, is apt to have moved to a point of behavior grossly unacceptable to those around her. In the United States, too, despite the different significance of female status, there are sex differences in patterns of hospital admission. In Maryland, for example, with metropolitan Baltimore and its approximately 450,000 blacks as a primary source, the total male admission rate to public mental hospitals is 36 per cent higher than for females. Differences in social attitudes are revealed in the 17 per cent higher admission rates to general and to private mental hospitals for females (Statistical Report, Maryland Department of Mental Hygiene, 1971).

GENERAL SYMPTOMATIC BEHAVIOR

The patients themselves reported subjective feelings and personal histories and exhibited behavior which often reflected difficulties other than those which most impressed their relatives and led immediately to hospitalization. The most frequently encountered awareness of change, as noted in Table 214, concerned sexual capacity, pleasure, or performance. Such changes related to the present illness, including for some, increased feelings of potency or pleasure, were reported by almost the entire group. While this observation fits those of practicing psychotherapists in Western countries, there is no epidemiological baseline against which to compare it. The discussion in Chapter X suggests that Brazilians are perhaps more overtly concerned and readier to speak of their sexual concerns than North American patients. The most frequent types of subjective suffering, reported by almost three-quarters of the entire group, were insomnia due to worries, and somatic pain or malfunction. These were followed by other reflections of anxiety, sufficiently intense to interfere with function. Closely related were other behaviors which may be regarded as depressive. These included for more than half the group, weakness, fatigue, and anorexia—all symptoms which could be increased by or represent psychological intensifications of problems associated with the realities of chronic physical illness, hard work, poor diet, and inadequate housing as well as chronic frustration. In short, the most prevalent complaints of this population, including anxiety to the point of interference with function, a variety of somatic complaints, feelings of depression and of being badly treated by others, appear to reflect the adaptive and coping struggles associated with abrasive and unmanageable life circumstances at least as much as ego-defensive mechanisms dealing with unconscious conflict. Aside from specific somatic or psychophysiological disturbance and facets of anxiety or depression, other categories reported by more than 40 per cent of the patients include obsessive concern with possible loss of control, anger and jealousy, problems in thinking and remembering, and sexual difficulties of various sorts.

These findings may be compared with those obtained from a large probability sample of the U.S. civilian noninstitutional population surveyed in 1960-1962 (Dupuy et al., 1970). The overall percentage of this group reporting having had a nervous breakdown was 4.9 with an additional 12.8 having felt an impending breakdown. The combined rate of 17.7 per cent, or almost one out of five, is roughly comparable to the 23.4 per cent of people classified as symptomatically "impaired" by Srole et al. (1962) in the Midtown Manhattan home survey. The most frequently encountered specific symptoms (in response to a limited set of questions) were nervousness in 58.5 per cent and insomnia in 32.4 per cent of the sample. Inertia, fainting, headaches, and perspiring hands were reported in that order by between 25.1 and 19.3 per cent. "Inertia" may include the fatigue, lack of energy, and weakness reported by the Brazilian patients. The relative frequency of these symptoms, headache, and fainting in a nonhospitalized, geographically nonconstrained United States sample suggests the possibility that they reflect the ordinarily encountered stresses of life rather than those of a particularly harsh environment.

Psychiatric symptom groups derived by Langner and Michael (1963) on the basis of specific questions in the noninstitutionalized Midtown population (slightly weighted in the direction of being white, adult, and childless) revealed some similarities. 70.8 per cent of the total were characterized as exhibiting symptoms of "mixed anxiety," and the next most frequent group, with 51.7 per cent of the respondents, was "psychosomatic." These two categories encompass insomnia and many other reflections of anxiety, including interference with function as well as most of the body-oriented complaints expressed by the Brazilian patients. "Free-floating anxiety" (in 15.1 per cent), "neurasthenia" (in 18.3 per cent), and "obsessive-compulsive" (in 8.1 per cent) symptom groups, which might include some of the symptoms in the patient population were, however, relatively far down the list. Even less evident (4.6 per cent or less) were groups which could conceivably include some of the problems in recall or thinking which concerned the patients. People called rigid, suspicious, passive-dependent, hypochondriacal, schizoid (6.4 per cent) or aggressive (4.9 per cent), but not hospitalized, are those who have managed to adapt to interpersonal demands and avoid serious conflict with the social control network despite an idiosyncratic view of the world. Such adaptation for most can logically be assumed to involve considerable limitations of self-expressive and instrumental behavior and a constrained life-style. Passive-dependency, depression, and hypochondria are also matrices in which many symptomatic behaviors leading to hospitalization may develop. Rigidity and suspiciousness sufficiently notable to be identified in approximately a third of this nonhospitalized population are precursors to paranoid complaints of the type present in slightly over half of the patients. Thus the general symptom reports of this nonhospitalized urban United States population and the hospitalized urban-rural Rio de Janeiro population appear to be more similar than different.

Another extensively studied nonhospitalized population is that of several small towns and semirural areas in Stirling County, Nova Scotia. Leighton and co-workers (1963) state in the third volume of their detailed report: ". . . our belief is that if the entire adult population of Stirling County were studied intensively by competent psychiatrists, approximately two-thirds would be found to have been suffering at some time during their lives from a psychiatric disorder (for the most part low grade and chronic) . . ." (p. 355). They believe that if the figure were limited to current disturbance-prevalence only in the case of the two most frequent types, psychoneurotic and psychophysiological, the estimates would be reduced by at most 10 per cent. The symptoms which they identify in this total population comprise ". . . on the one hand gastrointestinal, cardiovascular, and other bodily sensations and preoccupations, and on the other, chronic sentiments of anxiety, depression, self-depreciation, disgruntlement with one's life situation, apathy, lack of interest, hostility and suspiciousness . . ." in addition to a variety of reflections of emotional instability and self-defeating behavior patterns. It was estimated that Stirling County contains approximately as many cases of unhospitalized as hospitalized psychoses. As in most places, hospitalization depended not only on symptoms but on the availability of professional resources and attitudes toward them as well as home care. While the prevalence of symptoms was great, however, their degree in terms of individual impairment was not. The two categories of "most abnormal" (three per cent) and "psychiatric disorder with significant impairment" (17 per cent) totaled a fifth of the population, a figure comparable to those of the U.S. Health survey and the Midtown Manhattan study noted above. At the same time, while symptoms sometimes appeared to have adaptive roots as well as being reactive, they were largely and notably maladaptive. As seen in nonpatients they appeared to exhibit the same qualities of persistence observed in identified patients. In general, the significance of current social context was most striking in the production of impairment: "We think that the impairing aspect of the detailed symptom patterns is more than anything else under the immediate influence of noxious or benign environmental circumstances " (p. 355).

Symptomatic Behavior and Environment

BEHAVIOR INDICATING ANXIETY

The most frequently encountered indices of anxiety in the total patient group are listed in Table 215. These were mostly reported by the patients themselves as present at the moment of interviewing as well as historically. In many instances they were confirmed or added to by relatives, and in some cases objectively observed during interviews.

Insomnia was reported in almost three-quarters of the total study population followed in approximately two-thirds of the patients by discrete anxiety attacks and impaired work capacity. Anxiety about particular personal or situational issues occurred in from 25 to 40 per cent of the patients. These issues included body and organ functioning, jobs, families, the possibility of death, and of loss of control over one's actions. Aside from sex, sleeping and working appear the functions most vulnerable to disruption by anxiety. While cognitive functioning appeared vulnerable to disruption by anxiety, this was not true to as great an extent as had been expected. Impaired concentration and decision-making occurred with approximately the same frequency as intense worry about body malfunction.

Table 216 lists the comparative occurrence of anxiety indices according to sociocultural category whenever differences of 10 per cent or more were noted. Initial inspection suggests that within this population beset with many reality problems, a comparatively high frequency of a particular anxiety index reflects adaptive stress including the rigors of physical factors as well as frustration and ungratified wishes and needs, more than the presence of unconscious conflict. Clearly, however, these two roots of psychological tension and symptomatic behavior are not mutually exclusive.

Insomnia, the most frequent indicator, increases significantly with age. This is a finding reported in most Western cultures and one which may reflect biological factors as well as the social stresses of middle life. Among lower-class Brazilians however, people over 45 years old are in the upper age range of the population as a whole. They are increasingly vulnerable to discomfort and illness associated with inadequate living conditions, and those depending upon manual labor for a livelihood are at an increasing disadvantage relative to younger workers. Age status, especially for men, assumes special psychological significance in a socioculture which places unusual demands upon physical stamina and attributes particular emphasis to sexual performance and the importance of being a virile male. It confronts the mature man with the fact that passing the peak of his capacities he has remained powerless to master the social forces, which, for the lower-class patient in particular, have formed his constant and oppressive life context. The projective test data discussed in Chapter XII suggest that descriptively the symptom of insomnia is most often part of an anxious-depressive state. Psychodynamically, the material suggests (a) that for many of the patients this anxious-depressive state is related to the presence of aim-inhibited hostility generated in part by environmental circumstances which cannot be mastered; (b) insomnia reflects a failure of control of anxiety and hostility via the most regularly used defenses of denial, repression, and narrowing of attention; and, (c) insomnia reflects not only the less restrained emergence of previously defended against anxiety and hostility, but passive-dependent wishes most acute at night at sleep time, and intensified by the awareness of waning powers with age.

The only other statistically significant difference in insomnia incidence relates to color. Amost nine out of 10 browns, previously described as the most tense, hostile, upwardly striving, and frustrated of the color groups, suffered from insomnia attributable to worries. For this group, the proportionately higher frequency of insomnia appears part of the complex of tension indicators, particularly those involving the activation of angry feelings. While these feelings are symptomatically evident, it may be assumed that their expression and full subjective appreciation is inhibited and displaced. This is a culture in which, as noted previously, the free conscious awareness and expression of such feelings, especially toward parental figures (e.g., the dominant white power holders) has traditionally been frowned upon. The only sociocultural status in which browns are represented with notably greater frequency than either whites or blacks is that of being single, i.e., of having no consistent mate, either of a consensual or legal-religious nature. This difference, while not statistically significant, supports a view of their marginal social state as associated with restlessness, hostile tension, and impaired capacity to form long-term relationships, especially those requiring them to function in the parental (including husbandly) role. (As shown in Chapter IX, insomnia occurred slightly more often among the married than single.)

Insomnia varied directly, though not significantly, with illiteracy (which, as noted in Chapter V, occurred in similar proportions for browns and blacks) and was least frequent among those in nonmanual occupations (filled amost exclusively by whites). The preceding chapters indicate that being white in modern Brazil is most highly correlated with maximum psychological protection, the greatest likelihood of achieving aims and gratifying wishes, and with least environmental stress. More often than the nonwhite, the white is educated, literate, in nonmanual work, and better housed. The findings that insomnia was least prominent among nonmanual workers and literates and most prominent among the illiterate, brown, and older patients supports the supposition, then, that the symptom in this population reflects a variety of socioculturally imposed or mediated stresses (economic, physical, frustrated self-esteem, blocked upward mobility, marginality, information lack, etc.), leading to aim-inhibited hostility and intensified regressive passive-dependent wishes. It should be noted in this respect that none of these factors (color, occupation, literacy) vary systematically with age in this sample.

Discrete anxiety attacks, occurring in 67 per cent of the total group, also varied in frequency between subgroups although not to a statistically significant degree. The pattern of variation, however, is congruent with that noted for insomnia: attacks were most frequently reported for the unskilled manual workers and least often for the nonmanual group. Similarly, the recently migrant—still undergoing the stresses of separation and reintegration into a new community—reported more attacks than the settled. The recently migrant patient, as the others for whom insomnia and anxiety attacks occurred with greatest proportionate frequency, is one whose strivings for self-realization (c.f., for example, Karen Horney) are most obviously frustrated, and whose passive-dependent wishes have been defensively activated without hope of fulfillment. In fact, the high prevalence of these nonspecific reflections of anxiety in the total patient sample may be attributed to the prevalence of the aforementioned psychodynamic factors associated with actual powerlessness and helplessness.

The largest difference in incidence of anxiety attacks according to color was for the blacks who reported a markedly lower frequency. This pattern is consistent with that observed for most although not all of the other indices of anxiety. In most instances where differences of 10 per cent or more are present between groups, the browns and whites resemble each other. Except for a single category, anxious behavior is least often listed for the blacks. This despite the fact that, as summarized in Table 217, they were exposed to similar and sometimes greater degrees of deprivation than the browns in relation to illiteracy, lack of education, working at unskilled physical labor, and living in substandard housing. (There were no differences in incidence of recent migration according to color.) Nonspecific "stress" alone is evidently too crude a category to be useful in understanding symptomatic behavior. Deprivation without aspirations does not lead to frustration with its attendant anger and anxiety. If the aspirations are blocked at the source, the "stress" meaning of environmental circumstance can be minimized. Many of the several possibly protective elements operant among blacks discussed in Chapter V appear to be inherent in the persisting institutionalization of the dependent filial help-seeking relationship of blacks to whites in contrast to the browns' push for upward mobility. Other aids to anxiety control include religious participation with its relationship to a highly personal deity and its promise of immediate power and gratification. Belonging to a group unified by such beliefs also decreases social isolation. The relationship with the cult leader further gratifies passive-dependent needs and helps to dampen anxiety. While only 28 per cent of the blacks indicated that they participated in Afro-Spiritist services, this is more than twice the proportion for whites or browns.

Diminished evidence of anxiety because of greater use of alternative behaviors is also suggested by the larger proportion of blacks than whites or browns who are male. This proportion, as indicated in Table 222, is associated with a greater frequency or direct hostile expression and assaultive behavior (against friends and family) among blacks; expressed hostility as an alternative to anxiety or depression may have defensive value insofar as the mobilization of anger with its concomitant fantasy and preparation for outwardly directed destructive behavior can protect the person from awareness of his own disturbing feelings, fantasies, and memories.

Proportionally fewer blacks are in the youngest age category which, as indicated in Table 216, exhibits proportionately least insomnia and organ anxiety. This factor would therefore not appear responsible for the relatively low frequency of their anxious behavior. While fears of loss of control are most frequent for the youngest, constant diffuse anxiety is significantly least frequent for the oldest. There are no differences according to age for the other anxiety indices.

Work impairment due to worries was reported for 65 per cent of the total group, almost as many as suffered from anxiety attacks. This occurred, as did the above symptoms, with greatest frequency among the browns and least often for the blacks. Similarly, it was most frequent among the unskilled manual workers. In contrast, the similarly low frequency of such anxiety-induced impairment for those in the skilled manual and nonmanual categories probably reflects the relatively high degree of job satisfaction and stability for both. (The stability of occupational Class V, and the emerging sense of shared identity among those in this category, were discussed in Chapter VII.)

Religion was the only other factor revealing differences associated with work impairment due to worries. Afro-Spiritist participants showed considerably, though not statistically significant, less such impairment than the unaffiliated or those confining their religious observance to other forms. Table 218 summarizes the major sociocultural statuses of the patient population according to religious membership or observance. Those who belong to or acknowledge attendance at Afro-Spiritist centers are predominantly in the middle age range of the patients, include a slightly higher proportion of blacks than the other categories, and proportionately fewer with no schooling or who had not completed the primary grades. They were also significantly more stable in terms of residence (i.e., fewer were recent migrants), and significantly more were in Class V occupations. These protective factors, particularly membership in occupational Class V, are probably sufficient to account for the lower degree of work impairment among Afro-Spiritists. Beyond them, the data in Chapter XI suggest the central meaning of work and its possible vulnerability to emotional disturbance for the Protestants and to a lesser degree for the Catholics, as well as the unstable work adjustment of the unaffiliated. It seems likely that Afro-Spiritists are protected to some degree from adaptive stresses by their intimate and regular sense of connection with supernatural forces. These forces are more powerful than the usually white middle-class bosses for whom they work and who regulate their rewards. Supernatural forces provide a refuge; participation in Afro-Spiritist ceremonies offers immediate gratifications and the support of belonging to a system outside of the conventional work-oriented one which is often a source of frustration and alienation.

The feeling of being overwhelmed by many specific fears was present in over half of the patient population, but did not differ in frequency according to sociocultural status. This may reflect the universality of feeling "overwhelmed" in any population abandoning its autonomy for hospitalization.

Fear of loss of control, present in 50 per cent of the patients, varied considerably according to sociocultural status. Unlike most other indices of anxiety, this symptomatic fear was reported most often by the more privileged groups: occupationally nonmanual, better educated, and more adequately housed. Conversely, it was reported least often by the black, the unskilled, and uneducated, the illiterate, and the poorly housed. Either the nature of the stress provoking this type of symptom is different from the stress antecedent to insomnia, anxiety attacks, or work impairment, or the adaptive or defensive maneuvers activated by the stress are different. Privilege itself may constitute a stress for certain persons insofar as it activates guilt, anxiety about unacceptable wishes for dominance or power, or in relation to particular concomitants of success such as symbolically displacing the father. Common denominators for the more privileged are information, power, and responsibility. The patients with the most knowledge, social power, and responsibility more frequently fear loss of control over their words, feelings, or actions than those with less power and responsibility, for whom such loss of control would presumably be less consequential. The possible relationship of such fears to ambition, energy, or other aspects of a high generalized aggressive drive with unconscious destructive components is suggested by the finding that they are most frequent in the youngest and least in the oldest patients. The reports of projective testing in Chapter XII also suggest that these patients are troubled by ungratified passive-dependent wishes and repressed hostile impulses secondary to the frustration of upward social strivings less often than are the most deprived.

Aside from these considerations, education and literacy facilitate inward looking, self-awareness, rumination, and the use of thinking rather than action as a means of personal problem-solving. Information, mastery of verbal symbols, and relative access to societal power increase the availability of nonregressive defense mechanisms. Historically, the more integrated family structures and more systematic educational exposure of the most advantaged patients have presumably increased the likelihood of their developing self-scrutinizing and self-estimating functions and decreased the likelihood that externalizing defenses will be activated to deal with anxiety or guilt.

A seemingly incompatible finding is the highest frequency of fear of loss of control as compared with other religious groups among the predominantly poor and lowest-class Protestants. Table 218 shows that proportionately more Protestants than members of other religious categories were illiterate or partly literate, and unschooled or had not completed the primary grades. Along with the unaffiliated they were most heavily represented in occupational Class VI and among those with inadequate housing. They also included significantly more recent migrants. These factors are associated with lack of information, power, and responsibility and would thus be expected to reduce the frequency of fear of loss of control, and perhaps increase the frequency of such symptoms as insomnia, anxiety attacks, and interference with function. Protestants were not, however, proportionately overrepresented with respect to these symptoms. The opposite was in fact true; they were proportionately highest, as indicated in Table 216, in frequency of job and family worries. These symptoms, along with fear of loss of control, fit the Protestant conscientiousness, concern with values, standards, and achievements (as discussed in Chapter XI). Despite their lack of education and job status, the work and family ethic internalized along with their religious beliefs appears to have sensitized them to the importance of self-control and the maintenance of responsibility on the one hand, and the dangers of relinquishing such control and responsibility on the other.

In this instance, the influence of religious status upon symptom production appears to vary independent of the influence of educational, occupational, housing, and migratory status. SES-related factors would be expected to reduce the incidence of fear of loss of control. These elements were outweighed, however, by the acquisition of self-scrutinizing capacities and of standards against which personal behavior is measured.

One other factor listed in Table 218 may influence the relation of Protestant status to fear of losing control. Significantly fewer Protestants had no consistent mate, i.e., were free of family and marital responsibility. In this instance, current reality, that is, the presence of major responsibilities necessitating curbing personal wishes and delaying gratification, combined with a reinforcing social (religous) context and historically acquired moral standards and self-observing tendencies to produce a particular symptomatic behavior pattern. (It should be noted here that other classical features of obsessional neurosis, e.g., rituals, doubting, and maladaptive perfectionism, were not present to any notable degree in this predominantly lower-class population.)

Signs of direct anxiety, tension, and fear were observed during the interviews of 48 per cent of the patients. Recent migrants displayed anxious behavior significantly more often than the settled probably in consequence of their unfamiliarity with the setting, the urban communicative style, and the procedure. There was also proportionately more anxious behavior among the unskilled, the illiterate, the poorly housed, and the female patients. All are members of low status groups, minorities in the sense of distance from societal power, who may plausibly be regarded as apprehensive or at least unsure of themselves when closeted with an upper-class representative of medical authority. The possible influence of the psychiatrist's attitudes upon the relational behavior of patients is indicated in Table 230. The interviewers' self-ratings suggest less positive and more negative attitudes toward recent migrants, manual workers, the uneducated, nonliterate, and poorly housed.

In contrast to the verbal reports of anxiety or interference with function, no difference was observed in interview anxiety according to color. As previously indicated, the blacks appear to rely on institutionalized relational styles vis-à-vis the more powerful whites, and the browns, as noted below, seem more prone to exhibit hostile tension or depression than anxiety in direct conversation with whites or those of higher socioeconomic status. Table 230 shows, in contrast to their consistent attitudes regarding other categories, a mixed attitude by psychiatrists toward their patients according to color. They felt most involved and empathic with blacks and least optimistic and empathic and most anxious with browns. As expected, they found the whites most interesting and likeable and more often felt liked by them.

Aside from these considerations, it seems probable that lack of information associated with illiteracy and lack of communicative skills might hamper the development of adequate defense systems. An inadequate defensive repertory increases the probability of direct motor and autonomic expression of anxiety rather than of verbal reports which permit the patient some detachment from his concerns.

Restlessness due to worries, present in 45 per cent of the total, was significantly more prominent among the browns than the whites or blacks. This finding appears congruent with the characteristics of marginality and related features discussed above. The pattern here resembles that in other instances of anxiety interfering with function. This symptomatic behavior occurred most frequently among the unskilled, the poorly housed, and the female, and least often among the literate. As was true for the majority of anxiety indices, there was no differential occurrence according to education. This fits the impression (discussed in Chapter VI) that educational level in a mobility-blocked society is a less adequate index of functional capacity than literacy.

Difficulty in concentrating due to worries was present in 42 per cent of the total group. As was true for other indices of anxiety, the unskilled manual workers reported this problem with highest frequency. Concentration involves the capacity to shut out distractions and focus attention on the solution of particular problems. It would appear especially disruptible by high and persistent anxiety in people unaccustomed to such focusing and away from familiar supports. It is hence not surprising that recent migrants exhibited this symptom more often and significantly than the settled. At the same time, concentration and the capacity to exclude irrelevant stimuli, which would also seem important in decision-making capacity, showed no such differentiation. Decision-making involves preparation for action and discrimination between at least two choices, whereas concentration need not require committing oneself to a course of action. In this sense decision-making is more demanding, which makes it surprising that it did not differentiate more clearly between groups.

Major differences in decision-making problems, present in 37 per cent of the total, pertained to color and marital status. Blacks showed least difficulty. Singles had a significantly higher incidence of decision-making difficulty. Within the color category, the blacks are probably under less pressure to make life decisions since they have little societal power and appear for the moment to accept the institutionalized status quo. The singles, significantly more of whom are in the youngest age grouping, include fewer literate patients, more in Class VI, who have inferior housing, are brown, religiously unaffiliated, recently migrant, and male. In other words, the single state encompasses most of the conditions associated with high adaptive stress and poorly operating defense systems unable to keep anxiety at a manageable level. Singles might thus be expected to show high levels of interference with most tasks requiring persistent application in the face of distractions either from within or without. The sociocultural concomitants of single status are summarized in Tables 149 and 150.

Body or organ anxiety, present in 40 per cent of the total, follows the general pattern. It was most frequent in the deprived, the powerless, those with limited symbolic capacity, and those most subject to fatigue and illness. Anxiety about the integrity and capacity of one's body in contrast to psychosomatic symptoms is apparently related to low status and actual dependence for economic survival upon a body weakened by life stress. The singles, with a lower incidence of body anxiety, are not only younger but also do not bear the burden of dependents. The blacks, while poor and deprived, appear to have been more secure about their continuing physical stamina and prowess. Their relative lack of body anxiety (as discussed in Chapter V), is accompanied by a lower incidence (than in browns and whites) of guilty, depressive, and sexual complaints. This seems to be related to relative acceptance of their social status quo with less striving behavior than in the other two groups. In this population organ anxiety does not appear to be an alternative to other expressions of anxiety, concern, or depression. It co-exists with them, and actual impairment makes the body more available as a focus of concern.

The single finding which does not fit this pattern is a significantly higher incidence of organ or body anxiety among the Afro-Spiritists. Perhaps the apparent denial of anxiety and depression in other spheres may leave the body as the only acceptable focus. This finding may also reflect the patient selection process. The data in Chapter XI suggest that many regular devotees find relief for symptomatic behavior of a more obviously psychological nature in the Afro-Spiritist centers. Those who complain repeatedly of somatic discomfort are more apt, finally, to be sent by center leaders to conventional medical units.

Constant diffuse anxiety was present in 33 per cent of the patients. Its patterning contrasts with that of the much more commonly encountered discrete attacks, most frequent among the more deprived patients. Constant diffuse anxiety was more often encountered among the whites, the most educated, the literate, the non-manual workers, and the better housed. It was least among the black, the single, the poorly housed, the manual worker, and, to a significant degree, the least educated, the illiterate, and the oldest. Such constant, free-floating or unbound anxiety, in contrast to that occurring episodically and presumably in relation to eventually identifiable stimuli, was also most frequent among those reporting fear of loss of control, although not among the Protestants. Diffuse anxiety and fear of loss of control seem most prominent in patients who are less subject to the harsh rigors of lower-class life. In the present sample these were the more responsible, socialized, educated persons, more inclined to problem solving through thought than direct action. Unconscious conflict determined by past personal history apparently had greater relative importance for them as compared with lower SES patients in the maintenance of symptomatic behavior than ongoing interpersonal events. The possibility that diffuse anxiety reaching the point of intolerability is a major reason for their selection as patients (rather than, for example, assault or refusal to work) also fits these considerations. Females as a group, for whom hospitalization appears to be more a matter of last resort than it is for men, are also overrepresented in the population of patients with diffuse anxiety.

Phobic fears, present in 31 per cent of the group, are closely related to constant diffuse anxiety. These are also more frequent in the female patients, and significantly less so among blacks and Afro-Spiritists. Presumably these last two groups have other ways of more effectively binding anxiety.

Situational worries concerning jobs and concerning families were present in 27 per cent and 26 per cent of the patients respectively. Job anxiety sufficient to be noted by the interviewer was most frequent among the unskilled manual and least frequent among the nonmanual workers. This seems mainly a function of reality. It was highest, though not significantly so, among the browns, the recently migrant, and the oldest patients. For those geographically relocated and needing work, and for the older patients already less capable, the worries also appear realistic. For the browns, however, they seem related to social blocking of occupational aspirations and, inferentially, to anxiety-laden hostile feelings toward employers. Job anxiety was significantly least among the Afro-Spiritists, who, as noted above, also exhibited the lowest incidence of worries interfering with work.

Family worries appear to occur in relation both to realistic circumstances and to value systems. They were thus most marked among the Protestants, women, the recently migrant, and the married. They were least prominent among the whites, the better housed, and the literates, i.e., those with higher status and more resources.

In summary, the symptomatic expressions of anxiety did not vary in a unified manner; they do not readily lend themselves to generalization in terms of a unitary concept of social class or of culture. Many symptomatic behaviors appear directly related to the types of environmental circumstances impinging upon the patients. The stress value of such circumstances or of particular social contexts, however, varies with historically acquired, reinforced or muted factors such as strivings (e.g., for occupational status or political participation), values or standards, and self-observational functions. The behavioral consequence of environment also varies with protective factors available to the patient. The use of such social forms as religion, for example, in the service of defensive and adaptive needs evidently has significant protective value, reducing the occurrence of overt anxiety for some. Participation in other religious groups such as the Protestant, however, may promote the development of guilt or frustration. Similarly, conceptual and symbolic capacity, the ability to receive and transmit information through written language, familiarity with the city, integration into an interpersonal network, and other related factors, all determine the shape of symptomatic behavior, but not necessarily in a consistent or mutually complementary manner.

BEHAVIOR SUGGESTIVE OF DEPRESSION

Aside from insomnia, the most frequent depressive symptoms in the total patient group, as indicated in Table 219, were feelings of sadness, fatigue, weakness and anorexia. One or more of these four symptoms were reported for or observed in between 54 and 60 per cent of the patients. One or another of these symptoms may appear in the absence of demonstrable organic pathology as a reflection of a masked depressive process. Conversely, depression or realistic grief following loss or bereavement intensify ordinarily unemphasized symptoms of chronic illness or stress. Weakness and fatigue associated with undernutrition, overwork, or chronic minimal health impairment may also contribute to the development of depressed feelings, especially those associated with awareness of waning powers and inability to achieve life goals. Such awareness contributes to feelings of hopelessness, inadequacy, and self-disparagement; for many, failure can mean worthlessness, unlovability, and unconscious guilt over not meeting internalized standards.

As seen in Table 219, the females and the older patients with

few exceptions reported more depressive symptoms of every variety than the males and younger patients. This increase in depressive manifestations with age has been reported in all Western cultures.

Table 219 reveals significantly larger percentages of patients
suffering from fatigue among the recently migrant, the illiterate,
and the poorly housed, all of whom experienced chronic physical
stress and frustration. Migrants are by definition strivers, attempting actively to solve problems through geographical relocation
Brody (1969b). As indicated in Chapter IV, the recent migrants
who became patients are those whose striving was unsuccessful.
Fatigue is also more prominent within the oldest age group. For
these groups then, the symptom may be primarily a matter of
physical exhaustion, and it is indeed least often present among
the nonmanual workers. It seems probable, however, that beyond
the effect of physical vulnerability, the emotional consequences of
unsuccessful attempts at problem solving and upward mobility as
well as awareness of failure are important contributors to symptom formation. The significantly higher percentage of Protestants
suffering from fatigue probably reflects both their mobility strivings associated with a degree of self-deprivation, (as discussed in
Chapter XI), and the relatively higher representation among
them, as indicated in Table 218, of recent migrants, older people,
illiterates, and women.

Women complain significantly more than men of both fatigue
and anorexia. Whether this stems from the nature of their daily
activities, biological factors—including those associated with the
menstrual cycle—or a relative lack of constraint in admitting
physical symptoms is uncertain. In most societies women are
granted greater expressive freedom for both emotional and somatic complaints. Some observers of traditional societies have
linked womens' symptomatic behaviors to their social status. The
clear minority position of women in Brazil, as discussed in Chapter IX, can plausibly be implicated for the present sample.
Diaz-Guerrero (1955) has concluded, similarly, that women in
Mexico City had many more symptoms than men because of
their lower social position. Langner and Michael (1963), testing
this hypothesis, compared a group of married women from Mexico City with those of Tehuantepec whose status more closely

approximated that of their husbands. While the latter reported more psychophysiological symptoms than their mates, the difference was, indeed, less than for those in Mexico City. In Midtown, where female status is even closer to that of men, they still reported more symptoms than men, but the sex difference was less than in Mexico. Generally, the lower the income status of the woman, and her prestige position vis-à-vis men, the higher the level of reported psychological symptoms. In no instance, however, have men, regardless of income, reported more symptoms than women. Beyond this there is evidence, for example that of Hinkle et al., (1960), that women have higher morbidity rates for all types of illness than men, while the latter have higher mortality rates. The National Center for Health Statistics survey (Dupuy et. al., 1970) reported combined rates for nervous breakdowns and impending nervous breakdown in a noninstitutionalized population of 23.9 per cent for females, more than twice the 10.9 per cent found for males. Sex, age, and education appear to contribute cumulatively to the danger of nervous breakdown. The NCHS survey found the highest rate for nervous breakdown (14.6 per cent) among older, more poorly educated women and the lowest rate (0.9 per cent) among younger, better educated men and women.

The Stirling County Study (Leighton et al., 1963) reports a somewhat different picture, focusing on the relationship of gender status to level of community integration. A higher prevalence of psychiatric disorder was found among women than men, although their impairment level was only slightly higher. Women in Midtown, as noted by Langner and Michael, (1963) were more inclined to exhibit psychophysiologic and psychoneurotic and less inclined to sociopathic or "acting out" behavior patterns. Leighton and associates (1963) invoke contributory differences in respect to ". . .the definition of and means for attaining physical security, sexual satisfaction, expression of hostility, the giving and securing of love, recognition, expression of spontaneity, orientation regarding place in society, membership in a human group, and the sense of being right. . . ." In respect to these and other factors, however, ". . . it is not so much culture per se, but the extent and rate of acceleration in change of the sociocultural system that has a differential effect on the sexes . . ." (p. 366). In an

English Canadian fishing community, for example, while the men lived according to a relatively consistent, "integrated" sociocultural system centered on their work, the women, familiar with the changing ideas of the larger society, were ". . . beset by the conflicts and instability of transition" (p. 367). In a French Canadian Catholic community, however, characterized by a high degree of ". . . consistency and completeness of the role and sentiment network in which women live . . ." (p. 367), with comparatively little sense of relative deprivation, the women had a notably lower prevalence of psychiatric disorder in relation both to that of the fishing community and of Stirling County in general, as well as to the men of their own town. In the most disintegrated areas of the County, women presented a picture similar to men in terms both of general symptom prevalence and of quality, showing proportionately less psychoneurotic and more sociopathic manifestations than other women in the same County.

Langner and Michael's (1963) analysis of the Midtown Manhattan data reveals no difference in the average mental health risk of men and women. Their data also suggest that gender differences in the incidence of symptomatic behavior are less reflective of biological universals than of specific interactions between the social status, role, and integration of elements constituting the behavioral (community) context of women. Women in Midtown were more impaired than men by particular worries that might be expected to be exclusively male, including concern about work and socioeconomic status (getting ahead). In addition, proportionately more showed marital worries. Unlike the family-oriented Brazilians, parental worries were not significantly greater for Midtown Manhattan women than men.

Table 219 shows that despite their higher incidence of psychophysiological symptoms, female patients complained of weakness less frequently than men. Physical strength is less vital a concern for females than males. Its vicissitudes are not perhaps so closely monitored that they become primary foci for expressing or communicating anxiety, depression, or psychic discomfort. The distribution of weakness as a symptom, in general, is less clearly linked to socioeconomic position than is fatigue. Differences are generally not significant and in regard to education and literacy are ambiguous. Weakness, like fatigue, is more frequent among the older patients and the poorly housed. The prominence of this symptom among Protestants is not marked, but is, nonetheless, significantly greater than in the unaffiliated (and younger) patients.

Anorexia, even less clearly linked to deprived status, is also encountered most often among older patients. A related depressive complaint apparently consequent to reality conditions is the feeling that one's body is weak and inferior. As noted in Table 219, this complaint, present in less than a fifth of the total group, was most frequent among the illiterate and the unskilled. In general, depressive symptoms involving impaired bodily function, or a perception of one's body as weak, ineffective, or in some way inferior, are reported most often in patients whose bodies are actually subject to greater strain or have less stamina than the others. They are older, subject to greatest physical stress at work, and have the least adequate home environments. In addition, these patients are most excluded from the cultural (informational-symbolic) mainstream (Brody, 1966), depend more on their bodies for economic security and status, are unsuccessful strivers for a variety of goals, and are vulnerable because of social inequities associated with being female.

In contrast to the above, sadness and weeping are more prominent among the most privileged patients. These are the educated, literate, occupationally nonmanual, and better housed. Exceptions include the higher incidence of feelings of sadness among the recently migrant, who, presumably still suffering from separation and relative social isolation, may exhibit reality based grief. In view of the socioeconomic characteristics of recent migrants as indicated in Chapter IV and Table 221, the depressive effect of migration is probably greater than indicated by the data. Tables 219 and 220 show that sadness and weeping as well as feeling overwhelmed by criticism were also more often encountered in those residing in the transitional central urban slum and deteriorated areas (Area II), although not necessarily in the least adequate housing. It was suggested (in Chapter VIII) that these areas are characterized by greater social isolation, lack of community support, and anomic qualities. These findings are congruent with the impression that loss of interpersonal support, symbolizing loss of lovability and approval, is an important contributor to feelings of sadness, depression, rejection, and failure. Related are a higher incidence of feelings of loneliness among the recently migrant, residents of Area II, and the unmarried; a similar finding with a probable reality basis is the higher incidence among the recently migrant of guilt over failure in the parental role.

The wish for personal extinction or oblivion or the choice of unconsciousness as the only alternative to mental pain may represent yet another pattern. As noted in Table 219, death wishes, least prominent among the blacks, occur with greatest frequency in the more privileged, i.e., the nonmanual occupations and better housed. They were also most frequent in dwellers in Area II, however, the more transitory central urban regions including slums as well as expensive apartments. Suicidal threats occurred not at all among blacks and more among the nonmanual in comparison with manual workers. Suicidal attempts were reported least among the blacks—who also least often reported feeling sad, or being preoccupied with inadequacy—and most among Area II in comparison with Area I dwellers.

In short, suicide, as fantasy, threat, or attempt occurred most often in upper SES as compared with lower SES patients, and those living in center city areas often occupied by transients or new arrivals in comparison with the more stable suburbs. It is likely that the data on suicidal thoughts and attempts underrepresent the actual situation. As noted elsewhere, this is a society in which suicide, especially among adolescents, is not reported freely. The broadest relevant social framework in which to view the data is that delineated by Gibbs and Martin (1964). They review data supporting the postulate that the suicide rate of a population varies inversely with the degree of status integration in that population. "Status integration" is a function of the degree to which individuals occupy compatible statuses (e.g., age, sex, ethnic, occupational, etc.) and nonconflicting roles, the degree to which they conform to the patterned and sanctioned expectations of demands by others and engage in stable and durable social relationships. Data indicating a suicide rate among United States Negroes in the late 1940's and early 1950's approximately a third that of whites are interpreted by Gibbs and Martin as indicating the static social situation of United States blacks in that period. This may be compared with the institutionalized relationships of Brazilian blacks with whites, their apparent lack of upward mobility striving, and their apparently conflictless acceptance of a passive-dependent social role in comparison with browns or whites (as discussed in Chapter V).

The concept of status integration stems from Durkeim's (1951) imprecisely defined idea of social integration, which has by implication a social regulatory function; low degrees of status integration would appear also to occur in persons living under conditions described by Durkeim as anomic. Gibbs and Martin note the repeated employment by Durkeim of the idea of consensus in describing a socially integrated (nonanomic) population. Merton's (1938) redefinition describes an anomic situation as one emphasizing cultural goals without providing means to achieve them. The problems stemming from the acquisition of values from the dominant society without the tools for achieving them have been noted by Brody (1963) in studies of Negro children in Baltimore. The acquisition of new values and a new recognition of the possibilty of achieving them are aspects of recently accelerating social change among U.S. blacks which may be expected to occur in Brazil as the literacy and health of previously deprived populations improve. Butts (1969) believes that higher suicide rates in the middle- than in lower-class United States blacks reflect the former's move away from a tendency to deal with feelings through externally directed violence. This view accepts a general "violence-suicide" adaptation in which one or the other predominates. Hendin (1969), also considering the rising expectations of U.S. blacks and the obstacles to reaching their aspirations, noted that suicide becomes a problem at an early age for the black because of an early sense of despair that life can never be satisfying. This is contrasted to the waning hope of the older white in his possibilities for achievement. In recent years suicide has become recognized as a serious issue for blacks, at least for young adult urban males. Hendin (1969) noted, for example, that the suicide rate for black males aged 20-35 was twice that of whites in the same age group. In his psychoanalytic scrutiny of 25 suicidal black patients, he was impressed by the prominence, in contrast to white subjects, of unconscious murderous rage reflecting, in his opinion "the frustration and anger of the black ghetto" (p. 24). This, despite their essentially middle-class backgrounds. The higher incidence of suicide among the European wealthy than the poor was seen by Durkheim as a corollary of anomie: suicide vulnerability was greatest among those who had more that they could potentially lose.

In his work on Scandinavian suicide, Hendin (1964) outlines seven discrete patterns of fantasy and motivation leading to suicide: death as retaliatory abandonment, omnipotent mastery, retroflexed murder, reunion, rebirth, self-punishment or atonement, and a phenomenon that in an emotional sense has already taken place. Projective test findings (described in Chapter XII) suggest that for many of the present patients death as an emotionally significant phenomenon has already taken place. This was reflected in their perceptions of humans as "merely alive" and in the pervasive evidence of partly accepted passive-dependent wishes against which there was little struggle. Under these circumstances of emotional constriction and lack of available affectional resources, the suicidal fantasy and even the act may be viewed as the final step of a process already well advanced and requiring little new mobilization of energy. This formulation, while plausible for some patients, does not fit the observation that suicide was considered predominantly by the more privileged, educated, achievement-oriented patients. For these, the more active meanings of suicide may be valid and more congruent with the changes described in the Negro population of the U.S. These active types with clear-cut primary and secondary gains also include the "performance" type of suicide in Sweden described by Hendin, who believes it is becoming the rule in the modern world. This model is "based on rigid performance expectations with strong self-hatred for failure . . . also traceable to an early mother-child separation." Contrasted with this are the Danish "dependency loss" type of suicide based on ". . . passivity, over-sensitivity to abandonment, and an effective use of the technique of arousing guilt in others . . .", and the Norwegian "moral" form stemming from "aggressive anti-social behavior and strong guilt feelings aroused by such behavior, with the entire constellation cast in a puritanical setting" (p. 124). The first and third models appear applicable in the present population to the non-manual workers, more occupationally ambitious and sensitive to potential losses than the manual laborers, and to the Protestants. The second fits the traditional family orientation of the relatively well-to-do established Catholic population. Protestant patients, although the least educated and literate and almost entirely in manual occupations, did in fact show the highest prevalence of social role associated guilt and self-accusations. The impact of the Protestant ethic on the development of depressive symptoms is compounded by the higher proportion of Protestants who are female and older. The strikingly low incidence of suicidal behavior in blacks as compared to nonblacks suggests the protective value of "integrated" status. Religious affiliation may contribute another protective element for blacks; as noted in Table 217, significantly more than browns or whites engage in Afro-Spiritist observance. Such observance (as described in Chapter XI) offers a sense of connection with a suprahuman nurturant force, more powerful than the temporal determinants of low socioeconomic status. It provides a supportive community for otherwise isolated individuals and families. Afro-Spiritist participation thus appears to contibute significantly to personal security and the capacity to tolerate stress. As noted in Tables 219 and 220, Afro-Spiritists least frequently reported feelings of sadness, suicidal threats, self-accusations, feelings of guilt over failure in the role of parent, or social role failure in general.

In summary, the interpretation of depressive symptoms requires attention to a variety of vulnerability producing and protective factors. Complaints such as fatigue, weakness, anorexia, and bodily inferiority, all involving psychophysiological changes or the perception of somatic states and body image, seem to have important roots in physically stressful as well as frustration producing reality. The most apparent reality factors are those associated with lowest socioeconomic status and failure of upward mobility. These contribute to physical exhaustion and provide a legitimately reinforced somatic focus for anxiety and depression. Awareness of bodily inadequacy in vulnerable individuals is intensified by other factors producing a sense of powerlessness, hopelessness, and low self-esteem. In the low SES respondents described by Langner and Michael (1963) similar considerations appear to have contributed to a much larger proportion than among the middle or high SES of reports of "poor physical health." Complaints such as loneliness, feelings of inadequacy, and of being criticized, also have important reality roots in the interruption of supportive relationships through migration and residence in transitory anomic Area II. Similarly, more of the low- than high-SES Midtown residents felt life to be futile and complained of friendlessness and loneliness. The manual laborers among them, in particular with parents of low or migrant status, exhibited more indications of low self-esteem.

In contrast to the above, direct feelings of sadness, death wishes, and suicidal inclinations, along with guilt and self-critical and accusatory tendencies, occurred with greatest frequency among the better housed and those who had achieved higher occupational status. In this group, a sense of responsibility, an awareness of the need to preserve status and property, the need to bolster self-esteem by achievement, and sufficient freedom from the immediate necessities of survival to be concerned with the meaningfulness of life are suggested as vulnerability producing factors. Literacy and education with their associated symbolic facility, the responsibilities of supervisory work, the awareness of potential which should be utilized, and the standards and aspirations with their self-critical functions acquired while growing up in more educated families also increase the potential for feelings of guilt and inadequacy. This type of depression associated with being "dissatisfied with one's self" was most prevalent in the highest social class of Hollingshead and Redlich's (1958) New Haven patients and declined in frequency as the class ladder was descended.

Being female and older, statuses associated with an awareness of relative helplessness, also appear to contribute to depressive feelings. Perhaps the most striking gender-linked symptom, not reported in the United States, is the fear of being abandoned, present in more than a third of the female patients. This may be associated with their longer periods of prehospitalization illness and their generally dependent ("pre-modernization") status (discussed in Chapter IX). This fear also fits the unsystematically reported expulsion of chronically alcoholic and psychotic people from their homes. It seems probable that the experience of removal from home to mental hospital constitutes a more severe stress for the Brazilian woman than for her male counterpart.

The major factors protecting against depression, and particularly suicidal behavior, are associated with being black in a situation of apparently minimal role conflict and participating in

Afro-Spiritist activities. Youth, with its physical strength and optimism not yet foreclosed, may be plausibly regarded as having protective value before it is eroded by time and experience. Clearly, the protection from physical stress afforded by adequate housing and nonmanual occupations reduces the likelihood of body centered complaints.

HOSTILE OR IMPULSIVE BEHAVIOR

Direct anger or hostility were expressed during the interview by only 12 per cent of the patients. This conforms to a social context which does not sanction hostility by sons against fathers or by lower-class against upper-class adults. A past history of frequent arguments or identified attacks of rage or anger was, however, found in more than a third of the cases. This difference between immediate interview behavior in the hospital and past history is reminiscent of Schooler and Caudill's data (Caudill & Lin, 1969) on Japanese schizophrenics whose hospital behavior was relatively submissive and constrained. Compared with American patients in a Maryland state mental hospital, however, the Japanese had shown increased physical violence, especially toward family members—particularly the mother—and had been more emotionally impulsive in the year prior to their current admission to the hospital. These observations in a culture that emphasizes conformity suggest that maladaptive responses identified as mental illness stand out in contrast to the society's modal behavior patterns. The same may be said for the third of the Brazilian patients who had displayed repetitive argumentativeness or attacks of rage. These stood out in sharp relief in a society where interpersonal ends are achieved through elaborate circumlocution and avoidance of direct conflict. On the other hand, Draguns et al. (1966) suggest that psychopathological individuals express an exaggeration of prevailing cultural behavior patterns. They reported, for example, that Argentinian patients are relatively more passive and dependent than North American patients. These apparent differences may be resolved by recognizing, as have Katz et al. (1969), that the manner in which pathology is actually expressed may be quite different in the community and in the hospital—which appears to be true at least for the expression of hostile feelings within the present Brazilian patient group. As noted above, aggressive or other dramatic acts may be necessary for lowest-class persons with few available alternatives to communicate with the power holders. Beyond this, in a society placing a premium on courtesy and affectively toned interpersonal ritual, such behavior is more likely to be labeled deviant. The effects of the hospital subculture, combined with removal from former influences, modified symptom expression. Which behavior, in the hospital or in the community, most validly characterizes psychiatric illness in any ethnic or cultural group is open to question.

The incidence of aggressive behavior according to sociocultural status is seen in Table 222. While more males than females were admitted to the hospital because of immediate physical assault, the total number was only 22, and there were no gender differences of 10 per cent or more for the other forms of hostile or impulsive behavior listed in Table 222. Browns, who (as described in Chapter V) were characterized by the greatest tension and frustration of any color group, had the highest relative, though not significant, incidence of angry, argumentative, and impulsive behavior. Those partly literate also were more frequently aggressive than literates or illiterates. The youngest patients were consistently more aggressive and tense than their elders, although this did not account for a disproportionate number of their admissions. Afro-Spiritists and Catholics, the two most stable groups offering their participants greatest traditional and ritual support, showed the lowest proportionate incidence of arguments and attacks of anger. The religiously unaffiliated were high in these respects and significantly more so than the affiliated in regard to impulsive behavior. This is consistent with their relative youth and lack of capacity to relate to others. The similarly high incidence of impulsive behavior among the unmarried is congruent with this finding. Members of occupational Class V, who (as discussed in Chapter VII) appear most stable and least frustrated, showed proportionately less impulsive behavior than the others.

The single category in which blacks did not show the lowest incidence of aggressive behavior concerned assaults on others as a precipitant of admission. This may reflect the greater relative frequency of males among black patients. The data in Chapter V, however, suggest that this figure does not reflect the general characteristics of psychiatrically disturbed blacks so much as it does the nature of the entry system into mental hospitals. As in Baltimore, the black, uneducated, and poor of Rio de Janeiro must be more floridly disturbed or constitute a threat to the peace before hospitalization is considered.

In summary, impulsive or angry behavior as a leading symptom preceding hospitalization in this patient group appears to be associated with youth, lack of affiliation with organizations or individuals, and marginal status as regards both color and literacy. (The possibility that marginal literacy in this population might be associated with undiagnosed brain damage was discussed in Chapter VI.) Whether or not their symptomatic anger contributes to or is a consequence of lack of affiliation is uncertain. The marginal status of the browns, however, seems to have been consistently among the causes of their frustration and anger. Membership in a stable occupational group (Class V) representing achieved upward mobility, appears to diminish the likelihood of such behavior becoming prominent in a lower-class patient population. Class V occupational status appears consistently to have reduced frustration and anxiety as well as angry tension. In general terms, the data support a frustration-aggression hypothesis. They do not suggest that depressive feelings, as prominent among browns as whites, are a consequence of aggression turned against the self or that symptomatic anger is an effective defense against anxiety or depression.

Comparative North American data are available from the New Haven, Midtown, and Stirling County projects. Antisocial reactions were diagnosed most often in New Haven social Classes I–II, III and dropped sharply in Class IV, most comparable with the Brazilian skilled manual worker category. These antisocial diagnoses overlap with but are not identical with behaviors labeled hostile or "acting out" which most frequently precipitated mental hospitalization in the lowest-class New Haven patients. This last finding is perhaps comparable to the relatively high frequency of assaultive behavior among Rio blacks as a precipitant of hospitalization. Langner and Michael (1963) similarly observed a higher prevalence of aggressive behavior in their higher than lower SES Midtown nonpatient respondents, suggesting that such behavior may have adaptive value, as it appears to have had up to a point for Rio brown patients. They also found, as among New Haven patients, a much greater proportion of the "acting out" personality type in their lowest SES respondents. Broadly similar findings were also reported for Stirling County. Sociopathic behavior was slightly more frequent in highest occupational class nonpatient respondents, dropped in the next category, and rose again, so that prevalence was markedly highest among the least skilled or occupationally most disadvantaged persons. Sex status made a considerable difference, with a predominance of women showing psychoneurotic symptoms and men showing sociopathic behavior. As Leighton et al. (1963) put it: "This . . . matches common opinion: Women get nervous, while men get drunk and/or fight" (p. 261).

These data do not lend themselves to precise comparison with those from Rio. Specific sociocultural features of the Rio patients, i.e., color or lack of religious affiliation, do not correspond precisely with "social class" or "SES." The common denominator between aggressive, hostile, tensely argumentative, or impulsive patients or potential patients across sociocultures may be their lack of social integration. Another way of saying this is that they are not secure in their statuses, are not responsible, full participants in the culture, and are culturally excluded.

SOMATIC COMPLAINTS

As shown in Table 214, 74 per cent of the entire patient group complained of at least one type of pain or physical discomfort. These pains and discomforts represented such a wide range of organs, body regions, and qualities of malaise that, aside from the factors of occupation, age, and religion, there were no significant differences in distribution according to sociocultural status.

As expectable, the youngest and presumably most vigorous and unscarred patients least frequently reported physical discomfort. Those whose bodies were most used and abused by work demands, i.e., the unskilled manual laborers, more frequently reported physical discomfort than the skilled manual or nonmanual workers. This finding is congruent with that noted above regarding body or organ anxiety, although anxiety (in contrast to actual discomfort) was more closely linked to several indices of dependence upon bodily functions for socioeconomic survival. Such somatic anxiety or concern, in contrast to actual pain or discomfort, was present in 40 per cent of the total patient group. It was relatively more frequent in the deprived, culturally excluded segments of the population, as well as the unskilled. This last finding is also congruent with those for fatigue, although, as noted above, anorexia and weakness were less clearly aligned with SES related reality factors.

In contrast to both organ anxiety and bodily discomfort, specific reflections of autonomic nervous activity in the shape of psychosomatic symptoms were not clearly and consistently related to physical stress. As shown in Table 223, the most prevalent symptom was faintness or dizziness (the two being often indistinguishable by interview) present in almost half the patients. Palpitation was reported in almost a third and nausea or vomiting and dyspnea and related complaints in between a quarter and a third. All of these symptoms could plausibly be expected to occur most frequently in patients subject to hard manual labor, poor living conditions, and inadequate diet and health care. Literacy, however, was the only SES related factor yielding differences of 10 per cent for all of the symptom complexes, and symptoms occurred in a manner opposite to the expected direction, i.e., least often among the illiterates at the bottom of the socioeconomic ladder. This contrasts with their most frequent complaints of fatigue and weakness (as noted in Chapter VI). Illiterates (as discussed in the same chapter) probably constitute the most helpless minority group in Rio de Janeiro, without even the blacks' institutionalized ways of relating to those more powerful than themselves. The illiterates (presumably without the drive, competence, and family facilitation to overcome deficient education) include a disproportionate number of blacks, people of rural background, and recent migrants. Lack of literacy thus means low talent and drive plus cultural exclusion, unfamiliarity with the social context, added coping burdens, and absence of acquired skills and information—all leading to defective responsible participation in the symbolic-meaningful experience of the society. The illiterates are the psychiatrically most vulnerable patient subgroup. Their high prevalence of direct, sensory, nonsymbolic symptoms, i.e., hallucinations, present also among the recently migrant, uneducated, and black, suggests that the relatively subtle language of autonomic dysfunction displayed in psychosomatic symptoms may not be necessary for them. Of these other factors, however, only migration bears a similar relation to psychosomatic symptoms. Just as in the case of the illiterates, significantly fewer recent migrants complained of palpitation, dyspnea, or related difficulties.

The other factor revealing differences for all symptom groups in a manner similar to literacy is marital status. The married uniformly include more patients suffering from psychosomatic disturbance than the single. Factors contributing to this include their relatively older age. The single are somewhat more illiterate and more frequently in Class VI occupations. The major characteristics of the married are those of the literate, i.e., they are more economically stable, socially advantaged, have more information and are more responsibly participant in the symbolic-meaningful experience of the society.

The relative predominance of psychosomatic symptoms among the literate, married, and settled—all of whom have a lower prevalence of hallucinations and disorientation, a higher prevalence of fear of loss of control, of diffuse anxiety, and of feelings of weeping or sadness than the nonliterate, single, and recently migrant—suggests the possible importance of some denominator common to these groups. One such social denominator appears to be responsible informed participation in the socioculture, a condition opposite to that characterizing the most aggressive and impulsive patients. Associated psychological components may be inferred to include internalized self-critical standards, some inhibition of direct expression of feelings through action, fear of status loss, high value placed on rational, conscious control of behavior, and actively functioning defense mechanisms aimed at maintenance of such control. In support of this idea is the lower prevalence among browns than blacks and whites of faintness or dizziness.

In apparent contrast to the above, the distribution of psychosomatic symptoms according to occupation was in the totally opposite direction. The two symptom groups, faintness or dizziness and nausea or vomiting, for which occupation was a differential factor, occurred most often among the manual (skilled and unskilled) in comparison with nonmanual workers, as did most other somatic complaints. In other words, although there was a considerable overlap between unskilled manual and illiterate status (57 per cent of the illiterates were unskilled; 55 per cent of the unskilled were literate), the actual physical stress and dependence for survival upon an intact body of manual workers were overwhelming contributors to the production of all body-related symptoms including the psychosomatic.

Faintness or dizziness and dyspnea were both significantly more frequent among females than males. Females, as noted previously, also had a higher prevalence of fatigue, anorexia, weakness, and general organ anxiety.

Finally, there was a differential distribution according to religion for palpitation and dyspnea. In both instances, the unaffiliated (who tended to be younger) showed a lower prevalence than religiously affiliated patients. The higher prevalence of dyspnea among the Protestants and of palpitation among the Afro-Spiritists than other religious groups, as well as the unaffiliated, do not lend themselves to generalization. One specific factor possibly influencing the latter is their heavy use of cigar smoking during cultist ceremonies.

In summary, somatic symptoms of all kinds including those associated with autonomic dysfunction, i.e., the psychosomatic, were more prevalent among manual than nonmanual workers. Dependence upon an intact body for economic survival and regular exposure to physical stress appear to be, as indicated in preceding sections, the most important contributors to somatic concern, discomfort, feelings of inadequacy, and psychosomatic symptoms. Within the manual group physical aches and pains were more frequent among the unskilled than skilled, while, as previously noted, somatic anxiety was linked to several other indices of low SES as well. Psychosomatic symptoms, however, were as frequent among the skilled as unskilled, and aside from the broad division according to occupation, were distributed in the opposite direction, being most prevalent among the literate, married, and settled. This grouping is not confined to and does not include all of the higher "social class" or "SES" patients in the Rio sample, i.e., the most occupationally advanced, best housed, and best educated. It may best be defined as having been more able than the nonliterate to learn despite environmental limitations; more capable than the unmarried of relating responsibly to others over the long term; and more enculturated, socially connected, and part of a stable interpersonal network than the recently migrant. In comparison with their opposites, these patients showed not only a higher prevalence of psychosomatic symptoms, but of diffuse anxiety and fear of loss of control as well. They were, thus, despite their social differences, comparable in symptom formation to the upper-class New Haven patients. While these last showed the least association between class position and the frequency of psychosomatic reactions, prevalence rates were higher for Classes I-II (college educated, executives, or professionals) living in the most desirable neighborhoods. They did not, however, decline progressively in frequency as the class ladder was descended. After a mild trough in Class III (high school graduates, small managers, proprietors, white-collar workers), frequency increased slightly in Classes IV (employed, skilled workers with some high school) and V (irregularly employed, poorly connected with community institutions, elementary schooling). Phobic-anxiety reactions were also distributed among New Haven patients in a manner resembling that of diffuse anxiety and fear of loss of control in the Rio group, and opposite to the direction of somatic complaints and somatic anxiety. Phobic anxiety was most prevalent in Classes I-II, plateauing in III and IV, with a drop again in V. Obsessive-compulsive reactions, comparable to fear of loss of control, were markedly highest in New Haven Classes I-II, falling steeply to Class IV, and leveling out at V. Similarly, Langner and Michael found more compulsive symptoms among high than low SES Midtown nonpatients, with most in upwardly mobile (in relation to paternal SES) high SES respondents.

In Stirling County, as noted above, sociopathic symptom patterns increased in prevalence with increased occupational disadvantage (following a scale devised to fit local circumstances). Unlike Rio and New Haven patients, and urban Midtown nonpatients, however, the males among these rural and small town nonpatients also showed increasing rather than decreasing prevalence of psychoneurotic and psychophysiologic symptoms with increasing occupational disadvantage (although the last declined again in frequency at the lowest occupational level). Females exhibited a similar pattern except that their prevalence of psychophysiologic complaints continued to rise until it was highest among the occupationally most disadvantaged. Examination of specific symptom listings for the Stirling County respondents suggests that some of the difference between these observations and those in Rio may be associated with the inclusion of a broader variety of somatic discomforts under the rubric of "psychophysiologic" in Stirling County. That is, the relationship of occupational disadvantage to psychophysiologic symptoms in Stirling County is more similar to the relationship between occupation (manual versus nonmanual) and somatic symptoms in general than psychosomatic symptoms in particular in Rio patients. Apart from this, the pooling of symptoms under such broad headings as "psychoneurotic" may obscure differences in anxiety, obsessive-compulsive symptoms, or depression as such. It is also possible that in such semirural communities as those of Stirling County dominated, in contrast to pluralistic United States metropolitan centers, by particular ethnic and traditional groups, there is less opportunity for individual variation; disorder and symptom rates thus reflect the status of the total community more than the variability of the persons who make it up. Nonetheless, the use of broad categories revealed, as Leighton et al. indicated, that in Stirling County as in New Haven and Midtown proportionately more psychiatric disorder seems to exist within the most disadvantaged segments of the population.

SEXUAL BEHAVIOR

Table 224 shows that some change in sex behavior in association with the events leading to hospitalization was almost universally reported. This may be due in part to the general acceptance of sexual function as a significant part of life deserving no less attention than any other aspect of behavior. As discussed earlier, sexual capacity and performance are closely linked to self-concept and a sense of stable identity, at least in men.

Approximately half of the patients, including the largest proportions of whites, literates, and skilled manual workers in contrast to nonwhites, nonliterates, and both nonmanual and unskilled workers, reported a basically monogamous adult sex life. Less than a fifth reported casual relationships to have been their norm, and eight per cent had confined themselves to solitary masturbation. The remaining 26 per cent had had relatively stable relationships over varying periods with more than a single mate. As might be expected, the solitary masturbators were almost entirely in the youngest age group, and also predominated among those with primarily casual relationships. Browns were more heavily represented than other color groups among those with casual and nonmonogamous sexual patterns.

A relatively small proportion, less than a fifth, of the patients reported a preference for other than conventionally accepted heterosexual intercourse. Approximately a fifth (with no significant differences according to sex or other status) had engaged in anal intercourse, but this was not identified as preferred. It was most often described as a variant of heterosexual intercourse, sometimes as foreplay, occasionally associated with partial impotence, and sometimes used for contraceptive reasons. There are no reliable baseline data against which to compare this report, but Kinsey in his 1948 U.S. survey noted that ". . . anal activity in the heterosexual is not frequent enough to make it possible to determine the incidence of individuals who are specifically responsive to such stimulation" (p. 579).

Table 225 indicates the distribution according to sociocultural status of some of the most frequently reported sexual complaints. Conflict about sex, worry-induced impairment, impotence or frigidity, and increased or uncontrollable impulses were all less frequent among blacks than whites or browns. Whether (as discussed in Chapter V) these findings reflect a greater functional development of one of the few available sources of pleasure, or a relative lack of guilt and conflict secondary to the failure to acquire middle-class standards while growing up, is uncertain. A significant contributor to this color difference—not incompatible with the possibilities just noted—may be the relative rate of social change in regard to sexual standards within the various groups. As discussed in Chapter IX, Brazilian men have traditionally enjoyed a double standard permitting them considerable sexual freedom while the women have remained constrained. This standard is becoming more of an ideal than a practice, however, for those in the upper occupational brackets, especially with educated wives who are more "modernized." It seems likely that the men of this group, with less opportunity than in the past to affirm their masculinity via casual pickups or increasingly expensive mistresses, are more vulnerable to psychiatric interference with sexual capacity than are the men in the more static lower social classes. As noted above, social change of all kinds appears less prominent for the blacks than nonblacks; the relative role stability here appears to have contributed to a lower prevalence of sexual as well as anxious and depressive complaints.

Interference with function was most often reported by whites, who typically had a single mate over a long period. This finding is consistent with the considerable predominance among the married (responsible for meeting the expectations of regular partners), as compared with the single patients, of interference with sex by worries, sex difficulties as part of the present illness, and impotence or frigidity (this last being most common among the female patients, most of whom were married). Complaints of too intense or uncontrollable sex impulses, possibly compensatory as part of a pattern of grandiosity, were more often reported by the upwardly striving browns; because of their less stable marital condition they were also presumably more subject to sexual frustration. Intense or uncontrollable sexual desires were reported more frequently by males than females and singles than married.

The intensity and conflict surrounding sex for single males is also suggested by the finding that guilt or shame stemming from sexual performance were significantly more frequent for male than female and for unmarried than married patients. In fact, judging from the almost nonexistent reports of this kind among the married, the state of marriage and its social concomitants appear to grant significant protection from sexual guilt or shame, although the married, as noted above, reported more actual functional impairment.

Literacy, like whiteness, appears to be associated with a higher prevalence of impotence or frigidity; over a third of the literates, more than twice the number of illiterates, reported sexual difficulties as part of their psychiatric illness. Conversely, illiterates, like blacks, complained less often than literates and part literates of overly intense, fluctuating, or potentially uncontrollable sexual impulses. Some of the difference may be associated with the more rigid sexual standards espoused by the intact, literate, higher achieving families of literate patients. Another reason may be inherent in the process of selection for hospitalization. Literates had fewer reality breaks than illiterates, and their relatives (as those of white) considered hospitalization mainly because of anxious or depressed rather than dramatically disturbed behavior. The lack of equivalence between indices of socioeconomic status in this respect is suggested by the fact that occupation alone among them is significant with regard to the frequency of impotence and frigidity. These complaints are least frequent among the Class I-IV nonmanual workers who are mainly white and literate (although they are also less frequent among blacks than nonblacks). The major element here may be the statistically highest proportion of long-term monogamous relationships within the context in which these sexual complaints develop in occupational Class V rather than Class I-IV. This supposition is supported by the significantly lower incidence of impotence and frigidity among the younger patients, most represented in occupational Classes I-IV and VI.

Older age is also present as a contributor to the occurrence of sexual difficulties as part of the present illness. In contrast, sex is most frequently a source of guilt or shame for the youngest (and as noted above, the unmarried). The high prevalence of dysfunction among females, mainly married, is probably related to their submissive-dependent status vis-à-vis the males who often view them as nonparticipant sexual targets, as well as their lack of early sex education. Both of these are aspects of a double standard of morality granting considerable sexual freedom to the male while imposing traditional restraints on the female. The system is changing, however, as indicated above, especially for the educated classes.

Differences in reporting sexual complaints are not marked according to religion. Worries interfering with sex, sexual problems as part of the present illness, and impotence or frigidity occurred with somewhat greater frequency among the Protestants, who, (as described in Chapter XI) were more often monogamous, preoccupied with sexual morality, and more self-aware about these issues. Similarly, the first two symptom categories were least often re-

ported by the unaffiliated. The absence of sex-associated guilt or
shame in the Afro-Spiritists fits their previously reported lack of
tension about a number of other issues.

In summary, symptomatic sexual behavior appears to be divisible into at least three categories. The first includes tension produced functional impairment often related to the present illness, and such associated problems as impotence or frigidity. The second includes possibly compensatory symptoms and frustration-associated behavior such as too intense or uncontrollable sexual urges. The third, present in very few patients, is the occurrence of guilt or shame in association with sexual thoughts or acts. All categories were least frequent among blacks. The first appears most common among those who, married and monogamous, have the longest histories of sexual relations with a consistent partner and for whom sex presumably has the greatest communicative and interpersonal significance. This group includes whites, literates, Protestants, skilled manual workers, older patients, and females. Clearly, aside from the factor of monogamy, each sociocultural status contributes its own determinants to the final behavioral outcome.

The second category was most heavily represented among the marginal and unattached with the least stable sexual parterships. These were the brown, male, and the unmarried. Apparently inconsistent with other findings, the illiterate were least prominent in this group; this is probably because literacy was higher among the younger and unmarried patients, who having grown up in the urban setting had had more opportunity to learn.

The third category, sexual guilt or shame, was also most common among the young, the male, and the unmarried. These unmarried young men with emotional problems, i.e., those en route to psychiatric hospitalization, were those not yet successful in establishing a stable sexual identity. For them, sexual relations required initiative and interpersonal resourcefulness which they did not possess. Their masturbation was a reminder of frustration as well as a source of guilt at doing something religiously prohibited and shame for fear of being identified as unmanly. Attempts at heterosexual intercourse carried the threat of failure and humiliation.

While there is little information about sexual behavior in the major studies referred to above, a detailed description of its viscissitudes in schizophrenic families in Puerto Rico is provided by Rogler and Hollingshead (1965). As in Brazil, this is a double-standard culture in which masculine identity, especially in the slum dwellers among whom the study was conducted, requires frequent intercourse with as many partners as the man can obtain. Sex is a regular source of marital conflict, but in the well families the reluctant wives eventually grant or even initiate intercourse in an effort to keep their husbands from sexual adventures outside the home. When the husband becomes psychotic, marital sex conflict diminishes as the wife becomes the stronger one in the family, keeps him at home while she goes out to work, and allows him regular though less frequent intercourse perceived by her as therapeutically best for him. This is usually accepted by the husband, who has developed doubts about his strength and potency as part of his illness. If, on the other hand, the wife becomes mentally ill her capacity to control her repugnance is seriously impaired, she may violently refuse sex, and the husband increasingly looks elsewhere. These findings are consistent with the ubiquitousness of sexual change accompanying the onset of mental illness and the greater frequency of sexual complaints of female patients in the Rio sample. They do not, however, contain comparative material about sexual functioning in relation to SES or other sociocultural statuses.

ATTITUDES AND FEELINGS TOWARD OTHERS (PARANOID BEHAVIOR)

As seen in Table 226, more than half the patients felt that they were not being treated well by family, friends, or others. More than a third complained of being persecuted, harassed, talked about, or stared at by individuals or organized groups. Somewhat fewer exhibited behavior with grandiose elements, and from a fifth to over a quarter revealed other feelings of being influenced and a tendency to see unreliability, deprecation, and hostility in others.

Certain regularities in the distribution of these behaviors are immediately apparent. Thus, the browns, already described as marginal, tense, and sensitive, exhibit more paranoid behavior than others. For most indices, the whites reveal the lowest incidence of paranoid feelings. This contrasts to the distribution of depression, the incidence of which was similar among browns and whites. In this instance, the social group which is in fact a significant target of discrimination and is trying most vigorously to combat it, more often exhibits paranoid behavior which cannot be understood in adaptive terms. This is especially true for such complaints as being talked about or stared at, and the apparently compensatory feeling of being emulated or admired. Complaints of bad treatment, persecution, the untrustworthiness of others, being misjudged, and being regarded as inferior may have significant reality roots, but are expressed with inappropriate intensity and with regard to inappropriate persons or groups. The fact that these are more frequent among browns than blacks can be attributed both to the aspirations and actual upward mobility (sometimes evoking retaliation) of the former and the previously mentioned protective attitudes of the latter.

Paranoid complaints were more prevalent among recent migrants than settled patients. This was discussed in Chapter IV in respect to the loss of familiar supports and the impact of a new, unfamiliar, and possibly threatening environment. Again the adaptive need to be sensitive, wary, and cautious appears to increase the probability of more clearly pathological and maladaptive paranoid behavior. Unlike the incidence of depressive feelings, paranoid behavior in most of its symptomatic forms appears to occur more frequently among the most deprived and excluded patients. These include the unskilled and the poorly housed and also those who suffer from little information and disrupted personal relationships. Thus, depending upon the particular complaint, the prevalence of paranoid behavior was highest among the illiterate or lowest among the literate. The generally higher prevalence among patients living in urban transitional, slum, or deteriorated areas probably has similar significance to its occurrence among recent migrants.

Data on age and marital status suggest other factors stimulating or maintaining paranoid behavior. Such behavior, regardless of type, occurred more frequently among the single than the married. This may be most parsimoniously explained by assuming that paranoid or psychotic persons are unlikely to become married. It also seems likely that the relative isolation of the single perpetuates their fantasies about the attitudes of others toward them. As indicated in Chapter IX, the single are significantly younger than the married and more have been identified as behaviorally deviant since early life. This fits the age incidence noted in Table 222. In most instances, paranoid symptoms occur most often in the youngest age group and least frequently among the older patients. Paranoid symptom distribution according to religion is less consistent, but in general it seems to occur most frequently among the unaffiliated. Again, this fits the general impression of this type of symptomatic behavior as tending to develop in those who by choice or by circumstance are not securely anchored to social groups. Tendencies to suspiciousness, distrust, and concern with the motives of others, along with their associated needs for self-protection, are antithetical to affiliative tendencies.

PERCEPTUAL AND SENSORY EXPERIENCES—
HALLUCINATIONS AND ILLUSIONS

Apparent auditory hallucinations, as listed in Table 227, were present in approximately a third of the patients, and visual hallucinations in approximately a fifth: Of these latter, however, only approximately half reported hallucinations of people; the others stated that they had seen animals, ghostly, folkloric or other non-human entities, occasionally under circumstances suggesting that they might have included illusory phenomena. Not all of the patients reporting apparent auditory or visual hallucinations were steadfastly convinced of the significance of their experiences; a fifth of the total group insisted on the reality of what they had seen or heard, and somewhat fewer planned action on these bases. Experience easily interpretable as illusory was also reported by approximately a fifth of the patients.

While blacks did not most frequently report paranoid complaints, they exhibited a notably higher prevalence of hallucinations than the other two color groups. The lowest frequency was among whites. Auditory hallucinations were reported by almost two-thirds of the black patients. More than a third, four times the proportion of whites, also reported visual hallucinations of people. Similarly, blacks were considerably more insistent upon the reality of their experiences. The possible reasons for the consistent predominance of hallucinatory experience among blacks and, as noted in Table 227, of disorientation as well, are discussed in Chapter V. These include the probability that without prior psychiatric contact they were most often admitted for severely florid disturbance after repeated unsuccessful contacts with religious leaders. The whites and browns with shorter periods of prior illness did not require such dramatic symptomatology for admission. Forty-six per cent of blacks, approximately twice the proportion of whites and browns, admitted a history of excessive drinking, but none were admitted in an acutely intoxicated state or exhibited signs of delirium tremens.

The blacks' tendency to express psychological disturbance mainly in plastic sensory rather than symbolic terms, and in reference to the outer rather than inner world, seems most plausibly related to two factors. One is their relative lack of informational input about the modern urban world around them, a perceptual deprivation which can be linked to their comparative isolation (i.e., exclusion) from the complex symbolic-informational system, and the reduced likelihood of acquiring rational and achievement values reflected in the importance given to time, conscious planning, and control of oneself and others. To these may be added greater willingness to accept fantasy experience of various kinds as real and important. The suggestion that lack of information and cultural exclusion increase the frequency of symptomatic externalization (versus internalization) of conflictful elements in plastic form as a means of expressing anxiety and dealing with interpersonal and intrapsychic problems is supported by other data in Table 227: hallucinations, illusions, and disorientation are proportionately more frequent among those with rural backgrounds who have not yet learned about their new environment (the recently migrant), the symbolically least capable with the fewest sources of information (the uneducated and the illiterate), and, to a lesser degree, the inhabitants of transitory, anomic areas (Area II). The various symptomatic forms of plastic externalization were also most consistently frequent among the unskilled manual workers and the poorly housed.

A second factor contributing to the prevalence of hallucinations in black patients is suggested by their relatively infrequent display of hostile, tense, depressed, and to a lesser degree, paranoid behavior. As indicated in Chapter V, they appear to have achieved an adjustment to conditions of social deprivation and oppression which might (as in the case of the browns) be expected to evoke marked tension, anger, and sadness. A failure to have acquired unachievable aspirations is only part of the answer; this failure of itself may have psychological roots. It is plausible to assume that the blacks' adjustment, aided by the historical process (described in Chapter V), involves important elements of denial, repression, and other defense mechanisms, resulting in a manageable level of anxiety and relative conscious tranquility. With blocking of the expressive channels leading to conscious tension and significant awareness of reality problems, the only alternative is plastic sensory externalization in hallucinatory form embodying elements of wish fulfillment as well as of anger, tension, and depression.

The proportionately higher occurrence of hallucinations, illusions, and disorientation among single patients reflects in part that fact that, as indicated in Tables 149 and 150, they are proportionately more illiterate, unskilled, poorly housed, and nonwhite than the married. The prevalence of blacks among the singles is, however, similar to that among the married who hallucinated significantly less often. The singles' most striking characteristic is their relative youth. In them, hallucinations and disorientation reflect a chronic psychotic process with onset early in life more than the impact of social experience upon an already stablized personality.

OTHER SYMPTOMS REFLECTING IMPAIRED REALITY EVALUATION

The presence of hallucinations and particularly of disorientation may plausibly be attributed, at least in part, to the types of cerebral deficit (associated with alcoholism, head injury, or senility) reflected in cognitive dysfunction. Table 228 which lists the distribution of interview reports of impaired mental efficiency and of difficulties in recent or remote recall, does not, however, support this assumption. In no instance is cognitive dysfunction most frequent among the blacks who often had histories of excessive drinking and most frequently showed disorientation and hallucinatory behavior. Nor is it highest in the older age range. Impaired mental efficiency is most frequent among the young, the unmarried, and the female, the groups characterized by the most dramatically disturbed clearly psychotic behavior of longest duration. Impaired mental efficiency may be linked to realistic anxiety and lack of information which can contribute to a tendency to hallucinate. It is significantly more prevalent among recent migrants and the poorly housed than among the settled and the more adequately housed. The lack of a difference in impaired mental efficiency according to literacy or occupation suggests the importance of features associated with housing per se, such as frustration associated with inability to move or with abrasive surroundings, rather than with housing regarded only as an indication of low SES. Both these groups included proportionately high frequencies of hallucinating patients.

The low prevalence of memory difficulties among the Afro-Spiritists, as among the blacks, may reflect a lack of critical self-awareness and a relative lack of value placed upon accurate recall and precise thinking. Dreaming is another behavior with reality-evaluating significance. As noted in Table 229, only 30 per cent of the patients acknowledge remembered dreams with personal meaning. Most of these were unpleasant in nature. Significant differences according to sociocultural status were not obtained, in part because the total numbers involved were so small. There was no systematic relationship between the presence of hallucinatory or delusional symptoms and reports of dreaming.

RELATIONAL BEHAVIOR IN THE INTERVIEW

Since the major data-gathering locus was the interview of psychiatrist with patient, the attitudes and responses of both parties are relevant to the symptomatic data. Sixty-five percent of all patients were described by the psychiatrists as cooperative throughout. Table 231 summarizes differences of 10 per cent or more according to sociocultural status in patients' relational behavior. Significantly more of the better educated, literate, better housed, male, married and mid-age-range patients were regarded as cooperative. In general, these most resembled the interviewers in terms of social class and education. Presumably those in the middle-age group were most sure of themselves and prepared to meet the young physicians on a relatively egalitarian basis without anxiety or defiance. The trend was evident with regard to occupation as well. Insofar as skin color, migratory status, and religion are all related to economic status, as well as to similarity or difference of experience from the interviewers and experience in self-revelation to physicians, the lack of difference according to these statuses is unexpected. It suggests that interview cooperation is less a function of similarities associated with socioeconomic status or shared information than of a variety of factors including the security gained from long-institutionalized relationships or religious affiliation, the intelligent aggressiveness which may be part of conscious wishes for upward mobility, and the competence necessary for successful migration.

Cooperation was not always associated with behavior interpreted by the psychiatrists as courteous or friendly. While 60 per cent of the patients were so regarded, the males were significantly more courteous than the more anxious and disturbed females, and the presumably more interpersonally adept married were more courteous than the single. Least courteous and friendly were the religiously unaffiliated (who were, nonetheless, not notably uncooperative) in contrast to the affiliated, the youngest in comparison to both other age groups, the poorly housed and the illiterate in contrast to the literate and part literate. Again, those in the first two categories tended to have been disturbed since childhood and to have never developed easy relationships with others. Those in the last two categories were separated from the interviewers by broader social distances.

Related to both social form (courtesy, friendliness) and capacity to cooperate is anxiety-free attention to the interviewer. This means relative lack of distraction and tension and consistent participation in the interview process, even without a courteous bearing or unfailing cooperation. Approximately 65 per cent of patients were rated as paying attention comfortably. Again, those who did not were concentrated among the illiterates, the poorly housed, the unmarried, the young, and the religiously unaffiliated. Consistent with the conclusions of Chapter VII, members of the relatively stable skilled workers in Class V rather than of the nonmanual I-IV were most frequently rated as comfortable. Active seeking of advice was encountered in only 20 per cent of the patients. It seemed more frequent among the most secure, i.e., better educated, literate, and better housed but special factors were again suggested. The middle age-range patients (described in Chapter IX as more self-sufficient) were less prone to seek advice while the seeking of advice of the Protestants who were poor and anxious appears consistent with their ethic and their ambitiousness. Poverty and anxiety may thus be overridden in the final determination of behavior by ideologies and values, i.e., the patient's perceptions of what is right, necessary, and important. Further, seeking advice reflects a conscious choice of behavior which may require some effort on the patient's part to manage his anxiety or timidity.

The possible influence of the interviewer's attitudes on relational behavior is suggested in Table 230.

DISCUSSION AND SUMMARY

This discussion and summary is couched whenever possible in general and comparative terms aimed at creating a transcultural perspective. Most patterns of symptomatic behavior in the present patient population cannot be understood in terms of such inclusive categories as socioconomic status or social class. While some fit more easily under these rubrics than others, the significance of general categories and their components varies between countries and cultures. Some of the variance in symptomatic behavior in the Rio patient group as compared with United States populations lies, for example, in the difference between a developing and a fully industrialized society; it also lies in the difference between a traditionally Latin, Catholic socioculture with strong African influences and two historically separated socioeconomic classes, on the one hand, and, on the other, a traditionally English and Protestant socioculture with a number of historically discriminated-against racial, national, and religious minorities. The specific sociocultural statuses making up SES or social class are more significant. They elicit adaptive, coping, or defensive responses some of which lead to identifiable behavior defined as symptomatic. These statuses and their concomitants may be regarded as "stressful" although their stressful aspects may not be identical in all settings. Other statuses and concomitants appear to aid the coping or adaptive process in ways which reduce the occurrence of symptomatic behavior. They are to some degree, then, "protective." This varies for different individuals and in relation to different behavioral patterns, depending upon particular relationships to the environment and ways of participating in the social process. Creative adaptations and coping efforts as well as regressive, defensive, or symptomatic behavior may occur as part of interaction within particular contexts, acutely or, as implied by a status position, over the long term. Differences in symptomatic behavior in the present population suggest the varying evocative significance in a still industrializing and rapidly changing society with a unique cultural history of such unavoidable lifelong statuses as skin color and gender; of an unavoidable and progressively changing status such as age with its sequential crises; of rapid social and personal change as involved in migration; of statuses and capacities indicated by education and literacy which for many can be achieved only with great effort and motivation, but which for a few are a birthright reflecting family background more than individual talent or persistence; of work with its mobility satisfactions and frustrations as well as its correlated physical stress; of religion no longer so constrained by tradition as in the past and still an ascribed status for many, but for others a creative coping or adaptive participation.

All of the foregoing statuses involve characteristic participations in the social process. A sociocultural status such as age, skin color, occupation, or migratory phase implies the nature of a person's relationship with his current environment, i.e., his behavioral setting or context. This includes the ways in which he interacts with others and his centrality within the dominant culture, or a series of subcultures. It also implies a historically determined inner state, which influences the way in which he processes current information, i.e., perceives and responds to it. Together with such basic equipment as intelligence and talent, this inner state includes unresolved conflicts, a variety of self-and other regulating activities (sometimes referred to as ego functions), moral standards and self-punitive tendencies (sometimes subsumed under the concept of superego), acquired and innate though modified drive tendencies, and the memories contributing to his cognitive map or model of his world. In conjunction with current outer events, it determines the person's behavioral output, i.e., his

symptomatic, adaptive, coping, defensive, creative, or other behaviors. Dohrenwend (1961) conceptualized the relationship of
inner state and outer events as stress mediators in terms of "con-
straints." His concept of inner constraint appears clearly derived
from Freudian theory; it is related to drives, self-prescriptions,
and socialization practices. External constraint is related to status,
social relationships, family, similarity of inner goals of others, and
relative deprivation as compared with others. The intensity of a
stress varies directly with the strength of the external constraint
and that of the inner constraint associated with the stressor; the
adaptation syndrome represents efforts to reduce constraint.

A more general formulation, not concerned with the intensity
of "stress" but with adaptation as a process, is that of Lichtenberg
and Norton (1970). They extract from the literature on child development a series of basic themes beginning with the idea that
action is doubly directed, that is, the child relates to himself and
to others at the same time. More generally:

> A defining characteristic of action is that the organism is simulta-
> neously organizing its inner component parts into a unity, and at the
> same time forming a systematic relationship with things and people
> in the outer world. . . . As a unit . . . it is operative in organizing and
> regulating the elements that are within it. As a part of a context, it is
> operative in coming to terms with that which surrounds it . . . [p. 3].

They support from the literature the general contention, made
explicit by Piaget, that internal organization and adaptation to
the outer world are complementary aspects of a single process.
The comment which these reviewers make about infant and child
are also applicable to the adult patients in the Rio population:
"They are not simply responders to a conditioning, socializing
world, for they are dealing with themselves when they are attending to the world" (p. 8). This formulation is congruent with those
of Freud (1926) and Hartmann (1939) and with Barker's (1969)
idea of behavior settings (described in Chapter III).

APPRAISAL BEHAVIOR. PATHWAY TO THE MENTAL HOSPITAL

The world with which these patients have had to deal includes
family and community members. These people have responded

to the patients' cries for help, however disguised, in beginning the process of hospitalization. They have also initiated movement to a healer or social control agent in response to their own needs and anxieties. The process of appraisal by self or others as sick or deviant, and of acting upon this appraisal, reflect interacting-group and individual styles of dealing with long-term life situations and acute crises. Symptomatic behavior (of the "patient") and appraisal behavior (by self and of self by others) reflect norms, cognitive patterns, and expressive tendencies which are part of the socioculture and hence part of the external world; they are also acquired from the shared socioculture, and hence part of the inner states of the actors—patients and others. These norms, patterns, and tendencies include the shared symbol systems and sentiments in which patient and community participate with varying degrees of responsibility and involvement. They include institutionalized perceptual styles which determine, for example, what behavior is regarded as "sick" rather than criminal, immoral, immature, religiously inspired, nonconforming, or merely strange. They also include institutionalized ways of dealing with unacceptable, unpredictable, nonproductive behavior or behavior which inspires fear, anxiety, disgust, pity, or anger. In Talcott Parsons' (1952) words, institutionalized behavior provides "a mode of 'integration' of the actions of the component individuals" of society. Society's techniques for dealing with deviance involving variable degrees of collaboration by the labeled deviant include shunning, ridicule, nurturing, behavior change in place (as via outpatient treatment), extrusion from the system for punishment and deterrence (jail), or extrusion for behavior change (mental hospital). Such institutionalized ways of behaving represent unthinking conformity to cultural norms defining proper, legitimate, or expected modes of action or social relationship. They depend in part upon definitions and standards. As Parsons has noted ". . . moral standards constitute, as the focus of the evaluative aspect of the common culture, the core of the stabilizing mechanisms of the system of social interaction" (p. 22). These stabilize the ". . . cognitive definitions of what persons are in a socially significant sense." However ". . . all the components of the common culture are internalized as part of the personality structure . . ." (p. 23). Thus all cognitive-status definitions have cultural, hence normative significance; moral standards (key aspects of shared symbol systems) cannot be dissociated from the content of the orientation patterns which they regulate.

The institutionalized appraisal and response to deviance also depend upon the existence of "resources" or "facilities" such as mental hospitals, doctors, cult centers, and social agencies. As noted by Brody (1960) these undertake many of the social control functions once carried out by families. Facilities, as well as social norms and attitudes, reflect the developmental state of the behavior setting. The families of the Rio de Janeiro patients, socialized largely in preindustrial, semirural settings, often still living on the margin of the technological society, were more central decision-makers initiating the hospitalization process than often appears to be true for poor people in United States inner cities. While, as will be discussed later, the families responded nurturantly to behavior not central in the patients' own presentations, the patients did not as a rule resist the recommendation for psychiatric care. There was an apparently high degree of agreement between self-appraisal and the family or community decision that professional assistance was needed. Religious-spiritist centers rather than police stations were important relay points en route to the mental hospitals. Such centers are helping rather than disciplinary agencies and require the collaboration of the help-seekers. Their seemingly high viability in Brazil as institution-alized means for resolving psychological disturbance and keeping society comfortable is another suggestion that deviance here is viewed as a less severe threat to a highly differentiated social fabric than in the United States. Few of the patients appear to have evoked anger or fear in others. While the emphasis in the familial response and the religious-spiritist way-station was for behavior change—to reduce unpredictability, unproductivity, and evident mental pain—it was clearly nurturant as well. Thus, societal handling of the present population differed not only from that accorded lower SES United States patients, but also from that of many in Brazil who appear (on the basis of unsystematic data) to have been excluded from home and care to lead isolated lives at the margins of the social system.

Women and blacks (as in Baltimore's inner city) avoided hospitalization until their behavior became so florid or violent as to preclude further containment in the home or community. This reflects the subordinate status of women and greater tolerance by the power holders for their deviance as well as for the deviance of minority status blacks. Single, unemployed, residentially mobile males (alcoholic, chronically psychotic or brain-damaged but usually passive) were apt to have remained among the drifting homeless or to be picked up by a social service center rather than to have been hospitalized. Those who appeared in the present hospital population were mainly youthful and had been kept at home by more well-to-do and educated families until the complaints of neighbors made hospitalization inevitable. Thus nurturant behavior toward females, blacks, and youths (reflecting minority status in relation to the attitudes, values, and institutionalized behavior of paternalistic husbands, whites, or fathers) often delayed hospitalization until deviant patterns had become severe and/or habitual. It seems probable that industrialization and increased demands upon individuals to function at complex levels increase the social visibility of deviant persons. Intense social monitoring, the reduced protective capabilities of families and other naturally occurring sources of support, and the substitution of police and social agencies for families, combine with increased conventional hospital facilities to produce different patterns of mental hospitalization in the more highly industrialized countries than those encountered in Brazil.

Physical threats and assaults were more frequent precipitants of hospital admission for blacks than for browns and whites; for the less educated and nonliterate than for the more educated and literate. These people have the least capacity for verbal communication and the fewest opportunities for gaining self-esteem. Their deviant behavior tends to be tolerated by the white educated power holders, whose social distance from them is great and who regard blacks and lowest SES whites as primitive or childlike; it is also tolerated by their families, who know them as fellow sufferers from severe hardship and understandably variable in behavior. Tolerance reduces the communicative value of long-term behavior and requires an acute assault upon the feelings of others in order to effect change, e.g., removal from family or community to healer or hospital. When assaultive family members can no longer be easily appeased, or when others become tired of appeasement, the limits of tolerance are reached. It is, then, aggressive behavior past a certain level which becomes important in appraisal by members of the disadvantaged community. This idea is supported by Dohrenwend's (1963) finding that in New York City a sample of Negro and Puerto Rican leaders gave higher priority than a Jewish and Irish group to aggressive and antisocial behavior in their judgements about what constitutes a serious problem. These last were more likely to extend their judgements about what is serious beyond behavior regarded as threatening to others. Dohrenwend and Chin-Shong (1967) also found that once behavior was defined as seriously deviant, the low-status leaders were less tolerant than the high-status leaders.

Threats and assaults were also more frequent precipitants of hospitalization for males than females and for unmarried than married patients. The relative prominence of physically self-assertive responses (goal-seeking, adaptive, or defensive) among males as compared to females has been noted by observers in most cultures. Assault or threat as communication is congruent with the male's instrumental as compared with the female's expressive social role. Acceptance of almost totally dependent behavior in the deviant person is more common among families of mentally ill females than males.

For the unmarried yet other sets of circumstances seem important: their lack of affiliative capacity interfering with marriage in the first place makes anger and threats regular alternatives to withdrawal; the older unmarried are less closely monitored and, like the blacks, do not evoke action from the control system unless they become clearly dangerous; the younger unmarried, obviously sick from early adolescence, protected by parents who have abandoned expectations for growth and maturity, remain free until their behavior also is seen as clearly dangerous by the agents of social control.

Refusal or inability to work precipitated admission among the recently migrant more frequently than the settled, the nonliterate than the literate, and the uneducated than those with more schooling. The common denominator is inability to care for a nonproductive family member which may be associated with resentment at this further burden. The real threat, for which psychiatric care is the suggested cure, is to economic survival. This was reported by Brody et al. (1967) for Baltimore blacks. Rogler and Hollingshead (1965) in Puerto Rico, and Lewis and Zeichner (1960) in the continental United States reported diminished expectations of the patient leading at times to role substitution by family members which could delay hospital admission indefinitely. Refusal to work was also an issue for the browns. In this instance, however, economic survival may have been less important than their families' sensitivity to frustrated achievement strivings. Nonparticipation in the family striving culture, part of an atmosphere of relative rather than total deprivation, constituted the deviance perceived as requiring correction.

Paranoid or grandiose behavior more frequently precipitated admission of nonwhite (brown and black) than white, uneducated, and of illiterate than educated and literate, and of poorly housed than more adequately housed patients. In other words, this type of deviant behavior was perceived and appraised by a realistically oppressed population characterized by adaptively necessary mistrust and suspiciousness. This group includes both those at the bottom of the socioeconomic and cultural participation ladder and those (the browns) more characterized by marginality, relative deprivation, and the hope of upward mobility. The adaptive value of suspiciousness and hostile caution for this group suggests that the behavior of their patient members must have been extreme in order to surpass their limits of tolerance. Familial coping requires sufficient capacity for critical observation to diagnose illness before family integrity is threatened by the deviance, however rationalizable, of one of its members. Although paranoid behavior (feelings of being persecuted, misjudged, stared at, mistreated, etc.) was not regularly accompanied by retaliatory threats, the factors contributing to family and community appraisal resemble those involved in the appraisal of aggressive behavior. A key issue is the point beyond which paranoid behavior is no longer classified as rational or adaptive wariness, or as culturally accepted externalization, but as a problem requiring efforts at modification; if unmodifiable this problem is dealt with by extrusion from the system.

Anxious, depressed, or suicidal behavior most frequently stimulated admission procedures by the families of whites as compared to nonwhites, married as compared to unmarried, settled as compared to the recently migrant, and skilled manual workers as compared both to unskilled and nonmanual workers. While these were not uniformly the higher SES families, they were marked by relative social and interpersonal security, and more intact and reciprocally affective relationships. In these families individual deviance was regarded as serious and requiring attention before it became threatening to persons (assaultive or paranoid) or the family economy (nonproductive). The greater individual support evidently offered by these families to members suffering from obvious mental pain fits the conclusion of Dohrenwend and Dohrenwend (1970) about United States groups. They note that middle- and upper-class persons faced with stressful situations are more likely to receive emotional support from their families than are lower-class persons.

More of the least advantaged families (not including the division according to occupation) diagnosed their patient members as suffering from "mental illness." This may have been a recently learned way to label otherwise confusing behavior initially regarded as a reaction to stress or susceptible to religous cure. The more educated and socially secure families were more prone to regard the patients' behavior as resulting from life stress or to evaluate it in socially judgmental terms. The black, uneducated, illiterate, and poorly housed were less judgmental than the brown and white, more educated, literate and partly literate, and more adequately housed. The diagnosis of mental illness, then, is an alternative to social judgments which hold a person responsible for his own behavior. This suggests the possible role of actual powerlessness in behavioral appraisal. As noted in previous chapters, the most deprived patients in the present population often saw themselves as completely at the mercy of forces beyond their control. Dohrenwend and Dohrenwend, too, found that lower-class United States persons tended more often than members of the middle or upper class to regard themselves as powerless to manipulate their environment to their advantage.

Past histories of head injury were most common among the unskilled manual laborers, but not in other lowest SES groups. Past histories of disturbed behavior in general, including rages, were most common among the younger religiously unaffiliated and unmarried patients, i.e., those who had probably suffered from psychiatric illness from the earliest ages, and who, regardless of family SES, had achieved least social competence prior to hospital admission.

SYMPTOMATIC BEHAVIOR

In summary, the occurrence of symptomatic behavior reflects the variable operation of defensive, adaptive, and coping processes. Such processes, aspects of the integrative activity of the organism, result in characteristic distortions of function and exact costs in energy and discomfort. Their choice is related to a variety of vulnerability-producing and protective factors related both to historically influenced inner states and current external events of long or short duration.

Some of the vulnerability-producing factors are: defective informational inflow associated with illiteracy; unfamiliarity with the current behavioral setting; separation from previously accustomed persons, places, and norms; cultural discontinuities; sociocultural marginality; lack of supportive familial or extrafamilial groups; role incongruity; discrepancies between aspirations and achievements; lack of opportunity to realize personal potential; an emulative reference group which can never be entered; relative deprivation; awareness of economic and political powerlessness; limited channels for self-expression; being a target of discriminatory practices; persistent physical stress; regular reminders of one's low status; helplessness in the face of overwhelming environmental coercion and threat (lack of capacity for self-determination); lack of previous training for identity and for a variety of ego functions; awareness of declining physical and sexual prowess; intense attention to the adequacy of one's sexual performance; residence in an anomic area; lack of a stable occupational identity; the possibility of status loss; severe inner self-critical standards; and supervisory responsibility, especially in situations in which deviance is highly visible. Several of these factors are associated with or intensified by rapid social change. Others are associated with a feeling of the relative impossibility of such future change. Some are associated with lower and others with higher socioeconomic statuses.

Some protective factors which appear to reduce the probability of occurrence of particular types of symptomatic behavior include: a stable occupational identity (self-awareness as members of a newly visible group has both stressful and protective aspects); the satisfaction of achieved goals; secure identification with the power-holding, emulative reference group of the society; lack of responsibility for the performance or welfare of others; lack of decision-making responsibility; a stable, institutionalized passive relationship with societal holders of power; a passive-dependent orientation which can be gratified through magical solutions; lack of striving; role congruence; lack of severe self-critical standards; a stable supportive family; membership in supportive extrafamilial groups; membership in religious groups facilitating magical resolution of conflict; adequate housing; adequate physical health and opportunities for rest; regular incoming information; familiarity with persons, places, and norms; continuity of relationships; a feeling that change for the better is possible; and relative socioeconomic power to resist or to cope with environmental coercion (capacity for self-determination). These factors can be associated with both higher and lower socioeconomic status as well as with either social change or stability.

The vulnerability-producing and protective factors exert their behavioral effects through a range of intervening variables. These are transient inner cognitive-affective events and states. They include the following in variable degrees of intensity: feelings of self-esteem, guilt and self-criticism, shame, anxiety, direct and inhibited anger, subjective helplessness and hopelessness, strangeness and not belonging, loss and separation, isolation and alienation, fear of threats from others, frustration at not achieving or at not being granted opportunities, security of gender-identity and sexual potency, and others. Particular types of behavior identified as symptomatic can thus be related to particular vulnerability-producing and protective factors leading to intervening cognitive-affective events, leading in turn to the coping, adaptive, and defensive processes reflected in behavior.

CHAPTER 14

SOCIAL FORCES AND COMMUNITY
MENTAL HEALTH:
TRANSCULTURAL CONSIDERATIONS

THE PRECEDING chapters have focused upon the behavior of individuals within their communities. The nature of these communities—viewed as behavior settings or social contexts—has been clearly linked to the mental health of the persons constituting them. There has been, however, little discussion of the type of community change which might deliberately be induced in order to improve individual mental health. This type of focus, upon the social system rather than the individual, has not been a traditional concern of psychiatrists. In the years following the second World War, however, increasing population, urbanization, and public demand have forced the recognition that reparative or curative psychiatry carried out by a necessarily small corps of expensively trained specialists cannot stem the flow of casualties. In consequence, psychiatrists have vastly broadened their interprofessional contacts. Their new appreciation of social contexts, the variety of nonmedical persons and agencies involved in their maintenance and modification, and the need for interpersonal and political skills in implementing recommendations relevant to health has led to the substitution of the idea of community mental health for that of community psychiatry. Community mental health practitioners regard the behavioral setting (sometimes defined in terms of a "catchment area") as a primary concern. In contrast, other psychiatrists with concern for persons previously denied clinical attention (because of its financial, geographic, or psychological inaccessibility), still devote their major energies to providing that attention. The central role of consultation for community mental health rather than direct treatment, especially to the agencies of secondary socialization (such as the schools) and of social control (such as the courts and the police), has been delineated in two books by Gerald Caplan (1964, 1970).

If disordered as well as normatively acceptable behavior is regarded as a mode of participation in a social context, then the student or would-be modifier of such behavior must pay as close attention to the context as to the person. As noted in the preceding chapter, the sensitive interplay of person and context can be thought of in terms of the fluctuating relationship between "inside" and "outside" events. Both inner and outer events are aspects of the evolving socioculture, its nature and state of integration. They are part of the loose linkage of physiological, personality, social, and cultural systems described by Caudill (1958). All are to some degree involved in the process of coping, adaptation, and defense, leading to a relative behavioral steady state.

Many urban contexts, in spite of the label, "community," are in fact noncommunities. Their leaders and their institutions are weak and few in number; their communications are inadequate (Leighton et al., 1963). Their inhabitants do not constitute a collectivity in the sense of Parsons and Shils (1951), since they do not share a commitment to action based on a mutually held set of values. They are also characterized by little opportunity for self-determination, inadequate employment opportunities, racial and social class-based discrimination, a mobility blocking educational system, inadequate welfare agencies, little opportunity for realizing latent potential, poor information dissemination, lack of adequate housing and persistent exposure to severe physical (often occupational) stress with inadequate protective and reparative facilities. These features are prominent in the metropolitan centers of developing countries which are receiving and staging areas for large numbers of unacculturated migrants (Brody 1969a). These may be characterized, following Ortiz (1947), as in the process of "transculturation."

Lack of community also characterizes many United States "inner cities." These inner cities, although centers of a long-industrialized nation, are in a state of transition due in large part to the rise in numbers and expectations of populations previously excluded from full participation in the cultural experience and economic benefits of the society. They are marked by failures in transportation, housing, education, communications, social services, and political and administrative organization. In the United States as well as Latin America, they are the consequences in part of a legacy of laissez-faire capitalism which regarded human beings as a type of economically useful import. On both continents, metropolitan centers have accumulated increasing numbers of citizens who look, sound, and behave differently from the middle-class stereotype. In the great cities of the United States, these citizens are mainly black, and the most tension-laden social psychiatric issue of this country is the black ghetto. In Latin America, these "other citizens" are differentiated more by the stigmata of poverty and, to a lesser degree, of rural origin; here, too, however, descending socioeconomic status tends to be accompanied by increasing darkness of skin. In any case, the socially visible person at the bottom of the status scale is viewed in terms of the higher-status person's prejudice. He evokes discomfort and a series of defensively shaped perceptions and acts which tend to reinforce his own lower-status position and devalued perception of himself.

In both Americas, the failure of industry to grow concomitantly with populations as well as its increasing automation have led to chronic underemployment among the poor, the uneducated, the illiterate, and the dark-skinned; the experience of powerlessness and daily reminders of worthlessness and incapacity are commonplace. The people at the bottom of the scale are habituated to substandard housing and abrasive contacts with symbols of authority ranging from the police to the schoolteacher. Their family disorganization is fed by penalizing or inadequate welfare regulations and discriminatory hiring practices. They place special demands on urban institutions, which, unsupported by a proportionally increasing tax base, have begun to deteriorate. Most apparent are deterioration of agencies of secondary socialization, mainly the schools. This poses special problems when the primary socializing agency, the family, is fragmented by absent and deprecated fathers unable to find employment, with little self-esteem or much reactive rage because of discrimination, lack of education, and a sense of futility.

These phenomena may legitimately be considered reflections of sociocultural malfunction. They suggest that the society is not adequately fulfilling its function of organizing the human group and allocating its tasks and goods in such a way as to promote its survival. They also suggest that the culture—the historically rooted and socially transmitted design for living—does not promote effective social interaction. Under these circumstances, large numbers of individuals who constitute the society and might traditionally have been expected to behave as adequately enculturated and socialized group members are exposed to unusual stress. If their unpredictable responses are labeled "sick" they are funneled to the behavioral modification stations of the social control system. The muting, transformation, or obliteration of these responses by drugs, interviewing, or removal from society does not, however, change the conditions under which they develop.

Little doubt remains that these social factors can overload vulnerable individuals to the point of behavioral decompensation; further, those who are isolated, powerless, and without a meaningful social role are deprived of the support necessary for continued life outside of care-taking institutions. Together these elements form a social context promoting deviant behavior and increasing the burden on public mental institutions. They are the same factors which influence general health. Poverty, lack of information, and social isolation are the major contributors, for example, to malnutrition, injury, and illness in pregnant mothers and new infants. All of these increase later vulnerability to adaptive impairment or mental disorder.

Mental health consultation with the agencies of socialization and social control has been advanced as a partial answer to the problem of prevention. It is important to deal with the community where it has institutionalized connections with the developing young, and at points where it experiences definable pain. Consultation to the schools, the initiation, as described by Rafferty (1967), of diagnostic checkpoints through which all community members are required to pass at about the age of six, and work with teachers to make the system itself a more adequate socializing agency, represent a type of beginning. Consultation with the police and the courts which are the mental hospital gateways for the poor, the black, and the isolated may reduce the flow of those becoming socialized into a lifelong hospital or recidivistic career (Brody, Derbyshire & Schleifer, 1967). Crisis intervention, in the hospital emergency room or as far into the community and away from the hospital as possible, allows the solution of many problems which prove to be social or economic rather than narrowly psychiatric. Caplan's preventive series with crisis intervention at its core is equally relevant when manageable socioeconomic elements are not present.

Querido's (1968) experience in Amsterdam suggests that crisis intervention and consultation do indeed reduce the flow of patients into mental hospitals. Gruenberg (1968) has produced evidence that a reorganization of psychiatric services can reduce the incidence of social breakdown syndromes. These are measures which can reduce disability and chronicity. Yet, as Myers and Bean (1968) have indicated, a person's usual social context, the environment of his developmental period and adult life as indicated by social class characteristics, continue as crucial determinants of his capacity to resume productive and social living after the disruption of mental illness and hospital or office treatment.

There seems little doubt that a true preventive psychiatry with mass public health significance must go beyond consultation or modifying styles of child rearing. Even consultation with the schools, which represent the most massive national obligatory socialization experience outside of the family, will not touch the socioenvironmental roots of illness and malfunction. These require the establishment of health at all stages of life as a human right rather than a privilege. Beyond this they require the development of ways to bring people into meaningful relations with others and to reduce such ubiquitous social stresses as discrimination and joblessness. Support aimed at individual development and integration is, in the long run, support for community development and integration.

Support and intervention may begin in many areas. A mass preventive psychiatry, for example, would require attention to patterns of reproduction and human genetics. The most effective prevention would require the limitation of childbearing to healthy, eugenically sound parents who want and are capable of rearing children. It requires reducing what Pasamanick and Knobloch (1966) have called the cycle of reproductive insult.

The migratory process offers a place in the social system where preventive measures may be applied with some hope of reducing the number and severity of psychiatric casualties. Gateway centers in the large cities, anticipatory preparation in the communities of origin, improved communication with relatives and friends, preparation of the host community so that less hostility and more jobs' will be encountered, and the development of receptor networks may all improve the mental health of the community as well as that of its new arrivals.

Color in a white-dominated society is associated with frustrated striving, the need for vigilance concerning the motives of others, and the resisted or accepted temptation to surrender to the security of a passive-dependent relationship with powerful representatives of the paternalistic priveleged. Racial discrimination assumes particular importance insofar as the victim is placed at a disadvantage through characteristics over which he has no control. Ingrained prejudice by employers, expectations of failure by teachers, and constant though subtle deprecation by contemporaries will effectively block personal growth for all but the strongest and most talented of the target group. There is thus little possibility for constructive self-change through the usual means, and the major alternatives are aggressive action with the almost certain consequence of severe retaliation or resignation, passivity, and denial. Primary prevention may require that the group as a whole acquire a sense of ethnic identity (as fostered in the United States by the "black power" movement) and become able to develop its own institutions.

Although it has not been conclusively validated, it seems likely that the mental health of a total society, as well as that of its most discriminated against constituents, will suffer so long as it systematically deprives a significant segment of its members of their basic human rights. The minority group's inability to support itself, its high yield of welfare recipients, its regular production of poorly socialized citizens, and its psychiatric casualties, as well as the fears and prejudices supported by its presence in the members of the dominant system, constitute a massive drain on the resources and an obstacle to the potential growth of the society. Activities aimed at reducing racial discrimination might be legitimately regarded as having preventive value for psychiatric disturbance. The same could be said for any measures aimed at

increasing individual self-determination, the possibility of realizing individual talent and potential, participation in the cultural
process, and feelings of dignity, self-esteem, and personal worth.
Social factors which increase the likelihood and ease of self-
narcotization, denial, or disrupted reality-contact should be as important a focus for public health measures as mosquito-breeding
swamps, or inadequate and faulty nutritional intake.

Education and literacy are two indices most frequently employed to estimate the level of a society's development. Lack of
education is an ascribed state, a function of the person's childhood opportunities. In this sense it is akin to skin color or membership in a discriminated against ethnic group, blocking further
upward mobility in the system. The illiterate is automatically excluded from full participation in the cultural process of his society
since so much of this involves participating in its shared symbolic
experience. Action to deal with illiteracy as well as with racial
discrimination may be legitimately considered in the realm of
preventive or public-health psychiatry. Literacy, however, in the
presence of continued social and economic blocking on racial or
other ascribed grounds, or in the absence of economic opportunity, may have its own specific adverse effects on mental health.
The acquisition of new aspirations without the tools to achieve
them, or with denied access to the expected opportunity structure
can be more damaging than the previously depressed and passive
state. The findings of Parker and Kleiner (1966) in Philadelphia
appear to be congruent in this respect with the data on color in
Rio de Janeiro.

The deliberate development of groups which have protective
and supportive value and provide a sense of belonging and
self-determination may be regarded as yet another approach to
primary prevention of psychiatric breakdown. Membership in an
occupational category such as that of skilled factory operative
may offer little beyond personal reassurance of individual worth,
and freedom from economic anxiety. The sharing of common
concerns with others, however, and the demonstration that collective action is effective in moving the social power-holders may
have a significant effect in bolstering self-esteem and markedly reduce feelings of loneliness, lack of belonging, purposelessness, and
social impotence.

Other examples of group formation which also reduce social powerlessness include social workers' participation in the activities of a tenant's union aimed at promoting legislation to prevent retaliatory eviction by landlords, and the organization of a community to successfully resist disruption of its neighborhood by a crosstown expressway. Activities of this nature which may theoretically reduce individual psychiatric fallout may also be regarded as fostering the mental health of the community as a whole. Perhaps "integration" rather than "mental health" would be a more appropriate term, for such activities promote group formation and communication between individuals and groups. Beyond this, health workers who are visible to their clients as allies in the struggle for a better life may be psychologically more accessible to them as counselors and therapists. Experiences of successful self-determination and autonomy can certainly do much for personality growth and development.

The role of housing as a determinant of individual and community mental health requires further study. Participation of future occupants in planning and the imaginative use of vacant space within the city centers themselves offer possibilities. Many authors have recommended a halt in the blind progress of "urban renewal" and suggested instead effort to rehabilitate structures destined for removal.

Social change includes shifts in the meaning of age status. In Brazil, as in the Hispanic countries of Latin America, the respect accorded to age was transplanted from the Iberian peninsula and, at least among the upper classes, maintained with little change until the relatively recent acceleration of urbanization and industrialization. This, combined with the traditional importance granted to individual dignity and the maintenance of a person's inner sense of worth, has, with advancing age, led to increasing interpersonal security and some expectation of deference from others. Opposed to this tradition has been the rapid rise of younger people in the industrial occupational ladder, so that they have begun to surpass their elders in economic capacity as well as in literacy and their sense of orientation in a changing culture. This last phenomenon has, for obvious reasons, been limited for the most part to the lower classes in which the parents have been largely uneducated and engaged in manual labor. Any measure designed to insure the continuing recognition for older individuals of personal worth and to maintain their meaningful interpersonal contacts may be regarded as having primary preventive value.

Among the naturally occurring sources of support whose effectiveness varies with modernization is the church. Modernization implies a diminishing capacity to be comfortably dependent upon traditional authority, including both the *patrão* and the church. Patients who are Catholics still appear to conform most obviously to psychiatrist's expectations and hospital attitudes. In contrast, however, adherents of a younger church, the Protestants, are involved with here-and-now human issues, and less able to rely upon traditional forms. Further, in the presence of real illness, they have fewer alternatives to the mental hospital. For Afro-Spiritists, in contrast, the mental hospital is but one of many available mental health supporting resources. For them also, reflections of impaired reality contact were less often considered a reason for hospitalization than in subcultures attaching greater value to rational behavior control.

Cult membership and attendance provide a security system with more immediate value than the traditional church. One aspect of this is its crisis-intervention function. Others are the sense of belonging, together with the structure provided by regular attendance. Cult members (like Catholics), in contrast to Protestants, are less reinforced in the idea that problems should be met by individually responsible behavior and more inclined to relax in the belief that gods, saints, or spirits will make it unneccessary for them to assume individual responsibility for what happens to and around them. How professional mental health workers in developing regions might effectively utilize religious institutions and personnel is unclear. Collaboration between mental health professionals and folk-healers in general remains controversial. Psychiatric leaders in some developing countries, e.g., Henri Collomb in Dakar, Senegal, foster close working relationships with folk-healers; others remain more concerned with the possible dangers of such practices.

The major dilemma for mental health professionals lies in the fact that primary prevention of mental handicaps and the assurance of overall community health is total. It involves the whole social system and is thus beyond his power as well as his expertise. There is no reason to believe that most mental health professionals have the interests or capacities which would allow them to become expert or to develop the political power necessary for effective action regarding most of these issues. Many such actions were subsumed in the past under the heading of social engineering. Some may feel that, as in the case of malaria, the physician should not go beyond defining the etiological agent and its vector; swamp clearing should be left to other specialists. This has been a source of conflict within the staffs of some United States urban mental health centers (Brody, 1969e). Some have felt that more time and energy should be devoted to changing the casualty-producing aspects of society. Others, more oriented to illness, such as psychiatrically trained physicians, have been inclined to emphasize service to those already defined as patients or potential patients. This may be because psychiatrists see mental disturbances among the well-to-do and educated as well as the poor and deprived, and are not so ready to attribute most such suffering to social ills.

Psychological accessibility involves the use of people who can speak the "language" of the neighborhoods and who are able in their counseling to recognize the social and economic contributions to emotional disorder. Such neighborhood counselors or health aides have been trained and employed by a number of programs. They have been immensely useful, but centers such as that at the Lincoln Hospital in the Bronx, where studies have been made, also report significant difficulties. For example, their identification with local socioeconomic problems and their need to be part of the general upward thrust of previously deprived groups sometimes make it difficult for them to recognize signs of severe mental illness which they often tend to attribute to immediate circumstances. Also their close relationships with others in the neighborhood may make it difficult for them to be objective; conversely, it has sometimes inhibited people who might know them or their families, so they have not been able to talk as freely to them as to a more highly trained stranger.

As Brody (1967) pointed out, ". . . for better or for worse, the mental health center in a crowded urban area will become an agent of social change" (p. 372). The center itself can become a nucleus around which the population of an anomic area may coalesce to become, in fact, a community. Citizens' advisory groups, fostering new connections with sources of social power, participation in particular programs increasing the sense of self-determination, education with new roles fostering upward social mobility, and the simple existence of a new meeting place all contribute to the community building goal. Beyond this, increased information, skills, and health security contribute to the sense of self-esteem and personal dignity necessary to become fully human. The personnel of community mental health programs command experience and expertise far beyond that of the physician-psychiatrists assigned by custom and the need for medical responsibility to lead them. Perhaps a reconceptualization of the old idea of the mental health "team" might permit a new view of the legitimate social roles of its members (Brody, 1969c). All of them, regardless of discipline and preference, must inevitably deal with the stresses and human problems arising in the central cities. Without abandoning specific mental health expertise, the way is becoming open for new patterns of collaboration leading to a true public health psychiatry.

TABLES

TABLE 1
HEALTH DATA BY COUNTRY AND BRAZILIAN REGION (1964)

	Total Brazil	Brazil's 18 State Capitals	Brazil NE	Brazil Guanabara Surrounding	Brazil South	Mexico	USA
General mortality rate (per 1,000)	13	10.7	18	9	10	10.8	9.3
Infant mortality rate (per 1,000)	112	78.3	176	75	73	74.2	26
Average life expectancy at birth (yrs.)	54.8	—	48.9	60.7	58.6	59.6	70.9
Life expectancy at 1 yr. (yrs.)	60.7	—	58.3	64.6	61.5	63.4	71.8
Average life expectancy economically productive at 15 yrs. of age (yrs.)	40.2	—	39	41.3	39.6	40.5	43.3
Death rate by communicable disease (per 100,000)	506					473.5	45.4
Death rate by pulmonary tuberculosis (per 100,000)	67	57.2	—	—	—	23.5	5
Death rate by coronary atherosclerosis (per 100,000)	99	76.1	—	—	—		304.3

Adapted from Saúde e Saneamento Diagnostico Preliminar Ministerio do Planejamento e Coordenação Economica, Maio, 1966; and Campbell (1967).

TABLE 2

DEATH RATES PER 100,000 INHABITANTS ACCORDING TO TYPE OF ILLNESS AND LOCATION (STATE CAPITALS)

Causes of Death	Natal 1960–1965	Recife 1960–1966	Belo Horizonte 1960–1966	Rio de Janeiro 1955–1962	São Paulo 1960–1964
Groups					
Infectious disease and parasites	178–156	278–174	147–134	151–117	70–60
Diseases of respiratory apparatus	176–113	194–107	108–110	91–67	75–74
Diseases of digestive apparatus	871–745	326–263	170–118	158–78	72–48
Specific					
Pulmonary tuberculosis	71–61	92–60	85–64	79–69	22–20
Syphilis	12–5	29–18	9–4	12–6	4–3
Gastrointestinal infections and inflammations excepting diarrhea of the newborn	816–695	269–205	150–83	133–52	48–23

*Adapted from *Anuário Estatístico do Brasil* (1967), p. 56

TABLE 3
COMPARATIVE DEATH RATES

Location	General	Infant (less than one year)
Natal (Rio Grande do Norte)		
1960–65	19–17	363–223
Recife (Pernambuco)		
1960–1966	19–13	152–149
Belo Horizonte (Minas Gerais)		
1960–1966	11–12	74–87
Rio de Janeiro (Guanabara)		
1955–1962	11–10	112–65
São Paulo (São Paulo)		
1960–1964	8–9	63–68

Total death rates (per 1,000 inhabitants) and infant death rate (per 1,000 live births) in round numbers according to year and location in five state capitals. Other national infant mortality figures for 1967 include: Mexico, 75; Argentina, 61; United States, 25; Sweden, 16. Adapted from *Anuário Estatístico do Brasil* (1967), p. 40.

TABLE 4
DISTRIBUTION OF PHYSICIANS IN RELATION TO POPULATION

	Percentage of Population	Percentage of Physicians*	Total Number of Physicians***	Number per 100,000 population**
North	3.8	1.6	595	19.8
Northeast	30.0	13.5	2,979	22.8
Central West	4.6	2.4	1,065	27.8
Southeast	44	69.1 (East)***	16,195	58.2
South	17.6	13.4 (South)***	13,416	46.6
Total	100	100	34,250	42.1

*Data for 1963 from Associação Brasileira de Escolas Medicas, Ensino Medico do Brasil, Dadas Preliminares, 1966.
**Data for 1965 adapted from *Anuário Estatistico do Brasil* (1967) by Pinho (1968).
***Estimated percentage according to a geographical division of the overall "Southeast" category, placing São Paulo in the South: East, 30.6; South, 31.

TABLE 5
GENERAL HOSPITAL PERSONNEL

	Number of Hospitals	Average Number of beds per Hospital	Average Number Admissions per Hospital in 1964	Total Admissions in 1964	Average Number Graduate Physicians per Hospital	Average Number Graduate Nurses per Hospital	Average Number Nurses Aides, Practical Nurses and Attendants per Hospital
Rio Grande do Norte	17	39.2	951	16,166	5.1	.53	10
Pernambuco	53	83.3	1,160	87,971	7	1.8	14.6
Minas Gerais	316	62.1	967	305,643	6.2	1.8	6
Guanabara	89	148.8	2,492	221,819	29.2	9.6	34.3
São Paulo	400	73	1,878	751,439	11.9	1.7	14.8
Total Number for Brazil	2,145	129,473	2,654,413		15,649	3,165	24,709

Personnel associated with general hospitals for adults and children, December 31, 1964.
Data computed from *Anuário Estatístico do Brasil* (1967), pp. 455, 458.

TABLE 6
DISTRIBUTION OF PSYCHIATRIC HOSPITALS BY STATE
AND TERRITORY (1965)

| | Psychiatric Hospitals | |
	Neuropsychiatric	Mental Illness
Territories		
Rondonia	0	0
Acre	0	0
Amapa	0	0
Roraima	0	0
States		
Amazonaus	1	0
Para	0	1
Maranhao	1	0
Piaui	2	0
Ceara	1	2
Rio Grande do Norte	0	2
Paraiba	5	0
Pernambuco	5	4
Alagoas	2	3
Sergipe	2	2
Bahia	3	2
Minas Gerais	22	5
Espirito Santo	1	0
Rio de Janeiro	5	3
Guanabara	14	8
São Paulo	40	11
Parana	5	4
South Catarina	2	1
Rio Grande do Sul	5	3
Mato Grosso	0	0
Goias	3	2
Distrito Federal	0	0

Adapted from *Anuário Estatístico do Brasil* (1967), p. 454.

TABLE 7

REGIONAL DISTRIBUTION OF PSYCHIATRIC BEDS (1965) and DISPENSARIES (1966)

	Beds in public hospitals	Number per 100,000 inhabitants	Beds in private hospitals	Number per 100,000 inhabitants	Total beds	Number per 100,000 inhabitants	Public dispensaries	Number per 100,000 inhabitants	Private dispensaries	Number per 100,000 inhabitants	Total	Number per 100,000 inhabitants
North	1,048	35.1	0	0	1,048	35.1	2	.06	0	0	2	.06
Northeast	4,019	23.3	1,786	10.3	5,805	33.6	13	.07	5	.03	18	.10
East	16,720	60.1	5,813	20.9	22,533	81.0	130	.11	5	.01	35	.12
South	25,900	87.8	6,306	21.4	32,206	109.2	9	.03	1	.001	10	.03
Central West	946	24.7	344	9.0	1,290	33.7	4	.10	1	.03	5	.13
Total	48,633	59.8	14,249	17.5	62,882	77.3	58	.07	12	.01	70	.08

Adapted from *Anuário Estatistico do Brasil* (1967) by Pinho (1968).

TABLE 8
SOCIAL FEATURES OF PRIVATE AND PUBLIC MENTAL
HOSPITAL PATIENTS

	Public Hospital Percentage of Patients	Private Hospital Percentage of Patients
Color		
White male first admission	35	47
White female first admission	18	29
Nonwhite male first admission	28	17
Nonwhite female first admission	19	7
Age		
First admission, 60 or more	4	14
First admission, 19 or less	17	6
Hospitalization		
Readmission	60	32
Discharged as "cured"	18	29

Percentage distribution of hospital patients in Guanabara according to public or private status in 1966. Computations from unpublished data available in 1968 from Serviço Nacional de Doenças Mentais, Seção de Cooperação (Dr. Geraldo Junqueira Ribeiro, Chief), Courtesy of Dr. Jurandyr Manfredini, Director.

TABLE 9
AGE BY SEX AND COLOR OF 11,524 FIRST ADMISSIONS TO 10
PUBLIC AND 23 PRIVATE HOSPITALS IN GUANABARA IN 1966

Age	% White		% Nonwhite	
	Male	Female	Male	Female
0–19	11	17	15	16
20–39	53	45	58	50
40–59	28	30	22	26
60–80*	8	8	5	8

Computations from unpublished data available in 1968 from Serviço Nacional de Doencas Mentais, Seção de Cooperação (Dr. Geraldo Junqueira Ribeiro, Chief), courtesy of Dr. Jurandyr Manfredini, Director.

Data exclusive of 163 patients of unknown age. Numbers included in Computation: white male, 4,761; white female, 2,275; nonwhite male, 2,557; nonwhite female, 1,481.

* No patients over 80 years of age.

TABLE 10
DIAGNOSED FIRST ADMISSIONS TO GUANABARA
MENTAL HOSPITALS

	23 Private N = 5698 admissions %	10 Public N = 4611 admissions %	All 33 Hospitals N = 10,309 admissions %
Schizophrenias	15.5	38	25
Exotoxic psychoses	30	15	23
Neuroses	17	7	12
Manic-depressive psychoses	10	5	8.5
Mental illness associated with epilepsy	5	9	7
Psychoses associated with cerebral lesions	8	4	6.5
Oligophrenias	5	6	5
Psychogenic psychoses	2.5	5	3.5
Psychopathic personalities	3	3	3.5
Mixed and associated psychopathics	1.5	5	3
Syphilitic psychoses	1	1.5	1.5
Endotoxic psychoses	1.5	.5	1
Psychoses due to infection or parasitosis	.5	1	.5

Diagnostic distribution of mental hospital patients first admitted, in Guanabara, 1966. Computations from unpublished data available in 1968 from Serviço Nacional de Doenças Mentais, Seção de Cooperação (Dr. Geraldo Junqueira Ribeiro, Chief), courtesy of Dr. Jurandyr Manfredini, Director. An additional 1,203 of the public hospital patients or 20% of the total 5,919 first admissions for the year remained unclassified or had no diagnoses recorded while 105 or 2% of the total were listed as "without disease." In contrast, only 47 or .8% of the total 5,768 first admissions to private hospitals had no recorded diagnoses and only 23 or .4% were listed as "without disease."

TABLE 11

DIAGNOSED OUTPATIENTS IN GUANABARA PSYCHIATRIC CLINICS
N = 10,452

	%
Neuroses	36
Psychoses	25
Epilepsy	23
Oligophrenias	11
Alcoholism	4
Psychopathic personality	1

Diagnoses reported from 14 public (including medical school) plus 5 private psychiatric outpatient clinics in 1967. Computations from unpublished data available in 1968 from Serviço Nacional de Doenças Mentais, Seção de Cooperação (Dr. Geraldo Junqueira Ribeiro, Chief), courtesy of Dr. Jurandyr Manfredini, Director.

TABLE 12
DEMOGRAPHIC CHARACTERISTICS OF PATIENTS ADMITTED TO PRONTO SOCORRO PSIQUIATRICA PINEL IN 1967

	% Female	% Male
Age		
12–19	10	8
20–39	57	63
40–59	19	12
60–86	2	1
Unknown	12	16
Color		
White	55	57
Brown	24	22
Black	17	20
Unknown	4	1
Education		
No schooling	24	19
Primary	40	49
Secondary	10	14
Superior	3	6
Unknown	23	12
Marital State		
Never married	50	63
Married	35	29
Widowed	5	1.5
Desquitado	2	.5
Unknown	8	6

Computations based on unpublished data, courtesy of Dr. Oswaldo Moraes Andrade.

TABLE 13
BIRTHPLACE OF PATIENTS ADMITTED TO PRONTO SOCORRO PSIQUIATRICA PINEL IN 1967

	% Female	% Male
Guanabara	23	28
Minas Gerais	16	13
Rio State	12	13
Northeast	11	15
Other East	11	11
South	5	3
North	2	1.5
Foreign	2	2
Central West	1.5	.5
Unknown	16.5	13

Computations from unpublished data available in 1968 from Serviço Nacional de Doencas Mentais, Seção de Cooperação (Dr. Geraldo Junqueira Ribeiro, Chief), courtesy of Dr. Jurandyr Manfredini, Director.

TABLE 14
DIAGNOSTIC DISTRIBUTION OF PATIENTS AT PRONTO SOCORRO PSIQUIATRICA PINEL DURING 1967

	% Female N = 1,192	% Male N = 1,569
Schizophrenia	17	23
Alcoholic psychoses	3	16
Other exotoxic psychoses*	3	9
Neuroses	10	1
Manic-depressive psychoses	4	.5
Mental illness associated with epilepsy	7	9
Psychoses associated with cerebral lesions	1	0
Psychopathic personality	0	1
All other diagnoses combined	3	2.5
Unclassified	52	38

Computations based on unpublished data, courtesy of Dr. Oswaldo Moraes Andrade.
* Includes alcoholism in connection with other psychiatric illnesses.

TABLE 15
DIAGNOSES OF STUDY PATIENTS IN CASA EIRAS

Diagnoses Related to Schizophrenia	*No. of Cases*
Schizophrenia (unspecified)	19
Schizophrenia, paranoid and paraphrenic	2
Schizophrenia, simple	1
Schizophrenia, plus lues	1
Schizophreniform syndrome	8 (including 5 females)
Schizophrenic syndrome	1
Schizophrenic reaction	1
Schizopathic reaction	1
Schizomorphic picture	1
Paranoid syndrome plus psychogenic	5
Schizophreniform psychosis	1
Total diagnoses of psychotic behavior specified in some way as schizophrenic	41, or 26% of all diagnosed patients
Psychogenic psychosis	5 (including 3 females)

(If this were added to the schizophrenic group the total would be 29% of the diagnosed sample.)

Diagnoses Related to Alcoholism	
Exotoxic psychosis, alcoholism	21
Exotoxic psychosis, alcoholism plus neurosis	4
Exotoxic psychosis, alcoholism plus lues	2
Exotoxic psychosis, alcoholism plus epilepsy	1
Exotoxic psychosis, alcoholism plus depression	1
Exotoxic psychosis, alcoholism plus marihuana intoxication	1
Alcoholism, chronic	7
Total diagnoses of alcoholic psychosis or chronic alcoholism	37, or 23% of all diagnosed patients (21 or 13% with diagnoses of alcoholic psychosis alone)

TABLE 15 (continued)

Diagnoses Related to Neurosis	*No. of Cases*
Neurosis (unspecified)	20 (including 6 females)
Neurosis, compulsive	1
Neurosis, anxiety of war	1
Neurosis, anxious states	5
Neurosis, neurastheniform	1
Neurosis, vegetative exhaustion	3 (including 2 females)
Neurosis, hysterical states of conversion	1
Neurosis, phobic anxious	1
Neurosis, plus cerebral dysrhythmia	1
Total diagnoses of neuroses, exclusive of depression	34, or 21% of all diagnosed patients.

If 10 depressed patients were added, the total would be 28% of the diagnosed sample.)

Diagnoses Related to Depression	
Anxious depressive state	5 (including 3 females)
Depressive syndrome	4
Manic depressive psychosis, melancholic forms	4
Neurotic depression	3 (including 3 females)
Depressive anxious syndrome	1 (female)
Depressed state	1 (female)
Depression	1
Total diagnoses related to depression	19, or 13% of all diagnosed patients

Diagnoses Related to Epilepsy	
Epileptic psychosis	3
Epilepsy	1
Epilepsy, other forms	1
Epilepsy plus oligophrenia	1
Epilepsy plus neurosis, neurasthenic state	1
Cerebral dysrhythmia	1
Total diagnoses of epilepsy excluding one with exotoxic psychosis, alcoholism	8, or 5.5% of all diagnosed patients

Personality Diagnoses	
Psychopathic personality	3
Schizoid personality	2
Epileptic personality	1
Total personality diagnoses	6, or 5% of all diagnosed patients

TABLE 15 (continued)

Diagnoses not otherwise listed	*No . of Cases*
Manic-depressive psychosis, manic forms	2 (including 2 females)
Psycho-organic state	1 (female)
Hysteroepilepsy	1 (female)
Endotoxic psychosis because of metabolic deviation, anxious depressed	1
Mixed and associated psychopath	1
Drug addiction	1
General paresis	1
Total diagnoses not otherwise listed	8, or 5.5% of all diagnosed patients

Diagnoses applied to 158 of 183 patients. (In 3 cases, "no disease" was diagnosed; in 22 cases no diagnoses were available due to temporary loss of records, or none was made aside from "observation.") Wherever the official number was used in lieu of a written diagnosis, the official classification as stated in the diagnostic outline (Table 16) is recorded.

This tabulation was made from data collected by Dr. Jayme Bisker.

TABLE 16
BRAZILIAN SYSTEM OF PSYCHIATRIC CLASSIFICATION

I - *Psychoses due to infections and infestations*
    1A — Acute disorders
    1B — Successive mental states
II — *Psychoses due to syphilis*
    2A — General paresis
    2B — Other forms
III — *Exotoxic psychoses*
    3A — Alcoholism
    3B — Drug addiction
    3C — Occupational
    3D — Accidental
IV — *Endotoxic psychoses*
    4A — Due to functional visceral deviations
    4B — Due to metabolic deviations
    4C — Due to endocrine deviations
    4D — Other forms
V — *Psychoses due to cerebral lesions*
    5A — Senile dementia
    5B — Cerebral arteriosclerosis
    5C — Cranial trauma
    5D — In the course of intracranial tumors
    5E — Other forms (Alzheimer's disease, etc.)
VI — *Oligophrenias*
    6A — Feeble-mindedness
    6B — Imbecility
    6C — Idiocy

TABLE 16 (continued)

VII — *Epilepsies*
        7A — Epileptic psychosis
        7B — Other forms

VIII — *Schizophrenias*
        8A — Simple, hebephrenic, and catatonic forms
        8B — Paranoid and paraphrenic forms
        8C — Paranoia

IX — *Manic-depressive psychosis*
        9A — Manic forms
        9B — Melancholic forms
        9C — Mixed forms
        9D — Other forms (marginal, etc.)

X — *Mixed and Associated psychopathies*

XI — *Psychogenic psychoses* (situational psychosis, psychopathological reactions and developments)

XII — *Neuroses*
        12A — Hysterical states of conversion
        12B — Anxious states
        12C — Phobic states
        12D — Compulsive states
        21E — Neurasthenic states

XIII — *Psychopathic personality*

0 — *Unclassified mental states*
        OA — In observation
        OB — For lack of diagnostic elements

00 — *Without Mental Disturbances*

Direct Translation of the official Diagnostic System of the National Service for Mental Disease, which is the basis for statistical reporting throughout the country. Item I, 1B may also be taken to mean "chronic" mental states.

TABLE 17

Item 219. Patient's Approach to the Interview Situation

1. Attempts to leave area or avoid entering, with expressions of fear.
2. Attempts to leave area or avoid entering, with expressions of hostility.
3. Allows self to be escorted passively to area.
4. Actively cooperates in coming to area.
5. Comes to area with expressions of interest in interview.
6. Comes to area with expression of interest regarding interviewer or situation as culturally significant, or as possibly productive of culturally significant reward.
7. Comes willingly to area with expectation of receiving material reward or payment for cooperation.
8. Attempts to leave area or avoid entering, without clear motive.

TABLE 18

Item 378. Patient says he is persecuted, harassed, or attacked, primarily by:

1. no one; item does not apply
2. parents
3. spouse or mate
4. children
5. friends, peers, or colleagues
6. employers
7. the police or the law
8. religious figure
9. other culturally significant individuals
10. other culturally significant organizations
11. strangers
12. other relatives
13. dead people or ghosts
14. religious organizations or their representatives
15. others

    If positive answer, describe _____

TABLE 19

THE PATIENT'S SPECIFIC PERCEPTIONS OF THE ATTITUDES
AND BEHAVIOR OF OTHERS IN RELATION TO HIMSELF

384. Says that others are frightened by him. 1. yes 2. no
385. Says that others regard him as physically inferior to them. 1. yes 2. no
386. Says that others regard him as mentally or morally inferior. 1. yes 2. no
387. Says that others are inferior to him, and expresses contempt, disdain, or scorn toward them. 1. yes 2. no
388. Says that others can be attacked by his special powers. 1. yes 2. no
389. Says that others are not trustworthy. 1. yes 2. no
390. Says that others have wrong impressions about him or misjudge him in respect to particular roles. 1. yes 2. no
391. Says that others talk about him or stare at him. 1. yes 2. no
    If positive answer, or if other important perception of attitudes or behavior of others toward him, describe _____.

TABLE 20

POPULATION DISTRIBUTION BY REGION, STATE AND CAPITAL CITY ACCORDING TO THE 1960 CENSUS

Physiographic and Political Subdivisions	Capital Cities	% of National Population in States	% of State Population in Capital Cities
NORTH:			
Rondonia (territory)	Porto Velho	0.10	72.12
Acre	Rio Branco	0.23	29.89
Amazonas	Manaus	1.02	24.31
Roraima	Boa Vista	0.04	88.74
Pará	Belém	2.18	25.93
Amapá (territory)	Macapá	0.10	68.09
NORTHEAST:			
Maranhão	São Luiz	3.51	6.41
Piaui	Teresina	1.78	11.46
Ceara	Fortaleza	4.70	15.42
Rio Grande do Norte	Natal	1.63	14.56
Paraiba	João Pessoa	2.84	7.69
Pernambuco	Recife	5.83	19.27
Alagoas	Maceio	1.80	13.39
Fernando de Noronha		0.00	—

TABLE 20 (continued)

EAST:

		% of Total Population	% of Land Area
Sergipe	Aracajú	1.07	15.22
Bahia	Salvador	8.44	10.95
Minas Gerais	Belo Horizonte	13.81	7.08
Serra dos Aimores		0.54	
Espirito Santo	Vitoria	1.67	7.17
Rio de Janeiro	Niteroi	4.80	7.21
Guanabara (Identical with Rio city)	Rio de Janeiro	4.66	100.00

SOUTH:

São Paulo	São Paulo	18.28	29.48
Paraná	Curitiba	6.03	8.45
Santa Catarina	Florianopolis	3.03	4.59
Rio Grande do Sul	Pôrto Alegre	7.67	11.77

CENTRAL WEST:

Mato Grosso	Cuiaba	1.28	6.36
Goias	Goiania	2.76	7.85
Distrito Federal	Brasilia	0.20	100.00

SUMMARY:

	Total	% of Total Population	% of Land Area
North	2,601,519	3.67	42.00
Northeast	15,677,995	22.09	11.00
East	24,832,611	34.99	15.00
South	24,848,194	35.01	10.00
Central West	3,006,866	4.24	22.00
BRAZIL	70,967,185	100.00	100.00

TABLE 21
THE STRUCTURE OF METROPOLITAN RIO DE JANEIRO

Zones of Metropolitan or Greater Rio de Janeiro

1. City Center
2. Central Peripheral Zone
3. Urban Residential Zone

   a — South Zone
   b — Santa Tereza
   c — North Zone

4. Suburban Zone

   a — Central Suburbs
   b — Suburb of Rio Douro Railroad Line
   c — Suburb of Auxiliar Railroad Line
   d — Suburb of Leopoldina Railroad Line

5. Zone of Peripheral Suburbs (Rio State)

   a — Duque de Caxias
   b — São João de Meriti
   c — Nova Iguaçú
   d — Nilopolis
   e — Niteroi
   f — São Gonçalo

6. Urban Pioneer Zone: satellite towns, e.g., Itaguai, Mage, Itaborai, Petropolis, Teresopolis

Adapted from Geiger (1963).

TABLE 22
THE STRUCTURE OF GUANABARA

SEACOAST ZONE

Barra da Tijúca	Lagoa
Copacabana	Leblon
Gavea	Leme
Ipanema	Niemeyer
	Pedra de Guaratiba
	Sepetiba

GUANABARA BAY ZONE

North Border		*Central Border*	*Southern Border*
Benfica	Olaria	Centro	Botafogo
Bomsucesso	Penha	Gamboa	Catête
Bras de Pina	Ramos	Mangue	Flamengo
Cajú	São Cristovão	Santa Teresa	Laranjeiras
Cordovil	Vigario Geral		Urca
Higienopolis			

TABLE 22 (continued)

TIJÚCA ZONE

Alto da Boa Vista	Maracana
Andarai	Rio Comprido
Grajau	Tijúca
	Vila Isabel

MEIER ZONE

Abolição	Engenho da Rainha	Jacarezinho
Cachambí	Engenho de Dentro	Lins de Vasconcelos
Del Castilho	Engenho Novo	Meier
Encantado	Inhauma	Piedade
		Riachuelo

MADUREIRA ZONE

Bento Ribeiro	Marechal Hermes
Cascadura	Osvaldo Cruz
Cavalcante	Quinto Bocaluva
Guadalupe	Rocha Miranda
Madureira	

JACAREPAGUÁ ZONE

Freguesia	Taquara
Praca Seca	Val Queire

CAMPO GRANDE ZONE

Bangú	Padre Miguel
Campo Grande	Realengo
Cosmos	Santa Cruz
Magalhaes Bastos	Santissimo

IRAJÁ ZONE

Coelho Neto	Vicente de Carvalho
Irajá	Vila de Penha

ANCHIETA ZONE

Anchieta	Pavuna
Barros Filho	Ricardo de Albuquerque

ISLANDS

Governador e Cidade Universitária	Paqueta
	Outras

RURAL ZONE

Division of Guanabara according to census zones and tracts (1960).

TABLE 23
PERSONAL CHARACTERISTICS OF HOMELESS PEOPLE (LARGELY MIGRANT) SEEN AT ALBUERGUE XIII IN RIO DE JANEIRO

· *Average Figures for January, February and March*

		1967	1968
Total contacts		743	728
First admissions with identifying data		346	324
Admissions without identifying data**		146	137
Readmissions		251	267

		Average Percentages of Identified First Admissions	
Sex	Male	61	66
	Female	39	34
Marital State	No Legal Spouse	74	79
	Married	23	19
	Widowed	3	2
Age	Adult	91	94
	Child	9	6
Color	White	25	16
	Brown	45	60
	Black	30	24
*Literacy and Education***	Illiterate	34	32
	Partly literate	43	48
	Primary school	21	15
	Secondary school	2	5
Nationality	Brazilian	98	95
	Foreign	2	5

Percentages computed from *Boletim de Serviço*, No. 266 (1968), mimeographed. Estado de Guanabara: Secretaria de Serviços Sociais.

*Seen for disposition only.

**Literacy and schooling were included in the same continuum.

TABLE 24
MIGRATORY CHARACTERISTICS
OF THE TOTAL PATIENT SAMPLE (N = 254)

	% of Total Patient Sample
Total Native Patients	45
Born in Greater Rio de Janeiro	13
Born in Rio de Janeiro proper	32
Total Migrant Patients: born outside Greater Rio de Janeiro	55
Born in rural-provincial setting	46
Moved into Greater Rio de Janeiro within 10 years	40
Recently migrant patients: Moved into Greater Rio de Janeiro within 5 years	28
Moved into Greater Rio de Janeiro within 1 year	7*
Settled patients: Native and lived in Greater Rio de Janeiro more than 5 years	72
Lived in Greater Rio de Janeiro more than 10 years	55
Born in Greater Rio de Janeiro	44
Migrant since 5 years or more	27
Migrant into Greater Rio de Janeiro prior to 18, since 5 years or more	14

*24% of the recently migrant.

TABLE 25
MOBILITY CHARACTERISTICS OF MIGRANT AND SETTLED PATIENTS

	% of Total Patient Sample
Total migrant patients	55

	% of Total Migrant Patients
Born in rural-provincial settings	83
Moved into Greater Rio de Janeiro within 10 years	73
Moved into Greater Rio de Janeiro within 5 years: *Recently migrant*	51
Lived in Greater Rio de Janeiro more than 5 years: *Settled*	49

	% of Total Patient Sample
Total Settled Patients (all who resided in Rio more than 5 years)	72

	% of Total Settled Patients
Born in Greater Rio de Janeiro	62
Lived in Greater Rio de Janeiro more than 10 years	77
Migrant into Greater Rio de Janeiro since 5 years or more	38
Migrant into Greater Rio de Janeiro prior to age 18, since five years or more	19

TABLE 26
EDUCATION AND LITERACY ACCORDING TO MIGRATORY STATUS

	% Recently Migrant (28% of total sample)	% Settled (72% of total sample)
Education		
None	23	11*
Incomplete primary	45	44
Total, none or incomplete primary	68	55*
Complete primary	19	19
Beyond primary	13	27**
Total, complete primary and beyond	32	46
Literacy		
Illiterate	29	9***
Partly literate	16	13
Literate	52	74***

Significance of differences determined by chi-square:
*probability of chance occurrence, less than .05
**probability of chance occurrence, less than .01
***probability of chance occurrence, less than .001

TABLE 27
OCCUPATION ACCORDING TO MIGRATORY STATUS

Occupation*	% Recently Migrant (28% of total sample)	% Settled (72% of total sample)
Class I	1	3
Class II	1	2
Class III	10	13
Class IV	6	8
Class V	38	44
Class VI	38	25**
Unobtained	6	5

*Classification according to Hutchinson (1963).
**Significance of differences determined by chi-square: probability of chance occurrence, less than .01

TABLE 28
HOUSING ACCORDING TO MIGRATORY STATUS

Quality and Density of Housing	% Recently Migrant (28% of total sample)	% Settled (72% of total sample)
Barraco, under construction or unclassified	13	11
Has no essential services	20	10*
Has electricity and running water	65	73
Bedroom shared by others than mate	60	41**
Dwelling contains one room and kitchen and bathroom or less	35	14***

Significance of differences determined by chi-square:
*probability of chance occurrence, less than .05
**probability of chance occurrence, less than .01
***probability of chance occurrence, less than .001

TABLE 29
NATURE AND LOCATION OF LIVING AREA WITHIN GREATER RIO DE JANEIRO ACCORDING TO MIGRATORY STATUS

Living Area	% Recently Migrant (28% total sample)	% Settled (72% of total sample)
Combined suburban, industrial, and peripheral urban	46	61*
Combined (non-residential) urban	49	23**
Slum (favela), urban or suburban	7	6
Small town in Greater Rio de Janeiro	26	16

Significance of differences determined by chi-square:
*probability of chance occurrence, less than .05
**probability of chance occurrence, less than .001

TABLE 30

SOCIOECONOMIC STATUS AND ACCEPTANCE ACCORDING TO MIGRATORY STATUS

	% Recently Migrant (28% of total sample)	% Settled (72% of total sample)	% Total Migrant (55% of total sample)	% Native (45% of total sample)
Socioeconomic Status Compared with Father				
Patient feels is better than father	42	44	51	40
Patient feels worse than father	17	21	26	15
Socioeconomic Status Compared with Past Year				
Patient feels has improved	45	34	41	36
Patient feels has declined	29	31	30	33
Awareness of achievement/aspiration discrepancy	28	18	18	21
Migrated for personal-emotional rather than economic-rational reasons	63	30*	43	—

Significance of differences determined by chi-square:
*probability of chance occurrence, less than .001

TABLE 31
ORIGINS AND MOTIVES FOR MIGRATION
ACCORDING TO MIGRATORY STATUS

	% Recently Migrant (28% of total sample)	% Settled (72% of total sample)	% Total Migrant (55% of total sample)
Nature of Place of Origin			
Rural (village, hamlet, farm)	62	62	62
Small town	20	21	21
Combined: Rural-provincial	82	83	83
City of 70,000 +	18	17	17
Motive for Migration			
Undetermined	3	4	4
Lack of jobs economic	34	66**	50
Personal-emotional	47	26*	36
Psychiatric illness	16	4*	10
Combined: Personal and psychiatric	63	30**	46

Significance of differences determined by chi-square:
*probability of chance occurrence, less than .01
**probability of chance occurrence, less than .001

TABLE 32
PERSONAL RELATIONS AND INSTITUTIONAL PARTICIPATION
ACCORDING TO MIGRATORY STATUS

	% Recently Migrant (28% of total sample)	% Settled (72% of total sample)	% Total Migrant (55% of total sample)
Migratory Companions			
Conjugal family, sometimes plus others	40	17x****	24
Migrated alone	37	24x**	30
Family of origin, sometimes with others	20	41x***	37
Friends and Relatives in Area			
Has relatives other than nuclear family	94	90	92
Has close friends	42	54**	50
Has relatives near by	3	29*****	22
Hostile toward neighbors	17	5****	12
Knows nothing about neighbors	10	25****	24

TABLE 32 (continued)

Institutional Contact	% Recently Migrant (28% of total sample)	% Settled (72% of total sample)	% Total Migrant (55% of total sample)
Some contact with clergy	73	54*****	64
Friendly toward clergy	32	16*****	28
Some contact with social welfare workers	54	82*****	76
Friendly toward social workers	19	27	24
Frequently uses welfare services	10	19	20
Amusements			
Sometimes watches soccer	32	39	37
Watches soccer six times or more yearly	23	24	28
Sometimes goes to dances	42	24***	23
Goes to dances six times or more yearly	20	11	12

x refers to percentages of total migrants within settled group.
Significance of differences determined by chi-square:
    **probability of chance occurrence, less than .05
   ***probability of chance occurrence, less than .02
  ****probability of chance occurrence, less than .01
 *****probability of chance occurrence, less than .001

TABLE 33

RELIGIOUS PARTICIPATION ACCORDING TO MIGRATORY STATUS

Patient's Reported Religion	% Recently Migrant (28% of total sample)	% Settled (72% of total sample)	% Total Migrant (55% of total sample)
Catholic	70	68	71
Protestant	12	7	15
Spiritist-Afro-Other	1	8*	5
Supplemental Spiritist-Afro-Other	16	15	13
Total reported cult attendance	17	23	18
Deny any religious affiliation	16	13	14

Significance of differences determined by chi-square:
  *probability of chance occurrence, less than .05

TABLE 34
SOURCES OF INFORMATION ACCORDING TO MIGRATORY STATUS

	% Recently Migrant (28% of total sample)	% Settled (72% of total sample)
Media Attended or Owned		
Owns a radio	84	91
Radio only medium of information	45	34
Watches television	39	42
Owns television	26	42*
Owns one or more books	26	44**
Reads newspapers	38	43
Reads magazines	39	44
Reads newspapers, magazines, and books	39	47
Attends movies	57	56
Attends movies at least monthly	26	24
Never attends movies	43	44
Uses all media	35	31

Significance of differences determined by chi-square:
  *probability of chance occurrence, less than .05
  **probability of chance occurrence, less than .01

TABLE 35
CHILDHOOD INFLUENCES ACCORDING TO MIGRATORY STATUS

	% Recently Migrant (28% of total sample)	% Settled (72% of total sample)
Family Stability and Support		
Siblings by both parents	61	72
Father died before patient was 12	44	33
Earned money prior to age 14	27	13**
Financially independent by age 14	16	9
Discipline		
Disciplined mainly by beatings	43	34
Disciplined mainly by mother	12	24*

Significance of differences determined by chi-square:
  *probability of chance occurrence, less than .05
  **probability of chance occurrence, less than .01

TABLE 36
PATERNAL LITERACY AND OCCUPATION ACCORDING TO PATIENTS' MIGRATORY STATUS

	% Recently Migrant (28% of total sample)	% Settled (72% of total sample)
Paternal Literacy		
Illiterate	22	9**
Partly literate	36	33
Literate	22	32

	Recently Migrant	Settled	Total Migrant (55% of total sample)	Native (45% of total sample)
Paternal Occupation				
Class I	4	2	2	3
Class II	1	3	1	7
Class III	7	10	6	13
Class IV	13	9	14	7
Class V	27	27	13	37*
Class VI	39	39	54	27**

Occupation classifications according to Hutchinson (1963). Significance of differences determined by chi-square:

*probability of chance occurrence, less than .05

**probability of chance occurrence, less than .001

TABLE 37

EVENTS LEADING TO HOSPITALIZATION ACCORDING TO MIGRATORY STATUS

	% of Patients			
	% Recently Migrant (28% of total sample)	% Settled (72% of total sample)	% Total Migrant (55% of total sample)	Native (45% of total sample)
Acuteness of Illness				
Has had previous contact with psychiatrists	41	48	41	55*
Present illness duration 6 months or less	39	46	41	46
Present illness duration 1 month or less	14	20	21	17
Reasons for Hospital Admission				
Physical assaults or threats against people or property	15	15	15	11
Other bizarre or markedly peculiar behavior	13	17	13	17
Anxious, depressed, suicidal	11	23*	10	28**
Anxious about intent of others, paranoid, grandiose	8	10	21	12
Will not or cannot work	14	3*	8	5

Significance of differences determined by chi-square:
*probability of chance occurrence, less than .05
**probability of chance occurrence, less than .001

TABLE 38
FAMILY DIAGNOSIS ACCORDING TO MIGRATORY STATUS

	% Recently Migrant (28% of total sample)	% Settled (72% of total sample)
Family Diagnosis		
Reaction to persecution	25	12**
Reaction to life stress	76	72
A mental illness	45	33*
A physical illness	31	32
Strange behavior	30	40

Significance of differences determined by chi-square:
*probability of chance occurrence, less than .05
**probability of chance occurrence, less than .01

TABLE 39
RELATIONAL BEHAVIOR DURING PSYCHIATRIC INTERVIEW ACCORDING TO MIGRATORY STATUS

	% Recently Migrant (28% of total sample)	% Settled (72% of total sample)
Psychiatrist's Self-Ratings		
Feels interview to be interesting and rewarding	44	66***
Feels involved and empathic	44	57
Feels that patient liked him	38	57***
Feels remote or distant	32	24
Feels hostile or irritated	18	4****
Feels cheerful and optimistic	17	31*
Feels anxious or apprehensive	13	3***

Significance of differences determined by chi-square:
*probability of chance occurrence, less than .05
**probability of chance occurrence, less than .02
***probability of chance occurrence, less than .01
****probability of chance occurrence, less than .001

TABLE 39 (continued)

	% Recently Migrant (28% of total sample)	% Settled (72% of total sample)
Observations of Patient's Behavior		
Easily understood	77	88*
Cooperative throughout interview	54	71**
Actively cooperative approach	50	66*
Paid attention comfortably	49	67***
Request for direction, support and advice	41	28*
Obvious interview anxiety	40	57**
Less disturbed at end of interview	35	18***
Respectful, courteous, friendly	32	49**
Hypervigilant and distractible	24	10***
Expresses unsatisfied wish to be cared for	18	9*
Appropriate emotional expression throughout	16	34***

TABLE 40
TENSION, ANXIETY AND DISRUPTION OF FUNCTION ACCORDING TO MIGRATORY STATUS

	% Recently Migrant (28% of total sample)	% Settled (72% of total sample)
Report of Anxiety and Tension		
Worries about job	32	25
Worries about relatives	18	5***
Discrete anxiety attacks	76	65
Any type of organ anxiety	59	32***
Fear of disease in stomach	31	9***
Fear of disease in head	13	2***
Interference with Function		
Any feeling of impaired mental efficiency	64	39***
Difficulty in concentration due to worries	56	38**
Interview startles, anxious faces, ANS signs or anxious speech content	54	39*
Difficulty in clear thinking	31	8***

Significance of differences determined by chi-square:
  *probability of chance occurrence, less than .05
  **probability of chance occurrence, less than .02
  ***probability of chance occurrence, less than .001

TABLE 41
TENSION, SENSITIVITY AND FRUSTRATION
ACCORDING TO MIGRATORY STATUS

Report of Tension, Sensitivity and Frustration	% Recently Migrant (28% of total sample)	% Settled (72% of total sample)
Feels tense, uncomfortable or isolated with others	38	29
Feels others regard him as mentally-morally inferior	31	18**
Aspiration/achievement discrepancy	28	18*

Significance of differences determined by chi-square:
*probability of chance occurrence, less than .05
**probability of chance occurrence, less than .02

TABLE 42
AFFECTIVE SYMPTOMS AND BEHAVIOR ACCORDING TO
MIGRATORY STATUS

	% Recently Migrant (28% of total sample)	% Settled (72% of total sample)
Depressive Mood Indicators		
Often feels sad or like weeping	70	59*
Weeps frequently	47	40
Preoccupied with social inadequacy	36	27
Sees no humor in anything	31	22
Feels lonely	27	15*
Body feels slowed down	25	10**
Says body is weak and inferior	23	16
Feels generally inadequate	20	10
Generally self-accusatory and unworthy	27	19
Guilt re failure in social role	22	14
Guilt re failure in parental role	18	3***
Guilt re failure in filial role	14	7

Significance of differences determined by chi-square:
*probability of chance occurrence, less than .05
**probability of chance occurrence, less than .01
***probability of chance occurrence, less than .001

TABLE 43
PARANOID OR GRANDIOSE STATEMENTS ACCORDING TO
MIGRATORY STATUS

	% Recently Migrant (28% of total sample)	% Settled (72% of total sample)
Statements Concerning Others		
Complains about treatment by others	66	49***
Feels emulated or loved by certain others	53	27****
Expresses jealousy (usually of mate)	51	39*
Feels persecuted, harassed, or attacked	51	33***
Says others stare at or talk about him	43	30*
Says others are not trustworthy	38	22***
Others control his thoughts or actions	37	19***
Others know his inner thoughts and feelings	35	24*
Others regard him as mentally-morally inferior	31	18**

Significance of differences determined by chi-square:
*probability of chance occurrence, less than .05
**probability of chance occurrence, less than .02
***probability of chance occurrence, less than .01
****probability of chance occurrence, less than .001

TABLE 44
HALLUCINATORY AND ILLUSORY PHENOMENA
ACCORDING TO MIGRATORY STATUS

	% Recently Migrant (28% of total sample)	% Settled (72% of total sample)
Reports of Auditory and Visual Phenomena		
Hears voices in absence of other people	39	29*
Insists on reality of reported experience	29	16*
Plans action on basis of experience	27	11**
Sees people in absence of identifiable stimuli	24	14*
Sees religious, folkloric, or ghostly human figures	14	4**
Misinterpretations or Illusions		
Misinterprets communications and stimuli in all sensory spheres	26	17
Misinterprets or gives special meaning to auditory stimuli	13	7

Significance of differences determined by chi-square:
*probability of chance occurrence, less than .05
**probability of chance occurrence, less than .01

TABLE 45
DISORIENTATION ACCORDING TO MIGRATORY STATUS

	% Recently Migrant (28% of total sample)	% Settled (72% of total sample)
Orientation Problems		
Any disorientation	41	29*
Temporal disorientation	20	9**

Significance of differences determined by chi-square:
  *probability of chance occurrence, less than .05
 **probability of chance occurrence, less than .02

TABLE 46
SOMATIC AND PSYCHOPHYSIOLOGICAL COMPLAINTS
ACCORDING TO MIGRATORY STATUS

	% Recently Migrant (28% of total sample)	% Settled (72% of total sample)
Statements about Body Function		
Complains of fatigue	65	55*
Complains of weakness	59	51
Feels something strange inside the body	18	10*
Cardiopulmonary Complaints		
Faintness or dizziness	41	49
Palpitation	16	38***
Dyspnea	16	34**
Sweating or hot flashes	20	30*

Significance of differences determined by chi-square:
    *probability of chance occurrence, less than .05
   **probability of chance occurrence, less than .01
  ***probability of chance occurrence, less than .001

TABLE 47

MIGRATORY STATUS OF RIO DE JANEIRO MENTAL HOSPITAL PATIENTS, ACCORDING TO COLOR

	% White (64% of total sample)	% Brown (24% of total sample)	% Black (12% of total sample)
Total Migrants (non-native)	52	68	50
In present residence less than 1 year	13	14	4
In present residence more than 10 years	62	52	50

TABLE 48

MARITAL STATUS OF RIO DE JANEIRO MENTAL HOSPITAL PATIENTS, ACCORDING TO COLOR

	% Brown (24% of total sample)	% Black (12% of total sample)	% White (64% of total sample)
No consistant mate	41	32	30
Common-law, multiple, or undetermined status of mate	13	11	5
Both civil and religious marriage	28	25	46**
Civil marriage alone	18	29	18
Has children	45	36	34
All children are "legitimate"	45	46	56
Has children of different color than he	16	8	6*

Significance of differences determined by chi-square:
  *probability of chance occurrence, less than .05
  **probability of chance occurrence, less than .02

TABLE 49

INDICATIONS OF CHILDHOOD FAMILY STABILITY OR INSTABILITY OF
RIO DE JANEIRO MENTAL HOSPITAL PATIENTS, ACCORDING TO COLOR

Reports of Childhood Family Structure	% White (64% of total sample)	% Brown (24% of total sample)	% Black (12% of total sample)
Siblings by both natural parents	79	65	57**
Reared by parent-figures of both sexes	72	64	68
Describes home as not broken	63	51	43
Disciplined by both parents	56	57	46
Father died or status unknown prior to patient's age 12	26	27	36
Mother died or status unknown prior to patient's age 12	12	15	22
Independent prior to age 14	10	10	21
Parents divorced, separated, deserted, or relational status unknown	8	15	29***
Disciplined by others than parents, close relatives or institutions	10	22	4*
Reared by multiple individuals (relatives, friends, others)	5	20	8***

Significance of differences determined by chi-square:
  *probability of chance occurrence, less than .05
 **probability of chance occurrence, less than .02
***probability of chance occurrence, less than .01

TABLE 50

LITERACY AND EDUCATION OF RIO DE JANEIRO MENTAL HOSPITAL PATIENTS, ACCORDING TO COLOR*

	% White (64% of total sample)	% Brown (24% of total sample)	% Black (12% of total sample)
Literate	80	49	50*
Partly literate (can read and write with difficulty at a simple level)	11	21	20
Totally illiterate	2	13	18*
No schooling at all	8	23	32*
Incomplete primary (up to 5 yrs.)	37	51	54
Complete primary or partial secondary *ginasio* (up to 8 yrs.)	39	11	11*
Complete secondary, partial or complete *colegio* (up to 12 yrs.)	11	15	0*
Any university experience	4	0	0

No black person had gone past completed primary; no brown person had gone past *colegio.*
Significance of differences determined by chi-square:
*probability of chance occurrence, less than .001

TABLE 51

OCCUPATION, ACCORDING TO COLOR

Classification of occupation	% White (64% of total sample)	% Brown (24% of total sample)	% Black (12% of total sample)
Classes I and II: professionals, large and medium proprietors, managers, executives	6	0	0*
Class III: small administrators, proprietors, teachers, clergy	19	5	0**
Class IV: foremen, small farm owners, skilled technicians	8	5	7
Class V: skilled manual workers, drivers, chefs, policemen	45	41	39
Class VI: unskilled manual, garbage collectors, waiters	20	48	50***

Significance of differences determined by chi-square:
  *probability of chance occurrence, less than .01
 **probability of chance occurrence, less than .001
***Ten% white, 18% brown, 18% black are housewives. (Since most of latter also work, this further reduces the proportion of whites in class VI.)

TABLE 52

PARENTAL STATUS OF RIO DE JANEIRO MENTAL HOSPITAL PATIENTS, ACCORDING TO COLOR

	% White (64% of total sample)	% Brown (24% of total sample)	% Black (12% of total sample)
Father's status			
Father dead or status unknown	50	56	71
Father literate	38	17	18***
Father totally illiterate	8	20	25***
Father's occupation in class 1 or 2	9	0	0***
Father's occupation in class 6	33	49	57**
Mother's status			
Mother dead or status unknown	30	33	43
Mother has significant health problem	31	35	50
Mother literate	38	22	18**
Mother totally illiterate	6	15	18*

Significance of differences determined by chi-square:
*probability of chance occurrence, less than .05
**probability of chance occurrence, less than .02
***probability of chance occurrence, less than .01

TABLE 53

SELF-ESTIMATE OF SOCIOECONOMIC MOBILITY OF RIO DE JANEIRO MENTAL HOSPITAL PATIENTS, ACCORDING TO COLOR

	% White (64% of total sample)	% Brown (24% of total sample)	% Black (12% of total sample)
Estimate of socioeconomic status in comparison to father			
Considers present SES better than that of father	48	50	36
Considers present SES worse than that of father	20	19	32

TABLE 53 (continued)

	% White (64% of total sample)	% Brown (24% of total sample)	% Black (12% of total sample)
Estimate of socioeconomic status in relation to self			
Considers own SES better in comparison to one year ago	42	35	25*
Considers own SES worse in comparison to one year ago	27	37	46*

Significance of differences determined by chi-square:
*probability of chance occurrence, less than .05

TABLE 54

CONDITIONS OF MIGRATION OF RIO DE JANEIRO MENTAL HOSPITAL PATIENTS, ACCORDING TO COLOR

	% White (64% of total sample)	% Brown (24% of total sample)	% Black (12% of total sample)
Migrated because needed a job rather than for personal reasons	24	26	36
Migrated alone rather than with friends or family	9*	26	25
Migrated from a *fazenda* rather than a town or village	7*	18	25

Significance of differences determined by chi-square:
*probability of chance occurrence, less than .01

TABLE 55
HOUSING OF RIO DE JANEIRO MENTAL
HOSPITAL PATIENTS, ACCORDING TO COLOR

	% Black (12% of total sample)	% Brown (24% of total sample)	% White (64% of total sample)
Nature of Housing			
Sleeping room shared with others	52	52	39
Has no essential services	33	20	8***
House is *barraco*, unfinished or unclassified structure	32	21	6***
Has one room plus kitchen or bath, or less	30	35	13**
Includes a dining or living room	7	18	27*
Is in an apartment building	0	5	16**
Location of Housing			
In suburban neighborhood	50	38	43
In Rio State, part of metropolitan Rio de Janeiro	43	32	14***
In outlying small town, part of metropolitan Rio	29	26	15
In rural neighborhood	25	5	5***

Significance of differences determined by chi-square:
*probability of chance occurrence, less than .05
**probability of chance occurrence, less than .01
***probability of chance occurrence, less than .001

TABLE 56

SOURCES OF INFORMATION FOR RIO DE JANEIRO MENTAL HOSPITAL PATIENTS,
ACCORDING TO COLOR

	% White (64% of total sample)	% Brown (24% of total sample)	% Black (12% of total sample)
Owns a radio	94	90	75**
Reads newspapers, magazines, books	51	37	36
Watches television	49	42	16**
Owns a television set	49	27	7***
Owns one or more books (including religious)	47	34	11**
Goes occasionally to movies (less than one a month)	41	30	16*
Uses all media (radio, TV, newspapers, books, magazines, movies)	39	28	12**
Attends movies at least monthly	27	23	14
Radio alone is source of outside information	34	48	52*
Never attends movies	40	52	57

Significance of differences determined by chi-square:
  *probability of chance occurrence, less than .05
 **probability of chance occurrence, less than .01
***probability of chance occurrence, less than .001

TABLE 57

RELIGIOUS MEMBERSHIP AND OBSERVANCE OF RIO DE JANEIRO MENTAL HOSPITAL PATIENTS, ACCORDING TO COLOR

	% White (64% of total sample)	% Brown (24% of total sample)	% Black (12% of total sample)
Claims membership in Catholic church	71	68	68
Mother belonged to Catholic church	74	77	71
Claims membership in Protestant church	8	12	7
Mother belonged to Protestant church	9	16	7
Claims no formal membership in any church	13	17	14
Attends church only on holidays or special occasions	45	42	46
Attends church at least once weekly	9	12	7
Belongs to or (if member of other church) attends Spiritist or AfroBrazilian center	11	13	28*
Belongs to or attends "other" type of group	4	7	7
Probable minimum cultist attendance regardless of other membership	15	20	35*

Significance of differences determined by chi-square:
*probability of chance occurrence, less than .02

TABLE 58
PLACE OF HOSPITALIZATION OF RIO DE JANEIRO
MENTAL HOSPITAL PATIENTS, ACCORDING TO COLOR

	% White (64% of total sample)	% Brown (24% of total sample)	% Black (12% of total sample)
Casa Eiras	83	63	75*
Pronto Socorro	11	35	25**
Botafogo	6	2	0

Significance of differences determined by chi-square:
*probability of chance occurrence, less than .05
**probability of chance occurrence, less than .01

TABLE 59
DURATION OF ILLNESS OF RIO DE JANEIRO MENTAL
HOSPITAL PATIENTS, ACCORDING TO COLOR

	% White (64% of total sample)	% Brown (24% of total sample)	% Black (12% of total sample)
Ill only one week	8	8	20*
Ill six months or less	41	42	56

Significance of differences determined by chi-square:
*probability of chance occurrence, less than .05

TABLE 60
PHYSICAL VIOLENCE OF RIO DE JANEIRO MENTAL HOSPITAL
PATIENTS, ACCORDING TO COLOR

	% White (64% of total sample)	% Brown (24% of total sample)	% Black (12% of total sample)
Reason for admission to hospital:			
Damaged objects	4**	4	20
Attacked people	8	6	16
Past history reports:			
Frequent physical fights	4*	6	16

Significance of differences determined by chi-square:
*probability of chance occurrence, less than .05
**probability of chance occurrence, less than .01

TABLE 61

FAMILY ATTITUDES AND ACTIONS OF RIO DE JANEIRO
MENTAL HOSPITAL PATIENTS, ACCORDING TO COLOR

	% White (64% of total sample)	% Brown (24% of total sample)	% Black (12% of total sample)
Family expect willingly to take patient back home	94	92	81
Family brought patient to hospital	78	62	76
Family diagnosis: mental illness	35	39	46
Family diagnosis: defiant, immoral, immature or unacceptable	24	23	0*
Family does not identify specific behavioral problem	21	30	24
Brought to hospital by persons other than family	15	26	24
Came to hospital alone	7	12	0
Family brought patient because he would not work	3	16	4**

Significance of differences determined by chi-square:
*probability of chance occurrence, less than .01
**probability of chance occurrence, less than .001

TABLE 62

STATEMENTS OR ACTS LEADING TO HOSPITAL
ADMISSIONS OF RIO DE JANEIRO
MENTAL HOSPITAL PATIENTS, ACCORDING TO COLOR

	% White (64% of total sample)	% Brown 24% of total sample)	% Black (12% of total sample)
Verbal statements only	28	18	16
Acts only	30	14	28
Unspecified acts or statements*	35	48	40
Suicidal thoughts, fantasies, attempts; anxiety; depression	27	12	8**
Physical attacks against other people or objects	13	12	36**
Sexual complaints and acts	11	12	4
Paranoid behavior and anxiety about intent of others	10	20	20

TABLE 62 (continued)

	% White (64% of total sample)	% Brown (24% of total sample)	% Black (12% of total sample)
Somatic complaints	6	8	16
Failure to work	3	16	4***
Failure to eat	2	6	4
Other (obsessive fears, grandiose ideas)	4	8	4

*Since the figures in this category represent a summation and the presence of acts and statements is not mutually exclusive, the total exceeds 100%.
  Significance of differences determined by chi-square:
    **probability of chance occurrence, less than .01.
    ***probability of chance occurrence, less than .001.

TABLE 63

AFFECTIVE SYMPTOMS AND BEHAVIOR OF RIO DE JANEIRO
MENTAL HOSPITAL PATIENTS, ACCORDING TO COLOR

Reports of Depressed Mood	% White (64% of total sample)	% Brown (24% of total sample)	% Black (12% of total sample)
Frequently feels sad	63	62	46
Frequently feels like weeping	44	44	25
Problems in feeling intensity (low or high)	43	46	16*
Sees no humor in anything	28	24	12
Appears sad in interview	26	24	16
Has expressed suicidal threats	24	22	0**
Self-accusations	22	22	12
Wishes to be dead	21	14	4
Has had specific suicidal fantasies	19	20	0*
Feels lonely and friendless	19	22	8
Has made suicidal attempt	17	22	4
Feels inadequate	14	12	4
Feels guilty re failure as a child	10	8	4
Feels guilty re failure as a parent	6	10	4

Significance of differences determined by chi-square:
    *probability of chance occurrence, less than .05
    **probability of chance occurrence, less than .01

TABLE 64

TENSION, ANXIETY, AND DISTRIBUTION OF FUNCTION IN RIO DE JANEIRO MENTAL HOSPITAL PATIENTS, ACCORDING TO COLOR

	% White (64% of total sample)	% Brown (24% of total sample)	% Black (12% of total sample)
Reports of Tension and Anxiety			
Discrete anxiety attacks	69	71	56
Fear of loss of general control	43	40	32
Diffuse anxiety	39	34	20
Phobic fears	33	34	8**
Fear of loss of control over specific actions	28	25	16
Feeling of impending doom	19	24	8
Frightening dreams	17	18	8
Fear of disease in organ (stomach)	16	16	8
Interference with Function due to Tension			
Insomnia due to worries	71	86	76*
Worries interfere with work	65	74	56
Restlessness due to worries	41	64	37***
Worries make work impossible	49	58	37
Trouble concentrating due to worries	44	48	25
Problems in Thought Processes and Memory			
Lack of efficiency, clarity or precision in thinking	45	64	34**
Problems of recent, remote or fragmented recall	44	49	36
Obsessive, intrusive or controlled thinking	35	38	24
Difficulty in orderly decision making	36	36	20

Significance of differences determined by chi-square:
    *probability of chance occurrence, less than .05
    **probability of chance occurrence, less than .02
    ***probability of chance occurrence, less than .01

TABLE 65
ANGER AND FRUSTRATION OF RIO DE JANEIRO MENTAL HOSPITAL PATIENTS, ACCORDING TO COLOR

Reports of Angry, Frustrated, Inferior Feelings	% White (64% of total sample)	% Brown (24% of total sample)	% Black (12% of total sample)
Attacks of rage	43	48	32
Frequent arguments	33	38	28
Angry much of time	24	36	17
Worries about job	25	34	28
Worries about family	21	32	32
Marked aspiration/achievement discrepancy	19	26	16
Describes own body as unattractive and inferior	4	10	4

TABLE 66
IMPULSIVE BEHAVIOR IN RIO DE JANEIRO MENTAL HOSPITAL PATIENTS, ACCORDING TO COLOR

	% White (64% of total sample)	% Brown (24% of total sample)	% Black (12% of total sample)
Reports impulsive behavior	26	32	20
Reports unintended acts	20	28	16

TABLE 67
PARANOID OR GRANDIOSE STATEMENTS OF RIO DE JANEIRO
MENTAL HOSPITAL PATIENTS, ACCORDING TO COLOR

Statements Concerning Others	% White (64% of total sample)	% Brown (24% of total sample)	% Black (12% of total sample)
Complains about treatment by others	53	60	44
Others stare at or talk about him	28*	50	40
Feels self to be persecuted	34	44	44
Feels especially admired or loved by certain others	30	42	28
Others misjudge or misinterpret him	18*	38	24
Others are not trustworthy	23	34	28
Regarded as mentally inferior by others	10**	34	16
Reports persecutory dreams	10	14	4

Significance of differences determined by chi-square:
  *probability of chance occurrence, less than .01
  **probability of chance occurrence, less than .001

TABLE 68
RELATIONAL BEHAVIOR DURING PSYCHIATRIC INTERVIEW
OF RIO DE JANEIRO MENTAL HOSPITAL PATIENTS,
ACCORDING TO COLOR

Psychiatrists' Self-Ratings	% White (64% of total sample)	% Brown (24% of total sample)	% Black (12% of total sample)
Feels mild to moderate empathy with patient	58	46**	72
Estimates patient as emotionally neutral toward him	38	38**	68
Feels cheerful and optimistic during interview	31	14**	36
Feels neither sad nor cheerful but neutral	61	76	60
Feels remote and not empathetic with patient	25	34	20
Feels apprehensive or anxious during interview	9	22	16

TABLE 68 (continued)

	% White (64% of total sample)	% Brown (24% of total sample)	% Black (12% of total sample)
Feels pity for patient	19	20	8
Feels annoyance or slight anger toward patient	7	14	4
Regards interview as interesting and rewarding	66	56	40*
Felt liked by patient	58	52	32*
Feels a marked liking for the patient	19	6	4*
Observations of Patients' Behavior			
Actively cooperative	43	32	48
Respectful and courteous	32	22	36
Watches interviewer for cues	1	6*	12
Fluctuating attention to interviewer	35	50	40
Marked anxiety in relation to interviewer	48	52	40
Hand tremor	23	26	16
Active avoidance behavior, attempts to leave	8	22	8
Dull conformity	17	20	12
Asks for help about other life problems	7	20**	0

Significance of differences determined by chi-square:
*probability of chance occurrence, less than .05
**probability of chance occurrence, less than .01

TABLE 69

HALLUCINATORY AND ILLUSORY PHENOMENA IN RIO DE JANEIRO MENTAL
HOSPITAL PATIENTS, ACCORDING TO COLOR*

	% Black (12% of total sample)	% Brown (24% of total sample)	% White (64% of total sample)
Reports of Auditory Phenomena			
Hears voices in absence of other people	60	40	24***
Hears unexplained noises other than voices	21	34	17*
Hears voices which direct him to take action re others	12	4	1*
Hears voices which are religious in nature	8	6	1
Reports of Visual Phenomena			
Sees people in absence of identifiable outside stimulus	36	26	8***
Sees people only under certain circumstances	28	18	9***
Sees lights, colors, unformed entities	28	22	17
Sees animals	20	16	2***
Sees religiously meaningful nonhuman entities	16	12	1***
Sees religious, folkloric or ghostly human figures	9	12	2**
Insists on reality of reported experiences	42	37	11***
Plans action on basis of auditory or visual experiences	29	28	9***
Misinterpretations or Illusions			
Misinterprets communications and stimuli in all sensory spheres	28	32	14**
Misinterprets auditory stimuli	12	14	1***

Significance of differences determined by chi-square:
  *probability of chance occurrence, less than .02
  **probability of chance occurrence, less than .01
  ***probability of chance occurrence, less than .001

TABLE 70

DISORIENTATION IN RIO DE JANEIRO MENTAL
HOSPITAL PATIENTS, ACCORDING TO COLOR

Orientation Problems	% White (64% of total sample)	% Brown (24% of total sample)	% Black (12% of total sample)
Disoriented as to location	10	22	32*
Disoriented in all temporal spheres	5	22	28**

Significance of differences determined by chi-square:
*probability of chance occurrence, less than .01
**probability of chance occurrence, less than .001

TABLE 71

BODILY COMPLAINTS AND APPEARANCE OF RIO DE JANEIRO
MENTAL HOSPITAL PATIENTS, ACCORDING TO COLOR

	% White (64% of total sample)	% Brown (24% of total sample)	% Black (12% of total sample)
Somatic Complaints			
Head pain	16	20	32
Weakness	17	16	24
General discomfort	8	9	16
Physical Appearance			
Poorly nourished	24	35	36
Weak and not healthy	33	48	32
Emaciated	17*	31	28
Very neat and clean	23*	14	4

Significance of differences determined by chi-square:
*probability of chance occurrence, less than .05

TABLE 72

PSYCHOPHYSIOLOGICAL COMPLAINTS OF RIO DE JANEIRO
MENTAL HOSPITAL PATIENTS, ACCORDING TO COLOR

	% Brown (24% of total sample)	% Black (12% of total sample)	% White (64% of total sample)
Gastrointestinal Complaints			
Nausea or vomiting	28	24	21
Diarrhea	19	10	8
Feeling of something inside	19	10	8
Cardio-Pulmonary Complaints			
Faintness or dizziness	46	36	49
Dyspnea	29	20	32
Palpitation	26	36	33
Other			
Sweating or feelings of heat	20	40	28

TABLE 73

SEXUAL SYMPTOMS AND BEHAVIOR IN RIO DE JANEIRO MENTAL HOSPITAL PATIENTS, ACCORDING TO COLOR

Statements about Sexual Behavior	% Brown (24% of total sample)	% White (64% of total sample)	% Black (12% of total sample)
Sex a source of conflict (anxiety, shame, guilt)	64	58	44
Sex impulses too intense, uncontrollable or fluctuating	30	14	8***
Sex impulses absent or very weak	20	13	8
Solitary masturbation most frequent sexual activity	14	7	4
Claims exceptional sexual potency and desirability	12	2	4***
Reports polymorphous variable sexual practices	6	1	0*
Essentially monogamous sex relationship over most adult life	40	54	48
Worries interfere with sexual functioning	34	47	20**
Present sexual pattern associated with present illness	20	37	16**
Suffers from impotence or frigidity	20	37	10***
Says that engages in anal intercourse	12	20	4*

Significance of differences determined by chi-square:
*probability of chance occurrence, less than .05
**probability of chance occurrence, less than .02
***probability of chance occurrence, less than .01

TABLE 74
HISTORY OF PAST TRAUMATA. RIO DE JANEIRO MENTAL HOSPITAL PATIENTS, ACCORDING TO COLOR

Reports of Psychological Traumata or other Past Problems	% White (64% of total sample)	% Brown (24% of total sample)	% Black (12% of total sample)
Traumatic event(s) in adolescence or adulthood	49	50	32
Traumatic event(s) in childhood	26	28	20
Early problems in learning to relate to others	16	24	8
Problem in adjusting to work	20	18	12

TABLE 75
ALTERATION OR LOSS OF CONSCIOUSNESS ASSOCIATED WITH ILLNESS, INJURY OR NO IDENTIFIED CAUSE. RIO DE JANEIRO MENTAL HOSPITAL PATIENTS, ACCORDING TO COLOR

Reports of Past History of Altered Consciousness	% White (64% of total sample)	% Brown (24% of total sample)	% Black (12% of total sample)
Fainting or lapses of consciousness	27	22	16
Seizures, spells or fits	17	12	8
High fevers with altered consciousness	14	14	8
Deliria associated with fever, metabolic or other illness	11	14	4
Head injury with loss of consciousness	10	12	20

TABLE 76
SECONDARY SCHOOL ATTENDANCE ACCORDING TO URBANIZATION*

State	% of Population in Cities of 20,000 and Over	% of Youth Age 12 to 18 in Secondary Schools
Guanabara	97	29
Rio de Janeiro	36	12
Pernambuco	26	8
Pará	23	7
Minas Gerais	17	9
Bahia	16	6
Espirito Santo	15	10
Ceará	14	6
Maranhão	5	3

*Data from MEC—Serviço de Estatística da Educacao e Cultura—Sinopse Estatística da Ensimo Medio, 1960.

TABLE 77
DISTRIBUTION OF SCHOOL ACHIEVEMENT OF PATIENTS
COMPLETING PRIMARY GRADES OR ABOVE

Level of School Attained	% Completing Primary Grades or More
Completed primary school	44
Incomplete *ginásio* or equivalent	24
Completed *ginásio* or equivalent	12
Incomplete *colégio* or equivalent	4
Complete *colégio*	8
Incomplete university	3
Complete university	4
Undetermined	1

TABLE 78
RELATIONSHIP BETWEEN EDUCATIONAL LEVEL AND LITERACY

	% of Patients Educational Level*	
	Group I (57% of total sample)	Group II (43% of total sample)
Literacy		
Level I. Illiterate	25	0
Level II. Partly literate	24	0
Level III. Literate	50	98

	Illiterate (15% of total sample)	Partly Literate (14% of total sample)	Literate (71% of total sample)
Educational Level			
Group I. Incomplete primary	100	97	41
Group II. Primary and over	0	3	59

Significance of differences determined by chi-square:
*probability of chance occurrence, less than .001

TABLE 79

OCCUPATION ACCORDING TO EDUCATIONAL AND LITERACY LEVEL*

| | % of Patients** | | | | |
| | Educational Level | | | Literacy Level | |
Occupational Category	I (57% of total sample)	II (43% of total sample)	I (15% of total sample)	II (14% of total sample)	III (71% of total sample)
Class I. Professionals, large proprietors, executives	0	6	0	0	3
Class II. Medium proprietors, executives, managers	0	5	0	0	3
Class III. Small proprietors, administrators, clerks, salesmen, primary school teachers, clergy	4	25	0	0	18
Class IV. Foremen, skilled technicians, small farm owners	6	9	5	6	9
Class V. Skilled manual workers, drivers, policemen, conductors	45	38	38	36	46
Class VI. Unskilled workers, waiters	41	14	57	58	19

*Classifications according to Hutchinson (1963).
**Significance of differences determined by chi-square: probability of chance occurrence, less than .001

TABLE 80

HOUSING ACCORDING TO EDUCATIONAL AND LITERACY LEVEL

| | % of Patients | | | | |
| | Educational Level | | Literacy Level | | |
Quality and Density of Housing	I (57% of total sample)	II (43% of total sample)	I (15% of total sample)	II (14% of total sample)	III (71% of total sample)
Barraco, under construction, or unclassified	20	3*	30	20	5*
Has both electricity and running water	60	91***	35	60	84***
Has no essential services	23	2***	40	20	7***
Bedroom shared by others than mate	54	42	60	55	45
Dwelling contains one room and kitchen and bathroom or less	18	3**	46	43	18**

Significance of differences determined by chi-square.
  *probability of chance occurrence, less than .02
 **probability of chance occurrence, less than .01
***probability of chance occurrence, less than .001

TABLE 81

NATURE AND LOCATION OF LIVING AREA ACCORDING TO EDUCATIONAL AND LITERACY LEVEL*

	% of Patients				
	Educational Level		Literacy Level		
Living Area	I (57% of total sample)	II (43% of total sample)	I (15% of total sample)	II (14% of total sample)	III (71% of total sample)
Suburban or industrial	48	40	46	46	45
State of Rio de Janeiro (in greater Rio area)	34	13**	3?	40	16**
Central or peripheral urban or residential	30	52**	22	40	42
Small town	23	14	27	31	15*
Urban or suburban slum (favela)	10	1**	19	6	3**

Significance of differences determined by chi-square:
*probability of chance occurrence, less than .05
**probability of chance occurrence, less than .01

TABLE 82

SOCIOECONOMIC ACHIEVEMENT ACCORDING TO
EDUCATIONAL AND LITERACY LEVEL

	% of Patients				
	Educational Level		*Literacy Level*		
	I	II	I	II	III
	(57% of total sample)	(43% of total sample)	(15% of total sample)	(14% of total sample)	(71% of total sample)
Socioeconomic Status Compared with Father					
Patient feels is better than father	46	49	42	29	52
Patient feels is worse than father	21	21	22	29	20
Socioeconomic Status Compared with Past Year					
Patient feels has improved	33	46	27*	25	43
Patient feels has declined	34	27	40*	25	31

*Significance of differences determined by chi-square:
probability of chance occurrence, less than .05

TABLE 83

MIGRATORY STATUS ACCORDING TO EDUCATIONAL AND LITERACY LEVEL

| | % of Patients | | | | |
| | Educational Level | | Literacy Level | | |
	I (57% of total sample)	II (43% of total sample)	I (15% of total sample)	II (14% of total sample)	III (71% of total sample)
Length of Residence					
Lived in area for less than 10 years	49	37*	68	54	42**
Lived in present house for five years or less	49	29**	46	34	29
Migrated into area within past five years (recently migrant)	32	21	54	31	20**
Arrived in area after age 21	33	18**	51	33	20**
Where Born**					
East (Bahia, Espirito Santo, Minas Gerais, Rio State, Sergipe)	48	28	46	37	27
Area of present residence in greater Rio de Janeiro Guanabara	34	58	3	38	53
Northeast (Ceara, Maranhão, Paraiba, Pernambuco,	27	52	0	31	45
Piaui, Rio Grande do Norte)	20	14	41	9	13
Conditions of Migration (Percentage of Migrants Only)					
Migrated because of lack of jobs	58	31***	55	52	50
Changed type of occupation after move	52	20***	70	60	25***
Migrated from village, hamlet or *fazenda*	45	28**	64	60	37**
Migrated from some type of rural setting	70	40***	80	75	48**
Migrated alone	38	15**	37	35	27

Significance of differences determined by chi-square:

*probability of chance occurrence, less than .05

**probability of chance occurrence, less than .01

***probability of chance occurrence, less than .001

TABLE 84

COLOR AND FAMILY SIZE ACCORDING TO EDUCATIONAL
AND LITERACY LEVEL

	% of Patients				
	Educational Level		Literacy Level		
	I	II	I	II	III
	(57% of total sample)	(43% of total sample)	(15% of total sample)	(14% of total sample)	(71% of total sample)
Color					
White	51	82***	38	46	76**
Brown	32	15**	43	37	18
Black	17	3*	19	17	8
Number of Children					
None	31	43*	42	41	35
Three or less	36	43	25	24	44
Four or more	32	14**	34	35	21
Number of Siblings					
Three or less	22	37*	26	18	25
Four or more	77	63*	71	83	71

Significance of differences determined by chi-square:
*probability of chance occurrence, less than .05
**probability of chance occurrence, less than .01
***probability of chance occurrence, less than .001

TABLE 85

RELIGIOUS PARTICIPATION ACCORDING TO
EDUCATIONAL AND LITERACY LEVEL

	% of Patients				
	Educational Level		Literary Level		
	I	II	I	II	III
Patient's Reported Religion	(57% of total sample)	(43% of total sample)	(15% of total sample)	(14% of total sample)	(71% of total sample)
Catholic	72	69	73	76	68
Protestant	11	6	11	12	8
Spiritist-Afro-other cults	3	10	3	5	8
Supplemental Spiritist-Afro-other	18	13	27	12	14
Total reported cult Attendance	21	23	30	17	22

TABLE 86
CHILDHOOD INFLUENCES ACCORDING TO EDUCATION
AND LITERACY LEVEL

	% of Patients				
	Educational Level		*Literacy Level*		
	I	II	I	II	III
	(57% of total sample)	(43% of total sample)	(15% of total sample)	(14% of total sample)	(71% of total sample)
Family Stability					
Siblings by both parents	71	76	60	73	76
Reared by both parents	69	72	62	63	73
Father died prior to age 12	20	21	30	26	16
Discipline					
Disciplined mainly by beatings	41	31	40	50	34
Disciplined mainly by scoldings	38	43	29	32	44
Disciplined mainly by mother	18	27	11	14	26

TABLE 87
PARENTAL LITERACY ACCORDING TO PATIENT'S
EDUCATIONAL AND LITERACY LEVEL

	% of Patients*				
	Educational Level		*Literacy Level*		
	I	II	I	II	III
Parental Literacy	(57% of total sample)	(43% of total sample)	(15% of total sample)	(14% of total sample)	(71% of total sample)
Father illiterate	41	11	68	33	12
Father partly literate	24	29	5	23	26
Father literate	27	46	5	23	38
Mother illiterate	51	23	82	82	30
Mother partly literate	11	17	8	9	16
Mother literate	17	54	0	6	44

Significance of differences determined by chi-square:
   *probability of chance occurrence, less than .001

TABLE 88

OCCUPATION OF FATHER ACCORDING TO PATIENT'S EDUCATIONAL AND LITERACY LEVEL*

| | % of Patients* | | | | |
| | Educational Level | | Literacy Level | | |
Occupational Category of Father	I (57% of total sample)	II (43% of total sample)	I (15% of total sample)	II (14% of total sample)	III (71% of total sample)
Class I. Professionals, large proprietors, executives	0	6	0	0	4
Class II. Medium proprietors, executives, managers	1	6	0	0	4
Class III. Small proprietors, administrators, clerks, salesmen, primary school teachers, clergy	3	17	0	3	13
Class IV. Foremen, skilled technicians, small farm owners	3	14	6	6	13
Class V. Skilled manual workers, drivers, policemen, conductors	25	30	14	29	29
Class VI. Unskilled workers, waiters	54	20	72	60	30

Significance of differences determined by chi-square:
*Classifications according to Hutchinson (1963).
**probability of chance occurrence, less than .001

TABLE 89

SOURCES OF INFORMATION ACCORDING TO EDUCATIONAL
AND LITERACY LEVEL

	% of Patients				
	Educational Level		Literacy Level		
	I	II	I	II	III
	(57% of total sample)	(43% of total sample)	(15% of total sample)	(14% of total sample)	(71% of total sample)
Media Attended or Owned					
Owns a radio	87	95*	86	80	94*
Radio only medium of information	54	18***	78	48	28***
Watches television	31	62***	11	30	52***
Owns television	22	62***	3	11	51***
Owns one or more books	24	64***	3	23	52***
Reads newspapers	34	65***	8	21	54***
Reads magazines	32	62***	8	27	44***
Reads newspapers, magazines and books	28	58***	8	30	57***
Attends movies	24	53***	11	18	43***
Attends movies at least monthly	15	39***	16	17	9
Never attends movies	55	31**	59	50	41
Uses all media	22	50***	8	15	41***

Significance of differences determined by chi-square:
 *probability of chance occurrence, less than .05
 **probability of chance occurrence, less than .01
 ***probability of chance occurrence, less than .001

TABLE 90

PERSONAL RELATIONS AND INSTITUTIONAL PARTICIPATION
ACCORDING TO EDUCATIONAL AND LITERACY LEVEL

	% of Patients				
	Educational Level		Literacy Level		
	I	II	I	II	III
	(57% of total sample)	(43% of total sample)	(15% of total sample)	(14% of total sample)	(71% of total sample)
Friends and Relatives					
Has close friends	46	57	54	48	50
Relatives nearby	24	29	22	40	24
Knows nothing about neighbors	23	24	11	14	28

TABLE 90 (continued)

| | % of Patients | | | | |
| | Educational Level | | Literacy Level | | |
	I (57% of total sample)	II (43% of total sample)	I (15% of total sample)	II (14% of total sample)	III (71% of total sample)
Institutional Contact					
Has some contact with welfare workers	67	79*	51	67	87**
Frequently uses welfare services	16	18	8	17	18
Has some contact with clergy	60	57	68	66	54
Feels friendly toward clergy	23	19	32	26	16
Amusements					
Sometimes watches soccer	64	66	35	49	33
Watches soccer six times or more yearly	26	22	35	34	19*
Sometimes goes to dances	73	73	33	37	21
Goes to dances six times yearly or more	11	10	22	17	12

Significance of differences determined by chi-square:
*probability of chance occurrence, less than .05
**probability of chance occurrence, less than .001

TABLE 91

EVENTS LEADING TO HOSPITALIZATION ACCORDING TO EDUCATIONAL AND LITERACY LEVEL

% of Patients

	Educational Level		Literacy Level		
	I (57% of total sample)	II (43% of total sample)	I (15% of total sample)	II (14% of total sample)	III (71% of total sample)
Acuteness of Illness					
Has had previous contact with psychiatrists	41	58***	30	38	53**
Present illness duration six months or less	50	34**	60	39	42
Present illness duration one month or less	22	15	23	12	18
Reasons for Hospital Admission					
Physical assaults against people or property; threats	25	14*	21	19	11
Anxious, depressed, or suicidal	21	18	40	35	21*
Anxious about intent of others, paranoid; grandiose	20	10*	30	19	13*
Other bizarre or markedly peculiar behavior	12	22*	10	16	17
Will not or cannot work	9	1***	24	12	2****

Significance of differences determined by chi-square:
   *probability of chance occurrence, less than .05
  **probability of chance occurrence, less than .02
 ***probability of chance occurrence, less than .01
****probability of chance occurrence, less than .001

TABLE 92
FAMILY DIAGNOSIS ACCORDING TO EDUCATIONAL AND LITERACY LEVEL

	% of Patients				
	Educational Level		Literacy Level		
	I	II	I	II	III
	(57% of total sample)	(43% of total sample)	(15% of total sample)	(14% of total sample)	(71% of total sample)
Family Diagnosis					
An illness, mental or physical	68	55*	70	69	60
A mental illness	46	26**	65	49	31***
Behavior reflecting life stress—no illness	9	24**	7	4	19*
Strange behavior without value connotation	26	39*	8	30	37**
Religiously inspired behavior	8	5	13	3	6

Significance of differences determined by chi-square:
*probability of chance occurrence, less than .05
**probability of chance occurrence, less than .01
***probability of chance occurrence, less than .001

TABLE 93

RELATIONAL BEHAVIOR DURING PSYCHIATRIC INTERVIEW ACCORDING TO
EDUCATIONAL AND LITERACY LEVEL

| | % of Patients | | | | |
| | Educational Level | | Literacy Level | | |
	I (57% of total sample)	II (43% of total sample)	I (15% of total sample)	II (14% of total sample)	III (71% of total sample)
Psychiatrists' Self-Ratings					
Likes the patient	61	74*	57	73	67
Feels involved and empathetic	51	62	37	61	58
Feels interview to be interesting and rewarding	48	77****	33	65	64***
Feels that patient liked him	42	69***	27	46	59***
Felt cheerful and optimistic	21	37***	17	15	32*
Felt remote or distant	32	18**	40	15	26*
Felt hostility	—	—	23	12	5****
Observations of Patient's Behavior					
Cooperative throughout interview	62	74*	40	69	73****
Paid attention comfortably	60	65	33	65	66****
Appeared strong and healthy	58	71*	47	61	68*
Actively cooperative approach	57	69	38	65	66***
Respectful, courteous, friendly	49	57	40	58	53
No substantial behavioral change during interview	36	36	17	40	41**
Wet palms on handshake	23	17	30	27	17
Dramatic or attention seeking	22	32	20	27	27
Stated wish not to be helped	22	17	23	15	11
Actively advice seeking	19	38***	7	15	24
Voice faint or weak	15	8	23	19	9**
Hypervigilant and distractible	15	14	30	15	12*
Expresses unsatisfied wishes to be cared for	13	10	30	15	8***

Significance of differences determined by chi-square:
*probability of chance occurrence, less than .05
**probability of chance occurrence, less than .02
***probability of chance occurrence, less than .01
****probability of chance occurrence, less than .001

TABLE 94

TENSION, ANXIETY AND DISRUPTION OF FUNCTION ACCORDING TO LITERACY AND EDUCATIONAL LEVEL

| | % of Patients | | | | |
| | Educational Level | | Literacy Level | | |
	I (57% of total sample)	II (43% of total sample)	I (15% of total sample)	II (14% of total sample)	III (71% of total sample)
Reports of Anxiety and Tension					
Any type of organ anxiety	44	39	57	42	35*
Constant diffuse anxiety	26	41**	20	31	40*
Worry about relatives	26	23	36	31	22
Fear of loss of control over acts	20	33**	13	27	27
Interference with Function					
Insomnia due to worries	74	77	87	77	72
Restlessness due to worries	48	44	57	58	42
Interview startles, anxious facies, ANS signs or anxious speech content	42	47	60	50	44
Difficulty in clear thinking	22	12*	40	4	12***

Significance of differences determined by chi-square:
   *probability of chance occurrence, less than .05
  **probability of chance occurrence, less than .02
 ***probability of chance occurrence, less than .001

TABLE 95

ANGER AND FRUSTRATION ACCORDING TO LITERACY

Reports of Anger, Impulsivity, or Frustration	Partly Literate II (14% of total sample)	% of Patients Illiterate I (15% of total sample)	Literate III (71% of total sample)
Feels and expresses anger	54	37	49
Attacks of rage	54	23	44*
Feels tense, uncomfortable or isolated with others	46	27	31
Frequent arguments	46	40	29
Feels others regard him as mentally-morally inferior	46	33	15****
Impulsive acts	38	27	24
Achievement/aspiration discrepancy	26	25	19
Interview hostility	23	13	7**
Impulsive decision-making	19	3	4***
Denies or does not mention anger	42	60	48

Significance of differences determined by chi-square.
  *probability of chance occurrence, less than .05
 **probability of chance occurrence, less than .02
***probability of chance occurrence, less than .01
****probability of chance occurrence, less than .001

TABLE 96

AFFECTIVE SYMPTOMS AND BEHAVIOR ACCORDING TO LITERACY*

		% of Patients Literacy Level	
Depressive Mood Indicators	I (15% of total sample)	II (14% of total sample)	III (71% of total sample)
Weeps or appears sad during interview	30	27	23
Speech slow with silences	30	19	17
Says body is weak and inferior	30	23	15
Expresses fear of being abandoned	30	11	20
Expresses fear of impending doom	28	15	18
Says feelings are absent or dulled	20	11	9
Feels overwhelmed by criticism	33	46	22**
Generally self-accusatory	20	31	19
Guilty re failure in social role	13	31	13*
Guilty re failure in filial role	7	19	7*

Significance of differences determined by chi-square:
   *probability of chance occurrence, less than .05
 **probability of chance occurrence, less than .01

TABLE 97

PARANOID OR GRANDIOSE STATEMENTS ACCORDING TO LITERACY

| | % of Patients Literacy Level | | |
| | I | II | III |
	(15% of total sample)	(14% of total sample)	(71% of total sample)
Statements Concerning Others			
Complains about treatment by others	70	53	50
Feels persecuted, harassed or attacked	57	35	35*
Feels emulated or loved by certain others	50	50	26**
Says others stare at or talk about him	43	56	30**
Says others are not trustworthy	37	38	23
Says others misjudge or misinterpret him	33	35	19*
Says others know his inner thoughts and feelings	30	23	25
Says others control his thought reaction	13	23	22
Says others are inferior	13	16	4**

Significance of differences determined by chi-square:
*probability of chance occurrence, less than .05
**probability of chance occurrence, less than .01

TABLE 98

HALLUCINATORY AND ILLUSORY PHENOMENA ACCORDING TO EDUCATIONAL AND LITERACY LEVELS

% of Patients

	Educational Level		Literacy Level		
	I (57% of total sample)	II (43% of total sample)	I (15% of total sample)	II (14% of total sample)	III (71% of total sample)
Reports of Auditory Phenomena					
Hears voices in absence of other people	40	21***	57	39	27***
Hears unexplained noises other than voices	25	17	31	15	21
Hears voices which direct him to take action re others	13	1***	26	16	3****
Hears voices which are religious in nature	8	1**	17	11	2***
Reports of Visual Phenomena					
Sees people in absence of identifiable outside stimulus	25	2****	35	35	8****
Sees lights, colors, unformed entities	22	6***	25	19	17
Sees objects other than people	20	5***	24	27	9***
Sees religiously meaningful nonhuman entities	10	1***	17	11	4**
Sees religious, folkloric, or ghostly human figures	10	1***	14	19	2****
Sees figures which direct him to take action re others	7	2*	10	11	1***
Insists on reality of reported experiences	28	8****	45	32	14****
Plans action on basis of auditory or visual experiences	23	6***	38	27	9****
Misinterpretations or Illusions					
Misinterprets communications and stimuli in all sensory spheres	23	14	30	23	16*
Misinterprets or gives special meaning to auditory stimuli	11	5	20	11	5**.

Significance of differences determined by chi-square:
*probability of chance occurrence, less than .05
**probability of chance occurrence, less than .02
***probability of chance occurrence, less than .01
****probability of chance occurrence, less than .001

TABLE 99
DISORIENTATION ACCORDING TO EDUCATIONAL AND LITERACY LEVELS

	% of Patients				
	Educational Level		*Literacy Level*		
	I	II	I	II	III
	(57% of total sample)	(43% of total sample)	(15% of total sample)	(14% of total sample)	(71% of total sample)
Orientation Problems					
Disoriented as to location	21	7*	57	12	8**
Disoriented in time	39	10*	73	23	21**

Significance of differences determined by chi-square:
    *probability of chance occurrence, less than .01
    **probability of chance occurrence, less than .001

TABLE 100
SOMATIC AND PSYCHOPHYSIOLOGICAL COMPLAINTS ACCORDING TO EDUCATIONAL AND LITERACY LEVELS

	% of Patients				
	Educational Level		*Literacy Level*		
	I	II	I	II	III
Statements about body function	(57% of total sample)	(43% of total sample)	(15% total sample)	(14% of total sample)	(71% of total sample)
Any complaint of physical pain or discomfort	80	62**	70	81	73
Complains of fatigue	57	61	77	50	56
Complains of weakness	52	62	63	46	54
Complains of head pain	21	17	20	31	16
Feels that physical movements have slowed	15	16	30	23	15
Feels as though something strange is inside body	15	9	24	19	9*
Cardiopulmonary Complaints					
Faintness or dizziness			37	54	48
Palpitation			17	31	34
Dyspnea			17	27	31
Sweating or hot flashes			13	31	28
Gastrointestinal Complaints					
Anorexia			50	58	58
Nausea or vomiting			10	23	26
Diarrhea			10	8	18

Significance of differences determined by chi-square:
    *probability of chance occurrence, less than .02
    **probability of chance occurrence, less than .01

TABLE 101
SEXUAL SYMPTOMS AND BEHAVIOR
ACCORDING TO EDUCATIONAL AND LITERACY LEVELS

	% of Patients				
	Educational Level		Literacy Level		
	I	II	I	II	III
	(57% of total sample)	(43% of total sample)	(15% of total sample)	(14% of total sample)	(71% of total sample)
Statements about Sexual Behavior					
Worries interfere with sexual functioning	39	45	43	38	41
Present sexual problem associated with present illness	29	33	17	23	35*
Suffers from impotence or frigidity	28	33	23	27	33
Sex impulses too intense, uncontrollable, or fluctuating	15	21	3	19	20*

Significance of differences determined by chi-square:
*probability of chance occurrence, less than .05

TABLE 102
ITEMS OF PAST HISTORY ACCORDING TO LITERACY

	% of Patients		
	Partly Literate II	Illiterate I	Literate III
	(14% of total sample)	(15% of total sample)	(71% of total sample)
Reports of Past Events			
Psychological trauma in childhood	38	33	21
Fainting or lapses of consciousness	38	23	24
Problems in adjusting to work	38	20	15**
High fevers with altered consciousness	31	7	12**
Head injury with loss of consciousness	15	7	13
Childhood or adolescent rages	38	27	40
Childhood sleep disturbances	19	3	20*

Significance of differences determined by chi-square:
*probability of chance occurrence, less than .05
**probability of chance occurrence, less than .01

TABLE 103

LITERACY AND EDUCATION ACCORDING TO
OCCUPATIONAL LEVEL

| | *% of Patients*
*Occupational Group** | | |
	I–IV (25% of total sample)	V (43% of total sample)	VI (29% of total sample)
Illiterate	3	13	28
Partly literate	3	11	26
Literate	94	74	45
Incomplete primary education	24	61	80
Complete primary and beyond	76	38	20

Classifications according to Hutchinson (1963).
Significance of differences determined by chi-square:
*probability of chance occurrence, less than .001

TABLE 104

HOUSING ACCORDING TO OCCUPATIONAL LEVEL

| | *% of Patients*
Occupational Group | | |
	I–IV (25% of total sample)	V (43% of total sample)	VI (29% of total sample)
Quality and Density of Housing			
Barraco, under construction, or unclassified	2	6	28*
Has no essential services	3	9	31*
Has both electricity and running water	95	78	44*
Dwelling contains only 1 room plus kitchen and bathroom, or less	8	18	34*

Significance of differences determined by chi-square:
*probability of chance occurrence, less than .001

TABLE 105
NATURE AND LOCATION OF LIVING AREA ACCORDING TO OCCUPATIONAL LEVEL

	% of Patients Occupational Group		
Living Area	I–IV (25% of total sample)	V (43% of total sample)	VI (29% of total sample)
Urban, central and peripheral or residential	54	40	25***
State of Rio de Janeiro (Greater Rio)	13	21	31**
Small town	13	18	24
Rural area	8	6	10
Suburban or industrial	35	46	52*
Urban or suburban slum (favela)	2	5	12*

Significance of differences determined by chi-square:
  *probability of chance occurrence, less than .05
  **probability of chance occurrence, less than .01
  ***probability of chance occurrence, less than .001

TABLE 106
SOCIOECONOMIC ACHIEVEMENT ACCORDING TO OCCUPATIONAL LEVEL

	% of Patients Occupational Group		
	I–IV (25% of total sample)	V (43% of total sample)	VI (29% of total sample)
Socioeconomic Status Compared with Father			
Patient feels is better than father	55*	31	36
Patient feels is worse than father	18	20	26
Socioeconomic Status Compared with Past Year			
Patient feels has improved	45*	43	25
Patient feels has declined	24*	32	39

Significance of differences determined by chi-square:
  *probability of chance occurrence, less than .05

TABLE 107

MIGRATORY STATUS ACCORDING TO OCCUPATIONAL LEVEL

	% of Patients Occupational Group		
	I-IV (25% of total sample)	V (43% of total sample)	VI (29% of total sample)
Length of Residence			
Lived in area for less than 19 years	36	39	50*
Lived in present house for five years or less	38	42	54*
Migrated into area within past 5 years	19	24	35*
Arrived in area after age 21	17	26	32*
Where Born			
East (Bahia, Espirito Santo, Minas Gerais, Rio State, Sergipe)	21	34	40*
Area of present residence in Greater Rio de Janeiro	5	6	8
Guanabara	50	41	22**
Northeast (Ceará, Maranhão, Paraiba, Pernambuco, Piaui, Rio Grande do Norte)	13	13	26
Conditions of Migration (Percentage of Migrants only—55% of Total Sample)			
Migrated because of lack of jobs	37	50	59*
Migrated from village, hamlet or *fazenda*	30	40	66**
Migrated from some type of rural setting	37	50	79***
Migrated alone	12	30	38**
Occupational Changes (Percentage of Entire Group)			
Changed type of occupation after move	6†	22††	38†††****

Significance of differences determined by chi-square:
   *probability of chance occurrence, less than .05
  **probability of chance occurrence, less than .01
 ***probability of chance occurrence, less than .001

†Evenly divided between Classes V & VI before move.
††Prior to move, Class VI, 17%; Class V, 3%; Class IV, 2%.
†††Prior to move, Class VI, 37%; Class V, 1%.

TABLE 108
DEMOGRAPHIC FEATURES ACCORDING TO OCCUPATIONAL LEVEL

	% of Patients Occupational Group		
	I–IV (25% of total sample)	V (43% of total sample)	VI (29% of total sample)
Color			
White	85	66	42**
Brown	10	23	39**
Black	3	10	19**
Age			
15–25 or less	25	16	25
26–40 or less	48	51	52
41–60	25	33	23
Sex			
Male	63	62	75
Female	37	38	25
Marital Status			
No spouse or mate	43	21	38*
Both civil and religious ceremonies	40	45	30
Common-law mate	6	7	7
Number of Siblings			
Three or less	38	28	19*
Four or more	62	72	79
Number of Children			
None	46	26	42*
Three or less	40	45	30
Four or more	14	29	28*

Significance of differences determined by chi-square:
*probability of chance occurrence, less than .05
**probability of chance occurrence, less than .001

TABLE 109
RELIGIOUS PARTICIPATION ACCORDING TO
OCCUPATIONAL LEVEL

	% of Patients		
	Occupational Group		
	I–IV	V	VI
	(25% of total sample)	(43% of total sample)	(29% of total sample)
Patient's Reported Religion			
Catholic	76	73	63
Protestant	2	10	11*
Spiritist, Afro, other cults	3	13	14*
Supplemental Spiritist-Afro, other	14	18	14
Total reported cult attendance	17	31	28

Significance of differences determined by chi-square:
*probability of chance occurrence, less than .05

TABLE 110
CHILDHOOD INFLUENCES ACCORDING TO OCCUPATIONAL LEVEL

	% of Patients		
	Occupational Group		
	I–IV	V	VI
	(25% of total sample)	(43% of total sample)	(29% of total sample)
Family Stability and Economic Support			
Patient reports broken home	44	36	47
Patient reared by both parents	63	74	65
Financially independent prior to age 14	5	14	15*
Paternal Literacy			
Father illiterate	6	25	39***
Father partly literate	23	22	23
Father literate	49	27	19***
Paternal Occupation			
Father in Group I-IV	55	19	8***
Father in Group V	17	40	15**
Father in Group VI	16	35	70***

Significance of differences determined by chi-square:
*probability of chance occurrence, less than .05
**probability of chance occurrence, less than .01
***probability of chance occurrence, less than .001

TABLE 111
SOURCES OF INFORMATION ACCORDING TO
OCCUPATIONAL LEVEL

	% of patients Occupational Group		
	I–IV	V	VI
	(25% of total	(43% of total	(29% of total
Media Attended or Owned	sample)	sample)	sample)
Owns a radio	94	94	82
Radio only medium of information	19	39	56**
Watches television	62	47	24**
Owns television	69	38	13**
Owns one or more books	61	32	19**
Reads newspapers	67	38	32*
Reads magazines	67	38	35*
Reads newspapers, magazines and books	68	40	39*
Attends movies	54	36	20*
Attends movies at least monthly	45	15	24*
Never attends movies	23	50	55*
Uses all media	52	31	20*

Significance of differences determined by chi-square:
  *probability of chance occurrence, less than .01
  **probability of chance occurrence, less than .001

TABLE 112
PERSONAL RELATIONS AND INSTITUTIONAL PARTICIPATION
ACCORDING TO OCCUPATIONAL LEVEL

	% of Patients Occupational Group		
	I–IV	V	VI
	(25% of total	(43% of total	(29% of total
Friends and Relatives	sample)	sample)	sample)
Knows nothing about neighbors	29	18	26
Friendly to close neighbors	64	75	72
Institutional Contact			
Has some contact with welfare workers	77	88	65*
Friendly with welfare workers	26	31	18
Frequently utilizes services	11	24	11
Has some contact with clergy	56	67	48*
Friendly toward clergy	16	23	23
Amusement			
Watches soccer six times or more yearly	13	24	28*
Attends dances six times yearly or more	18	14	12

Significance of differences determined by chi-square:
  *probability of chance occurrence, less than .05

TABLE 113
EVENTS LEADING TO HOSPITALIZATION ACCORDING TO OCCUPATIONAL LEVEL

	% of Patients Occupational Group		
	I–IV (25% of total sample)	V (43% of total sample)	VI (69% of total sample)
Acuteness of Illness			
Has had previous contact with psychiatrist	54	49	44
Present illness duration 6 months or less	40	47	42
Present illness duration 1 month or less	24	15	19
Reason for Hospital Admission			
Bizarre or markedly peculiar behavior	22	11	15
Anxious, depressed, or suicidal	15	25	18
Physical assaults or threats	13	16	15
Anxious about intent of others, paranoid, grandiose	7	15	24*
Will not or cannot work	5	5	9

Significance of differences determined by chi-square:
*probability of chance occurrence, less than .05

TABLE 114
FAMILY DIAGNOSIS ACCORDING TO OCCUPATIONAL LEVEL

	% of Patients Occupational Group		
Family Diagnosis	I–IV (25% of total sample)	V (43% of total sample)	VI (29% of total sample)
An illness, mental or physical	51	70	61*
A mental illness	27	30	34
Behavior reflecting life-stress —no illness	27	15	6**
Religiously inspired behavior	0	3	9
Bad behavior	4	0	4

Significance of differences determined by chi-square:
*probability of chance occurrence, less than .05
**probability of chance occurrence, less than .001

TABLE 115
RELATIONAL BEHAVIOR DURING PSYCHIATRIC INTERVIEW
ACCORDING TO OCCUPATIONAL LEVEL

	% of Patients by Occupational Group		
	I–IV	V	VI
	(25% of	(43% of	(29% of
	total	total	total
Psychiatrist's Self-Ratings	sample)	sample)	sample)
Feels interview interesting and rewarding	78	51	54*
Likes the patient	76	60	63
Feels involved and empathic	68	51	49
Feels liked by patient	64	58	37*
Feels cheerful and optimistic	39	24	21
Feels remote or distant	15	31	31*
Feels hostile toward patient	2	9	15*
Observations of Patient's Behavior			
Cooperative throughout interview	76	66	60
Stream of speech unremarkable	71	76	58
Actively cooperative approach	63	52	51
Paid attention comfortably	56	69	54
No evidence of marked anxiety	53	59	45
Exhibited appropriate emotional expression	36	32	27
Hypervigilant or distractible	25	7	15*

Significance of differences determined by chi-square:
*probability of chance occurrence, less than .05

TABLE 116
TENSIONS, ANXIETY, AND DISRUPTION OF FUNCTION
ACCORDING TO OCCUPATIONAL LEVEL

	% of Patients by Occupational Group		
	I–IV	V	VI
	(25% of	(43% of	(29% of
	total	total	total
Reports of Anxiety and Tension	sample)	sample)	sample)
Specific attacks of anxiety	64	68	75
Constant diffuse anxiety	42	34	33
Any type of organ anxiety	35	39	45
Fear of loss of control over acts	34	25	18*
Worries about job	13	31	37**
Interference with Function			
Insomnia due to worries	69	77	79
Worries interfere with work	65	62	72
Startle reactions, anxious facies, ANS	44	37	53
Restlessness due to worries	42	42	56
Difficulty concentrating due to worries	40	41	48

Significance of differences determined by chi-square:
*probability of chance occurrence, less than .05
**probability of chance occurrence, less than .02

TABLE 117

ANGER AND FRUSTRATION ACCORDING TO OCCUPATIONAL LEVEL

Reports of Anger, Impulsivity, or Frustration	% of Patients by Occupational Group		
	I–IV (25% of total sample)	V (43% of total sample)	VI (29% of total sample)
Feels and expresses anger	47	51	52
Attacks of rage or anger	42	40	43
Frequent arguments	31	29	37
Feels tense, uncomfortable, or isolated with others	39	25	36
Impulsive acts	29	20	31
Feels others regard him as mentally-morally inferior	20	15	30*
Interview hostility	11	5	18*
Achievement/aspiration discrepancy	24	13	25

Significance of differences determined by chi-square:
*probability of chance occurrence, less than .05

TABLE 118

AFFECTIVE SYMPTOMS AND BEHAVIOR ACCORDING TO OCCUPATIONAL LEVEL

	% of Patients by Occupational Group		
	I–IV (25% of total sample)	V (43% of total sample)	VI (29% of total sample)
Depressive Mood Indicators			
Often feels sad	64	65	56
Often feels like weeping	47	42	36
Rigid, flat or apathetic during interview	25	15	27
High-intensity feelings are a problem	22	34	30
Weeps or appears sad during interview	18	30	22
Says feelings are absent or dulled	18	8	10
Says body is weak and inferior	16	14	22
Suicidal Thoughts or Acts			
Expresses death wishes	29	16	7*
States specific suicidal fantasies	27	11	15*
Makes suicidal threats	27	17	16
Has made an actual suicidal attempt	16	19	13

TABLE 118 (continued)

	% of Patients by Occupational Group		
	I-IV (25% of total sample)	V (43% of total sample)	VI (29% of total sample)
Guilt Feelings			
Is generally self-accusatory	29	19	15
Feels generally inadequate	24	7	10*
Guilty re failure in social role	25	11	13
Guilty re failure in filial role	13	6	9
Guilty re failure in parental role	11	4	6

Significance of differences determined by chi-square:
*probability of chance occurrence, less than .05

TABLE 119

PARANOID STATEMENTS ACCORDING TO OCCUPATIONAL LEVEL

	% of Patients by Occupational Group		
	I–IV (25% of total sample)	V (43% of total sample)	VI (29% of total sample)
Statements Concerning Others			
Complains about treatment by others	51	50	57
Feels persecuted, harassed, or attacked	36	30	45
Others stare at or talk about him	26	31	43*
Others know inner thoughts and feelings	24	24	31
Others are not trustworthy	22	19	37*
Others misjudge him	22	21	27
Others control inner thoughts and feelings	20	23	27

Significance of differences determined by chi-square:
*probability of chance occurrence, less than .05

TABLE 120

HALLUCINATORY AND ILLUSORY PHENOMENA ACCORDING TO OCCUPATIONAL LEVEL

	% of Patients by Occupational Group		
	I–IV (25% of total sample)	V (43% of total sample)	VI (29% of total sample)
Reports of Auditory Phenomenon			
Hears voices in absence of other people	26	21	51**
Hears unexplained noises other than voices	14	26	23
Hears voices which are religious in nature	6	0	12*
Hears voices which direct him to take action re others	4	0	21**
Reports of Visual Phenomena			
Sees people in absence of identifiable outside stimuli	6	10	35***
Sees lights, colors, unformed entities	16	17	27
Sees objects other than people	6	9	27**
Sees religious, folkloric, or ghostly human figures	0	1	16**
Sees religious, folkloric, or ghostly nonhuman entities	2	1	16**
Sees figures which direct him to take action re others	4	0	9
Insists on reality of experience	13	11	37*
Plans specific action on basis of experience	7	6	33**
Misinterpretations or Illusions			
Misinterprets communications and stimuli in all sensory spheres	16	16	24

Significance of differences determined by chi-square   **probability of chance occurrence, less than .01
*probability of chance occurrence, less than .05   ***probability of chance occurrence, less than .001

TABLE 121
DISORIENTATION ACCORDING TO OCCUPATIONAL LEVEL

	% of Patients Occupational Group		
	I–IV	V	VI
	(25% of total	(43% of total	(29% of total
Orientation Problems	sample)	sample)	sample)
Disoriented as to location	7	14	25*
Disoriented in time	18	25	42**

Significance of differences determined by chi-square:
*probability of chance occurrence, less than .05
**probability of chance occurrence, less than .01

TABLE 122
SOMATIC AND PSYCHOPHYSIOLOGICAL COMPLAINTS ACCORDING TO OCCUPATIONAL LEVEL

	% of Patients Occupational Group		
	I–IV	V	VI
	(25% of	(43% of	(29% of
	total	total	total
Statements About Body Function	sample)	sample)	sample)
Any complaint of physical pain or discomfort	66	73	81*
Headaches	54	61	70*
Anorexia	53	63	56
Complains of fatigue	49	62	64*
Faintness or dizziness	33	52	51*
Sweating or hot flashes	25	22	35
Nausea or vomiting	15	26	25
Complains of head pain	13	19	24
Feels as though something strange is inside body	8	9	19

Significance of differences determined by chi-square:
*probability of chance occurrence, less than .05

TABLE 123
SEXUAL SYMPTOMS AND BEHAVIOR ACCORDING TO OCCUPATIONAL LEVEL

| | % of Patients Occupational Group | | |
| | I–IV | V | VI |
Statements about Sexual Behavior	(25% of total sample)	(43% of total sample)	(29% of total sample)
Basically monogamous pattern	61	75	57*
Suffers from impotence or frigidity	33	36	24
Sex impulses absent or weak	20	12	12

Significance of differences determined by chi-square:
*probability of chance occurrence, less than .05

TABLE 124
PAST PSYCHIATRIC HISTORY ACCORDING TO OCCUPATIONAL LEVEL

| | % of Patients Occupational Group | | |
| | I–IV | V | VI |
	(25% of total sample)	(43% of total sample)	(29% of total sample)
Developmental Problems			
Difficulty in attaining bladder control	33	30	24
Psychological trauma in childhood	29	27	19
Childhood sleep disturbances	27	15	12*
Institutional Adjustment			
School adjustment problems	38	30	34
Work adjustment problems	18	12	23
Medical History			
Past history of seizures or fainting spells	24	21	33
Past history of head injury with loss of consciousness	5	10	23**

Significance of differences determined by chi-square:
*probability of chance occurrence, less than .05
**probability of chance occurrence, less than .001

TABLE 125

LIVING AREAS OF TOTAL PATIENT POPULATION

Districts or Zones	% of Total Population
Urban Total	44
Central urban	17
Residential urban	14
Peripheral urban	9
Deteriorated or slum urban	4
Suburban Total	49
Suburban, general	42
Suburban, slum	4
Suburban, industrial	3
Total Rural	7

TABLE 126

HOUSING CHARACTERISTICS OF TOTAL PATIENT POPULATION

	% of Total Population
Services in Home	
Both electricity and running water	70
Neither electricity nor running water	13
Electricity only	11
Running water only	4
Undetermined	2
Privacy of Sleeping Quarters	
Alone or with mate	51
With children or other family members	43
Undetermined	6
Distribution of Rooms	
No separate sleeping room	21
Separate sleeping room plus kitchen and bath	24
More than one room plus kitchen and bath	55
Nature of Structure	
Separate housing unit	54
Vila or house grouping around a single courtyard	14
Apartment house	11
Rented room in tenement or home	9
Barraco	9
Non-residential building, incomplete structure or unclassified	3

TABLE 127
SOCIAL AND HOUSING CHARACTERISTICS
ACCORDING TO LIVING AREA

% of Patients

	Area I (65% of total sample)	*Area II* (21% of total sample)
Nature of Housing		
Has both electricity and running water	81	65**
Has neither electricity nor running water	9	19*
Lives in *barraco* or unclassified structure	7	23***
Lives in *favela* or slum	0	22****
Social characteristics		
Literate	73	61
Reads newspapers, magazines, and books	49	39
Owns TV	46	34
In house five years or less	41	52
Migrated in preceding 5 years	21	43****
Has four or more children	19	33*
Father illiterate	15	30**

Significance of differences determined by chi-square:
*probability of chance occurrence, less than .05
**probability of chance occurrence, less than .02
***probability of chance occurrence, less than .01
****probability of chance occurrence, less than .001

TABLE 128
INTERPERSONAL PARTICIPATION ACCORDING TO LIVING AREA

% of Patients

	Area I (65% of total sample)	*Area II* (21% of total sample)
Relations with Others		
Has had some contact with welfare workers	83	66**
Has close friends	57	34**
Has had some contact with clergy	54	71*
Knows nothing about neighbors	27	14*
Friendly with clergy	17	30*
Participation in Amusements		
Sometimes watches soccer games	32	46
Sometimes attends dances	24	36
Watches soccer at least six times yearly	21	31
Attends dances at least six times yearly	11	21

Significance of differences determined by chi-square:
*probability of chance occurrence, less than .05
**probability of chance occurrence, less than .01

TABLE 129

SOCIOECONOMIC INDICATORS ACCORDING TO
ADEQUACY OF HOUSING

	% of Patients with Electricity and Running Water in Dwelling	
	Have One or Neither (28% of total sample)	Have Both (70% of total sample)
Housing Area, Quality, Size		
Favela	21	1**
Other urban including residential area	15	48**
Barraco or unclassified structure	36	3**
One room with kitchen and bath or less	42	13**
Sleeping room shared by others than mate	59	43*
*Education***		
No or incomplete primary school	84	45
Complete primary or beyond	14	55
*Literacy***		
Literate	43	80
Illiterate	36	8
Partly literate	21	12
*Occupation***		
Classes I and II	0	6
Classes III and IV	4	27
Class V	34	46
Class VI	58	17
Socioeconomic Mobility		
Regards SES as better than father's	38	51
Feels SES worse in past year	42	29

Significance of differences determined by chi-square:
*probability of chance occurrence, less than .05
**probability of chance occurrence, less than .001

TABLE 130
DEMOGRAPHIC CHARACTERISTICS ACCORDING TO ADEQUACY OF HOUSING

	% of Patients with Electricity and Running Water in Dwelling	
Age	Have One or Neither (28% of total sample)	Have Both (70% of total sample)
25 or less	18	28
41 or more	28	20
Marital Status		
Unmarried	39	29
Married (civil and religious)	19	46*
Common-law	11	5
Color		
White	43	72*
Brown	35	21*
Black	22	6*
Family Size		
4 or more siblings	80	68
3 or fewer siblings	19	32
No children	43	34
3 or fewer children	29	43

Significance of differences determined by chi-square:
*probability of chance occurrence, less than .001

TABLE 131
CHILDHOOD INFLUENCES ACCORDING TO ADEQUACY OF HOUSING AS ADULTS

	% of Patients with Running Water and Electricity in Dwelling	
Parental Literacy	Have One or Neither (28% of total sample)	Have Both (70% of total sample)
Father illiterate	47	16*
Father literate	19	36*
Father partly literate	17	26*
Mother literate	19	39*

Significance of differences determined by chi-square:
*probability of chance occurrence, less than .001

TABLE 132

INFORMATION AND SOCIAL PARTICIPATION ACCORDING TO
ADEQUACY OF HOUSING

	% of Patients with Electricity and Running Water in Dwelling	
	Have One or Neither	*Have Both*
Media Utilized or Owned		
Owns radio	77	94***
Radio only medium	67	28***
Never attends movies	59	39**
Reads newspapers, magazines and books	30	53**
Reads newspapers	25	50***
Owns book(s)	23	47**
Attends movies monthly or more	18	28
Watches TV	15	53***
Owns TV	2	52***
Relations with People/Institutions		
Some contact with welfare workers	64	85***
Knows nothing about neighbors	17	27
Friendly to welfare workers	15	30*
Frequently uses welfare organization	8	20*
Participation in Amusements		
Sometimes watches soccer	65	36***

Significance of differences determined by chi-square:
*probability of chance occurrence, less than .05
**probability of chance occurrence, less than .01
***probability of chance occurrence, less than .001

TABLE 133

MIGRATORY STATUS ACCORDING TO ADEQUACY OF HOUSING

	% of Patients with Electricity and Running Water in Dwelling	
	Have One or Neither (28% of total sample)	Have Both (70% of total sample)
Birthplace		
East (Sergipe, Bahia, Minas Gerais, Espirito Santo, Rio State outside Greater Rio)	48	28**
Northeast (Maranhao, Piaui, Ceara, Rio Grande do Norte, Paraiba, Pernambuco)	24	13*
Guanabara	16	46**
Rio State (in Greater Rio area)	13	4
Length of Residence		
5 years or less in present dwelling	55	41*
Less than 10 years in present area	47	39
Migrated in past 5 years	33	24
Conditions of Migration (Percentage of migrants only— 55% of total sample)		
Came from a rural setting	55	23**

Significance of differences determined by chi-square:
  *probability of chance occurrence, less than .05
  **probability of chance occurrence, less than .001

TABLE 134
HOSPITALIZATION AND FAMILY DIAGNOSIS ACCORDING TO ADEQUACY OF HOUSING

	% of Patients with Electricity and Running Water in Dwelling	
	Have One or Neither (25% of total sample)	Have Both (70% of total sample)
Hospital Contact		
Previous psychiatric contact	38	52
Seen in Pronto Socorro	37	11**
Admitted because of paranoid or grandiose behavior	23	13
Family Diagnosis		
A mental illness	56	31**
Religiously inspired behavior	12	5
Strange behavior	6	21*
Life stress	4	10
Bad behavior	3	8

Significance of differences determined by chi-square:
  *probability of chance occurrence, less than .01
 **probability of chance occurrence, less than .001

TABLE 135

COMPLAINTS ACCORDING TO PRIVACY OF SLEEPING QUARTERS

% According to Sleeping Privacy

	Alone or with Mate (51% of total sample)	With Children or Other Family (43% of total sample)*
Anxiety attacks	73	63
Worries interfere with work	70	59
Fatigue	65	47**
Any organ anxiety	43	33
Sweating or hot flashes	32	19*
Fear of head disease	20	7**

Significance of differences determined by chi-square:
  *probability of chance occurrence, less than .05
 **probability of chance occurrence, less than .01
 †6% other arrangements or undetermined.

TABLE 136

INTERVIEW BEHAVIOR ACCORDING TO ADEQUACY OF HOUSING

	% of Patients with Electricity and Running Water in Dwelling	
	Have One or Neither (28% of total sample)	Have Both (70% of total sample)
Psychiatrists Self-Rating During Interview		
Involved and empathic	46	59
Remote	35	24
Interview interesting and rewarding	28	69****
Apprehensive	25	8****
Hostile	18	5***
Cheerful	15	33**
Patient's Interview Behavior		
Stream of speech unremarkable	60	73
Cooperative approach	53	69*
Pays attention comfortably	48	69***
Preoccupied with one or two themes	38	54*
Dramatic, attention seeking	30	44
Wet palms on handshake	27	17
Expresses unsatisfied wish to be cared for	17	9
Weeps, seems sad	15	25
Actively advice-seeking	14	25

Significance of differences determined by chi-square:
*probability of chance occurrence, less than .05
**probability of chance occurrence, less than .02
***probability of chance occurrence, less than .01
****probability of chance occurrence, less than .001

TABLE 137

COMPLAINTS ACCORDING TO ADEQUACY OF HOUSING

	% of Patients with Electricity and Running Water in Dwelling	
	Have One or Neither (28% of total sample)	Have Both (70% of total sample)
Anxiety, Tension and Interference with Function		
Restless due to worries	57	46
Any problem in thought process	57	40*
Anxious speech content, facies and startle	52	42
Any worry about relatives	37	23*
Fear of loss of control	34	44
Diffuse anxiety	30	39
Somatic Complaints		
Fatigue	71	54*
Weakness	62	53
Any type of organ anxiety	54	37*
Diarrhea	23	14
Feels something change inside body	18	10

Significance of differences determined by chi-square:
*probability of chance occurrence, less than .05

TABLE 138

DEPRESSION ACCORDING TO AREA OF RESIDENCE AND PRESENCE OF ESSENTIAL SERVICES

	% of Patients Essential Services			
	Area I (65% of total sample)	Area II (21% of total sample)	Both (70% of total sample)	One or Neither (28% of total sample)
Depressive Mood Indicators				
Often feels sad	57	70	65	48***
Often feels like weeping	38	47	48	28***
Feels overwhelmed by criticism	22	45***	27	26
Generally self-accusatory	17	30*	22	19
Feels lonely	15	26*	20	17
Has specific suicidal fantasies	15	26*	18	15
Says body is weak or inferior	15	24	16	19
Has made a suicide attempt	12	24*	17	12
Expresses wish to die	13	24*	20	10
Feels guilty re failure in social role	11	26**	16	15
Feels generally inadequate	9	24**	13	14
Feels guilty re failure as parent	3	17***	7	12

Significance of differences determined by chi-square:
  *probability of chance occurrence, less than .05
 **probability of chance occurrence, less than .01
***probability of chance occurrence, less than .001

TABLE 139

IMPAIRED REALITY TESTING

ACCORDING TO ADEQUACY OF HOUSING

	% of Patients with Electricity and Running Water in Dwelling	
	Have One or Neither (28% of total sample)	Have Both (70% of total sample)
Statements Concerning Others		
Complains about treatment from others	62	49
Feels persecuted	60	32****
Grandiose—feels emulated	43	26**
Others stare at or talk about him	40	32
Others know his inner thoughts and feelings	34	20*
Others control his inner thoughts and feelings	27	20
Auditory Phenomena		
Hears voices in absence of others	50	24****
Voices direct him to take action	20	3****
Voices are religious or folkloric in nature	11	3**
Visual Phenomena		
Sees people in absence of others	36	11****
Sees objects other than people	27	9****
Sees religious or folkloric nonhuman figures	21	3****
Sees religious or folkloric human figures	14	3***
Reality of Experience		
Insists on reality of experience	33	14****
Plans specific action on basis of experience	27	10***
Misinterpretations and Illusions		
Misinterprets or attributes special meaning to all stimuli and communications	30	13***
Orientation		
Disoriented in time	31	8****
Disoriented in place	47	20****

Significance of differences determined by chi-square:
    *probability of chance occurrence, less than .05
    **probability of chance occurrence, less than .02
    ***probability of chance occurrence, less than .01
    ****probability of chance occurrence, less than .001

TABLE 140

IMPAIRED REALITY TESTING ACCORDING TO AREA OF RESIDENCE

	% of Patients	
	Area I (65% of total sample)	Area II (21% of total sample)
Statements Concerning Others		
Feels persecuted	33	51**
Grandiose, feels emulated	29	42
Others are not trustworthy	24	34
Others misjudge him	22	32
Others control his thoughts	19	32*
Others regard him as mentally or morally inferior	18	34**
Others regard him as physically inferior	8	21***-
Visual and Auditory Phenomena		
Says he hears voices (in absence of appropriate stimuli)	34	81****
Says he sees people (in absence of appropriate stimuli)	13	25*
Misinterpretations and Illusions		
Misjudges or attributes special meaning to stimuli and communications of all kinds	16	27
Temporal Disorientation	26	38

Significance of differences determined by chi-square:
   *probability of chance occurrence, less than .05
  **probability of chance occurrence, less than .02
 ***probability of chance occurrence, less than .01
****probability of chance occurrence, less than .001

TABLE 141
PAST MEDICAL HISTORY ACCORDING TO HOUSING ADEQUACY

	% of Patients with Electricity and Running Water in Dwelling	
	Have One or Neither (28% of total	Have Both (70% of total
Past History of Loss of Consciousness	sample)	sample)
Lapses or fainting spells	30	24
Head injury with consciousness loss	19	10
Seizures	18	12
High fevers with altered consciousness	17	12

TABLE 142
SOCIOECONOMIC INDICATORS ACCORDING TO SEX

	% of Patients	
	Female (35% of total sample)	Male (65% of total sample)
Education		
None or incomplete primary	51	59
Complete primary or more	48	39
Occupation		
Class V	47	40
Classes I, II and III	23	14
Class VI	21	34*
Class IV	3	10
Housing		
Both electricity and running water	77	68
Only one room, kitchen and bath or less	17	22
No essential services	9	16
Barraco or unclassified structure	9	13
Socioeconomic Mobility		
Feels has improved in past year	51	30**
Feels has declined in past year	16	38**
Feels is better than father	54	40
Feels is worse than father	13	24

Significance of differences determined by chi-square:
*probability of chance occurrence, less than .02
**probability of chance occurrence, less than .001

TABLE 143

SOME SOCIOCULTURAL FEATURES ACCORDING TO SEX

	% of Patients	
	Female (35% of total sample)	Male (65% of total sample)
Information and Participation		
Contact with clergy	78	50***
Belongs to Catholic church	72	68
Owns books	53	33**
Attends services of major religious affiliation monthly or more often	39	17***
Sometimes attends spiritist or Afro-Brazilian centers	32	23
Friendly with clergy	31	16**
Attends movies often	28	47**
Belongs to Protestant church	13	7
Attends soccer games sometimes	10	50***
Attends soccer games often	5	33***
Family and Background		
Married, both civil and religious ceremonies	44	36
Was disciplined mainly by beatings	29	41
Independent prior to age 14	7	14
Migratory Status		
Arrived after age 21	25	42**
Migrated alone	8	20*

Significance of differences determined by chi-square:
*probability of chance occurrence, less than .02
**probability of chance occurrence, less than .01
***probability of chance occurrence, less than .001

TABLE 144
HOSPITALIZATION AND INTERVIEW BEHAVIOR
ACCORDING TO SEX

	% of Patients	
	Female (35% of total sample)	Male (65% of total sample)
Hospitalization		
Had previous psychiatric contact	57	44*
Duration of illness one month or less	13	22
Admitted because of assaultive behavior	4	18***
Interview Behavior		
Silly, hostile, or fearful	58	43**
Speech content irrelevant or bizarre	57	45
Cooperative throughout	57	72**
Actively cooperative approach	48	69****
No obvious anxiety	44	57*
Respectful, courteous, friendly	43	57*
Weeps or appears sad	40	16****
Dramatic, attention-seeking	29	20
Expresses unsatisfied wishes to be cared for	18	9*
Voice faint or weak	18	9*
Hand tremor	16	26
Wet palms on handshake	12	24*
Doctor feels liked by patient	11	54****

Significance of differences determined by chi-square:
  *probability of chance occurrence, less than .05
  **probability of chance occurrence, less than .02
  ***probability of chance occurrence, less than .01
  ****probability of chance occurrence, less than .001

TABLE 145
ANXIOUS AND HOSTILE TENSION ACCORDING TO SEX

	% of Patients	
	Female (35% of total sample)	Male (65% of total sample)
Anxiety Symptoms		
Difficulty in concentrating	56	36***
Anxious speech, facies, startles	53	41
Restless due to worries	51	42
Difficulty in thinking clearly	51	41
Any type of organ anxiety	46	36
Constant diffuse anxiety	46	30***
Phobic fears	40	26**

TABLE 145 (continued)

	% of Patients	
	Female (35% of total sample)	Male (65% of total sample)
Often feels tense and isolated when with others	37	29
Worries about relatives	37	19***
Fear of dying	35	23*
Hostile Tension and Impulsivity		
Attacks of rage or anger	37	45
Past history of adult or adolescent rages	31	42
Impulsive acts	21	29

Significance of differences determined by chi-square:
  *probability of chance occurrence, less than .05
  **probability of chance occurrence, less than .02
  ***probability of chance occurrence, less than .01

TABLE 146
DEPRESSION ACCORDING TO SEX

	% of Patients	
	Female (35% of total sample)	Male (65% of total sample)
Depressive Indicators		
Often feels sad	76	53****
Often feels like weeping	59	32****
Weeps or appears sad	40	16****
Expresses fear of being abandoned	37	12****
Feelings are intense and unpleasant	36	24*
Has made suicidal attempts	29	10****
Says body is weak or inferior	26	14**
Has expressed wish to die	26	13***
Has made suicidal threats	25	14*
Has expressed specific suicidal fantasies	25	14*
Feels lonely	24	16
Feelings are absent or dulled	19	8***
Expresses guilt about failure as a parent	13	4**

Significance of differences determined by chi-square:
  *probability of chance occurrence, less than .05
  **probability of chance occurrence, less than .02
  ***probability of chance occurrence, less than .01
  ****probability of chance occurrence, less than .011

TABLE 147

IMPAIRED REALITY TESTING ACCORDING TO SEX

| | % of Patients | |
	Female (35% of total sample)	Male (65% of total sample)
Paranoid Behavior		
Grandiose, feels emulated by others	40	29
Others are not trustworthy	34	24
Disorientation		
Temporal	38	24*
Spatial	26	11**

Significance of differences determined by chi-square:
*probability of chance occurrence, less than .02
**probability of chance occurrence, less than .01

TABLE 148

SOMATIC AND SEXUAL COMPLAINTS ACCORDING TO SEX

| | % of Patients | |
	Female (35% of total sample)	Male (65% of total sample)
Somatic Complaints		
Fatigue	71	53***
Anorexia	71	50***
Weakness	60	78***
Dizziness or faintness	59	43
Dyspnea	40	23***
Headaches	28	59****
Physical movements slowed	26	10***
Something strange inside body	18	9*
Sweating or hot flashes	16	32***
Sexual Complaints		
Suffers from impotence or frigidity	40	25***
Sex impulse absent or weak	24	9***
Masturbates only—no relationship with sexual partners	13	4**
Sex impulses too intense or uncontrollable	9	19*
Sex a source of anxiety, guilt, or shame	5	16***
Usual sex relationship casual or transitory	0	26****

Significance of differences determined by chi-square:
*probability of chance occurrence, less than .05
**probability of chance occurrence, less than .02
***probability of chance occurrence, less than .01
****probability of chance occurrence, less than .001

TABLE 149
SOCIOECONOMIC INDICATORS ACCORDING TO
MARITAL STATUS†

	% of Patients	
	Married (39% of total sample)	Single (32% of total sample)
Education and Literacy		
Literate	82	62***
Illiterate	6	15***
Incomplete primary school or less	56	46
Complete primary or beyond	43	53
Occupation		
Class V	49	28**
Class VI	23	34*
Classes I, II, III	22	23
Class IV	4	11
Housing		
Electricity and running water	88	67***
One room, kitchen and bath or less	14	22
Barraco or unclassified	6	11
No electricity or running water	5	17**
Living Area		
Suburban or industrial	54	37*
All urban except slum	39	51
Small town	12	23
Rio State (in Greater Rio)	12	24*
Socioeconomic Mobility		
SES worse during past year	37	21**
SES better than that of father	59	31***
SES worse than that of father	15	27***

---

† Percentages for married and single on Tables 149 through 159 do not include 20% who reported civil ceremonies alone; 7% who reported consensual or common-law unions; and 20% who had undetermined marital status.

Significance of differences determined by chi-square:

*probability of chance occurrence, less than .05

**probability of chance occurrence, less than .02

***probability of chance occurrence, less than .01

TABLE 150
SOME DEMOGRAPHIC FACTORS ACCORDING TO
MARITAL STATUS

| | % of Patients | |
	Married (39% of total sample)	Single (32% of total sample)
Age		
15–25	6	54***
26–40	57	37**
41–60	38	10**
Sex		
Male	61	71
Female	39	29
Color		
White	75	59*
Brown	17	30*
Black	7	11
Religion		
Catholic	78	67
All others	10	6
Unaffiliated or undetermined	12	27*
Total affiliated	88	73*
Migratory Status		
Born in Greater Rio (nonmigrant)	48	59
Arrived within 5 years	13	24
Arrived after age 21	31	16*

Significance of differences determined by chi-square:
*probability of chance occurrence, less than .05
**probability of chance occurrence, less than .02
***probability of chance occurrence, less than .01

TABLE 151

INFORMATION AND PARTICIPATION ACCORDING
TO MARITAL STATUS

	% of Patients	
	Married (39% of total sample)	Single (32% of total sample)
Media of Information and Communication		
Owns radio	95	84**
Owns TV	51	34**
Reads newspapers, magazines, and books	45	58
Reads magazines	42	58*
Owns books	34	54***
Uses all media	32	45
Attends movies monthly or more	16	40***
Institutional and Social Contact		
Some contact with welfare workers	93	68****
Never attends movies	53	32***
Friendly with welfare workers	37	19***
Knows nothing about neighbors	32	19
Sometimes attends dances	16	37***
Attends dances six times or more yearly	6	20***

Significance of differences determined by chi-square:
*probability of chance occurrence, less than .05
**probability of chance occurrence, less than .02
***probability of chance occurrence, less than .01
****probability of chance occurrence, less than .001

TABLE 152

CHILDHOOD INFLUENCES ACCORDING TO MARITAL STATUS

	% of Patients	
Childhood Influences	Married (39% of total sample)	Single (32% of total sample)
Siblings by both parents	79	67
Reared by both parents	77	62*
Disciplined mainly by both parents	59	47
Broken home	35	45
Father literate	27	40
Mother literate	29	46**

Significance of differences determined by chi-square:
*probability of chance occurrence, less than .05
**probability of chance occurrence, less than .02

TABLE 153
HOSPITALIZATION AND MENTAL ILLNESS ACCORDING TO MARITAL STATUS

Hospitalization	% of Patients (39% of total sample)	(32% of total sample)
Had previous contact with a psychiatrist	57	44
Duration of illness, 6 months or less	47	31*
Hospitalized because of depressed or suicidal behavior	24	7***
Hospitalized because of assaultive behavior	14	24
Seen at Pronto Socorro	3	29****
Family Diagnosis		
A mental illness	19	44***
Strange behavior	27	11***
Life stress	21	8**

Significance of differences determined by chi-square:
*probability of chance occurrence, less than .05
**probability of chance occurrence, less than .02
***probability of chance occurrence, less than .01
****probability of chance occurrence, less than .001

TABLE 154
INTERVIEW BEHAVIOR ACCORDING TO MARITAL STATUS

Psychiatrists' Self-Ratings	% of Patients Married (39% of total sample)	Single (32% of total sample)
Cheerful and optimistic	33	24
Pity for patient	15	24
Hostile to patient	4	16**
Patients Interview Behavior		
Pays attention comfortably	77	35***
Stream of speech unremarkable	77	53**
Cooperative throughout	73	59*
Respectful, courteous, friendly	62	35**
Has appropriate emotional expression	41	13**
Silly, hostile, fearful or apathetic	38	65**
Tremor of hand	26	14
Expresses unsatisfied wish to be cared for	8	19*
Hypervigilant or distractible	5	26**

Significance of differences determined by chi-square:
*probability of chance occurrence, less than .05
**probability of chance occurrence, less than .01
***probability of chance occurrence, less than .001

TABLE 155
TENSIONS, ANXIETY, SENSITIVITY AND FRUSTRATION

	% of Patients	
	Married	Single
	(39% of total	(32% of total
Anxiety Symptoms	sample)	sample)
Insomnia	79	69
Any type of organic anxiety	46	35
Constant diffuse anxiety	41	31
Worries about relatives	30	11**
Tension and Sensitivity		
Engages in impulsive acts	19*	32
Feels others regard him as morally/ mentally inferior	14**	30
Achievement-aspiration discrepancy	9***	34
Others regard him as physically inferior	6*	17
Interference with Function		
Any difficulty in thinking efficiently	35**	57
Any difficulty in making decisions	30**	49

Significance of differences determined by chi-square:
*probability of chance occurrence, less than .05
**probability of chance occurrence, less than .01
***probability of chance occurrence, less than .001

TABLE 156
DEPRESSION ACCORDING TO MARITAL STATUS

	% of Patients	
	Married	Single
	(39% of total	(32% of total
Depressive Mood Indicators	sample)	sample)
Often feels like weeping	51	28**
Weeps, or face and gestures sad	28	15
Has made a suicidal attempt	18	8
Impassive, detached or flat	11***	42
Feels overwhelmed by criticism	21	31
Guilty *re* failure in social role	6**	24
Expresses wish to be dead	11	22
Feels lonely	10*	22
Feelings are absent or dull	8*	18
Feels generally inadequate	8*	18
Guilty *re* failure as a son or daughter	0***	18
Is unrealistically optimistic	1**	11

Significance of differences determined by chi-square:
*probability of chance occurrence, less than .05
**probability of chance occurrence, less than .01
***probability of chance occurrence, less than .001

TABLE 157

REALITY CONTACT ACCORDING TO MARITAL STATUS

| | % of Patients | |
	Single (32% of total sample)	Married (39% of total sample)
Statements about Others		
Complains about treatment from others	63	43***
Feels persecuted	45	25***
Others stare at or talk about him	44	27**
Grandiose, feels emulated	42	16***
Others know his inner thoughts	39	14***
Others control his inner thoughts	35	14***
Others misjudge him	35	14***
Others are not trustworthy	34	18**
Auditory Phenomena		
Hears voices in absence of others	41	20***
Voices direct him to take action	15	1***
Visual Phenomena		
Sees objects other than people in absence of stimuli	17	6*
Sees religious or folkloric nonhuman figures	13	1***
Reality of Experiences		
Insists on reality of experience	27	9***
Plans specific action on basis of experience	24	6***
Orientation		
Disoriented in time	31	21
Disoriented in place	20	6***
Misinterpretations or Illusions		
Misinterprets or sees special meaning in visual or auditory stimuli or communications	28	9***

Significance of differences determined by chi-square:
*probability of chance occurrence, less than .05
**probability of chance occurrence, less than .02
***probability of chance occurrence, less than .01

TABLE 158
SOMATIC AND SEXUAL COMPLAINTS ACCORDING TO MARITAL STATUS

| | % of Patients | |
	Married	Single
Somatic Complaints		
Anorexia	59	46
Faintness or dizziness	49	37
Palpitations	35	18**
Nausea or vomiting	35	4****
Dyspnea	32	20
Sweating or hot flashes	30	14**
Sexual Problems		
Suffers from impotence or frigidity	42	17***
Worries interfere with sexual functioning	48	32*
Present sexual pattern is part of present illness	43	19***
Sex a source of anxiety, guilt or shame	3****	27
Sex impulse too intense or uncontrollable	14	25
Sex impulses absent or weak	13	22
Masturbation only sexual activity	0****	21

Significance of differences determined by chi-square:
*probability of chance occurrence, less than .05
**probability of chance occurrence, less than .02
***probability of chance occurrence, less than .01
****probability of chance occurrence, less than .001

TABLE 159
PAST HISTORY ACCORDING TO MARITAL STATUS

| | % of Patients | |
	Single (32% of total sample)	Married (39% of total sample)
Past Psychiatric History		
School adjustment problems	45	24**
Work adjustment problems	32	9**
Problems in learning to relate	24	10*
Childhood temper tantrums	17	8

Significance of differences determined by chi-square:
*probability of chance occurrence, less than .02
**probability of chance occurrence, less than .01

TABLE 160
AGE DISTRIBUTION OF RESIDENTS OF GUANABARA
AND OF FAVELAS IN GUANABARA (1960)

	% of Total Residents of	
Age	All Guanabara	Guanabara Fevelas
0–14	31	43
15–24	18	17
25–39	26	24
40–59	18	13
60–80+	6.5	3

Percentages computed from *Censo Demografico. Estado do Guanabara* (1968)

TABLE 161
Percentage of Total Residents of Guanabara (1960) by
Age Group for Each Sex and Color Category

Age	White Males	White Females	Black Males	Black Females	Brown Males	Brown Females
0–14	30	30	39	32	37	37
15–24	16	16	18	20	20	15
25–39	28	26	25	25	25	28
40–59	20	19	15	18	15	15
60–80+	6	8	3	5	3	5

Percentages computed from *Censo Demografico (1968)*

TABLE 162
SOCIOECONOMIC INDICATORS ACCORDING TO AGE

	% of Patients		
	Age 15–25 (22% of total sample)	26–40 (63% of total sample)	41–60 (15% of total sample)
Education			
Completed primary school or beyond	50	41	40
Housing			
Both electricity and running water	64	74	81**
Neither electricity nor running water	21	12	7**
Bedroom shared by others than mate	59	49	28*
Occupation			
Class V	35	45	50
Class VI	34	28	24

TABLE 162 (continued)

	% of Patients		
	Age 15–25 (22% of total sample)	26–40 (63% of total sample)	41–60 (15% of total sample)
Socioeconomic Status			
SES better than father	36	51	56**
SES worse in past year	26	39	33

Significance of differences determined by chi-square:
*probability of chance occurrence, less than .01
**probability of chance occurrence, less than .05

TABLE 163

DEMOGRAPHIC AND MIGRATORY CHARACTERISTICS
ACCORDING TO AGE

	% of Patients		
	Age 15–25 (22% of total sample)	26–40 (63% of total sample)	41–60 (15% of total sample)
Religion			
Catholic	76	64	70
Marital State			
Single	64	17	11***
Married: civil and religious	21	47	52**
Number of Children			
Four or more	4	32	42***
Migratory Status			
Born in East (Sergipe, Bahia, Minas, Espirito Santo, Rio State)	35	34	25
Born in Northeast (Maranhao, Piauni, Ceara, Rio Grande do Norte, Paraiba, Pernambuco)	13	13	24
Considers self a non-migrant	52	47	41
Migrated in past 5 years	32	22	30
Arrived after age 21	13	28	41*
Lived in present house 5 years or less	51	43	38

Significance of differences determined by chi-square:
*probability of chance occurrence, less than .02
**probability of chance occurrence, less than .01
***probability of chance occurrence, less than .001

TABLE 164
CHILDHOOD INFLUENCES ACCORDING TO AGE

Family Stability	% of Patients		
	Age 15–25 (22% of total sample)	26–40 (63% of total sample)	41–60 (15% of total sample)
Has siblings by both parents	67	74	77
Disciplined mainly by scoldings	51	30	38*
Disciplined mainly by beatings	32	37	42
Father no longer living	29	56	70**
Independent prior to age 14	8	11	18
Parental Literacy			
Father literate	37	30	21
Mother literate	45	36	24

Significance of differences determined by chi-square:
*probability of chance occurrence, less than .05
**probability of chance occurrence, less than .001

TABLE 165
INFORMATION AND SOCIAL PARTICIPATION ACCORDING TO AGE

Relations with Neighbors	% of Patients		
	Age 15–25 (22% of total sample)	26–40 (63% of total sample)	41–60 (15% of total sample)
Friendly with close neighbors	79	62	76*
Knows nothing about neighbors	19	34	15**
Relations with Institutions and Activities			
Some contact with welfare workers	71	85	80
Some contact with clergy	62	49	69*
Friendly with clergy	21	17	27
Frequently uses welfare services	9	21	22
Sometimes goes to dances	36	27	17*
Watches soccer six times yearly or more	19	26	28
Informational Media			
Owns radio	86	91	98
Reads magazines	57	34	41***
Reads newspapers, magazines and books	57	38	43*
Reads newspapers	51	36	43

TABLE 165 (continued)

	% of Patients		
	Age 15–25 (22% of total sample)	26–40 (63% of total sample)	41–60 (15% of total sample)
Watches TV	49	38	45
Owns books	45	35	41
Attends movies	45	29	29
Uses all media	43	25	32*
Attends movies at least monthly	34	18	21*
Never attends movies	34	54	45*

Significance of differences determined by chi-square:
*probability of chance occurrence, less than .05
**probability of chance occurrence, less than .02
***probability of chance occurrence, less than .01

TABLE 166

HOSPITALIZATION AND FAMILY ATTITUDE ACCORDING TO AGE

	% of Patients		
	Age 15–25 (22% of total sample)	26–40 (63% of total sample)	41–60 (15% of total sample)
Acuteness of Illness			
Previous contact with psychiatrists	40	56	43
Reason for Admission			
Paranoid or grandiose	24	10	11*
Other bizarre acts	18	17	5
Refuses to work	11	4	2
Anxious, depressed, or suicidal	8	21	10*
Family Diagnosis			
A mental illness	40	26	22*
Life stress	11	14	22
Hospitalization			
Seen in Pronto Socarro	26	13	17
Seen in Casa Eiras	68	84	76*

Significance of differences determined by chi-square:
*probability of chance occurrence, less than .05

TABLE 167
INTERVIEW BEHAVIOR AND PSYCHIATRIST'S RESPONSES ACCORDING TO AGE OF PATIENT

	% of Patients		
	Age 15–25 (22% of total sample)	26–40 (63% of total sample)	41–60 (15% of total sample)
Psychiatrist's Self-ratings			
Likes patient	69	56	70
Interview interesting and rewarding	63	53	65.
Feels pity	23	10	20*
Feels remote	23	34	20
Interview Behavior			
Silly, hostile, fearful, apathetic	52	33	43***
Dramatic, attention seeking	48	25	40***
Actively advice seeking	21	14	29*
Actively cooperative approach	53	73	61**
Respectful, courteous, friendly	34	64	58****
Appropriate emotional expression	24	35	32
Unremarkable stream of speech	56	74	74
Pays attention comfortably	50	62	72*
Hand tremor	13	26	29
Speaks slowly with silences	30	18	16

Significance of differences determined by chi-square:
*probability of chance occurrence, less than .05
**probability of chance occurrence, less than .02
***probability of chance occurrence, less than .01
****probability of chance occurrence, less than .001

TABLE 168
TENSIONS, ANXIETY, ANGER, AND SENSITIVITY
ACCORDING TO AGE

	% of Patients		
	Age 15–25	26–40	41–60
	(22% of total sample)	(63% of total sample)	(15% of total sample)
Anxiety Symptoms			
Fear of loss of control	47	42	31
Constant diffuse anxiety	37	42	22*
Worries about job	23	27	32
Insomnia	65	75	85*
Any organ anxiety	31	44	47
Fear of stomach disease	9	17	20
Fear of head disease	1	3	13*
Interference with Function			
Worries interfere with work	61	66	70
Any change in thought processes	57	41	35*
Frustration, Anger, Impulsivity			
Feels and expresses anger	55	52	32*
Feels tense and isolated with others	55	23	25**
Has attacks of rage or anger	45	44	32
Has frequent arguments	37	31	29
Acts impulsively	33	26	16*
Feels others regard him as inferior	33	14	14**
Has marked achievement-aspiration discrepancy	28	10	18
Denies or does not mention angry feelings	43	48	56

Significance of differences determined by chi-square:
*probability of chance occurrence, less than .05
**probability of chance occurrence, less than .01

TABLE 169
DEPRESSION ACCORDING TO AGE

	% of Patients		
Depressive Mood Indicators	Age 15–25	26–40	41–60
High intensity of affective feelings a problem	21	27	40*
Body is weak or inferior	18	10	27**
Weeps, or faces and gestures sad	17	22	34*
Rigid, flat, apathetic	30	18	13*
Feels guilty re failure in social role	23	10	13
Feels generally inadequate	19	9	9
Feels guilty re failure as a child	18	3	4***
Feelings absent or dulled	16	6	11

Significance of differences determined by chi-square:
*probability of chance occurrence, less than .05
**probability of chance occurrence, less than .02
***probability of chance occurrence, less than .001

TABLE 170

IMPAIRMENT IN REALITY TESTING ACCORDING TO AGE

	% of Patients		
	Age 15–25 (22% of total sample)	26–40 (63% of total sample)	41–60 (15% of total sample)
Statements Concerning Others			
Complains about treatment from others	60	58	39*
Feels persecuted	42	45	24*
Others stare at or talk about him	42	30	27
Others are not trustworthy	33	18	24
Others regard him as mentally-morally inferior	33	14	14**
Others know his inner thoughts and feelings	32	27	21
Others regard him as physically inferior	18	5	9**

Significance of differences determined by chi-square:
　*probability of chance occurrence, less than .05
　**probability of chance occurrence, less than .01

TABLE 171

SOMATIC AND SEXUAL PROBLEMS ACCORDING TO AGE

	% of Patients		
	Age 15–25 (22% of total sample)	26–40 (63% of total sample)	41–60 (15% of total sample)
Somatic Complaints			
Any physical discomfort	62	79	80*
Fatigue	47	57	72*
Weakness	42	53	67*
Anorexia	45	60	63
Sweating or hot flashes	16	31	36
Nausea or vomiting	11	27	32*
Something strange inside body	19	7	9*
Sexual Problems			
Present sexual patterns part of present illness	28	25	41
Suffers from impotence or frigidity	20	33	39*
Sexual impulse absent or weak	11	9	23
Most sexual contacts casual or transitory	32	9	7***
Sex a source of anxiety, guilt or shame	19	8	11
Masturbation only form of sexual activity	14	5	0**

Significance of differences determined by chi-square:
　*probability of chance occurrence, less than .05
　**probability of chance occurrence, less than .01
　***probability of chance occurrence, less than .001

TABLE 172

PAST PSYCHIATRIC HISTORY ACCORDING TO AGE

	% of Patients		
	Age 15–25 (22% of total sample)	26–40 (63% of total sample)	41–60 (15% of total sample)
Reports of Developmental Problems			
School adjustment problems	50	27	16**
Adolescent rages	47	35	27*
Problems in bladder control	38	29	20*
Work adjustment problems	33	9	9**
Childhood traumatic experiences	24	27	13
Traumatic experiences in adulthood	46	43	56
High fevers with altered consciousness	11	20	7
Deliria	8	18	5*

Significance of differences determined by chi-square:
*probability of chance occurrence, less than .05
**probability of chance occurrence, less than .001

TABLE 173

RELIGIOUS OBSERVANCE ACCORDING TO AFFILIATION

	% of Patients			
	Unaffiliated (13% of total sample)	Catholic (57% of total sample)	Protestant (8% of total sample)	Afro-Spiritist (22% of total sample)
Attends services once or more monthly	0	23	75	44*
Occasionally attends other Afro-Spiritist services	3	18	15	68*
Though unaffiliated has personal convictions	14	—	—	—
Member of a Spiritist center	0	0	0	19*
Member of Umbanda or Macumba center	0	0	0	56*
Member of some other Afro-Spiritist center	0	0	0	25*

Significance of differences determined by chi-square:
*probability of chance occurrence, less than .001

TABLE 174

AGE, SEX, COLOR, AND MARITAL STATUS ACCORDING TO RELIGIOUS AFFILIATION AND ATTENDANCE

	% of Patients			
	Unaffiliated (13% of total sample)	Catholic (57% of total sample)	Protestant (8% of total sample)	Afro-Spiritist† (22% of total sample)
Age				
15–25	17	25	25	15
26–40	57	49	40	65
41–60	26	26	35	20
Sex				
Male	85	65	50	61**
Female	15	35	50	39**
Color				
White	57	67	53	64
Brown	29	23	35	19
Black	14	10	10	21
Marital Status				
Unmarried-no mate	54	32	15	24**
Civil-religious ceremony	26	44	35	32*

Significance of differences determined by chi-square:
*probability of chance occurrence, less than .05
**probability of chance occurrence, less than .01

†In tables 174 through 180, this category refers to the sum of those patients who (1) list any form of spiritism or any African-derived religion or cult such as Macumba or Umbanda as their primary affiliation, and (2) acknowledge occasional attendance at such services or ceremonies in spite of nominal unaffiliation or membership in some other group.

TABLE 175

MIGRATORY STATUS AND SOCIOECONOMIC MOBILITY ACCORDING TO RELIGIOUS AFFILIATION AND ATTENDANCE

	% of Patients			
	Unaffiliated (13% of total sample)	Catholic (57% of total sample)	Protestant (8% of total sample)	Afro-Spiritist (22% of total sample)
In present region 5 years or less	34	26	40	15*
In area less than 10 years	43	43	65	31*
Relatives nearby	11	28	15	35*
Arrived after age 21	28	25	40	15*
Came from rural setting	23	30	55	22*
SES better than father's	34	52	30	49*
SES worse than father's	29	23	15	28
SES improved in past year	26	40	50	31*
SES worse in past year	46	31	15	31*

Significance of differences determined by chi-square:
*probability of chance occurrence, less than .05

TABLE 176

BIRTHPLACE ACCORDING TO RELIGIOUS AFFILIATION OR ATTENDANCE

	% of Patients			
Birthplace	*Unaffiliated* (13% of total sample)	*Catholic* (57% of total sample)	*Protestant* (8% of total sample)	*Afro-Spiritist* (22% of total sample)
Northeast	11	17	15	15
Present area, Greater Rio	17	4	10	3*
East	20	32	70	26**
Guanabara	31	41	5	52**
Other	21	6	0	4**

Significance of differences determined by chi-square:
*probability of chance occurrence, less than .01
**probability of chance occurrence, less than .001

TABLE 177

HOUSING QUALITY ACCORDING TO RELIGIOUS AFFILIATION OR ATTENDANCE

	% of Patients			
	Unaffiliated (13% of total sample)	*Catholic* (57% of total sample)	*Protestant* (8% of total sample)	*Afro-Spiritist* (22% of total sample)
Barraco, under construction, or unclassified	9	11	20	9
No essential services	25	9	25	16
Both electricity and running water	66	78	55	77
1 room plus kitchen and bath or less	20	20	25	16
Bedroom shared by other than mate	48	45	65	46

TABLE 178

LITERACY, EDUCATION, AND OCCUPATION ACCORDING TO RELIGIOUS AFFILIATION AND ATTENDANCE

	% of Patients			
	Unaffiliated (13% of total sample)	Catholic (57% of total sample)	Protestant (8% of total sample)	Afro-Spiritist (22% of total sample)
Illiterate	14	14	20	14
Partly literate	6	16	20	12
Literate	77	68	60	75
No school or incomplete primary	54	58	60	47
Complete primary or more	46	42	20	41*
Education undetermined	0	0	20	12***
Occupational class I–IV	26	29	5	22**
Occupational class V	26	46	45	55**
Occupational class VI	46	26	40	22*

Significance of differences determined by chi-square:

*probability of chance occurrence, less than .05

**probability of chance occurrence, less than .01

***probability of chance occurrence, less than .001

TABLE 179

OWNERSHIP OR USE OF INFORMATIONAL MEDIA ACCORDING TO RELIGIOUS
AFFILIATION AND ATTENDANCE

	% of Patients			
	Unaffiliated (13% of total sample)	Catholic (57% of total sample)	Protestant (8% of total sample)	Afro-Spiritist (22% of total sample)
Reads newspapers, magazines, and books	60	45	70	38**
Watches TV	46	46	30	38
Attends movies	40	36	30	31
Attends movies once monthly or more	40	23	15	15*
Radio only source of information	31	40	40	37
Never attends movies	31	45	60	55**
Owns TV	29	44	30	45*

Significance of differences determined by chi-square:
   *probability of chance occurrence, less than .05
   **probability of chance occurrence, less than .01

TABLE 180

INSTITUTIONAL AND AMUSEMENT ACTIVITY ACCORDING TO RELIGIOUS AFFILIATION AND ATTENDANCE

	% of Patients			
	Unaffiliated (13% of total sample)	Catholic (57% of total sample)	Protestant (8% of total sample)	Afro-Spiritist (22% of total sample)
Some contact with welfare workers	71	83	60	77*
Friendly with workers	23	30	15	21
Some contact with clergy	26	62	90	60**
Friendly with clergy	3	20	65	19**
Sometimes watches soccer	40	37	25	51*
Watches soccer six times yearly or more	77	74	20	61**
Sometimes dances	19	25	25	33
Dances six times yearly or more	19	11	15	17

Significance of differences determined by chi-square:
  *probability of chance occurrence, less than .05
  **probability of chance occurrence, less than .001

TABLE 181

REASON FOR BEING REGARDED ILL (AND SENT TO HOSPITAL) AND DURATION OF ILLNESS, ACCORDING TO RELIGIOUS AFFILIATION

Reason for Being Regarded Ill		% of Patients		
	Unaffiliated (13% of total sample)	Catholic (57% of total sample)	Protestant (8% of total sample)	Afro-Spiritist† (5% of total sample)
Suicidal, depressed or anxious statements	21	20	25	28
Paranoid-persecutory statements	9	15	31	21*
Threatening or assaultive behavior	16	17	13	7
Other bizarre acts	28	15	0	28**
Duration of illness 6 months or less	28	49	56	14*

†From this point on, this category includes only those who are affiliated with a group.
Significance of differences determined by chi-square:
   *probability of chance occurrence, less than .01
   **probability of chance occurrence, less than .001

TABLE 182
FAMILY DIAGNOSIS ACCORDING TO
RELIGIOUS AFFILIATION AND ATTENDANCE

	% of Patients			
	Unaffiliated (13% of total sample)	*Catholic* (57% of total sample)	*Protestant* (8% of total sample)	*Afro-Spiritist* (5% of total sample)
Family Diagnosis				
An illness	50	65	75	65
A mental illness	40	35	45	45
Behavior is strange or bad	31	24	10	9*
Behavior is religiously inspired	9	5	10	16

Significance of differences determined by chi-square:
*probability of chance occurrence, less than .01

TABLE 183
PARENTAL LITERACY ACCORDING TO RELIGIOUS AFFILIATION

	% of Patients			
	Unaffiliated (13% of total sample)	*Catholic* (57% of total sample)	*Protestant* (8% of total sample)	*Afro-Spiritist* (5% of total sample)
Father				
Illiterate	11	26	40	18*
Partly literate	31	21	30	28
Literate	26	31	20	34
Undetermined	32	22	10	20*
Mother				
Illiterate	23	46	70	44**
Partly literate	20	13	5	16*
Literate	40	34	15	34**
Undetermined	17	7	5	6*

Significance of differences determined by chi-square:
*probability of chance occurrence, less than .05
**probability of chance occurrence, less than .01

TABLE 184

CHILDHOOD INFLUENCES AND FAMILY SIZE ACCORDING TO RELIGIOUS AFFILIATION

	% of Patients			
	Unaffiliated (13% of total sample)	Catholic (57% of total sample)	Protestant (8% of total sample)	Afro-Spiritist (5% of total sample)
Had siblings by both parents	75	73	70	77
Came from a broken home	49	41	30	64*
Reared by both parents	63	71	85	77*
Disciplined by beatings	37	37	40	51
Father died before patient was 12	26	21	15	20
Four or more siblings	74	72	65	67
Three or less siblings	23	28	30	31
Has no children	60	35	20	28**
Four or more children	14	23	40	21*
Three or less children	26	41	30	53*

Significance of differences determined by chi-square:
  *probability of chance occurrence, less than .05
  **probability of chance occurrence, less than .01

TABLE 185

ITEMS OF PAST PSYCHIATRIC HISTORY ACCORDING TO RELIGIOUS AFFILIATION

% of Patients

	Unaffiliated (13% of total sample)	Catholic (57% of total sample)	Protestant (8% of total sample)	Afro-Spiritist (5% of total sample)
Problems in learning to relate to others	19	16	25	7*
History of psychological trauma in childhood	28	28	19	7*
History of psychological trauma in adulthood	59	48	50	7**
Adult or adolescent rages	62	37	38	21**
School adjustment problems	31	37	38	21*
Head injury with loss of consciousness	22	12	6	7*
Lapses or fainting episodes	28	29	6	14*

Significance of differences determined by chi-square:
  *probability of chance occurrence, less than .05
  **probability of chance occurrence, less than .001

TABLE 186
INTERVIEW BEHAVIOR ACCORDING TO RELIGIOUS AFFILIATION

	% of Patients			
	Unaffiliated	Catholic	Protestant	Afro-Spiritist
Psychiatrist's Self-Ratings				
Feels liked by patient	59	54	56	28*
Feels involved and empathic	56	53	60	33*
Regards interview as interesting or rewarding	53	62	56	44
Feels pity for patient	19	20	5	0**
Patients Observed Interview Behavior				
Alert and wakeful	81	74	81	50*
Silly, hostile, fearful or apathetic	62	47	44	36*
Pays attention comfortably	44	67	69	64*
Respectful, courteous, friendly	41	60	63	64*
Dramatic or attention seeking	41	38	50	36
Speech and ANS signs of anxiety	41	45	50	28
States wish not to be helped	19	9	25	28
Actively advice seeking	12	23	31	14

Significance of differences determined by chi-square:
*probability of chance occurrence, less than .05
**probability of chance occurrence, less than .01

TABLE 187

TENSIONAL AND ANXIETY SYMPTOMS ACCORDING TO RELIGIOUS AFFILIATION

	% of Patients			
	Unaffiliated (13% of total sample)	Catholic (57% of total sample)	Protestant (8% of total sample)	Afro-Spiritist (5% of total sample)
Any situational anxiety	59	60	81	69*
Worries about job	31	28	38	14*
Worries about relatives	19	22	50	23*
Fear of loss of control	31	26	50	43*
Phobic fears	41	30	25	14*
Work interfered with by worries	69	68	69	50

Significance of differences determined by chi-square:
*probability of chance occurrence, less than .05

TABLE 188

ANGER, IMPULSIVITY, AND FRUSTRATION ACCORDING TO RELIGIOUS AFFILIATION

| | Unaffiliated (13% of total sample) | % of Patients | | |
		Catholic (57% of total sample)	Protestant (8% of total sample)	Afro-Spiritist (5% of total sample)
Denies or doesn't mention anger	34	53	38	64**
Feels and expresses anger	56	48	69	39*
Acts impulsively	44	12	19	21**
Has attacks of rage or anger	59	39	56	28*
Frequent arguments	41	30	44	36
Complains of achievement/aspiration discrepancy	25	16	25	28

Significance of differences determined by chi-square:
*probability of chance occurrence, less than .05
**probability of chance occurrence, less than .01

TABLE 189

DEPRESSIVE MOOD INDICATORS ACCORDING TO RELIGIOUS AFFILIATION

	Unaffiliated (13% of total sample)	Catholic (57% of total sample)	Protestant (8% of total sample)	Afro-Spiritist (5% of total sample)
		% of Patients		
Often feels sad	59	61	75	43*
Flat, apathetic	31	20	13	36*
High intensity feelings a problem	28	28	50	28**
Generally self-accusatory	28	18	38	0***
Speech slow with silences	25	19	13	14
Suicidal threats	25	20	19	7*
Suicidal attempts	22	15	19	28
Feeling of impending doom	16	16	31	21*
Guilty re failure as child	16	8	0	0**
Guilty re failure in social role	16	14	25	7*
Guilty re failure as parent	3	7	13	0*

Significance of differences determined by chi-square.
  *probability of chance occurrence, less than .05
 **probability of chance occurrence, less than .01
***probability of chance occurrence, less than .001

TABLE 190
INDICATIONS OF A BREAK WITH REALITY ACCORDING TO RELIGIOUS AFFILIATION

	% of Patients			
	Unaffiliated (13% of total sample)	Catholic (57% of total sample)	Protestant (8% of total sample)	Afro-Spiritist (5% of total sample)
Complains of treatment from others	59	48	50	50
Others know inner thoughts	31	20	31	29
Others control inner thoughts	31	19	25	22
Others stare at or talk about him	44	33	31	28*
Hears voices	34	33	31	15*
Voices direct him to take action	19	4	19	0***
Sees people	25	16	19	8**
Sees objects other than people	22	15	0	8***
Sees religious nonhuman figures	16	6	6	0***
Sees lights, colors or unformed entities	19	19	19	28
Plans action on basis of experience	22	13	31	0***
Insists on reality of experiences	25	17	38	14**
Misinterprets auditory stimuli	9	7	13	7
Misinterprets all stimuli	19	20	19	8

Significance of differences determined by chi-square:
  *probability of chance occurrence, less than .05
  **probability of chance occurrence, less than .01
  ***probability of chance occurrence, less than .001

TABLE 191

MEMORY, THINKING, AND ORIENTATION ACCORDING TO RELIGIOUS AFFILIATION

	% of Patients			
	Unaffiliated (13% of total sample)	Catholic (57% of total sample)	Protestant (8% of total sample)	Afro-Spiritist (5% of total sample)
Any memory problem	44	41	31	22*
Any decision making problem	25	39	31	15*
Temporal disorientation	28	25	44	22*
Spatial disorientation	19	12	25	28

Significance of differences determined by chi-square:
*probability of chance occurrence, less than .05

TABLE 192

SOMATIC COMPLAINTS ACCORDING TO RELIGIOUS AFFILIATION

	% of Patients			
	Unaffiliated (13% of total sample)	Catholic (57% of total sample)	Protestant (8% of total sample)	Afro-Spiritist (5% of total sample)
Any type of organ anxiety	38	38	56	78**
Any complaint of physical pain or discomfort	63	78	56	72*
Feels something strange inside body	9	13	31	0***
Physical movements are slowed	9	14	25	14
Complains of fatigue	59	55	81	64**
Complains of weakness	49	53	69	64*
Complains of palpitations	31	33	25	50*
Complains of sweating or hot flashes	37	27	38	7**
Complains of dyspnea	16	24	38	21**
Complains of anorexia	53	56	75	49*

Significance of differences determined by chi-square:
  *probability of chance occurrence, less than .05
  **probability of chance occurrence, less than .01
  ***probability of chance occurrence, less than .001

TABLE 193

SEXUAL BEHAVIOR ACCORDING TO RELIGIOUS AFFILIATION

	% of Patients			
	Unaffiliated (13% of total sample)	Catholic (57% of total sample)	Protestant (8% of total sample)	Afro-Spiritist (5% of total sample)
Suffers impotence or frigidity	32	32	38	28
Worries interfere with sex functioning	34	42	50	43
Sex impulses absent or weak	6	18	0	14**
Sex impulses too intense, uncontrollable or fluctuating	31	14	31	14
Sex a source of anxiety, guilt or shame	16	13	6	0*
Basically monogamous	44	76	88	77***
Most sex contacts casual	41	14	0	21***
Sex pattern part of present illness	22	31	44	36*

Significance of differences determined by chi-square.
   *probability of chance occurrence, less than .05
   **probability of chance occurrence, less than .01
   ***probability of chance occurrence, less than .001

TABLE 194
INTELLECTUAL POTENTIALITIES AND GENERAL LEVEL
OF COGNITIVE-INTELLECTUAL EFFICIENCY
REVEALED BY RORSCHACH TESTING

Rorschach Results	
	% of Test Sample
Low or undeterminable (8%) level of innate capacity	68
Inferior level of intellectual-cognitive efficiency	89
Functional weaknesses potentially affecting efficiency	100

      32 Impaired reality testing
      30 Narrowed interest
      21 Mobility of resources impaired by emotions
      12 Weakness of integration and related problems
       5 Miscellaneous

TABLE 195
IDEATIONAL DRIVE REPRESENTATION REVEALED
IN RORSCHACH RESPONSES, DRIVES WITH LIBIDINAL AIMS

		% of Test Sample			
	Oral	*Phallic-Genital*	*Anal*	*Sexual Ambiguity*	*Exhibitionistic-Voyeuristic*
Nature of Rorschach Response					
One or few	44	8	8	6	8
Several or many	11	6	2	5	0
Overwhelming	2	3	0	8	0
Libidinal theme involved, but without clear reference to the particular bodily channel of expression	13	37	21	8	0
None	30	46	69	81	92

TABLE 196
PSYCHOLOGICAL DERIVATIVES OF DRIVES REVEALED IN RORSCHACH RESPONSES. RESPONSES REVEALING DEPENDENT AND SADOMASOCHISTIC THEMES

% of Test Sample

Predominant Aspects of Dependency Drive Derivatives		*Predominant Aspects of Sadomasochistic Drive Derivatives*	
Aggressive Dependency	38	Sado-Masochistic Themes, Unspecified	38
Oral Dependency Themes, Unspecified	28	Sadistic Drive Derivatives	33
Receptive Dependency	24	Masochistic Drive Derivatives	16
Mixed Receptives and Aggressive Dependency	10	Mixed Sadistic and Masochistic Drive Derivatives	11

TABLE 197
IDEATIONAL DRIVE REPRESENTATION REVEALED IN RORSCHACH RESPONSES, DRIVES WITH AGGRESSIVE AIMS

% of Test Sample Showing

Nature of Rorschach Response	*Potential Aggression*	*Active Aggression*	*Results of Aggression*	*Direct Mutual Aggression*
One or few	22	16	27	6
Several or many	3	0	2	0
Overwhelming	2	0	0	0
None	73	84	61	94

TABLE 198
HOMOSEXUAL THEMES REVEALED IN RORSCHACH RESPONSES

	% of Test Sample	
	Males: Attitudes Toward Masculine Identity	Females: Attitudes Toward Feminine Identity
Presenting 2 or more subthemes	14	14
Feelings of being part male and part female, or implicit denial of sexual identity	9	9
Castration themes	5	9
Feminine emphasis	2	—
Hostile or fearful conceptions of male role	2	—
Reference to perversions	—	5

TABLE 199
RORSCHACH INDICATORS OF EGO FUNCTION

% of Test Sample

1. The ties with reality are good: a good and flexible kind of reality testing and a more active form of mastery function are indicated 0
2. The ties with reality are apparently good, but rigid and inflexible. Reality testing is uncreative, tedious, banal: reaction formation against distortions of reality—DS; dr; perfectionistic approach; $F+$ % 100 with above average intellectual potentiality; defense rigidity 9
3. The ties with reality are weakened: few P's, especially in Card V; unbalanced use of locations, especially a low D percentage and a poor form level; O-; F % below 20, poor form level and not plenty of control factors; weak contamination, emergence of confabulation, confabulatory combination or even minor perceptual distortions if the subject is not aware of them 11
4. The ties with reality are seriously weakened (several or all of the above signs) 17
5. There is a loosening of ties with reality: interspersing of some responses in a chain of perseverations; the rejection of most of the cards with a somewhat appropriate response to a few cards; the combination of two or three chains of perseverations, minus form level; M-; complex or strong contamination; reality index form -4; autistic logic; etc. 60
6. There is the emergence of a primitive form of mastery of a puzzling reality testing (magic perseveration) which indicates the depth of regression 3

TABLE 200
CRITERIA FOR TAT CODING

Scores from 0 to 5 were used according to the following criteria:

*Attitudes and traits; forces of the
central character's environment*

0. no information or none applicable
1. apparently free of that trait or attitude
2. with occasional feelings, but mostly
   expressing the opposite attitude
3. ambivalent, with no definite pattern
4. fairly manifest attitude, but showing
   some degree of the opposite feeling
5. openly manifest attitude; no signs of
   the opposite feeling

Inner states or emotions

0. no information or none applicable
1. apparently free of that emotion or inner state
2. with occasional or just implicit signs

3. mildly explicit signs
4. fairly manifest signs

5. overemphasis of signs

After scoring each story all scores were added. The total points for each subject were summed to arrive at a total for the whole sample. On the
basis of these totals the percentage of frequency of appearance of each variable was calculated.

TABLE 201
ATTITUDE OR TRAIT: TAT THEMES AND CONTENT

% of Test Sample

Abasement		5
Achievement		9
	Emotional and verbal	7
	Physical, social	1
Aggression	Physical, asocial	5
	Destruction	0
Dominance		1
Intraggression		11
Nurturance		4
Passivity		29
Sex		9
Succorance		17
Other		2

TABLE 202
INNER STATES OR EMOTIONS: TAT THEMES AND CONTENT

% of Test Sample

Conflict	16
Emotional change	17
Dejection	34
Anxiety	26
Other	7

TABLE 203
FORCES OF THE HERO'S ENVIRONMENT: TAT THEMES AND CONTENT

Variables		*% of Test Sample*
Affiliation	Associative	4
	Emotional	22
	Emotional and verbal	6
Aggression	Physical, social	4
	Physical, asocial	2
	Destruction of property	1
Dominance	Coercion	2
	Restraint	3
	Inducement, seduction	8
Nurturance		18
Rejection		6
Lack, loss	Lack	8
	Loss	11
Physical danger	Active	1
	Insupport	0
Physical injury		4

TABLE 204
INTERACTION PATTERN: TAT THEMES AND CONTENT

	% of Test Sample
Social engagement	72
Social breakdown	15
Interpersonal impairment	13

TABLE 205
ORIENTATION EMPHASIS: TAT THEMES AND CONTENT

	% of Test Sample
Systemic	13
Individual	51
Sub-systems (pairs, etc.)	35
Role assignment	1
Social: value oriented	0

TABLE 206
DOMINANT VALUES: TAT THEMES AND CONTENT

Values	% of Test Sample
Economic	1
Theoretical	1
Political	0
Social	0
Religious	9
Aesthetic	3
Ethical	7
Absent	79

TABLE 207

OUTCOME: TAT THEMES AND CONTENT

% of Test Sample

Undetermined or the story has not
gone beyond the descriptive level 67
Happy end, success 8
Unhappy end, failure 10
Ambivalent outcome   15

TABLE 208

REPORTED REASONS FOR BRINGING PATIENT
FOR HOSPITAL ADMISSION

Interview reports by family (72%), friends or authorities	*% of Patients*
Engaged in overtly deviant behavior in presence of family	64
Made disturbing or symptomatic statements in presence of family	57
Admitted because of combination of acts and statements	50
Admitted because of overt behavior only	25
Admitted because of verbal statements only	25
Made anxious, depressed, or suicidal statements	20
Engaged in bizarre acts	14
Attacked or threatened others	8
Made paranoid or grandiose statements	7
Destroyed objects or property	6
Would not work	6
Engaged in suicidal or self-mutilating behavior	6

TABLE 209

DIFFERENCES IN REPORTED REASONS FOR COMING TO HOSPITAL ACCORDING TO SOCIOCULTURAL STATUS

% of Patients

Behavior Leading to Hospitalization	Color	Education	Literacy	Sex / Marital	Age	Migration	Occupation	Housing	Religion
Physical assaults or threats	Bl 36** Br 12 W 13	I 25* II 14	I 21 II 19 III 11	Sex: M 18**, F 4 Marital: S 24, M 14					
Will not or cannot work	Bl 4 Br 16** W 3	I 9 II 1**	I 24*** II 12 III 2		I 11 II 4 III 2	Recent 14* Settled 3			
Anxious, depressed, suicidal	Bl 8** Br 12 W 27		I 40 II 35 III 21*	Marital: S 7**, M 24		Recent 11* Settled 23	I-IV 15 V 25 VI 18		
Paranoid or grandiose	Bl 20 Br 20 W 10	I 20* II 10	I 30* II 19 III 13		I 24* II 10 III 11		I-IV 7 V 15 VI 24*	−23* +13	U 9** C 15 P 31 AS 21
Other bizarre acts		I 12* II 22			I 18 II 17 III 5				U 28 C 15 P 0*** AS 28

Significance of differences determined by chi-square:
*probability of chance occurrence, less than .05
**probability of chance occurrence, less than .01
***probability of chance occurrence, less than .001

TABLE 210
FAMILY OR COMMUNITY DIAGNOSIS

Interview reports by family (72 percent), friends or authorities	*Percentage of patients*
Patient is mentally ill	31
Patient is physically ill	31
Patient is not ill but suffering from life stress (including persecution by others, physical and emotional stress)	15
No diagnosis or opinion	10
Patient has no problem, the wrong diagnosis has been made	6
Patient is suffering from religious influences, possession, etc.	4
Patient is eccentric, immoral, bad, or unacceptably deviant	3

TABLE 211
FAMILY-COMMUNITY DIAGNOSIS

% of Patients

Family or Community Diagnosis

Mental illness

Migration	Color	Education	Literacy	Housing	Marital	Age	Religion
Recent 45*	Bl 46	I 46***	I 65****	−56****	S 44***	I 40*	U 40
Settled 33	Br 39	II 26	II 49	+31	M 19	II 26	C 35
	W 35		III 31			III 22	P 45
							AS 45

Reaction to life stress

Education	Literacy	Occupation	Marital	Age
I 9***	I 7	I-IV 27	S 8**	I 11
II 24	II 4	V 15	M 21	II 14
	III 19*	VI 6***		III 22

Strange, eccentric or undesirable

Color	Migration	Education	Literacy	Housing	Marital	Religion
Bl 0***	Recent 30	I 26*	I 8***	−6	S 11***	U 31
Br 23	Settled 40	II 39	II 30	+21	M 27	C 24
W 24			III 37			P 10
						AS 9***

Significance of differences determined by chi-square:
   *probability of chance occurrence, less than .05
  **probability of chance occurrence, less than .02
 ***probability of chance occurrence, less than .01
****probability of chance occurrence, less than .001

TABLE 212
DURATION OF DEFINED PRESENT ILLNESS

Duration of Present Illness	% of Patients
1 month or less	18
1–6 months	24
6–12 months	12
1–5 years	21
5 years or more	12
Undetermined	13

Evaluation by Psychiatrists of Interview Reports of Patients and Relatives

TABLE 213
PAST HISTORY EVENTS OCCURRING IN 15% OR MORE OF THE ENTIRE PATIENT POPULATION

Interview Reports by Patients and/or Relatives	% of Patients
Previous contact with psychiatrists	47
Serious psychological trauma in adult life	47
Marital conflict	40
Adult or adolescent rages	38
School adjustment problems	34
Problems in developing bladder control	30
Serious psychological trauma in childhood	25
Fainting spells or lapses	25
Unusual age (late) of menarche	22
A serious accident	19
Work adjustment problems	18
An episode of altered consciousness accompanying high fever	17
An apparent convulsion	15

TABLE 214
SYMPTOMATIC BEHAVIOR PRESENT IN 40% OR
MORE OF THE ENTIRE PATIENT POPULATION

Interview Reports by Patients	*% of Patients*
Any decrease, increase or other change in sexual desire, capacity, pleasure, or performance possibly related to present illness	95
Insomnia due to worries	74
Any complaint of pain or specific malfunction of some body organ or region	74
Discrete attacks of anxiety	67
Worries interfere with work	65
Headache	62
Feels sad, now or frequently	60
Feels overwhelmed by many, specific fears	58
Marked fatigue or lack of energy	57
Lack of appetite or inability to eat	57
General physical weakness	54
Complains about treatment from specific others	53
Fears loss of control of thoughts, feelings, and actions	50
Anxious, tense, or fearful behavior in interview	48
Complains of a specific sexual problem	47
Faintness or dizziness	47
Some problems in mental efficiency or clarity of thought	45
Restless due to worries	45
Expresses jealousy of some person or group	43
Attacks of rage or anger	43
Difficulty concentrating due to worries	42
Feels like weeping, now or frequently	41
Any problem in remembering	41
Worries interfere with sexual behavior	41
Frequent or intense worry about body malfunction or illness	40

TABLE 215
INDICATORS OF ANXIETY OCCURRING IN 15% OR
MORE OF THE ENTIRE PATIENT POPULATION

Interview Reports and Observations	% of Patients
Insomnia due to worries	74
Discrete anxiety attacks	67
Worries interfere with work	65
Overwhelmed by many specific fears	58
Fears of loss of control of thoughts, feelings or actions	50
Interview anxiety, tension, fear	48
Restlessness due to worries	45
Difficulty concentrating due to worries	42
Any body or organ anxiety	40
Difficulty in making decisions due to worries	37
Constant diffuse anxiety	35
Phobic fears	31
Frequent or intense job worries	27
Frequent or intense family worries	26
Frequent fear of dying	27
Fears loss of control of acts alone	25
Tremor of hand during interview	23
Wet, clammy palms on handshake	20
Frequent feeling of impending doom	19
Tense and fidgety psychomotor behavior during interview	17
Tic-like motions during interview	15

TABLE 216

INDICATORS OF ANXIETY OCCURING IN 15% OR MORE OF THE ENTIRE

Interview Reports and Observations	Color	Migration	Occupation	Education
Insomnia due to worries	Br 86* Bl 76 W 71	——	I-IV 69 V 77 VI 79	——
Discrete anxiety attacks	Br 71 Bl 56 W 69	Recent 76 Settled 65	I-IV 64 V 68 VI 75	——
Worries interfere with work	Br 74 Bl 56 W 65	——	I-IV 65 V 62 VI 72	——
Fears loss of control of thoughts, feelings and actions	Br 40 Bl 32 W 43	——	I-IV 34* V 25 VI 18	I 20 II 33*
Interview anxiety, tension, fear	——	Recent 54** Settled 39	I-IV 44 V 37 VI 53	——
Restlessness due to worries	Br 64*** Bl 37 W 41	——	I-IV 42 V 42 VI 56	——
Difficulty concentrating due to worries	——	Recent 56** Settled 38	I-IV 40 V 41 VI 48	——
Any body or organ anxiety	——	Recent 59**** Settled 32	I-IV 35 V 39 VI 45	——
Difficulty in making decisions due to worries	Br 36 Bl 20 W 36	——	——	——
Constant diffuse anxiety	Br 34 Bl 20 W 39	——	——	I 26 II 41**
Phobic fears	Br 34 Bl 8** W 33	——	——	——
Frequent or intense job worries	——	——	I-IV 13 V 31 VI 37**	——
Frequent or intense family worries	Br 32 Bl 32 W 21	Recent 18 Settled 5	——	I 36 II 31 III 22

Significance of differences determined by chi-square: | **probability of chance occurrence,
*probability of chance occurrence, less than .05   less than .02

PATIENT POPULATION ACCORDING TO SOCIOCULTURAL STATUS

% of Patients

Literacy	Housing	Religion	Sex	Marital	Age
I 87 II 77 III 72	—	—	—	—	I 65 II 75 III 85*
—	—	—	—	—	—
		P 69 U 69 C 68 AS 50	—		
I 13 II 27 III 27	+44 –34	P 50 U 31 C 26 AS 43	—	—	I 47 II 42 III 31
I 60 II 50 III 44	+42 –52	—	F 53 M 41	—	—
I 57 II 58 III 42	+46 –57	—	F 51 M 42	—	—
	—	—	F 56*** M 36	—	—
I 57 II 42 III 35	+37 –54	P 56 U 38 C 38 AS 78***	F 46 M 36	M 46 S 35	I 31 II 44 III 47
—	—	—	—	M 30 S 49***	—
I 20 II 31 III 40*	—	—	F 46 M 36	M 41 S 31	I 37 II 42 III 22*
—	—	P 25 U 41 C 30 AS 14*	F 40** M 26	—	—
—	—	P 38 U 31 C 28 AS 14*	—	—	—
—	+23 –37	P 50* U 19 C 22 AS 23	F 37*** M 19	M 30*** S 11	—

*probability of chance occurrence, less than .01   ****probability of chance occurrence, less than .001

TABLE 217
DIFFERENCES OF 10% OR MORE IN SOCIOCULTURAL STATUS
ACCORDING TO COLOR

| | | % of Patients | |
Other Sociocultural Indices	*White*	*Brown*	*Black*
Literate (Level III)	80	49	50****
Illiterate (Level I)	2	13	18****
No education or			
incomplete primary (Level I)	8	23	32****
Completed primary (Level II)	37	51	54
Single	30	41	32
Married (civil and religious)	46	28	25**
Occupation VI	20	48	50****
Occupation I–IV	33	10	7***
Inferior housing	8	20	33*****
Afro-Spiritist observation	11	13	28**
Male sex	65	60	78*
Age 15–25	36	39	28

Significance of differences determined by chi-square:
*probability of chance occurrence, less than .05
**probability of chance occurrence, less than .02
***probability of chance occurrence, less than .01
****probability of chance occurrence, less than .001

TABLE 218
DIFFERENCES OF 10% OR MORE IN SOCIOCULTURAL
STATUS ACCORDING TO RELIGIOUS
MEMBERSHIP OR OBSERVANCE (AFRO-SPIRITIST)

% of Patients

Other Sociocultural Indices	*Unaffiliated*	*Catholic*	*Protestant*	*Afro-Spiritist*
Age 15–25	17	25	25	15
26–40	57	49	40	65
41–60	26	26	35	20
Male	85	65	50	61***
Female	15	35	50	39***
White	57	67	55	62
Brown	29	23	35	18
Black	14	10	10	20
Single	54	32	15	24***
Married (civil and religious)	26	44	35	32**
Recent Migrant	34	26	40	15*
Housing	25	9	25	16
Illiterate	14	14	20	14
Partly literate	6	16	20	12
Literate	77	68	60	75
Education Level I				
Incomplete primary or no education	54	58	60	47
Occupation I–IV	26	29	5	25***
V	26	46	45	55***
VI	46	26	40	22*

Significance of differences determined by chi-square:
  *probability of chance occurrence, less than .05
  **probability of chance occurrence, less than .02
  ***probability of chance occurrence, less than .01

TABLE 219
SELECTED INDICATORS OF DEPRESSION
ACCORDING TO SOCIOCULTURAL STATUS

Interview Reports and Observations	Total	Color	Migration	Occupation	Religion
Feels sad now or frequently	60	W 44 Br 44 Bl 25	Recent 70 Settled 59*	——	U 59 C 61 P 75 AS 43*
Marked fatigue or lack of energy	57	——	Recent 65 Settled 55*	I-IV 49 V 62 VI 64*	U 59* C 55 P 81*** AS 64
Lack of appetite	57	——	——	——	——
General physical weakness	54	——	——	——	U 49* C 53 P 69 AS 64
Feels like weeping now or frequently	41	——	——	I-IV 47 V 42 VI 36	——
Has made suicidal threats	20	W 24 Br 22 Bl 0***	——	I-IV 27 V 17 VI 16	U 25 C 20 P 19 AS 7*
Feels lonely now or frequently	18	——	Recent 27 Settled 15*	——	——
Death wishes	17	W 21 Br 14 Bl 4*	——	I-IV 29* V 16 VI 7	——
Has made a suicidal attempt	16	W 17 Br 22 Bl 4*	——	——	——
Guilty over social role failure	15	——	——	——	U 16 C 14 P 25* AS 7
Preoccupied with inadequacy	13	W 14 Br 12 Bl 4	——	I-IV 24* V 7 VI 10	——

Significance of differences determined by chi-square:
*probability of chance occurrence, less than .05
***probability of chance occurrence, less than .01
****probability of chance occurrence, less than .001

% of Patients

Literacy	Housing	Sex	Marital	Age	Education
——	+ 65**** − 48 Area II 70 I 57	F 76**** M 53	——	——	——
III 56 II 50 I 77	+ 54 − 71*	F 71 M 53***	——	III 72* II 57 I 47	——
——	——	F 71*** M 50	M 59 S 46	III 63 II 60 I 45	——
III 54 II 46 I 63	+ 53 − 62	F 60 M 78***	——	III 67 II 53 I 42	II 62 I 52
——	+ 48**** − 28 Area II 47 I 38	F 59**** M 32	M 51 S 28***	III 34* II 22 I 17	——
——	——	F 25* M 11	——	——	——
——	Area II 26* I 15	——	M 10 S 22*	——	——
——	+ 20 − 10 Area II 24* I 13	F 26*** M 13	M 11 S 22	——	——
——	Area II 24* I 19	F 29 M 10****	M 18 S 8	——	——
III 14 II 31* I 13	——	——	M 6 S 24***	III 13 II 10 I 23	——
——	Area II 24*** I 9	——	M 8 S 18*	III 9 II 9 I 19	——

TABLE 220

SELECTED INDICES OF DEPRESSION DIFFERING ACCORDING TO
SOCIOCULTURAL STATUS

		% of Patients			
Reports and Interview Observations	*Total*	*Literacy*	*Housing*		
Feels overwhelmed by criticism	26	III 22 II 46 I 33	Area II 45*** Area I 22		
		Religion			
Accuses self of wrong doing or unworthiness	21	P 38 U 28 C 18 AS 0***			
		Age			
Intense feelings about a problem	21	III 40* II 27 I 21			
		Sex			
Has fears of being abandoned	20	F 37*** M 12			
		Literacy	*Occupation*		
Feels body weak or inferior	17	III 15 II 23 I 30	I–IV 16 V 14 VI 22		
		Migration	*Sex*	*Religion*	
Guilt over failure as a parent	7	Recent 18*** Settled 3	F 13** M 4	P 13 C 7 U 3 AS 0*	

Significance of differences determined by chi-square:
*probability of chance occurrence, less than .05
**probability of chance occurrence, less than .02
***probability of chance occurrence, less than .001

TABLE 221

DIFFERENCES OF 10% IN MIGRATION ACCORDING TO
SOCIOCULTURAL STATUS

	% of Patients	
	Recently Migrant	Settled
Education I		
None or incomplete primary	68	55*
Education II		
Complete primary and beyond	32	46
Illiterate	29	9***
Partly literate	16	13
Literate	52	74***
Occupational Class I–IV	18	26
V	38	44
VI	38	25**
Housing		
No essential services	20	10*
Electricity and running water	65	73

Significance of differences determined by chi-square:
*probability of chance occurrence, less than .05
**probability of chance occurrence, less than .01
***probability of chance occurrence, less than .001

TABLE 222

HOSTILE OR IMPULSIVE BEHAVIOR ACCORDING TO DIFFERENCES OF 10% OR MORE IN SOCIOCULTURAL STATUS

Interview Report and Observations of Patients and Relatives

Sociocultural Statuses

	Total	Color	Literacy	Occupation	Age	Marital	Sex	Education	Religion
History of attacks of rage or anger	38	Brown 48, White 43, Black 32	III 49, II 54, I 37		III 32, II 44, I 45				U 59, P 56, C 39, AS 28*
History of frequent arguments	33	Brown 38, White 33, Black 28	III 29, II 46, I 40						P 44, U 41, AS 36, C 30
History of impulsive behavior	26	Brown 32, White 26, Black 20	III 24, II 38, I 27	I–IV 29, V 20, VI 31	III 16, II 26, I 33*	S 32*, M 19			U 44*, AS 21, P 19, C 12
Feels tense and isolated with others	26		III 31, II 46, I 27	I–IV 39, V 25, VI 36	III 25, II 23, I 55**				
Admitted because attacked people or objects	8	Black 36, Brown 12, White 13	III 11, II 19, I 21			S 25, M 14	M 18**, F 4	II 14, I 24*	C 17, U 16, P 13, AS 7

Significance of differences determined by chi-square:
*probability of chance occurrence, less than .05
**probability of chance occurrence, less than .01

TABLE 223
SOMATIC COMPLAINTS ACCORDING TO SOCIOCULTURAL STATUS

Interview Reports and Observations — *% of Patients*

Interview Reports and Observations	Total					
Any physical pain or discomfort	75	*Occupation* I-IV 66 V 73 VI 81*	*Age* I 62 II 79 III 80*	*Religion* U 63 C 78 P 56* AS 72	*Occupation* I-IV 33* V 51 VI 52	*Marital* M 49 S 37
Faintness or dizziness	47	*Color* Black 46 Brown 36* White 49	*Sex* F 53* M 43	*Literacy* I 37* II 54 III 48	*Religion* U 31 C 33 P 25 AS 50*	
Palpitation	31	*Migration* Recent 15 Settled 38****	*Literacy* I 17 II 31 III 34	*Marital* M 35** S 18		
Dyspnea or related complaints	29	*Migration* Recent 15*** Settled 34	*Literacy* I 17 II 27 III 31	*Sex* F 40*** M 23	*Marital* M 32 S 20	*Religion* U 16*** C 24 P 38 AS 21
Nausea or vomiting	24	*Literacy* I 10 II 23 III 26	*Occupation* I-IV 15 V 26 VI 25	*Marital* M 35 S 4		*Age* I 11* II 27 III 32

Significance of differences determined by chi-square:
*probability of chance occurrence, less than .05
**probability of chance occurrence, less than .02
***probability of chance occurrence, less than .01
****probability of chance occurrence, less than .001

TABLE 224

SEXUAL BEHAVIOR IN THE ENTIRE PATIENT POPULATION

Interview Reports by Patients and/or Relatives	*% of Patients*
Any decrease, increase, or other change in desire, capacity, pleasure, or performance possibly related to present illness	95
Sexual behavior a source of conflict	50
Has been part of a monogamous heterosexual relationship most of adult life	49
A specific sexual problem	47
No change in sexual behavior since adulthood	46
Worries interfere with sexual behavior	41
Sexual behavior labeled as sick, disturbed, or impaired occurring in clear relationship to present illness or within the year preceding hospitalization	31
Impotence (males) or frigidity (females)	30
Erectile or orgasmic impotence, premature or retarded ejaculations	18
Painful intercourse	17
Any basic preference other than conventional heterosexual relations with other adults	17
Most sexual relations with casual partners	17
Has engaged on more than a single occasion in anal intercourse	16
Sexual impulses are intense or uncontrollable depending upon the presence of a female (reported only by males)	16
No interest or markedly low interest in sex	14
Sexual activity confined to solitary masturbation	8

TABLE 225
SEXUAL COMPLAINTS ACCORDING TO SOCIOCULTURAL STATUS

Interview Report and Observations	Total	Color				% of Patients								

Interview Report and Observations	Total	Color							
Sex a source of conflict	50	Brown 64 White 58 Black 44							

Interview Report and Observations	Total	Color	Marital	Religion					
Worries inter- fere with sex	40	Brown 34 White 47** Black 20	M 48* S 32	U 34 C 42 P 50 AS 43					

Interview Report and Observations	Total	Literacy	Marital	Religion	Age
Sex problems are part of present illness	31	I 17 II 23 III 35*	M 43**** S 19	U 22* C 31 P 44 AS 36	I 28 II 25 III 41

Interview Report and Observations	Total	Color	Marital	Religion	Age	Literacy	Occupation	Sex
Impotence or frigidity	30	Brown 20 White 37*** Black 10	M 42*** S 17	U 32 C 32 P 38 AS 28	I 20 II 33 III 39*	I 23 II 23 III 33	I-IV 24* V 36 VI 33	M 25**** F 40

Interview Report and Observations	Total	Sex	Marital	Religion	Age
Sex a source of guilt or shame	14	M 16*** F 5	M 3 S 27****	U 16 C 13 P 6 AS 0*	I 19 II 8 III 11

Interview Report and Observations	Total	Color	Marital	Religion	Sex	Literacy
Sex impulse too strong, fluctuating or uncontrollable	16	Brown 30 White 14 Black 8	M 14 S 25	U 31 C 14 P 31 AS 14	M 19 F 9*	I 3* II 19 III 20

Significance of differences determined by chi-square:
*probability of chance occurrence, less than .05
**probability of chance occurrence, less than .02
***probability of chance occurrence, less than .01
****probability of chance occurrence, less than .001

TABLE 226
ATTITUDES AND FEELINGS TOWARD OTHERS (PARANOID BEHAVIOR)

Interview Reports and Observations	Total	Color		Migration		Literacy	
Complains about treatment by others	53	Br	60	Recent	66***	III	50
		W	53	Settled	49	II	53
		Bl	44			I	70
Feels persecuted, harassed or attacked by person or group	38	Br	44	Recent	51***	III	35
		W	34	Settled	33	II	35
		Bl	44			I	57*
Says others talk about or stare at him	34	Br	50	Recent	43*	III	30*
		W	28	Settled	30	II	56
		Bl	40			I	43
Feels especially emulated, admired or loved by person or group (grandiose)	30	Br	42	Recent	53****	III	26***
		W	30	Settled	27	II	50
		Bl	28			I	50
Others know inner thoughts, feelings or problems	27			Recent	35		——
			——	Settled	24		
Feels others are not trustworthy	26	Br	34	Recent	38	III	23
		W	23	Settled	22	II	38
		Bl	28			I	37
Others control his inner thoughts and feelings	24		——	Recent	37***	III	22
				Settled	19	II	23
						I	13
Others misjudge him	23	Br	38***		——	III	19*
		W	18			II	35
		Bl	24			I	30
Others regard him as mentally or morally inferior	21	Br	34****	Recent	31*	III	15*
		W	10	Settled	18	II	46
		Bl	16			I	33

†Approximately 10% of the patients reporting this feeling or belief attributed the admiration or love, or knowledge of inner feelings to a relative or loved one. The majority attributed the feeling or knowledge to unrelated persons or to culturally significant, often quasi-religious or cultist, organizations.

Significance of differences determined by chi-square:
　　*probability of chance occurrence, less than .05
　**probability of chance occurrence, less than .02
　***probability of chance occurrence, less than .01
****probability of chance occurrence, less than .001

BY SOCIOCULTURAL STATUS WITH DIFFERENCES OF 10% OR MORE

Occupation	Housing	Sex	Marital	Age	Religion
___	−62 +49	___	S 63*** M 43	III 39* II 58 I 60	U 59 P 50 AS 50 C 48
I-IV 36 V 30 VI 45	−60**** +32 Area II 51** I 33	___	S 45*** M 25	III 24* II 45 I 42	___
I-IV 26 V 31 VI 43*	−40 +32	___	S 44** M 27	III 27 II 30 I 42	U 44* P 31 AS 28 C 33
___	43** +26 Area II 42 I 29	F 40 M 29	S 42*** M 16	___	___
___	−34* +20	___	S 39*** M 14	III 21 II 27 I 32	U 31 P 31 AS 29 C 20
I-IV 22 V 19 VI 37*	___ Area II 34 I 24	F 34 M 24	S 34** M 18	III 18 II 24 I 33	___
___	___ Area II 32 I 19	___	S 35*** M 14	___	U 31 P 25 AS 22 C 19
___	___ Area II 32 I 22	___	S 35*** M 14	___	___
I-IV 20 V 15 VI 30*	Area II 34 I 8	___	S 30*** M 14	III 14 II 14 I 33***	___

TABLE 227
HALLUCINATORY, ILLUSORY, AND DISORIENTATION

% of Patients

Interview Reports and Observations	Total	Color		Migrant	Education	
Hears voices in absence of others	33	Bl	60****	Recent 39*	I	40****
		Br	40	Settled 29	II	21
		W	24			
Has auditory and visual illusory experiences	21	Bl	28	Recent 26	I	23
		Br	32	Settled 17	II	14
		W	14****			
Sees people in absence of others	16	Bl	36****	Recent 24*	I	25****
		Br	26	Settled 14	II	2
		W	8			
Sees animals or nonhuman entities	15	Bl	20****	——	I	20***
		Br	16		II	5
		W	2			
Insists on reality of what has seen or heard	20	Bl	42****	Recent 29*	I	28****
		Br	27	Settled 16	II	8
		W	11			
Plans action on basis of what has seen or heard	17	Bl	29	Recent 27*	I	23***
		Br	28	Settled 11	II	6
		W	9****			
Temporal disorientation of any degree or duration	16	Bl	28***	Recent 20**	I	39****
		Br	22	Settled 9	II	10
		W	5			
Spatial disorientation of any degree or duration	12	Bl	32***	——	I	21***
		Br	22		II	7
		W	10			

Significance of differences determined by chi-square:
*probability of chance occurrence, less than .05
**probability of chance occurrence, less than .02
***probability of chance occurrence, less than .01
****probability of chance occurence, less than .001

EXPERIENCES ACCORDING TO SOCIOCULTURAL STATUS

Literacy		Occupation		Housing	Area		Marital		Religion	
I	57***	I-IV	26	−50	I	34	S	41***	U	34
II	39	V	21	+24	II	81**	M	20	C	33
III	27	VI	51***						P	31
									AS	15*
I	30	——		−30****	I	16	S	28***	U	19
II	23			+13	II	27	M	9	C	20
III	16*								P	19
									AS	8
I	35	I-IV	6	−36****	I	13	S	17*	U	25
II	35	V	10	+11	II	25*	M	6	C	16
III	8****	VI	35***						P	19
									AS	8****
I	21	I-IV	6	−27****	——		——		U	22****
II	27	V	9	+9					C	15
III	9***	VI	27***						P	0
									AS	8
I	45****	I-IV	13	−33****	——		S	27***	U	25
II	32	V	13	+14			M	9	C	17
III	14	VI	37*						P	38****
									AS	14
I	38****	I-IV	7	−27***	——		S	21***	U	22
II	27	V	6	+10			M	6	C	13
III	9	VI	33***						P	31
									AS	0****
I	73****	I-IV	18	−31***	I	26	S	31	U	28
II	23	V	25	+8	II	38	M	21	C	25
III	21	VI	42***						P	44*
									AS	22
I	57****	I-IV	7	−47****	——		S	20***	U	19
II	12	V	14	+20			M	6	C	12
III	8	VI	25*						P	25
									AS	28

TABLE 228

SUBJECTIVE REPORTS OF COGNITIVE DIFFICULTIES ACCORDING TO SOCIOCULTURAL STATUS

Interview Reports by Patient

% of Patients

	Total	Color	Migration	Housing	Sex	Marital	Age
Impaired mental efficiency	45	Brown 64* White 45 Black 34	Recent 64*** Settled 39	−57* +40	F 51 M 41	S 57** M 35	I 57* II 41 III 35*
		Color	*Religion*				
Any memory difficulty	41	Brown 49 White 44 Black 36	U 44 C 41 P 31 AS 22*				

Significance of differences determined by chi-square:
  *probability of chance occurrence, less than .05
  **probability of chance occurrence, less than .01
  ***probability of chance occurrence, less than .001

TABLE 229
DREAMING IN THE ENTIRE PATIENT POPULATION

Interview Reports		*% of Patients*
Admits dreaming, but regards dreams as unimportant and cannot recall them		42
Denies dreaming		21
Presence or absence of dreaming not determinable		7
Does not Acknowledge Significant Dreams:	Total	70
Has fearful dreams		16
Has persecutory dreams		10
Has sexual dreams		4
Acknowledges Significant Dreams:	Total	30

TABLE 230

RELATIONAL ASPECTS OF THE INTERVIEW: PSYCHIATRISTS'

% of Patients

Psychiatrists' Self-Ratings

	Migration	*Color*	*Occupation*
Feels interview interesting and rewarding	Recent 44*** Settled 66	Br 56 Bl 40* W 66	I-IV 78* V 51 VI 54

	Migration	*Color*	*Occupation*
Feels involved and empathic	Recent 44 Settled 57	Br 46 Bl 72*** W 58	I-IV 68 V 51 VI 49

	Migration	*Color*	*Occupation*
Feels liked by patient	Recent 38*** Settled 57	Br 52 Bl 32* W 58	I-IV 64 V 58 VI 37*

	Migration	*Color*	*Occupation*
Feels cheerful and optimistic in interview	Recent 17* Settled 31	Br 14*** Bl 36 W 31	I-IV 39 V 24 VI 21

	Migration	*Occupation*	*Literacy*
Feels hostile or irritated at patient	Recent 18**** Settled 4	I-IV 2 V 9 VI 15*	I 23**** II 12 III 5

	Migration	*Color*	*Housing*
Feels anxious or apprehensive in interview	Recent 13*** Settled 3	Br 22 Bl 16 W 9	−25**** +8

	Color	*Sex*	*Age*
Feels a marked liking for patient	Br 6 Bl 4 W 19*	F 11 M 54	I 69 II 56 III 70

	Occupation	*Education*	*Literacy*
Feels remote or distant	I-IV 15* V 31 VI 31	I 32** II 18	I 40* II 15 III 26

Significance of differences determined by chi-square:
*probability of chance occurrence, less than .05
**probability of chance occurrence, less than .02
***probability of chance occurrence, less than .01
****probability of chance occurrence, less than .001

SELF-RATINGS ACCORDING TO PATIENT'S SOCIOCULTURAL STATUS

Education	Literacy	Housing	Age	Religion
I 48****	I 33***	28****	I 63	U 53
II 77	II 65	+69	II 53	C 62
	III 64		III 65	P 56
				AS 44

Education	Literacy	Housing	Religion	
I 51	I 37	−46	U 56	
II 62	II 61	+59	C 53	
	III 58		P 60	
			AS 33*	

Education	Literacy	Religion		
I 42***	I 27***	U 59		
II 69	II 46	C 54		
	III 59	P 56		
		AS 28*		

Education	Housing			
I 21***	−15**			
II 37	I 33			

Housing				
−18***				
+5				

Housing	Age			
−35	I 23			
+24	II 34			
	III 20			

TABLE 231
RELATIONAL BEHAVIOR IN THE INTERVIEW

% of Patients

Interview Reports	Education	Literacy	Occupation	Housing	Sex	Marital	Age	Religion
Cooperative throughout	I 62 II 74*	I 40 II 69 III 73*	I-IV 76 V 66 VI 60	−53 +69*	F 57 M 72**	M 73 S 59*	I 53 II 73 III 61**	U 41 C 60 P 63 AS 64*
Courteous, friendly	—	I 40 II 58 III 53	—	−30 +44	F 43 M 57*	M 62 S 35***	I 34 II 64 III 58*	U 44 C 67 P 69 AS 64*
Paid attention comfortably	—	I 33 II 65 III 66****	I-IV 56 V 69 VI 54	−48 +69***	—	M 77 S 31****	I 50 II 62 III 72*	
*Actively advice seeking	I 19 II 38*	I 7 II 15 III 24	—	−14 +25*	—	—	I 21 II 14 III 29*	U 12 C 23 P 31 AS 14

Significance of differences determined by chi-square:
  *probability of chance occurrence, less than .05
  **probability of chance occurrence, less than .02
  ***probability of chance occurrence, less than .01
  ****probability of chance occurrence, less than .001

REFERENCES

Adrados, I. (1967), *Teoria e Pratica do Teste de Rorschach.* Rio de Janeiro: Fundação Getulio Vargas.

Antonovsky, A. (1956), Toward a refinement of the "marginal man" concept. *Social Forces,* 35:57.

Anuário Estatistíco do Brasil (1967), Hospitals and Beds in 1964, p. 479.

Anuário Estatistíco do Brasil. IBGE, Conselho Nacional de Estatística, XVIII and XXI. Rio de Janeiro, 1957 and 1960.

Augras, M. (1967), Estudas para padrões Brasileiros de Rorschach. *Arquinos Brasileiros de Psicotecnica.* Rio de Janeiro: Fundação Getulio Vargas.

Auld, F. (1952), *The Influence of Social Class on Tests of Personality.* Drew University Studies, No. 5, December, pp. 1-16.

Azoubel, D. (1967), Estado actual de la epidemiologia del alcoholismo y problema del alcohol en algunos paises de America Latina, Brazil. *Epidemiologia,* 1:72-77.

Back, K. W. (1962), *Slums, Projects, and People: Social Psychological Problems of Relocation in Puerto Rico.* Durham, N.C.: Duke University Press.

Balandier, G. (1951), The colonial situation: A theoretical approach. In: *Social Change: The Colonial Situation,* ed. I. Wallerstein. New York: Wiley, pp. 34-61.

Banco da Providencia (1968), 7 Relatorio de Ativadades 1967.

Banfield, E. C. (1958), *The Moral Basis of a Backward Society.* Glencoe: The Free Press.

Barker, R. G. (1968), *Ecological Psychology.* Stanford: Stanford University Press.

———(1969), Wanted: an eco-behavioral science. In: *Naturalistic Viewpoints in Psychological Research,* ed. E. P. Willems & H. Raush. New York: Holt, Rinehart & Winston.

Bastide, R. (1959), *Brasil, Terra de Contrastes*. São Paulo: Diffusão Europeia do Livro.

——— (1960), *Les Religions Africaines au Brasil*. Paris: Presses Universitares de France, p. 443.

——— (1961), Messianism and social and economic development. In: *Social Change, the colonial situation*, ed. I. Wallerstein. New York: Wiley, 1966, pp. 467–477.

——— & Van den Berghe, P. (1959), Estereótipos, normas e comportamento inter-racial em São Paulo. In: *Brancos e Negros em São Paulo*, ed. R. Bastide & F. Fernandes. São Paulo: Companhia Editôra Nacional.

Beck, S. J. (1945), *Rorschach's Test. Vol. II, A Variety of Personality Pictures*. New York: Grune & Stratton.

Benedict, P. K. & Jacks, I. (1954), Mental illness in primitive societies. *Psychiat.*, 17:377–389.

Beyer, G. H. (1967), *The Urban Explosion in Latin America*. Ithaca: Cornell University Press.

Blay, E. A. (1967), A participação da Mulher na industria Paulista. *Amer. Latina*, 10:81–95.

Bonilla, F. (1961), *Rio's Favelas*. American Universities Field Staff Reports Service, August, 1961.

Bosco, Santa Helena (1965), Perfil socioeconomico da mulher migrante nordestina. *Sociologia*, 27:67–61.

Brandão Lopes, J. R. (1961), Aspects of the adjustment of rural migrants to urban industrial conditions in Sao Paulo, Brazil. In: *Urbanization in Latin America*, ed. P. Hauser. New York: Columbia University Press, pp. 234–248.

——— (1964), *Sociedade Industrial no Brasil*. Editôra da Universidade de São Paulo. São Paulo: Difusão Europeia do Livro.

——— (1966), Some basic developments in Brazilian politics and society. In: *New Perspectives of Brazil*, ed. E. N. Baklanoff. Nashville, Tenn.: Vanderbilt University Press.

——— (1967), *Crise do Brasil Arcaíco*. São Paulo: Difusão Europeia do Livro.

Brasil-Medico (1923), Um caso de Loucura collectiva. September 29.

Brazil Herald (1966), January 14.

——— (1968), August.

Briggs, A. (1963), Technology and economic development. *Sci. Amer.*, 209(3).

Brody, E. B. (1960), The public mental hospital as a symptom of social conflict. *Maryland State Med. J.*, June, pp. 330–334.

——— (1961), Social conflict and schizophrenic behavior in young adult Negro males. *Psychiat.*, 24:337–346.

———— (1963), Color and identity conflict in young boys: Observations of Negro mothers and sons in urban Baltimore. *Psychiat.,* 26:188–201.

———— (1964a), Color and identity conflict in young boys. II Observations of white mothers and sons in urban Baltimore. *Arch. Gen. Psychiat.,* 10:354–360.

———— (1964b), Some conceptual and methodological issues involved in research on society, culture and mental illness. *J. Nerv. Ment. Dis.,* 139:62–74.

———— (1965), Cultural exclusion, character and illness. *Amer. J. Psychiat.,* 122:852–857.

———— (1966), Recording cross-culturally useful psychiatric interview data: Experience from Brazil. *Amer. J. Psychiat.,* 123:446–456.

———— (1967), Mental health planning and directed social change. In: *Psychiatric Epidemiology and Mental Health Planning,* ed. R. R. Monroe, G. D. Klee & E. B. Brody. American Psychiatric Association Research Report, No. 22.

———— (1968), Culture, symbol and value in the social etiology of behavioral deviance. In: *Social Psychiatry,* ed. J. Zubin. New York: Grune & Stratton, pp. 8–33.

———— Ed., (1969a), *Mental Health in the Americas.* Report of the First Hemisphere Conference. Washington, D.C.: The American Psychiatric Association.

———— (1969b), Migration and adaptation. In: *Behavior in New Environments,* ed. E. B. Brody. Beverly Hills: Sage Publications.

———— (1969c), Psychiatry's continuing identity crisis: Confusion or growth? *Psychiat. Digest,* 30:12–17.

———— (1969d), Socio-cultural influences on vulnerability to schizophrenic behavior. In: *The Origins of Schizophrenia,* ed. J. Romano. Excerpta Medica International Congress Series No. 151, pp. 228–238.

———— (1969e), Urban disintegration and the psychiatrist's dilemma. Editorial. *Amer. J. Psychiat.,* 125:1719–1721.

———— ed. (1970), *Behavior in New Environments: Adaptation of Migrant Populations.* Beverly Hills: Sage Publications.

———— Derbyshire, R., & Schleifer, C. (1967), How the young adult Baltimore Negro male becomes a mental hospital statistic. In: *Psychiatric Epidemiology and Mental Health Planning,* ed. R. R. Monroe, G. D. Klee, & E. B. Brody. American Psychiatric Association Research Report, No. 22.

———— & Fishman, M. (1960), Therapeutic response and length of hospitalization of psychiatrically ill veterans. *Arch. Gen. Psychiat.,* 2:174–181.

Burgess, E. W. (1955), Mental health in modern society. In: *Mental Health and Mental Disorder: A Sociological Approach,* ed. A. M. Rose. New York: Norton.

Butts, H. (1969), Discussion of Hendin, H. *Bull. Assn. Psychoanal. Med.,* 9:26.

Camargo, C. P. (1961), *Ferreira de Kardecismo e Umbanda.* São Paulo: Livaria Pioneira Editôra.

Campbell, E. P. (1967), Health and Development—Brazil. Paper prepared for Health Service Office, USAID/Brazil.

Caplan, G. (1964), *Principles of Preventive Psychiatry.* New York: Basic Books.

————(1970), *Mental Health Consultation.* New York: Basic Books.

Carli, G. de (1940), Aspectos Açucareiros de Pernambuco. Rio de Janeiro.

Carlson, R. (1952), A normative study of Rorschach responses of eight-year-old children. *J. Proj. Tech.,* 16:56–65.

Carneiro, E. (1967), *Candomblés de Bahia (1948).* Rio de Janeiro: Coleção Brasileira de Ouro.

Carothers, T. C. (1959), Culture, psychiatry and the written word. *Psychiat.,* 22:307–320.

Caudill, W. (1958), *Effects of Social and Cultural Systems in Reactions to Stress.* New York: Science Rev. Council, Pamphlet 14.

Caudill, W. and Lin, T., eds. (1969), *Mental Health Research in Asia and the Pacific.* Honolulu: East-West Center Press.

Censo Demografico de 1960 (1968). Favelas do estado da Guanabara, VII recenseamento géral do Brasil, Vol. 4 (serie especial); Guanabara, Vol. 1, No. 12, part 1 (serie regional). Rio de Janeiro: Fundação IBGE.

Costa Pinto, L. A. (1952), *O Negro no Rio de Janeiro.* São Paulo: Companhia Editôra Nacional.

Cunha, J. A. (1969), *Rorschach: Inventário de Dados Significativos.* Rio de Janeiro: Edicões CEPA.

———— & Maraninchi, S. (1968), A dimensão clinica do criterio de realidade ('reality testing') no teste do Rorschach. *Bol. Psicol.* (São Paulo) 15:SS/56, 81–86.

Da Costa Eduardo, O. (1948), *The Negro in Northern Brazil. A Study in Acculturation.* Monographs of the American Ethnological Society. Seattle: University of Washington Press.

Damboriena, P. (1963), *El Protestantismo en America Latina.* Oficina International de Investigaciones Sociales. Bogotá.

Davis, A. (1948), *Social Class Influences Upon Learning.* Cambridge: Harvard University Press.

Davis, W. A. & Havighurst, R. J. (1946), Social class and color difference in child rearing. *Amer. Sociol. Rev.,* 11:698–710.

deCastro, C. L. M. (1966), Caracterização socio-economica do estudante universitário: dados gerais. *Rev. Bras. Estudos Pedagog.*, 46:282–400.

de Castro, J. (1966), *Death in the Northeast.* New York: Random House.

de Onis, J. (1968), *New York Times.*

Derbyshire, R. & Brody, E. B. (1964), Marginality, identity and behavior in the American Negro: A functional analysis. *Internat. J. Social Psychiat.*, 10:7–13.

————Brody, E. B., & Schleifer, C. (1963), Family structure of young adult Negro male mental patients: Preliminary observations from urban Baltimore. *J. Nerv. Ment. Dis.*, 136:245–251.

Desenvolvimento e Conjuntura (1966), Caracteristicas da mão-de-obra na Guanabara, 10:65–74.

Desenvolvimento e Conjuntura (1967), Conjunctura social em 1966, 11:97–104.

Dias, H. (1968), Disniveis sociais na baixada fluminense sao cada vez maiores. *Jornal do Brasil,* August 25.

Diaz-Guerrero, R. (1955), Neurosis and the Mexican family structure. *Amer. J. Psychiat.*, 112:411–417.

Diegues, Jr., M. (1960), *Regiões Culturais do Brasil.* Rio de Janeiro: Centro Brasileiro de Pesquisas Educacionais.

————(1963), *Etnias e Culturas do Brasil.* Rio de Janeiro: Editôra Letras e Artes, 3rd ed.

Dietz, A. G. H., Koth, M. N. & Silva, J. A. (1965), *Housing in Latin America.* MIT Report No. 1. Cambridge: MIT Press.

Dohrenwend, B. & Dohrenwend, B. P. (1970), Class and race as status-related sources of stress. In: *Social Stress,* ed. S. Levine & N. Scotch. Chicago: Aldine Press.

Dohrenwend, B. P. (1961), The social psychological nature of stress: A framework for causal inquiry. *J. Abnorm. & Soc. Psychol.*, 62:294–302.

————(1963), Urban leadership and the appraisal of abnormal behavior. In: *The Urban Condition.* New York: Basic Books, pp. 259–299.

———— & Chin-Shong, E. (1967), Social status and attitudes toward psychological disorder: The problem of tolerance of deviance. *Amer. Sociol. Rev.*, 32:417–433.

Dollard, J. (1937), *Caste and Class in a Southern Town.* New Haven: Yale University Press.

Douvan, E. (1956), Social status and success striving. *J. Abnorm. Soc. Psychol.*, 52:219–223.

Draguns, J. G.; Knobel, M.; de Fundia, T. A.; Broverman, I. K.; & Phillips, L. (1966), Social competence, psychiatric symptomatology and culture. In: *Proceedings of the Ninth Interamerican Congress of Psychology,* ed. M. B. Jones, Miami: Interamerican Society of Psychology.

Dupuy, H. J.; Engel, A.; Devine, B. K.; Scanlon, J.; & Querec, L. (1970),

Selected symptoms of psychological stress. *National Center for Health Statistics.* Series 11, No. 37. Rockville, M.: U.S. Department of Health, Education and Welfare.

Durkeim, E. (1951), *Suicide.* Glencoe, Ill.: The Free Press.

Eichler, R. (1951), Experimental stress and alleged Rorschach indices of anxiety. *J. Abnorm. Soc. Psychol.,* 46:344–355.

Ellenbogen, B. L. (1964), *Rural Development in Brazil: Persepectives and Paradoxes.* Multilithed pamphlet. Based on material compiled in June, 1964. Department of Rural Sociology, New York State College of Agriculture at Cornell University, Ithaca, New York.

Faris, R. E. L. & Dunham, H. W. (1960), *Mental Disorders in Urban Areas.* New York: Hafner.

Fernandes, F. (1965), *A Integração do Negro na Sociedade de Classes.* Vol. II. São Paulo: Dominces Editôra S.A.

———— (1969), *The Negro in Brazilian Society.* New York: Columbia University Press.

Field, M. J. (1960), *Search for Security: An Ethno-psychiatric Study of Rural Ghana.* Evanston, Ill.: Northwestern University Press.

Fleiss, J., Spitzer, R. L., & Burdock, E. I. (1965), Estimating accuracy of judgment using recorded interviews. *Arch. Gen. Psychiat.,* 12:562–567.

Frazier, E. F. (1942), The Negro family in Bahia, Brazil. *Amer. Sociol. Rev.,* 7:465–478.

Freud, S. (1926), Symptom, inhibition and anxiety. *The Standard Edition,* 20:87–169. London: Hogarth Press, 1959.

Freyre, G. (1964), *The Masters and the Slaves.* New York: Knopf.

Fried, J. (1962), Social organization and personal security in a Peruvian hacienda Indian community, Vicos. *Amer. Anthrop.* 64:771–780.

Furtado, C. (1963), The development of Brazil. *Sci. Amer.,* 209(3).

———— (1964), O processo revolucionário no Nordeste, In: *Dialectica de Desenvolvimento.* Rio de Janeiro: Editôra Fundo de Cultura.

Geiger, P. (1960), Ensaio para a estrutura urbana do Rio de Janeiro. *Rev. Brasileira Geografia,* 22:4–45.

———— (1963), *Evolução da Rede Urbana Brasileira.* Rio de Janeiro: Centro Brasileiro de Pesquisas Educacionais, I.N.E.P.

Gibbs, J. & Martin, W. (1964), *Status Integration and Suicide: A Sociological Study.* Portland: University of Oregon Books.

Green, A. A. (1947), Re-examination of the marginal man concept. *Social Forces,* 26:167–171.

Goldberg, M. (1941), A qualification of the marginal man theory. *Amer. Sociol. Rev.,* 6:52–58.

Goldenberg, H. (1953), The role of group identification in the personality organization of schizophrenic and normal Negroes. Unpublished Ph.D. thesis, University of California, Los Angeles.

Golovensky, D. (1952), The marginal man concept: an analysis and critique. *Social Forces,* 30:333–339.

Gordon, E. B. (1965), Mentally ill West Indian immigrants. *Brit. J. Psychiat.,* 111:877–887.

Gough, H. G. (1948), A new dimension of status, II. *Amer. Sociol. Rev.,* 13:401–409.

Gouveia, A. J. (1957), Inequalities in Brazilian secondary education. *Amer. Latina,* 10(3).

Gruenberg, E. M. (1968), Can the reorganization of psychiatric services prevent some cases of social breakdown? In: *Psychiatry in Transition: 1966–1967,* ed. A. B. Stokes. Toronto: University of Toronto Press, pp. 95–109.

Haggard, E. (1954), Social status and intelligence: An experimental study of certain cultural determinants of measured intelligence. *Genet. Psychol. Monogr.,* 49:145–185.

Haller, A. O. (1967), Urban economic growth and changes in rural stratification, Rio de Janeiro 1953–1962. *Amer. Latina,* 10:48–67.

Hallowell, A. I. (1955), *Culture and Experience.* Philadelphia: University of Pennsylvania Press.

Harrington, M. (1962), *The Other America.* New York: Macmillan.

Harris, L. (1968), Living sick. *Sources:* 21–36. Blue Cross Association.

Harris, M. (1956), *Town and Country in Brazil.* New York: Columbia University Press.

Hartmann, H. (1939), *Ego Psychology and the Problem of Adaptation.* New York: International Universities Press, 1958.

Hemsi, L. (1967), Psychiatric morbidity of West Indian immigrants. *Soc. Psychiat.,* 2:95–100.

Hendin, H. (1964), *Suicide and Scandinavia.* New York: Grune & Stratton.
——— (1969), *Black Suicide.* New York: Basic Books.

Herskovits, M. (1937), African gods and Catholic saints in new world Negro belief. *Amer. Anthropol.,* 39:635–643.
——— (1938), *Dahomey: An Ancient West African Kingdom,* Vol. 2. New York: Augustin.
——— (1941), *The Myth of the Negro Past.* New York: Harper.
——— (1943), The Negro in Bahia, Brazil: A problem in method. *Amer. Sociol. Rev.,* 8:394–402.
——— (1944), Drums and drummers in Afro-Brazilian cult life. *Musical Quart.,* 30:477–492.
——— & Herskovits, F. (1943), The Negroes of Brazil. *Yale Rev.,* 32: 263–279.

Hertz, M. R. (1951), Current problems in Rorschach theory and technique. *J. Proj. Tech.,* 15:307–338.

Hinkle, L. E., Jr.; Redmond, R.; Plummer, N.; & Wolff, H. G. (1960),

An examination of the relations between symptoms, disability and serious illness in two homogenerous groups of men and women. *Amer. J. Pub. Health,* 50:1327–1339.

Hollingshead, A. B. & Redlich, F. C. (1958), *Social Class and Mental Illness: A Community Study.* New York: Wiley.

Holmberg, A. & Whyte, W. F. (1956), From company camps to open cities. *Human Organiz.,* 15:22–26.

Holt, E. R. & Havel, J. (1961), A method for assessing primary and secondary process in Rorschach. In: *Rorschach Psychology,* ed., Rikhers-Ovsiankina. New York: Wiley.

Holtzman, W. H.; Thorpe, J. S.; Swartz, J. D.; Herron, E. W. (1961), *Inkblot Perception and Personality.* Austin, Tex.: University of Texas Press.

Horwitz, J., Marconi, J., & Adis Castro, G., eds. (1967), *Alcoholismo.* Buenos Aires: Fundacion Acta.

Hunt, G. J. & Butler, E. W. (1970), Migration, participation and anomie. Unpublished. Presented at annual meeting of American Sociology Association, San Francisco, 1970.

Hutchinson, B. (1959), Social status and social mobility in Leopoldinha and Cataguases, Minas Gerais. Unpublished study for Brazilian Center of Educational Research.

———— (1960), *Mobildade e Trabalho.* Rio de Janeiro: Instituto Nacional de Estudos Pedagogicos, Centro Brasileiro de Pesquisas Educacionais.

– ———— (1963), Urban social mobility rates in Brazil related to migration and changing occupational structure. *Amer. Latina,* 3:47–62.

———— (1965), Colour, social status and fertility in Brazil. *Amer. Latina,* 4:3–25.

Ignace, E. (1908), Le fetichesime des Negres du Bresil. *Ontheropes,* 3: 881–904.

Instituto Brasileiro de Geographia (1967). Rio de Janeiro.

Iutaka, S. (1966), Social status influence in differential distribution of illness in urban Brazil. Paper prepared for 60th Anniversary Conference, Milbank Memorial Fund.

Jaco, E. (1960), *The Social Epidemology of Mental Disorders.* New York: Russell Sage Foundation.

Jaeger, C. & Selznick, P. (1965), A normative theory of culture. *Amer. Sociol. Rev.,* 29:653–669.

Jesus, M. C. (1963), *Child of the Dark.* New York: Signet.

Jornal do Brasil (1968), August 4, 1°, p. 18.

Jornal do Brasil (1968), August 8, 1°, p. 15.

Jornal do Brasil (1968), August 19, p. 4.

Jornal do Brasil (1968), August 30.

Jornal do Brasil (1968), September 1, 1° Cod.

Kahl, J. A. (1965), A study of career values in Brazil and Mexico. Mimeographed manuscript.

———— (1966), Mimeographed manuscript.

———— (1967), Modern values and fertility ideals in Brazil and Mexico. *J. Soc. Issues,* 23:99–114.

Katz, M. M.; Gudeman, H.; & Sanborn, K.; (1969), Characterizing differences in psychopathology among ethnic groups: A preliminary report on Hawaiian, Japanese and Mainland-American schizophrenics. In: *Mental Health Research in Asia and the Pacific,* ed. W. Caudill, and T. Lin. Honolulu: East-West Center Press, pp. 148–163.

Kimble, G. A. (1945), Social influences on Rorschach records. *J. Abnorm. Soc. Psychol.,* 40:89–93.

Kinsey, A. C.; Pomeroy, W.; & Martin, C. E. (1948), *Sexual Behavior in the Human Male.* Philadelphia: Saunders.

Klatskin, E. (1952), An analysis of the effect of the test situations upon the Rorschach record. *J. Proj. Tech.,* 16:193–198.

Klein, R. (1966), *The Self-Image of Adult Males in an Indian Culture.* Ann Arbor, Mich.: University Microfilms.

Klopfer, B.; Ainsworth, M. D.; Klopfer, W. G.; & Holt, R. R. (1954), *Developments in the Rorschach Technique,* Vol. I. New York: Harcourt, Brace & World.

———— & Davidson, H. H. (1966), *Tecnica del Rorschach: Manual Introdutario,* Buenos Aires: Editorial Paidos, 2nd edition.

———— & Kelly, D. M. (1956), *The Rorschach Technique,* Vol. II. New York; Harcourt, Brace & World.

Kluckhohn, C. (1944), *Mirror for Man.* New York: McGraw-Hill.

Knobloch, H. & Pasamanick, B. (1966), Prospective studies on the epidemiology of reproductive casualty. *Merrill-Palmer Quart.,* 12:127–143.

Korchin, S. J., Mitchell, H. E., & Meltzoff, J. A. (1950), Critical evaluation of the Thompson TAT. *J. Proj. Tech.,* 14:445–452.

Kornhauser, A. (1962), Toward an assessment of the mental health of factory workers: A Detroit study. *Human Organization,* 21:43–47.

Kramer, M. (1967), Epidemiology, biostatistics and mental health planning. In: *Psychiatric Epidemiology and Mental Health Planning,* ed. R. R. Monroe, G. D. Klee & E. B. Brody. American Psychiatric Association Research Report, No. 22.

Kroeber, A. L. & Parsons, T. (1958), The concept of culture and of social system. *Amer. Sociol. Rev.,* 23:582–583.

Krupinsky, J., Schaechter, F., & Cade, J. F. (1965), Factors influencing the incidence of mental disorders among migrants. *Med. J. Australia,* 52:269–277.

Langner, T. & Michael, S. (1963), *Life Stress and Mental Health*. Glencoe: Free Press.

Lanternari, V. (1963), *The Religions of the Oppressed*. New York: Knopf.

Leiby, G. M. & Figueira, F. A. (1964), Community health challenge— Northeast Brazil. *Amer. J. Pub. Health*, 54:1207–1221.

Leighton, A. H. (1968), Some propositions regarding the relationship of sociocultural integration and disintegration to mental health. In: *Social Psychiatry*, ed. J. Zubin & F. Freyham. New York: Grune & Stratton, pp. 1–7.

———Lambo, T., Hughes, C., Leighton, D., Murphy, J., & Macklin, D. (1963), *Psychiatric Disorder among the Yoruba*. Ithaca: Cornell University Press.

Leighton, D. C.; Harding, J. S.; Macklin, D. B.; Macmillan, A. M.; & Leighton, A. H. (1963), *The Character of Danger—Psychiatric Symptoms in Selected Communities*. New York: Basic Books.

Leite, C. B. & Velloso, L. P. (1963), *Previdencia Social*. Rio de Janeiro: Zahar Editôres.

Levy, L. & Rowitz, L. (1970), The spatial distribution of treated mental disorder in Chicago. *Social Psychiat.*, 5:2–11.

Lewis, V. S. and Zeichner, A. (1960), Impact of admission to a mental hospital on the patient's family. *Ment. Hygiene*, 44:503–510.

Lichtenberg, P. & Norton, D. (1970), *Cognitive and Mental Development in the First Five Years of Life: A Review of Recent Research*. Public Health Service Publication, no. 2057. Rockville, Md.: National Institute of Mental Health.

Lindzey, G. (1961), *Projective Techniques and Cross-Cultural Research*. New York: Appleton-Century-Crofts.

Listwan, I. A. (1959), Mental disorders in migrants: Further study. *Med. J. Australia*, 43:776–777.

Madalena, J. C., de Mello, N. B., Curzio, J. L. F., Pairao, T. (1968), Incidence of alcoholism according to religious affiliation in a Guanabara psychiatric hospital population. Unpublished. Presented at Symposium, Salvador do Bahia, July 24, 1968.

Malzberg, B. & Lee, E. S. (1956), *Migration and Mental Disease, 1939–41*. New York: Social Science Research Council.

Manchete, Special English language issue on Brazil (1968). Rio de Janeiro.

Mason, B. and Ammons, R. B. (1956), Note on social class and the Thematic Apperception Test. *Percept. & Motor Skills*, 6:88.

Matta da Silva, W. W. (1964), *Segredos da Magia de Umbanda e Quimbanda*. Rio de Janeiro: Livraria Freitas Bastos.

McGregor, P. (1966), *The Moon and Two Mountains*. London: Souvenir Press.

McMahon, J. T. (1963), The working class psychiatric patient: a clinical view. In: Reissman, F. et al., eds. (1964), pp. 283–302.

Medeiros, J. (1957), *Candomblé*. Rio de Janeiro: Edicôes O Cruzeiro.

Mendonca, L. de (1966), Nupcialidade no Rio de Janeiro: Alguns resultados preliminarès. *Amer. Latina*, 9:103–137.

Merton R. (1938), Social structure and anomie. *Amer. Sociol. Rev.*, 3:672–682.

———— (1952), *Social Theory and Social Structure*. Glencoe, Ill.: The Free Press.

Miller, S. M. (1964), The American lower classes: A typological approach. In: Reissman, F. et. al., eds. '(1964), pp. 139–154.

Mischel, W. & Mischel, F. (1958), Psychological aspects of spirit possession. *Amer. Anthropol.*, 60:249–260.

Moraes, A. O. (1967), Organização e functionamento hospitalar como fator terapeutico. *O Hospital*, 72:1757–1760.

Munoz, L.; Marconi, J.; Horwitz, J.; & Naveillan, P. (1966), Cross-cultural definitions applied to the study of functional psychoses in Chilean Mapuches. *Brit. J. Psychiat.*, 112:1205–1215.

Mutchler, D. E. (1965), *Roman Catholicism in Brazil: Studies in Comparative International Development*, Vol. 1. St. Louis; The Brazilian Social Science Institute, Washington University, pp. 103–117.

Myers, J. K. & Bean, L. L. (1968), *A Decade Later: A Followup of Social Class and Mental Illness*. New York: Wiley.

Nogueira, O. (1955), Preconçeito de Marca e Preconçeito Racial de Origem. In: *Anais do XXXI: Congresso de Americanista*, Aug. 23–28, 1955, ed. H. Baldus, São Paulo: Editôra Anhembi, pp. 409–434.

O Cruzeiro, no. 37, September 14, 1968.

O Jornal (1968), Sept. 8.

Opler, M. K. (1956), *Culture, Psychiatry and Human Values*. Springfield, Ill.: Charles C Thomas.

Ortiz, F. (1947), *Cuban Counterpart*. New York: Knopf.

PAHO/WHO (1961), *Summary of Four Year Reports on Health Conditions in the Americas, 1957–1960*. Washington, D.C.

Parker, S. & Kleiner, R. J. (1966), *Mental Illness in the Urban Negro Community*. New York: The Free Press.

Parsons, T. (1952), The superego and the theory of social systems. In: *Social Structure and Personality*. Glencoe, Ill.: The Free Press.

———— and Shils, E. (1951), *Toward a General Theory of Action*. Cambridge: Harvard University Press.

Pasamanick, B. and Knobloch, H. (1966), Retrospective studies on the epidemiology of reproductive casualties: Old and new. *Merrill-Palmer Quart.*, 12:7–26.

Pearse, A. (1958), Notas sobre a organização social de uma favela do Rio de Janeiro. *Educacao e Ciencias Sociais,* 3, no. 7.

————(1961), Some characteristics of urbanization in the city of Rio de Janeiro. In: *Urbanization in Latin America,* ed. P. M. Hauser. New York: Columbia University Press (International Documents Service), pp. 191–205.

Peattie, L. R. (1968), *The View from the Barrio.* Ann Arbor: University of Michigan Press, p. 147.

Pereira, L. (1965), *Trabalho e Desenvolvimento no Brasil.* São Paulo: Difusão Europeia do Livro.

Pierson, D. (1942), *Negroes in Brazil: A Study of Race Contact at Bahia.* Chicago: University of Chicago Press.

Pinho, R. A. (1968), Mental Health Resources in Brazil. Paper prepared for Conference on Mental Health in the Americas, San Antonio.

Pinto, C. & Contreras, L. (1969), *Nordestinos Criam Entidade Contra o "Trabalho Escravo."* Rio de Janeiro: O Globo.

Pinto, T. de S. (1964), *New York Times,* September 20, p. 40.

Pollin, W. and Stabenau, J. R. (1968), Biological, psychological and historical differences in a series of monozygotic twins discordant for schizophrenia. In: *The Transmission of Schizophrenia,* ed. D. Rosenthal, & S. S. Kety. New York: Pergamon Press, pp. 317–332.

Ponte, V. M. (1966), Algunas consideraciones sobre la participacion de la mujer de guanabara en la vida moderna. *Amer. Latina,* 9:81–95.

Poppino, R. E. (1968), *Brazil, the Land and the People.* New York: Oxford University Press.

Prado, Caido, Jr. (1964), Marcha de questão agraria no Brasil. *Revista Brasiliense,* 51:1–9.

Prince, R. (1966), Possession cults and social cybernetics. In: *Trance and Possession States,* ed. R. Prince. Canada: Bucke Memorial Society, pp. 157–165.

Querido, A. (1968), The shaping of community mental health care. *Brit. J. Psychiat.,* 114:293–302.

Queiroz de Pereira, I. (1952), Classification de messianismes bresiliens. *Arch Soc. Rel.,* 5:111–120.

Rafferty, F. (1967), Child psychiatry service for a total population. *J. Amer. Acad. Child Psychiat.,* 6:295–308.

Ramos, A. (1934), *O Negro Brasileiro: Ethnographia, Religiosa e Psychanalyse.* Rio de Janeiro: Civilização Brasileiro.

Ribeiro, J. G. (1968), Data prepared for Serviço Nacional de Doenças Mentais, Rio de Janeiro.

Ribeiro, L. & de Campos, M. (1931), *O Espiritismo no Brasil.* São Paulo: Companhia Editôra Nacional.

Ribeiro, R. (1945), On the amaziado relationship and other aspects of the family in Recife (Brazil). *Amer. Sociol. Rev.*, 10:44–51.

———(1952), Cultos afrobrasileiros do Recife. *Boletin do Instituto Joaquim Nabuco.* Numero Especial, Grafica Editôra do Recife J/A.

———(1959), Analisis socio-psicologico de la posesion en los cultos Afro-brasilenos. *Acta Neuropsiquiat. Arg.*, 5:249–262.

———(1969), Estudo comparativo dos problemas de vida em duas culturas afins: Angola-Brasil. *J. Interamer. Stud.*, 11:2–15.

Richardson, A. (1957), Some psycho-social characteristics of satisfied and dissatisfied British immigrant skilled manual workers in Western Australia. *Human Relations,* 10: 235–248.

Riessman, F.; Cohen, J.; & Pearl, A. eds. (1964), *Mental Health of the Poor.* Glencoe, Ill.: The Free Press.

———and Miller, S. M. (1958), Social Class and projective tests. In: *Riessman et al. eds. (1964).*

Rodrigues, N. (1901), La folie des foules. *Annales Medico-Psychol.* (Paris), Jan.-Aug.

Rogler, L. H. & Hollingshead, A. B. (1965), *Trapped: Families and Schizophrenia.* New York: Wiley.

Rosen, B. C. (1962), Socialization and achievement motivation in Brazil. *Amer. Sociol. Rev.*, 27:612–624.

Rosenberg, M. (1949), The social roots of formalism. *J. Soc. Issues,* 5:14–23.

Rotondo, H. (1961), Psychological and mental health problems of urbanization based on case studies in Peru. In: *Urbanization in Latin America,* ed. P. M. Hauser. New York: Columbia University Press, International Documents Service, pp. 249–257.

Roxo, H. de B. B. (1918), Delirio espirita episodico. In: *Manual de Psiquiatria,* ed. 4. Livraria-Guanabara, 1946.

Sanua, V. D. (1970), Immigration, Migration and Mental Illness: A Review of the Literature with Special Emphasis on Schizophrenia. In: *Behavior in New Environments,* ed. E. B. Brody. Beverly Hills; Sage, pp. 291–352.

Schaechter, F. A. (1962), A study of psychoses in female migrants. *Med. J. Australia,* 49:458–461.

Schleifer, C. B., Derbyshire, R. L., & Martin, J. (1968), Clinical change in jail-referred mental patients. *Arch. Gen. Psychiat.,* 18:42–46.

Schooler, S. and Caudill, W. (1969), Symptom patterns and background characteristics of Japanese Psychiatric Patients. In: W. Caudill and T. Lin, ed. (1969), pp. 114–147.

Segadas Soares, M. T. de (1965), Fisionomia e estrutura do Rio de Janeiro. *Rev. Brasileira Geografia,* 27:329–387.

Serrana, G. (1967), *A Prece Segundo O Espiritismo.* Rio de Janeiro: Editôra Eco.

Singer, J. (1962), Cognitive, social and physiological determinants of emotional state. *Psychol. Rev.,* 69:379–399.

Smith, T. L. (1963), *Brazil: People and Institutions.* Baton Rouge, La.: Louisiana State University Press.

Souza de Andrade, C. (1952), Migrantes nacionais no Estado de São Paulo. *Sociologia,* 14:123–127.

Spitzer, R. L. (1965), Immediately available record of mental status exam. *Arch. Gen. Psychiat.,* 13:76–78.

———— Fleiss, J. L., Burdock, E. I., & Hardesty, A. S. (1964), The mental status schedule: rationale, reliability and validity. *Compr. Psychiat.,* 5:384–395.

———— ————Kernohan, W., Lee, J. C., & Baldwin, I. T. (1965), Mental status schedule. *Arch. Gen. Psychiat.,* 12:448–455.

SPLAN (Sociedade de Pesquisas e Planejamento) (1968), O Conselho do Reitores das universidades Brasileiras. Reported in "Quem sao os estudantes Universitários." *J. Brasil,* 10 Cad., August 18, 1968.

Srole, L., Langner, R. S., Michael, S. T., Opler, M. K., & Rennie, T. A. C. (1962), *Mental Health in the Metropolis.* New York: McGraw-Hill.

Stainbrook, E. (1952), Some characteristics of the psychopathology of schizophrenic behavior in Bahian society. *Amer. J. Psychiat.,* 109:330–335.

Statistical Report (1971), Maryland State Department of Health and Mental Hygiene, 1st Quarter.

Stone, L. J. & Fiedler, M. F. (1956), The Rorschachs of selected groups of children in comparison with published norms. II. The effect of socioeconomic status on Rorschach performance. *J. Proj. Tech.,* 20:276–279.

Teixeira, A. A. (1967), *O Livro dos Médiuns.* Rio de Janeiro: Editôra Eco.

Tejo, L., Brejos ed Carrascaes do Nordeste em São Paulo, 1937. Quoted in Smith (1963).

Tewfik, G. I. & Okasha, A. (1965), Psychosis and immigration. *Postgrad. Med. J.,* 41:603–612.

Treitas, B. Torres de, and da Silva Pinto, T. (1951), *Doutrina e Ritual de Umbanda.*

Turner, R. J. & Wagenfeld, M. O. (1967), Occupational mobility and schizophrenia: An assessment of the social causation and the social selection hypotheses. *Amer. Sociol. Rev.,* 32:104–122.

United Nations Demographic Yearbook (1961), UN, New York.

Useem, J.; Tangent, P.; & Useem, R. (1942), Stratification in a prairie town. *Amer. J. Sociol.,* 7:331–342.

Van den Berghe, P. L. (1967), *Race and Racism.* New York: Wiley.

Verrissimo, E. (1946), *O Tempo e O Vento.* Porto Alegre: Globo Press.

Wagley, C. (1953), *Amazon Town: A Study of Man in the Tropics.* New York: Macmillan.

————(1963), *An Introduction to Brazil.* New York: Columbia University Press.

Willems, E. (1949), Racial Attitudes in Brazil. *Amer. J. Sociol.,* 54:402–408.

————(1966), Religious mass movements and social change. In: *New Perspectives of Brazil,* ed. E. Baklanoff. Nashville, Tenn.: Vanderbilt University Press, pp. 205–232.

————(1967), *Followers of the New Faith.* Nashville, Tenn.: Vanderbilt University Press.

Wilson, A. W., Saver, G., & Lachenbruch, P. A. (1965), Residential mobility and psychiatric help-seeking. *Amer. J. Psychiat.,* 121:1108–1109.

Wittkower, E. (1967), Perspectives of transcultural psychiatry. Proceedings of the IV World Congress of Psychiatry. *Excerpta Medica Foundation,* I:228–234.

————& Fried, J. (1959), Some problems of transcultural psychiatry. In: *Culture and Mental Health,* ed. M. K. Opler. New York: Macmillan.

Yap, P. M. (1951), Mental diseases peculiar to certain cultures: A survey of comparative psychiatry. *J. Ment. Sci.,* 97:313–327.

Xavier, F. C. (1938), *Brasil, Coração do Mundo, Patria do Evangelho.* Rio de Janeiro: Federação Espirita Brasileira.

INDEX